D1825448

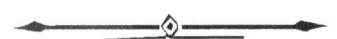

ISBN 978-0-260-10310-9
PIBN 10928156

SIXTH INTERNATIONAL

OTOLOGICAL CONGRESS,

LONDON,

AUGUST 8TH TO 12TH, 1899.

SIXTH INTERNATIONAL

OTOLOGICAL CONGRESS, 6

LONDON,

AUGUST 8th to 12th, 1899.

PRESIDENT - PROFESSOR URBAN PRITCHARD.

TRANSACTIONS

EDITED UNDER THE DIRECTION OF THE EDITORIAL COMMITTEE,

BY

E. CRESSWELL BABER,

HON. SECRETARY-GENERAL.

London:

THE SOUTHERN PUBLISHING COMPANY, LIMITED,
62, FLEET STREET.

1900.

PREFACE.

In preparing these Transactions for publication, accuracy has, as far as possible, been attained by submitting the proofs of the foreign papers to the authors themselves. The unread papers have been arranged alphabetically under the authors' names.

I have to acknowledge my considerable indebtedness to Mr. Arthur J. Hutchison, M.B., for valuable help in correcting the proofs and in preparing the Index, also to Dr. E. Hobhouse for assistance with the Italian papers.

E. C. B.

TABLE OF CONTENTS.

PAGE.

Preface ... ... v.
List of Illustrations ... ... xiii.
International Organization Committee ... ... xv.
Sub-Committees ... ... xvii.
Invitation to the Sixth International Otological Congress ... xix.
Programme ... . xxi.
List of Delegates ... ... xxii.
Regulations ... ... xxii.
General Discussion ... ... xxii.
Communications Announced ... ... xxiii.
Museum ... ... xxviii.
List of Members ... ... xxix.
Officers of the Congress ... ... xxxvi.

INAUGURAL MEETING:—
    Tuesday, August 8th 1-10
Opening Address 1
Letters of Apology for Absence 7
List of Delegates 7
Vote of thanks to the Royal Colleges of Physicians and Surgeons 8
Address by the President of the last Congress 8
Telegram to H.M. The Queen 10
Appointment of Officers 10

SECOND MEETING:—
    Tuesday, August 8th 11-60
DR. E. SCHMIEGELOW. On a new method of measuring the
    quantitative hearing power by means of tuning forks... 11
Discussion 15
    Remarks by: Prof. Politzer—Dr. Dundas Grant.
PROF. G. GRADENIGO. A scheme for the uniform notation of
    the results of the investigation of hearing power ... 15
PROF. G. GRADENIGO. A new optical method of acoumetry 16
DR. R. KAYSER. Experimentelle Untersuchungen über acus-
    tische Phänomene in flüssigen Medien 17

PAGE.

Discussion   20
   Remarks by : Prof. Lucae.
DR. O. BRIEGER. Ueber Tuberculose des Mittelohrs   ...   20
DR. MILLIGAN. Tuberculous disease of the middle ear   ...   34
Discussion   39-40
   Remarks by : Prof. Kümmel — Prof. Politzer — Dr.
   McBride—Dr. Brieger.
DR. ARTHUR HARTMANN. Angeborenes Fehlen des äusseren
   Gehörganges und erworbener Verschluss desselben   ...   40
Discussion   42-43
   Remarks by : Dr. Holinger—Mr. Cresswell Baber.
DR. F. ROHRER. Ueber blaue Diaphanität am Trommelfell
   und über Varixbildung an Demselben   43
DR. T. BOBONE. L'involution précoce du tissu adénoïdien
   sur la Riviera   47
DR. ALLEN T. HAIGHT. Naso-pharyngeal adenoids as a
   causative factor in ear diseases   54
Discussion   59-60
   Remarks by : Prof. Grazzi—Prof. Eeman—Dr. H. Knapp—
   Prof. Gradenigo.

THIRD MEETING :—
   Wednesday, August 9th   61-106
GENERAL DISCUSSION ON INDICATIONS FOR OPENING THE
   MASTOID IN CHRONIC SUPPURATIVE OTITIS MEDIA.
Opening Addresses by :
   PROF. A. POLITZER   61
   PROF. WILLIAM MACEWEN   66
   DR. LUC...   72
   DR. HERMAN KNAPP   84
PROF. LUCAE. Zur Radicaloperation bei chronischer puru-
   lenter Mittelohrentzündung   92
Discussion   94-106
   Speeches by : Prof. Guye—Dr. Moure—Dr. McBride—Dr.
   Jansen—Prof. Gradenigo—Dr. Noyes—Prof. Kümmel—
   Prof. Eeman—Dr. Brieger—Dr. Barr—Prof. G. Faraci—
   Dr. Suarez de Mendoza—Dr. Milligan—Mr. T. Mark
   Hovell—Dr. Holmes—Prof. Dench—Mr. Cresswell Baber
   —Dr. Holinger—Mr. De Santi—Mr. Faulder White—Dr.
   Lederman—Prof. Urban Pritchard.

FOURTH MEETING :—
   Wednesday, August 9th   107-125
DR. ARTHUR HARTMANN. Die Anatomie des Sinus frontalis,
   und der vorderen Siebbeinzellen. Mit Projektion   ...   107

PAGE.

DR. ALDREN TURNER. Lantern-slide demonstration ... 108
MR. R. DWYER JOYCE. The topography of the facial nerve
in its relation to mastoid operations... 108
Discussion 114
Remarks by : Prof. Eeman.
DR. L. KATZ. Demonstration microscopischer und macro-
scopischer Präparate des Gehörorgans 114
DR. P. RUDLOFF. The operation of the removal of adenoid
growths with the head hanging over the table while the
patient is under the influence of chloroform 116
Discussion 120-121
Remarks by : Dr. Herman Knapp—Dr. Lederman.
PROF. UCHERMANN. Rheumatic diseases of the ear 121
Discussion 124
Remarks by : Dr. Hartmann.

FIFTH MEETING :—
Thursday, August 10th 126-198
DR. E. MÉNIÈRE. Traitement des suppurations chroniques
de l'attique 126
DR. MARCEL LERMOYEZ. La contagion des otites moyennes
aiguës 127
PROF. E. J. MOURE. Deux cas de complications encéphaliques
(abcès-cérébraux) d'origine otique 138
Discussion 145-147
Remarks by : Prof. Luc—Prof. Gradenigo—Dr. Heiman—
Dr. Brieger—Dr. Lermoyez.
DR. E. BRADFORD DENCH. The operative treatment of
mastoid inflammation 147
Discussion 151
Remarks by : Dr. Knapp.
DR. DELIE. Panotite avec complication cérébrale. Opéra-
tion. Mort. Autopsie 151
MR. ARTHUR CHEATLE. The petro-squamosal sinus : its
anatomy and pathological importance 160
Discussion 170
Remarks by : Dr. Knapp.
PROF. V. GRAZZI. Nouveau traitement des inflammations
chroniques catarrhales du pharynx en rapport aux
maladies de l'oreille 170
DR. ARISTIDE MALHERBE. Traitement chirurgical de l'otite
moyenne chronique sèche par l'évidement petro-mastoïdien
avec et sans tubage 176
Discussion 186-187
Remarks by : Prof. Faraci—Dr. Suarez de Mendoza.

PAGE.

PROF. AVOLEDO. Ascessi della faccia   187
DR. LOUIS BAR. Abcès antérieurs de la mastoïde et furoncu-
    lose du conduit auditif externe (Etude de diagnostic) ...   188
DR. A. COSTINIU. Résultat des exercices acoustiques chez les
    sourds-muets   195
Discussion   198
    Remarks by : Dr. Didsbury—Dr. Heiman—Prof. Grazzi—
    Dr. Garnault.

SIXTH MEETING :—
    Friday, August 11th   199-269
DR. M. A. GOLDSTEIN. Therapy of the tympanic mucous
    membrane   199
Discussion   207-208
    Remarks by : Dr. Lederman—Dr. William Ballinger.
DR. THEODORE HEIMAN. De l'inflammation primitive de
    l'apophyse mastoïde   208
DR. P. LACROIX. Complications otiques de l'ozène   217
DR. RUTTEN. Exostose du conduit auditif droit   219
PROF. POLITZER. Extraction of the stapes   221
Discussion   223
    Remarks by : Prof. Lucae.
PROF. OSTMANN. Ueber die Heilerfolge der Vibrationsmassage   223
Discussion   234-237
    Remarks by : Dr. F. Rohrer—Prof. Politzer—Dr. Felix
    Cohn—Dr. Dundas Grant—Prof. Lucae—Dr. M. A. Gold-
    stein—Dr. J. M. E. Scatliff.
Resolution regarding the representation of Otology and
    Laryngology by separate and full Sections at all General
    Medical Congresses   237
PROF. EEMAN. Des bourdonnements provoqués par l'insuffi-
    sance aortique   238
Discussion   240
    Remarks by : Dr. Dundas Grant.
PROF. G. FARACI. Sulla possibilità di riaprire la finestra
    ovale nei casi di anchilosi ossea dell'articolazione stapedio-
    vestibolare. Tyridanoixi-ovalis   240
Discussion   245-246
    Remarks by : Dr. Garnault—Prof. Politzer—Dr. Nuvoli—
    Dr. Knapp.
DR. FR. FISCHENICH. Ueber die Behandlung der katar-
    rhalischen Adhaesivprocesse im Mittelohre, mittelst intra-
    tympanaler Pilocarpininjectionen   246
Discussion   250-251
    Remarks by : Prof. Gradenigo.

PAGE.

DR. P. J. MINK. Pneumomassage unter höherem Drucke ... 251

Discussion 254
    Remarks by : Dr. Chevalier Jackson.

DR. G. NUVOLI. On pneumatic treatment of diseases of the ear 254

DR. SARGENT SNOW. Twentieth century prognosis in chronic
    catarrhal deafness 257

Discussion 260-261
    Remarks by : Dr. Lewis Taylor—Dr. C. R. Holmes.

DR. PAUL GARNAULT. Sur la mobilisation et l'extraction de
    l'étrier 261

DR. LAURENS. Otite moyenne chronique suppurée avec
    thrombose du sinus latéral et abcès du cervelet 265

CLOSING MEETING :—
    Friday, August 11th 270-275

Next Place of Meeting ... ..., ... 270

Organization Committee for the next Congress... 270

The Lenval Prize Award 272

Concluding Speech by Prof. Urban Pritchard 273

Remarks by : Prof. Grazzi—Dr. Benni—Prof. Politzer—Mr.
    Cresswell Baber—Mr. Arthur Cheatle 274-275

Termination of Proceedings 275

COMMUNICATIONS NOT READ:—

DR. FERDINAND ALT. Experimentelle Untersuchungen über
    das corticale Hörcentrum 276

DR. BARATOUX. De l'unité de mensuration de l'ouïe 281

DR. THOMAS BARR. Case of extensive purulent thrombosis of
    lateral sinus—septic pneumonia—pulmonary abscess and
    gangrene consequent upon chronic purulent otitis media.
    Gradual improvement after clearing out the lateral sinus
    and ligaturing the internal jugular vein 286

DR. PIERRE BONNIER. Acoumétrie 290

DR. ADOLPH BRONNER. On the local application of remedies in
    the treatment of non-suppurative catarrh of the middle ear 293

MR. ARTHUR H. CHEATLE. Adeno-carcinoma of meatus with
    chronic middle ear suppuration. Operation 294

DR. J. GALBRAITH CONNAL. Sarcoma of the external auditory
    canal 295

DR. E. COOSEMANS. L'audition chez les Beetlers 296

DR. A. COSTINIU. L'état des oreilles, du larynx, et du nez
    chez les vieillards 304

DR. JEHANGIR J. CURSETJI. Some aspects of aural practice
    in India, ancient and modern, with special reference to
    Bombay 306

PAGE.

DR. H. J. DADYSETT. The various domestic remedies with their effects used by the people of India for certain diseases of the ear 328

MR. PHILIP R. W. DE SANTI. The radical cure of chronic purulent otorrhœa by antrectomy and attico-antrectomy, based on the results of twenty-six operations 331

MR. PHILIP R. W. DE SANTI. Some cases illustrating the intracranial complications of neglected otorrhœa 340

PROF. GIUSEPPE FARACI. Mobilizzazione precoce della catena degli ossicini nel periodo sub-acuto di alcune otiti medie non suppurative 343

PROF. GIUSEPPE FARACI. Importanza acustica e funzionale della mobilizzazione della staffa 351

PROF. GRADENIGO. The amplified bibliographical otological notation, according to the decimal system of Melvil Dewey 366

PROF. GRADENIGO. Sui mezzi più opportuni per promuovere un conveniente incremento degli studi otologici nelle università e nella legislazione sociale 373

DR. DUNDAS GRANT. Diminished bone-conduction as a contra-indication for ossiculectomy 375

DR. ALBERT A. GRAY. A case of tumour of the medulla and pons, causing deafness and other remarkable symptoms 378

PROF. HESSLER. Ueber einen Fall von Hirntumor bei acuter Mittelohreiterung, und über die Differentialdiagnose zwischen Hirntumor, Hirnabscess, und Hydrocephalus internus 384

DR. JOBSON HORNE. The formation of a circumscribed intra-dural abscess at the site of the saccus endolymphaticus ... 392

MR. HUGH E. JONES. Cases of mastoid and intracranial extension of suppuration from the tympanum, with remarks and queries respecting the chronology of complications, and its bearing upon treatment 394

MR. HUGH E. JONES. A case of malformation of the left auricle, with atresia of the meatus, etc. Operation ... 403

DR. G. F. KEIPER. Description of a set of mastoid gouges ... 406

DR. KOEBEL. Ueber Combination von Otitis Media "mit rhinogenem Gehirnabscess" 406

DR. M. LANNOIS. Epilepsie ab aure laesa 407

DR. URBANO MELZI. A case of nasal hydrorrhœa 410

DR. URBANO MELZI. A case of endothelial fibro-angioma of the external auditory meatus 412

DR. URBANO MELZI. A case of retropharyngeal abscess of auricular origin 414

PAGE.

DR. SUAREZ DE MENDOZA. Sur le traitement des obstructions de la trompe d'Eustache et de la surdité consécutive, par l'emploi méthodique des bougies régulièrement graduées... 415

DR. FRANK S. MILBURY. Diseases of the mastoid, their course and treatment 418

PROF. CAMILLO POLI. Le vie nasali e auricolari dell'infezione endocranica 429

DR. G. D. COHEN TERVAERT. A case of thrombosis of both sinus cavernosi, as a complication of chronic mastoiditis ex otorrhœa, which ended in recovery 446

DR. LAURENCE TURNBULL. Some of the most important discoveries in Otology, many of which have stood the test of thirty-five years 452

DR. VEYRAT. Des améliorations de l'ouïe obtenues par le tympan artificiel dans l'otite moyenne sèche ou sclérose tympanique 459

DR. VEYRAT. Des injections interstitielles de sublimé corrosif dans le traitement des lupus du nez 464

MR. F. FAULDER WHITE. Curability of chronic suppurative otitis media 467

LIST OF ILLUSTRATIONS.

Outer surface of temporal bone, showing line of projection of facial canal 110

Outer aspect of a temporal bone of a Cebus monkey, showing the external opening of petro-squamosal sinus 161

Inner aspect of preceding 161

Superior aspect of left temporal bone of a child in whom the anterior opening persisted, showing well-marked groove, and the inner aspect of the anterior opening 163

External aspect of same bone showing opening between an unusually large post-glenoid tubercle and the meatus, with a groove running outwards 163

Right temporal bone of a child showing the valve-like opening in lateral sinus 163

Superior surface of left temporal bone of a young adult with dura mater thrown back to show groove for sinus ... 163

Outer surface, showing perforation in the zygoma 164

Posterior surface of same showing opening under bridge into sigmoid groove ... ... :.. 165

Superior surface of left adult temporal bone, dura mater thrown back, showing partly-bridged-over groove ... 165

PAGE.

Section through front of preceding showing canal in the
zygoma   166
Posterior aspect of same showing the opening of the sinus
into the lateral sinus   166
Adult bone showing deep partly-bridged-over groove opening
into sigmoid groove under bridge   167
Adult bone, showing shallow groove partly-bridged-over
opening into sigmoid groove   167
Adult bone, showing the bridge behind   168
Section of mucous membrane of pharynx   171
Ditto   172
Instruments of Prof. Grazzi   173

PLATES.

Plates illustrating Dr. Schmiegelow's paper on a new method
of measuring the quantitative hearing power by means of
tuning forks   15
Plate illustrating Prof. Gradenigo's paper on a new optical
method of acoumetry   16
Charts illustrating Prof. Ostmann's paper on the results of
vibratory massage   234
Charts illustrating Dr. Costiniu's paper on the condition of the
ears, larynx, and nose in old age   306
Chart illustrating Mr. de Santi's paper on the radical cure of
chronic purulent otorrhœa, by antrectomy and attico-
antrectomy   337-339
Plate illustrating Dr. Jobson Horne's paper on the formation
of a circumscribed intra-dural abscess at the site of the
saccus endolymphaticus   394
Temperature Chart illustrating Case 1 in Mr. Hugh Jones'
paper   402
Plate illustrating Mr. Hugh Jones' case of malformation of the
auricle   405
Plate illustrating Prof. Poli's paper   442
Charts illustrating ditto   443-445

6TH INTERNATIONAL OTOLOGICAL CONGRESS.

INTERNATIONAL ORGANIZATION COMMITTEE:

PRESIDENT · URBAN ·PRITCHARD, London.

AMERICA.

CLARENCE BLAKE,	Boston.	RANDALL,	Philadelphia.
ORNE GREENE,	,,	C. H. BURNETT,	,,
A. H. BRECH, ·	New York.	HOLMES,	Chicago.
ST. JOHN ROOSA,	,,	DALY,	Pittsburg.
H. KNAPP,	,,	BARKAN,	San Francisco.
LAURENCE TURNBULL,	Philadelphia.	ROALDES,	New Orleans.

AUSTRIA-HUNGARY.

POLITZER,	Vienna.	SZENES,	Buda-Pesth.
MORPURGO,	Trieste.	ZAUFAL,	Prague.
BÖKE,	Buda-Pesth.		

BELGIUM.

DELSTANCHE,	Brussels.	DELIE,	Ypres.
CAPART,	..	SCHIFFERS,	Liege.
HUGUET,		EEMAN,	Ghent.
GORIS,			

DENMARK.

SCHMIEGELOW,	Copenhagen.	HOLGER MYGIND,	Copenhagen.

FRANCE.

GELLÉ,	Paris.	NOQUET,	Lille.
MÉNIÈRE,	..	LERMOYEZ,	Paris.
HELME,		LUBET-BARBON,	,,
BARATOUX,	,,	GOUGENHEIM,	,,
MOURE,	Bordeaux.	LANNOIS,	Lyons.

GERMANY.

LUCAE,	Berlin.	KIRCHNER,	Wurzburg.
HARTMANN,	,,	BRIEGER,	Breslau.
BEZOLD,	Munich.		

·HOLLAND.

GUYE,	Amsterdam.	VAN HOEK,	Nymwegen.
ZWAARDEMAKER,	Utrecht.	MOLL,	Arnheim.

ITALY.

GRAZZI,	Florence.	FERRERI,	Rome.
AVOLEDO,	Milan.	COZZOLINO.	Naples.
BOBONE,	San Remo.	GRADENIGO,	Turin.
BRUNETTI,	Venice.	MASINI,	Genoa.
CHIUCINI,	Rome.	PUTELLI,	Venice.
DE ROSSI,	..	SECCHI, .	Bologna.

RUSSIA AND POLAND.

RÜHLMANN.	St.Petersburg.	STEPANOFF,	Moscow.
BENNI,	Warsaw.	STEIN,	..

SPAIN.

SUNE-Y-MOLIST,	Barcelona.	BOTEY,	Barcelona.
GONZALEZ ALVAREZ,	Madrid.	VERDOS.	,,
URUÑELA,	,,	MORESCO,	Cadiz.
SOTA-Y-LASTRA,	Sevilla.	CASANOVA,	Valencia.

SWEDEN.

SWANBERG,	Stockholm.	CETERBLAD,	Stockholm.

SWITZERLAND.

SECRETAN,	Lausanne.	COLLADON,	Geneva
ROHRER,	Zurich.		

BRITISH EMPIRE.

J. B. BALL,	London.	W. MILLIGAN,	Manchester.
C. A. BALLANCE,	..	SECKER WALKER,	,,
J. W. BOND,		WALTER RIDLEY,	Newcastle-on-Tyne.
W. C. BULL,			
ARTHUR CHEATLE,	,,	A. BRONNER,	Bradford.
SIR W. DALBY,		H. A. BALLANCE,	Norwich.
G. P. FIELD,		W. H. HARSANT,	Clifton.
DUNDAS GRANT,		WATSON WILLIAMS,	,,
F. G. HARVEY,		F. W. BENNETT,	Leicester.

BRITISH EMPIRE—*Continued.*

W. Hill,	London.	J. M. E. Scatliff,	Brighton.
Jobson Horne,	..	D. R. Paterson,	Cardiff.
Mark Hovell,		Mackenzie Booth,	Aberdeen.
Percy Jakins,		P. McBride,	Edinburgh.
Macnaughton Jones,	,,	Mackenzie Johnston,	,,
R. Lake,		Logan Turner,	,,
E. Law,		Thos. Barr,	Glasgow.
L. A. Lawrence,		Brown Kelly,	,,
Matheson,		Johnston McFie,	,,
Stephen Paget,		Taylor Guild,	Dundee.
H. Pegler,		A. W. Sandford,	Cork.
Bilton Pollard,		Walton Browne,	Belfast.
Marmaduke Sheild,	,,	A. H. Benson,	Dublin.
Scanes Spicer,		E. B. Story,	..
W. R. H. Stewart,	,,	R. H. Woods,	
St. Clair Thomson,	,,	C. E. Fitzgerald,	,,
H. Tilley,		H. R. Swanzy,	,,
E. Waggett,		W. C. Scholtz,	Cape Town, Africa.
E. Woakes,		J. W. Barrett,	Melbourne, Aus.
P. M. Yearsley,	,,	A. Brady,	Sydney, Aus.
C. J. Lewis,	Birmingham.	Hope Lewis,	Auckland, N.Z.
F. Marsh,	·,,	Ferguson,	Dunedin, N.Z.
J. M. Hunt,	Liverpool.	Birkett,	Montreal.
Edgar Browne,	..	Buller,	,,
H. E. Jones,		W. K. Hatch,	Bombay.
George Stone,	,,	J. J. Cursetji,	,,
G. C. Wilkin,	West Coker.	P. M. Nair,	Madras.

Hon. Treasurer:

A. E. CUMBERBATCH,

80, Portland Place, London, W.

Hon. Secretary General:

E. CRESSWELL BABER,

46, Brunswick Square, Brighton.

SUB-COMMITTEES.

RECEPTION :—

GEORGE P. FIELD, Vice-Chairman.
H. MACNAUGHTON JONES.   EDWARD LAW.
RICHARD LAKE, Hon. Sec.

EXCURSIONS :—

DUNDAS GRANT, Vice-Chairman.
WILLIAM HILL.   W. R. H. STEWART.   E. WAGGETT.
P. MACLEOD YEARSLEY, Hon. Sec.

DINNER :—

T. MARK HOVELL, Vice-Chairman.
J. B. BALL.   J. W. BOND.
L. A. LAWRENCE, Hon. Sec.

MUSEUM :—

CHAS. A. BALLANCE, Vice-Chairman.
THOMAS BARR.   F. W. BENNETT.   C. E. FITZGERALD.
A. BROWN KELLY.   P. MCBRIDE.   W. MILLIGAN.
H. TILLEY.   A. LOGAN TURNER.   H. R. WOODS.
ARTHUR H. CHEATLE, Hon. Sec.

INVITATION

TO THE

SIXTH INTERNATIONAL OTOLOGICAL CONGRESS,

LONDON,

August 8th to August 12th, 1899.

46, BRUNSWICK SQUARE,

BRIGHTON.

MY DEAR SIR,

By direction of the British Organization Committee, I have much pleasure in informing you that the Sixth International Otological Congress will take place from August 8th to 12th, 1899, and in inviting you to take part in its proceedings.

On Monday evening, August 7th, a preliminary Reception will be held by the President Elect, Dr. Urban Pritchard (Professor of Aural Surgery at King's College, London). On August 8th, 9th, 10th, 11th, the Congress will be in session, and will be followed on Saturday, August 12th, by an excursion for members and their lady friends. Shorter excursions will also be arranged during the week.

By kind permission of the Royal College of Physicians of London, and of the Royal College of Surgeons of England, the Congress will meet in the Examination Hall, Victoria Embankment.

The official languages of the Congress are English, French, German, and Italian.

The subscription, including a copy of the Transactions, is fixed at £1, which must be paid to the Treasurer, Mr. A. E. Cumberbatch, 80, Portland Place, London, W., before the Opening of the Congress.

The subject chosen for special discussion is "Indications for opening the Mastoid in Chronic Suppurative Otitis Media."

A Museum of Specimens and Instruments relating to Otology, shown by Members, will be held during the Meeting. Communications regarding the Museum should be addressed to Mr. A. H. Cheatle, 117, Harley Street, London, W.

I trust that you will honour the Committee with a favourable reply, by signifying to me as soon as possible, and in any case not later than May 1st, your intention to take part in the Congress, in order that I may be able to send you a more detailed programme.

I shall also be glad to receive, not later than May 1st, the title of any paper you may wish to read, together with a short abstract of the same. I may mention that one of the Rules of the Congress is, that no paper shall exceed fifteen minutes in reading, so that all long communications should be read in abstract.

To facilitate the necessary arrangements, I shall feel obliged if you will kindly inform me at the same time whether you propose to attend the Congress alone, or in company with one or more ladies.

I have the honour, Sir, to remain,
Yours very truly,

E. CRESSWELL BABER,
Hon. Secretary General.

December, 1898.

PROGRAMME.

MONDAY, AUGUST 7TH.

9-11 p.m.—Opening Reception by the President of the Organization Committee at the Examination Hall of the Royal Colleges of Physicians and Surgeons, Victoria Embankment.

TUESDAY, AUGUST 8TH.

10 a.m.—Opening Meeting in the Examination Hall, Victoria Embankment.

    1.   Address by the President of the Organization Committee.

    2.   Address by the President of the last Congress.

    3.   Election of Officers.

3-6 p.m.—Meeting for papers and discussions at the Examination Hall.

9-12 p.m.—Public reception of the Members of the Congress by the British Otologists at King's Hall, Holborn, W.C.

WEDNESDAY, AUGUST 9TH.

10-1.30.—Meeting for general discussion on "Indications for opening the Mastoid in Chronic Suppurative Otitis Media," and for papers, at the Examination Hall.

3 p.m.—Demonstrations at the Examination Hall.

7.30 p.m.—Dinner given by the President to the foreign Otologists at the Hotel Cecil, Strand.

THURSDAY, AUGUST 10TH.

10-1.30.—Meeting for papers and discussions at the Examination Hall.

FRIDAY, AUGUST 11TH.

10-1.30—Meeting for papers and discussions at the Examination Hall.

3-6 p.m.—Closing meeting of the Congress.

7.30 p.m.—Dinner given by the British Organization Committee to their foreign guests at the Whitehall Rooms, Hotel Metropole.

SATURDAY, AUGUST 12TH.

Excursion to Windsor Castle, and to Luncheon at Bray, by kind invitation of Mr. George P. Field.

LIST OF DELEGATES.

THE CHICAGO OPHTHALMOLOGICAL AND OTOLOGICAL SOCIETY appointed Dr. Allen T. Haight, of Chicago, Delegate to the Congress, and he also represented the CHICAGO MEDICAL SOCIETY.

THE AMERICAN LARYNGOLOGICAL, RHINOLOGICAL, AND OTO-LOGICAL SOCIETY was represented by Dr. Lederman, of New York, and Dr. M. A. Goldstein, of St. Louis. The latter also represented the WESTERN OPHTHALMOLOGIC AND OTO-LARYNGOLOGIC ASSOCIATION, of which he is Vice-President.

DIE DEUTSCHE OTOLOGISCHE GESELLSCHAFT appointed as Delegates, Prof. Lucae (Berlin), President of the Society; Dr. Arthur Hartmann (Berlin); and Prof. Stacke (Erfurt).

REGULATIONS.

1. The Official Languages are French, English, German, and Italian. If special request is made, one of the members present will be asked to give in abstract a translation of each communication.
2. No paper shall exceed 15 minutes in reading, so that all long communications should be read in abstract. Any speech in the subsequent discussions shall not exceed 5 minutes.
3. The communications will be published in the Transactions which will appear after the Congress, and be sent gratuitously to each Member.
4. All papers read, and all communications made to the Congress are to be *immediately* sent to the Editorial Committee.
5. All speakers taking part in the discussions are requested to send to the Editorial Committee *before the end of the Meeting* a written abstract of their remarks.
6. The Subscription, entitling to Membership of the Congress, is fixed at £1.
7. The Officers reserve to themselves the right of fixing the order of communications each day.

GENERAL DISCUSSION.

A general discussion on "Indications for opening the Mastoid in Chronic Suppurative Otitis Media" will be opened by Prof. Knapp (New York), Dr. Luc (Paris), Prof. William Macewen (Glasgow), and Prof. Politzer (Vienna).

* COMMUNICATIONS ANNOUNCED.

I.—NORMAL AND PATHOLOGICAL ANATOMY
(Anatomie Normale et Anatomie Pathologique).

1. JOYCE, Mr. R. (Dublin).—"The topography of the facial nerve in its relation to mastoid operations, with specimens and lantern demonstration."
2. CHEATLE, Mr. A. H. (London).—"The Petro-Squamosal Sinus."
3. COSTINIU, Dr. (Bucharest).—"L'état des oreilles, du larynx, et du nez observé chez les vieillards."
4. COZZOLINO, Prof. Vincenzo (Naples).—"Contribution à l'histologie du squelette des cornets pour la pathogénèse de l'ozène." (avec demonstration).
5. DENKER, Dr. (Hagen).—"Zur Anatomie des Gehörorgans der Säugethiere, mit Demonstration von Präparaten und Zeichnungen."
6. RUTTEN, Dr. (Namur).—"Présentation d'une exostose du conduit auditif droit."

II.—PHYSIOLOGY AND METHODS OF EXAMINATION
(Physiologie et méthodes d'exploration).

7. BARATOUX, Dr. J. (Paris).—"L'unification et la mesure de l'ouïe."
8. BONNIER, Dr. Pierre (Paris).—"Un procédé d'acoumétrie."
9. GRADENIGO, Prof. G. (Turin).—"Sur l'examen fonctionnel de l'organe de l'ouïe, et sur la notation uniforme des résultats."
10. KAYSER, Dr. Richard (Breslau). — "Experimentelle Untersuchungen über acustische Phaenomene in flüssigen Medien." (mit Demonstration).
11. SCHMIEGELOW, Dr. E. (Copenhagen).—"On a new method of measuring the quantitative hearing power by means of tuning forks."

III.—PATHOLOGY AND THERAPEUTICS
(Pathologie et Thérapeutique).

12. AVOLEDO, Prof. (Milan).—"Due casi di complicazioni patologiche della faccia in seguito a propagazione di un processus suppurativo acuto dell'Orecchio Medio e Esterno."

* Some of the Communications were subsequently withdrawn.

13. AVOLEDO, Prof. (Milan).—"Risultati della chirurgia intra-timpanica nei riguardi della funzione acustica, ma solo per la forma suppurativa."

14. BABER, Mr. Cresswell (Brighton).—"Turbinotomy in nasal obstruction."

15. BAR, Dr. Louis (Nice).—"Abcès antérieurs de la mastoïde et furonculose du conduit auditif externe."

16. BOBONE, Dr. T. (San Remo).—"L'involution précoce du tissu adénoïdien sur la Riviera."

17. BRIEGER, Dr. O. (Breslau).—"Ueber Tuberculose des Mittelohrs."

18. CHEATLE, Mr. A. H. (London).—"A case of Adenoma of the meatus in a patient suffering with chronic middle ear suppuration."

19. COSTINIU, Dr. (Bucharest).—"Résultats des exercises-acoustiques chez les sourds-muets."

20. COZZOLINO, Prof. Vincenzo (Naples). — "Statistiques des mastoïdotomies simples et radicales, et des opérations de chirurgie oto-endocrânienne pratiquées dans ma Clinique universitaire depuis l'an 1883."

21. COZZOLINO, Prof. Vincenzo (Naples).—"Pseudo-actinomycosis auriculaire externe avec ostéomiélite diffuse à la zone mastoïdienne, causée par un nouveau bacille filamenteux pyogénique" (avec demonstration).

22. CURSETJI, Dr. J. J. (Bombay).—"Some aspects of aural practice in India, with special reference to Bombay."

23. DADYSETT, Dr. H. J. (Bombay).—"A paper on various domestic remedies with their effects, used by the people of India for certain diseases of the ear."

24. DELIE, Dr. (Ypres).—"Panotite avec complication cérébrale—opération—mort—autopsie."

25. DENCH, Dr. E. B. (New York).—"The Operative Treatment of Mastoid Inflammation."

26. DE SANTI, Dr. P. (London).—"The Radical Cure of chronic suppurative Otitis Media by Antrectomy and Attico-Antrectomy, with notes of thirty cases."

27. DE SANTI, Dr. P. (London).—"Some cases illustrating the intra-cranial complications of neglected Otorrhœa."

28. EEMAN, Prof. (Ghent).—"La sclérose de la caisse tympanique."

29. FARACI, Prof. Giuseppe (Palermo).—"Sulla possibilita di riaprire la finestra ovale nei casi di anchilosi ossea della articolazione stapedo-vestibolare."

30. FARACI, Prof. Giuseppe (Palermo).—"Importanza acustica e funzionale della mobilizzazione della staffa."

31. FARACI, Prof. Giuseppe (Palermo).—"Utilita della miringectomia temporanea e consecutiva mobilizzazione di tutta la catena

degli ossicini nel periodo sub-acuto di un otite catarrale decorsa senza perforazione timpanica."

32. FISCHENICH, Dr. Fr. (Wiesbaden).—" Die Behandlung der katarrhalischen Adhaesivprocesse im Mittelohre, durch intratympanale Pilocarpininjectionen."

33. GARNAULT, Dr. Paul (Paris).—"Mobilisation (two years ago and extraction (one year ago) of the Stapes, in the same patient) with great improvement in hearing and typical phenomena."

34. GARNAULT, Dr. Paul (Paris).—" Mobilisation (three years ago) of the Stapes, in a man seventy-two years of age, deaf for forty years, absolutely so for fifteen, with great and permanent improvement in hearing."

35. GARZIA, Dr. Vincenzo (Naples).—" Experimental study of the influence of malaria in diseases of the ear."

36. GOLDSTEIN, Dr. M. A. (St. Louis, U.S.A.).—"Therapy of the Tympanic Mucous Membrane."

37. GRANT, Dr. Dundas (London).—" Diminished 'Bone-conduction' as a Contra-Indication for Ossiculectomy."

38. GRAY, Dr. Albert (Glasgow).—"A case of unilateral Deafness caused by a Tumour of the Medulla, producing other remarkable symptoms—Post Mortem " (with microscopic slides of the medulla).

39. GRAZZI, Prof. V. (Florence).—" Nuova cura delle faringiti catarrali croniche in rapporto specialmente alle malattie dell'orecchio."

40. HAIGHT, Dr. Allen T. (Chicago).—" Naso-Pharyngeal Adenoids as a causative factor in Ear Diseases."

41. HARTMANN, Dr. Arthur (Berlin).—"Angeborener und erworbener Fehler des äusseren Gehörganges mit Demonstration von Präparaten."

42. HEIMAN, Dr. Th. (Warsaw).—" De l'inflammation primaire de l'apophyse mastoïde."

43. KEIPER, Dr. Geo. F. (La Fayette, Ind.).—" A Description of a set of Mastoid Gouges."

44. LACROIX, Dr. P. (Paris).—"Complications otiques de l'ozène."

45. LAURENS, Dr. (Paris).—"Otite moyenne chronique suppurée avec thrombose du sinus latéral et abcès du cervelet."

46. LERMOYEZ, Dr. Marcel (Paris).—"La Contagiosité des Otites moyennes aiguës."

47. LUBET-BARBON, Dr. (Paris).—" Note sur les abcès aigus de l'apophyse mastoïde sans abcès de la caisse."

48. LUCAE, Prof. A. (Berlin).—" Zur Radicaloperation bei chronischer purulenter Mittelohrentzündung."

49. MALHERBE, Dr. (Paris).—" Traitement chirurgical de l'Otite moyenne chronique sèche par l'évidement petro-mastoïdien, avec et sans tubage."

50. MELZI, Dr. Urbano (Milan).—"A case of retropharyngeal abscess of auricular origin."

51. MELZI, Dr. Urbano (Milan).—"A case of nasal hydrorrhœa."

52. MELZI, Dr. Urbano (Milan).—"A case of endothelial fibro-angioma of the external auricular canal."

53. MÉNIÈRE, Dr. E. (Paris).—"Traitement des suppurations chroniques de l'attique."

54. MILLIGAN, Dr. W. (Manchester).—"Some observations upon the diagnosis and treatment of tuberculous disease of the middle ear and adjoining mastoid cells."

55. MINK, Dr. P. J. (Zwolle).—" Pneumomassage unter höherem Drucke."

56. MOURE, Dr. E. J. (Bordeaux).—" Sur quelques cas de complications endocrâniennes d'origine otique."

57. MOURE, Dr. E. J. (Bordeaux).—" Sur quelques points de technique à propos de la trépanation de l'apophyse mastoïde."

58. NUVOLI, Dr. G. (Rome).—" Sulla cura pneumatica nelle malattie dell'orecchio."

59. OSTMANN, Prof. (Marburg).—" Ueber die Heilbarkeit bisher unheilbarer Schwerhörigkeit durch Vibrationsmassage des Schallleitungsapparates."

60. PASSOW, Prof. (Heidelberg).—"Chirurgische Eingriffe bei Sklerose und bei Ménièreschen Symptomen."

61. POLITZER, Prof. Adam (Vienna).—"On the extraction of the stapes, with demonstrations of histological preparations."

62. ROHRER, Dr. F. (Zurich).—"On blue ear drums, 'tympanum cœruleum.' "

63. ROHRER, Dr. F. (Zurich).—"The appearance of varices on the ear drums."

64. RUDLOFF, Dr. P. (Wiesbaden).—"The operation of the removal of adenoid growths with the head hanging over the table, while the patient is under the influence of chloroform."

65. RYERSON, Dr. G. Sterling (Toronto).—"Objective noises in the ears."

66. SNOW, Dr. S. F. (Syracuse, N.Y.).—"Twentieth Century Prognosis in Chronic Catarrhal Deafness."

67. SZENES, Dr. (Budapest).—"Zur primärer Erkrankung des Warzenfortsatzes."

68. TANSLEY, Dr. J. Oscroft (New York).—"Shall we use cold in acute Middle Ear or Mastoid Affections—if so, *how long?*

69. TANSLEY, Dr. J. Oscroft (New York).—"Additional Remarks upon Ear Diseases caused by Deflected Septa."

70. TERVAERT, Dr. G. D. Cohen (The Hague).—"A case of thrombosis of both sinus cavernosi as a complication of chronic mastoiditis ex otorrhœa, which ended in recovery."

71. TURNBULL, Dr. Laurence (Philadelphia).—"Some of the most important discoveries in Otology : many of which have stoop the test of 35 years."

72. UCHERMANN, Prof. V. (Christiana).—"Rheumatic diseases of the ear."

73. VEYRAT, Dr. Ernest (Chambéry).—"Des améliorations de l'ouïe obtenues par le tympan artificiel, dans l'otite moyenne chronique sèche, ou sclérose tympanique."

74. VEYRAT, Dr. Ernest (Chambéry).—"Des Injections interstistielles de subliné dans le traitement des lupus du nez."

75. WHITE, Mr. F. Faulder (Coventry).—"The Curability of Suppurative Otitis Media, without operation."

IV.—DEMONSTRATIONS.

76. HARTMANN, Dr. Arthur (Berlin).—"Lantern-slide demonstration on the Anatomy of the Frontal Sinus."

77. KATZ, Dr. L. (Berlin).—"Demonstration microscopischer und macroscopischer Präparate des Gehörorgans."

78. SZENES, Dr. S. (Budapest).—"Demonstration pathologisch-anatomischer Präparate : (*a*) 'Melanosarcoma auriculae et meatus.' (*b*) 'Osteoma liberum meatus auditorii externi.' "

79. TURNER, Dr. Aldren (London).—"Lantern-slide demonstration on the course and connections of the Central Auditory Tract."

ADDITIONAL COMMUNICATIONS.

(Received since the issue of the first edition of the Programme).

80. BARR, Dr. Thomas (Glasgow).—"Otitic pyœmia *with pneumonia* —recovery after clearing out the lateral sinus, and ligaturing the internal jugular vein."

81. BRONNER, Dr. A. (Bradford).—"Local medication in the treatment of non-purulent catarrh of the middle ear."

82. CALAMIDA, Dr. (Turin).—"On the nerves of the enlarged pharyngeal and faucial tonsils."

83. CONNAL, Mr. Galbraith (Glasgow).—"A case of sarcoma of the ear in a girl six years of age." (With photograph and microscopic sections).

84. COOSEMANS, Dr. (Brussels).—"L'audition chez les Beetlers."

85. GRADENIGO, Prof. G. (Turin).—"On the amplified Otological Bibliographical notation according to the decimal systems of Melvil Dewey."

86. GRADENIGO, Prof. G. (Turin).—"On the opportune means for pro-
    moting a congruous increment of otological study in the
    Universities and in the social legislation."
87. HESSLER, Prof. (Halle, a/S.).—"Hirntumor bei Mittelohreite-
    rung."
88. HORNE, Dr. Jobson (London).—"The conversion of the saccus
    endo-lymphaticus into an abscess sac which ruptured and caused
    septic lateral sinus thrombosis and death" (a preliminary com-
    munication).
89. JONES, Dr. Hugh E. (Liverpool).—"Cases of mastoid and
    intracranial extension of suppuration from the tympanum with
    remarks and queries respecting the chronology of complications,
    and its bearing on treatment."
90. JONES, Dr. Hugh E. (Liverpool).—"A case of malformed auricle."
91. KOEBEL, Dr. (Stuttgart).—"Ueber Combination von Otitis media
    mit rhinogenem Gehirnabscess."
92. LANNOIS, Dr. M. (Lyons).—"L'oreille et l'Epilepsie."
93. OSTINO, Dr. G. (Turin).—"On the experiment of Egger."
94. POLI, Prof. Camillo (Genoa).—"Cinque casi di sinuflebite otitica
    trattati colla disinfezione del sinu e la legatura della giugulare."
95. POLI, Prof. Camillo (Genoa).—"Rapporti tra le vie nasali e le vie
    auricolari dell'infez˙one endocranica."
96. MILBURY, Dr. F. S. (Brooklyn, N.Y.).—"Mastoiditis, course and
    treatment."
97. ˙ALT, Dr. Ferdinand (Vienna).—"Experimentelle Untersuchungen
    über das corticale Hörcentrum."

MUSEUM.

A Museum of about five thousand Specimens, illustrating the
Comparative and Human Anatomy and Diseases and Injuries of the
Ear, Nose, and Naso-Pharynx, and Instruments, was held at the
Examination Hall during the Congress.

A full descriptive Catalogue (published by Adlard and Son), has
been issued, copies of which have been supplied to Foreign and
Colonial Members of the Congress. Price to other Members, 5/-, to
Non-Members, 7/6.

For copies apply to Messrs. Adlard and Son, Bartholomew Close,
London, E.C.

LIST OF MEMBERS.

* Signifies those present.

*Dr. FERDINAND ALT, ix. Alserstrasse 4,   Vienna.
*Dr. VAN ANROOIJ, 27, Withstraat,   Rotterdam.
Dr. RICHARD ARTHUR, Military Road, Mosman,   Sydney, N.S.W.
*Surgeon ASANO,   Japanese Navy.
*Prof. PIETRO AVOLEDO, 15, Via Agnello,   Milan.
Dr. AYRES, 14, East Seventh Street,   Cincinnati, Ohio.

*Mr. E. CRESSWELL BABER, 46, Brunswick Square, Brighton.
*Dr. J. B. BALL, 12, Upper Wimpole Street, W.,   London.
*Mr. CHARLES BALLANCE, 106, Harley Street, W., London.
*Mr. H. A. BALLANCE, 46, Prince of Wales' Road,   Norwich.
*Dr. WILLIAM BALLINGER,   Chicago.
*Dr. LOUIS BAR, 22, Boulevard Dubouchage,   Nice.
Dr. J. BARATOUX, 13, Avenue de l'Opéra,   Paris.
*Dr. BARCK, 2715, Locust Street,   St. Louis, U.S.A.
*Dr. BARK, 54, Rodney Street,   Liverpool.
*Prof. A. BARKAN, 14, Grant Avenue,   San Francisco.
*Dr. THOMAS BARR, 13, Woodside Place, Charing
    Cross,   Glasgow.
Dr. J. W. BARRETT, 127, Collins Street,   Melbourne.
*Dr. BECO, 4, Rue Larnelle,   Liege.
*Dr. OLIVER BELT, 922, Farragut Square,   Washington, D.C.
Dr. F. W. BENNETT, 25, London Road,   Leicester.
*Dr. C. H. BENNI, 16, Bracka,   Warsaw.
Dr. A. H. BENSON, 42, Fitzwilliam Square,   Dublin.
*Dr. BIRKETT, 123, Stanley Street,   Montreal.
*Dr. T. BOBONE, 15, Via Vittorio Emanuele,   San Remo.
*Dr. J. W. BOND, 26, Harley Street, W.,   London.
Dr. PIERRE BONNIER, 166, Faubourg St., Honoré, Paris.
Dr. MACKENZIE BOOTH, 367, Union Street,   Aberdeen.
*Dr. BOUCHERON, 11, Rue Pasquier,   Paris.
Dr. A. BRADY, 3, Lyons Terrace, Hyde Park,   Sydney, Aus.
*Dr. O. BRIEGER, 2, Königsplatz,   Breslau.
*Dr. A. BRONNER, 33, Manor Row,   Bradford.
*Dr. J. E. BROWN, 239, East Town Street,   Columbus, Ohio.
*Dr. W. L. BROWN, 103, Fortress Road, N.W.,   London.

Mr. EDGAR BROWNE, 39, Rodney Street,   Liverpool.
Dr. J. WALTON BROWNE, 10, College Square North, Belfast.
*Dr. J. H. BRYAN, 818, Seventeenth Street,   Washington.
Dr. J. SANTIUSTE BUEGA, 5, Wad-Ras,   Santander, Spain.
*Mr. W. C. BULL, 5, Clarges Street, Mayfair, W., London.
Dr. BULLER, 123, Stanley Street,   Montreal.
*Mr. HAMILTON BURT, 34, West Hill Road,   Brighton.

*Dr. A. CAPART, 5, Rue Egmont,   Brussels.
*Dr. CAPART (fils), Chateau de Dielighem,   Jette-Saint-Pierre,
                                                 Belgium.
*Dr. GEORGE CATHCART, 35, Harley Street, W.,   London.
*Dr. TALBOT CHAMBERS, 293, York Street,   Jersey.
*Mr. ARTHUR CHEATLE, 117, Harley Street, W.,   London.
*Dr. FELIX COHN, 717, Madison Avenue,   New York City.
*Mr. GALBRAITH CONNAL, 4, Burnbank Terrace,   Glasgow.
*Dr. J. CARDEEN COOPER,   Philadelphia.
*Dr. E. COOSEMANS, 12, Avenue du Midi,   Brussels.
*Dr. A. COSTINIU, 48, Str. Fontanei,   Bucharest.
Prof. COZZOLINO,   Naples.
*Mr. A. E. CUMBERBATCH, 80, Portland Place,. W., London.
Dr. J. J. CURSETJI, 10, Churchgate Street,   Bombay.

Dr. H. J. DADYSETT, Church Gate Medical Hall Fort, Bombay.
*Dr. GIOVANNI D'AJUTOLO, 16, Via Marsala,   Bologna.
Sir WILLIAM DALBY, 18, Savile Row, W.,   London.
*Dr. DELIE,   Ypres, Belgium.
*Dr. V. DELSAUX, 250, Avenue Louise,   Brussels.
*Dr. E. B. DENCH, 17, West 46th Street,   New York.
Dr. DENKER, 49, Bahnhofstrasse,   Hagen, Westphalia.
*Dr. ERNEST DELSTANCHE,   Brussels.
*Dr. G. M. DIDSBURY, 6, Rue Saint Florentin,   Paris.
Mr. JAMES DONELAN, 2, Upper Wimpole Street, W.,   London.
*Dr. L. DUBAR, Rue de Dunkerque,   Armentières, France
*Dr. DUCHESNE, 1, Rue St. Adalbert,   Liege.

Dr. WELLS EAGLETON, 121, Orange Street,   Newark, N.J.
*Prof. EEMAN, 8, Quài des Récollets,   Ghent.
*Dr. EULENSTEIN,   Frankfort, a/M.
*Dr. F. C. EWING,   St. Louis, U.S.A.

Mr. C. H. FAGGE, 22, St. Thomas' Street, S.E.,   London.
*Prof. GIUSEPPE FARACI,   Palermo, Sicily.
Dr. FERGUSON, Waimona, High Street,   Dunedin, N.Z.

*Mr. GEORGE P. FIELD, 34, Wimpole Street, W.,   London.
*Dr. FR. FISCHENICH, 20, Taunusstrasse,   Wiesbaden.
Dr. C. E. FITZGERALD, 27, Upper Merrion Street, Dublin.
Dr. W. JONES FREER, 2, Chepstow Road,   Newport, Mon.
*Dr. FREW,   Kilmarnock.
*Dr. ROBERT FULLERTON, 24, Newton Place,   Glasgow.

*Dr. PAUL GARNAULT, 15, Rue Manomemil,   Paris.
*Dr. L. R. GASPAR,   Funchal, Madeira.
Dr. GEORGES GELLÉ, 4, Rue Ste. Anne,   Paris.
*Dr. CHARLES GEVAERT, 3, Quai des Moines,   Ghent.
*Dr. M. A. GOLDSTEIN, 3702, Olive Street,   St. Louis, U.S.A.
*Prof. GIUSEPPE GRADENIGO, 44, Corso Vittorio
    Emanuele,   Turin.
*Dr. DUNDAS GRANT, 8, Upper Wimpole Street, W., London.
*Dr. ALBERT A. GRAY, 16, Berkley Terrace,   Glasgow.
*Prof. VINCENZO GRAZZI, 8, Borgo dei Greci,   Florence.
*Mr. CHARLES D. GREEN, The Ferns, South Street, Romford.
Dr. ORNE GREEN, 182, Marlborough Street,   Boston, Mass.
Dr. G. TAYLOR GUILD, 164, Nethergate,   Dundee.
*Prof. A. A. GUYE, 314, Herrengracht,   Amsterdam.

*Dr. ALLEN T. HAIGHT, 103, State Street,   Chicago.
*Dr. HAIKE, 33, Wilhelmstrasse,   Berlin.
*Dr. DAVID HARROWER,   Worcester, Mass.
Mr. W. H. HARSANT, Tower House, Clifton Road, Clifton, Bristol.
*Dr. ARTHUR HARTMANN, 8, N.W. Roonstrasse,   Berlin.
Mr. F. G. HARVEY, 4, Cavendish Place, W.,   London.
Dr. W. K. HATCH, Breachcandy,   Bombay.
*Dr. A. E. HAYES, 201, Providence Road,   Rhode Island,
     U.S.A.
*Dr. TH. HEIMAN, 127, Marszalkowska,   Warsaw.
*Dr. C. HENNEBERT, 27, Rue de la Pépinière,   Brussels.
*Prof. HESSLER, 44, Mühlweg,   Halle a/S.
*Dr. JULES HIGUET,   Brussels.
*Dr. W. HILL, 28, Weymouth Street, W.,   London
*Dr. F. WHITEHILL HINKEL,   Buffalo, U.S.A.
*Dr. HIRSCHLAND, 63, Linden-Allée,   Essen a/R.
*Dr. HOCKE,   Nymwegen, Holland
*Dr. C. R. HOLMES, 8 & 10, East Eighth Street,   Cincinnati, Ohio.
*Dr. J. HOLINGER, 103, Randolph Street,   Chicago.
*Dr. W. JOBSON HORNE, 27, New Cavendish St., W., London.
*Mr. T. MARK HOVELL, 105, Harley Street, W.,   London.
*Prof. A. A. HUBBELL, 212, Franklin Street,   Buffalo, N.Y.
*Dr. A. HUIJSMAN,   Utrecht.

*Dr. JOHN M. HUNT, 55, Rodney Street,   Liverpool.
*Dr. ARTHUR J. HUTCHISON, Throat & Ear Hospital, Brighton.

*Dr. CHEVALIER JACKSON, 63, Sixth Avenue,   Pittsburg, Pa.
*Dr. PIERRE JACQUIN, 4ᴵᴵ, Rue des Consuls,   Rheims.
 Dr. PERCY JAKINS, 120, Harley Street, W.,   London.
*Dr. JANSEN, 11, N.W. Neustädt-Kirchstrasse,   Berlin.
*Mr. RAYMOND JOHNSON, 11, Wimpole Street, W.,   London.
*Dr. MACKENZIE JOHNSTON, 2, Drumsheugh Gardens, Edinburgh.
*Dr. HUGH E. JONES, 7, Rodney Street,   Liverpool.
*Dr. MACNAUGHTON JONES, 131, Harley Street, W., London.
*Dr. H. M. MACNAUGHTON JONES, 12, Sandwell
     Mansions, West End Lane, N.W.,   London.
 Mr. R. JOWERS, 55, Brunswick Square,   Brighton.
*Dr. ROBERT JOYCE, Medical School, Cecilia Street, Dublin.

*Dr. KARUTZ, 5, Mühlenstrasse,   Lübeck.
*Dr. L. KATZ, 43, Jerusalemerstrasse,   Berlin.
*Dr. RICHARD KAYSER, 1, Tauentzienstrasse,   Breslau.
*Dr. GEORGE F. KEIPER, Cor. 6th & South Streets, La Fayette, Ind.
*Dr. A. BROWN KELLY, 26, Blythswood Square,   Glasgow.
 Dr. W. H. KELSON, 96, Queen St., Cheapside, E.C., London.
 Dr. A. L. KENNY, 87, Collins Street,   Melbourne.
*Dr. CHARLES J. KIPP, 534, Broad Street,   Newark, N.J.
*Dr. STAFFAN KLINGSPOR,   Stockholm.
*Dr. HERMAN KNAPP, 26, West 40th Street,   New York.
*Dr. KOEBEL, 16ᴵᴵ, Langestrasse,   Stuttgart.
*Prof. KUEMMEL,   Breslau.

*Dr. P. LACROIX, 41, Rue de Berlin,   Paris.
*Dr. C. B. LAGERLOEF, 13, Drottninggatan,   Stockholm.
*Mr. RICHARD LAKE, 19, Harley Street, W.,   London.
*Dr. W. LAMB, 41, Newhall Street,   Birmingham.
*Dr. M. LANNOIS, 14ᵎ Rue St. Dominique,   Lyons.
*Dr. LAUBI, 37, Bahnhofstrasse,   Zurich.
*Dr. LAURENS, 60, Rue de la Victoire,   Paris.
*Dr. EDWARD LAW, 35, Harley Street, W.,   London.
*Mr. L. A. LAWRENCE, 4, Queen Anne Street, W.,   London.
*Mr. A. B. LAZARUS, 77, Wimpole Street, W.,   London.
*Dr. LEDERMAN, 38, East 60th Street,   New York.
*Mr. CHARLES J. LEE, 73, Rodney Street,   Liverpool.
*Dr. G. A. LELAND, 669, Boylston Street,   Boston, U.S.A.
*Dr. LENHARDT, 25, Rue de l'Orangerie,   Le Havre.
*Dr. MARCEL LERMOYEZ, 20ᵇⁱˢ, Rue La Boétie,   Paris.
*Dr. C. J. LEWIS, 72, Newhall Street,   Birmingham.

*Dr. F. H. LEWIS, 46, Weymouth Street, W., London.
*Dr. F. P. LEWIS, Buffalo, N.Y.
Dr. HOPE LEWIS, Auckland, N.Z.
*Dr. MOORE LINDSAY, Salt Lake City, Utah.

Dr. HANAU LOEB, 3559, Olive Street, St. Louis, U.S.A.
Dr. LUBET-BARBON, 110, Boulevard Haussmann, Paris.
*Prof. LUC, 54, Rue de Varenne, Paris.
*Prof. A. LUCAE, 9, Lützow-Platz, Berlin.

*Prof. WILLIAM MACEWEN, 3, Woodside Crescent,
 Charing Cross, Glasgow.
Dr. JOHNSTON MACFIE, 45, Ashton Terrace,
 Hillhead, Glasgow.
*Dr. F. MADEUF, 10, Rue Fontaine-au-Roi, Paris.
*Dr. HUDSON MAKUEN, 1419, Walnut Street, Philadelphia.
*Dr. MALHERBE, 12, Place Delabórde, Paris.
*Monsieur MALHERBE, ,, ,, Paris.
Mr. F. MARSH, 34, Paradise Street, Birmingham.
Dr. D. JOSÉ A. MASIP, 58-1°, Pelayo, Barcelona.
*Dr. MATHESON, 11, Soho Square, W., London.
*Dr. P. McBRIDE, 16, Chester Street, Edinburgh.
Prof. URBANO MELZI, 4, Via Silvio Pellico, Milan.
*Dr. SUAREZ DE MENDOZA, 22, Avenue Friedland, Paris.
*Dr. E. MÉNIERE, 3, Place de la Madeleine, Paris.
*Dr. W. POSTHUMUS MEYJES, 582, Keizersgracht, Amsterdam.
Dr. F. S. MILBURY, 215, Jefferson Avenue, Brooklyn, N.Y.
*Dr. W. MILLIGAN, 28, St. John Street, Manchester.
*Dr. P. J. MINK, Zwolle, Holland.
*Dr. A. C. H. MOLL, 81, Steenstraat, Arnheim.
*Dr. E. J. MOURE, 25, Cours du Jardin Public, Bordeaux.
*Mr. GEORGE MURRAY, 34, Wimpole Street, W., London.

Dr. NAIR, Royapettah, Madras.
Dr. NELSON, Belfast.
*Dr. CHICHELE NOURSE, Abchurch House, Sher-
 borne Lane, King William Street, E.C., London.
*Dr. HENRY T. NOYES, 233, Madison Avenue, New York.
*Dr. G. NUVOLI, 47, Piazza del Gesü, Rome.

*Dr. OKADA, The University, Tokio, Japan.
*Prof. OSTMANN, Marburg a/L.
 Cassel.

*Mr. STEPHEN PAGET, 70, Harley Street, W., London.

*Dr. PATERSON, 18, Windsor Place,	Cardiff.
*Dr. H. PEGLER, 27, Welbeck Street, W.,	London.
*Dr. NORVAL H. PIERCE, 31, Washington Street,	Chicago.
Dr. B. PIETKOWSKI, 235, Bernardyńska,	Lublin, Poland.
*Prof. CAMILLO POLI, 12, Via Assaroti,	Genoa.
*Prof. ADAM POLITZER, 19, Gonzagagasse,	Vienna.
*Dr. JOSEPH POLLAK, 1, Kärnthnerstrasse 39,	Vienna.
Mr. BILTON POLLARD, 24, Harley Street, W.,	London,
*Prof. URBAN PRITCHARD, 26, Wimpole Street, W.,	London.
*Dr. A. PROEBSTING,	Wiesbaden.
*Dr. CHALLINOR PURCHAS,	Auckland, N.Z.
*Dr. F. PUTELLI,	Venice.
*Dr. RICHARD A. REEVE, 22, Shuter Street,	Toronto.
*Mr. ST. GEORGE REID,	Thornton Heath, Surrey.
*Dr. C. W. RICHARDSON, 1102, L. Street,	Washington, D.C.
*Dr. WALTER RIDLEY, 6, Ellison Place,	Newcastle-on-Tyne.
Dr. A. W. DE ROALDÈS, 203, North Rampart Street,	New Orleans, U.S.A.
*Dr. W. ROBINSON, 214-216, East 34th Street,	New York City.
*Dr. W. L. ROGERS, c/o J. D. Rogers and Co.,	Galveston, Texas.
*Dr. F. ROHRER, 9, Münsterhäuser,	Zurich.
*Dr. ROEPKE,	Solingen, Germany.
*Dr. R. ROUSE, Winter Palace,	Monte Carlo.
*Dr. P. RUDLOFF, 2a, Wilhelmstrasse,	Wiesbaden.
*Dr. RUTTEN,	Namur.
Dr. RICHARD SACHS, 13, Colonnaden,	Hamburg.
*Dr. A. W. SANDFORD, 13, St. Patrick's Place,	Cork.
*Mr. P. DE SANTI, 91, Harley Street, W.,	London.
*Dr. PAUL J. SARTAIN, 212, W. Logan Square,	Philadelphia.
*Dr. ROBERT SATTLER,	Cincinnati, Ohio.
*Dr. J. M. E. SCATLIFF, 11, Charlotte Street,	Brighton.
*Dr. E. SCHMIEGELOW, 18, Nórregade,	Copenhagen.
*Dr. DONALD SCHOKMAN,	Ceylon.
*Dr. E. SCHWARTZ, 1, Gartenstrasse,	Gleiwitz a/S.
*Prof. LOUIS SECRÉTAN,	Lausanne.
Mr. MARMADUKE SHEILD, 4, Cavendish Place, W.,	London.
*Dr. SARGENT F. SNOW, 204, E. Jefferson Street,	Syracuse, N.Y.
*Dr. GUIDO SONNENKALB, 1, Innere Johannisstrasse,	Chemnitz.
Dr. J. A. SPENCER, 91, Merrimack Street,	Haverhill, Mass.
*Dr. FREDERICK SPICER, 57, Devonshire Street, W.,	London.
*Dr. SCANES SPICER, 28, Welbeck Street, W.,	London.
*Dr. STANISLAS VON STEIN, 3, Grosser Afanasjewsky Pereulok,	Moscow.

Mr. W. R. H. STEWART, 42, Devonshire Street, W., London.
*Mr. GEORGE STONE, 88, Rodney Street,   Liverpool.
*Dr. STOERMANN,   Oberhausen, Rhein-
     land.
*Dr. J. B. STORY, 6, Merrion Square,   Dublin.
*Dr. GRAHAM STREET, 207-208, Norcross Building, Atlanta, Ga.
*Dr. SUNE-Y-MOLIST, 8, Calle del Carmen,   Barcelona.
Dr. H. R. SWANZY, 23, Merrion Square,   Dublin.

*Fleet Surgeon TAKEDA,   Japanese Navy.
*Dr. LEWIS TAYLOR,   Wilkes Barri, Pa.
Dr. COHEN TERVAERT, 10, Parkstraat,   The Hague.
*Dr. TEXIER, 8, Rue Jean Jacques Rousseau,   Nantes.
*Dr. SAMUEL THEOBALD, 304, Monument Street,   Baltimore, Md.
*Dr. ST. CLAIR THOMSON, 28, Queen Anne St., W., London.
*Mr. ATWOOD THORNE, 10, Nottingham Place, W., London.
Dr. A. B. THRASHER, "The Groton," N.E. Cor.
     7th and Race,   Cincinnati, Ohio.
*Dr. H. TILLEY, 101, Harley Street, W.,   London.
Dr. LAURENCE TURNBULL, 1933, Chestnut Street, Philadelphia.
*Dr. LOGAN TURNER, 20, Coates Crescent,   Edinburgh.

*Prof. V. UCHERMANN, 26B, Prinsens Gade,   Christiana.

Dr. PEDRO VERDÓS, Caspe-71-pràl,   Barcelona.
*Dr. ERNEST VEYRAT, Rue Juiverie,   Chambéry.
*Dr. B. VINCENT,   Copenhagen.
*Dr. DENNIS VINRACE, 24, Alexander Square,
     South Kensington,   London.

*Dr. E. WAGGETT, 45, Upper Brook Street, W.,   London.
*Mr. H. SECKER WALKER, 45, Park Square,   Leeds.
*Dr. F. H. WESTMACOTT, 8, St. John Street,   Manchester.
*Mr. F. FAULDER WHITE, The White House,   Coventry.
Mr. G. C. WILKIN,   West Coker,
     Somerset.
Dr. P. WATSON WILLIAMS, 1, Victoria Square,   Clifton, Bristol.
Dr. F. H. WILSON,   Brooklyn, N.Y.
*Mr. WYATT WINGRAVE, 11, Devonshire Street, W., London.
Dr. EDWARD WOAKES, 78, Harley Street, W.,   London.
Dr. ROBERT H. WOODS, 39, Merrion Square East, Dublin.

*Mr. P. MACLEOD YEARSLEY, 33, Weymouth St., W., London.

Prof. ZWAARDEMAKER,   Utrecht.

OFFICERS OF THE SIXTH CONGRESS.

President :

URBAN PRITCHARD.

Treasurer :

A. E. CUMBERBATCH.

Secretary-General :

CRESSWELL BABER.

Secretaries :

BARR,	HARTMANN,
BENNI,	LERMOYEZ,
BOBONE.	

The same will form the Editorial Committee.

NOTE.—The Seventh International Otological Congress will be held in 1902, at Bordeaux, under the Presidency of Dr. E. Moure.

SIXTH INTERNATIONAL OTOLOGICAL CONGRESS.

INAUGURAL MEETING.

CHAIRMAN   -   PROF. URBAN PRITCHARD.

The Inaugural Meeting of the Sixth International Otological Congress was held in the Theatre of the Examination Hall of the Royal Colleges of Physicians and Surgeons, on the Victoria Embankment, on Tuesday, August 8th, at 10 a.m.

The proceedings commenced with the following Address by

PROF. URBAN PRITCHARD,

President of the Organization Committee :—

In the name of the British Organization Committee, and in the name, indeed, of all British Otologists, I wish to offer a very hearty welcome to our foreign colleagues and to their ladies.

We thank you most sincerely for coming here, in many cases, hundreds—nay, even, I may say, thousands—of miles, in order to assist at this, the Sixth International Otological Congress, and I trust that your visit to London will be a very pleasant one ; at any rate, I may certainly promise that we will do all in our power to make it so.

There is, however, one serious difficulty which, with all the good-will in the world, cannot be removed. I refer to the fact that, owing to the immense size of this London of ours, so much loss of time is entailed in getting from place to place. When I remember how conveniently we were located during the pleasant gatherings of the Congress at Basle, at Brussels, and at Florence, and the ease with which we were enabled to find our way about, I cannot help regretting that our vast metropolis cannot be, for the moment, brought within more manageable compass; but as that is impossible, we must content ourselves with doing the best we can under the circumstances.

In bidding you welcome I have used the word "foreign" to our guests; but I do not like that designation in connection with our

Congress.   For SCIENCE acknowledges no differences of nationality; she is, herself, all in all; and faithfulness to her is the sole condition of citizenship in her kingdom.

Therefore let us regard ourselves, not as under our national flags, but as assembled in common brotherhood, marching together under the banner of Otology, and forming one part of that army, commanded by Science, which is engaged in overthrowing the foes of humanity, those foes which have Ignorance, Vice and Prejudice, for their leaders.

Personally, I feel a thrill of pleasure in seeing so many valued friends assembled again for conference ; and of these may 1 be permitted to mention the names of Politzer, Guye, Hartmann, Knapp, Benni, Ménière, Lucae, and that of our last President, Prof. Grazzi.

But it is a real grief to miss some old familiar faces.   The genial President at Basle, Burkhardt-Merian, dear old Sapolini of Milan, Moos of Heidelberg, and Delstanche (père) of Brussels, these bear honoured names which will long be remembered in the annals of Otology, though they themselves have passed "behind the veil."

Again, since our meeting in Florence, our branch of medical science has lost another faithful servant ; I allude to Dr. Meyer, of Copenhagen, whose name in connection with the discovery of postnasal adenoids is so justly renowned.   Lastly, among other names that must occur to each one of us, I will only refer to those of Prof. Colladon, of Geneva, and Hewetson of Leeds, who were both to have taken an active part in our proceedings this week.

We deeply regret also to note the absence, from unavoidable circumstances, of several friends whom we should so gladly have welcomed among us to-day ; and I am especially grieved that ill-health has prevented Dr. Charles Delstanche, our hospitable President at Brussels, from being in his accustomed place on this occasion,—I believe that it is the first time that our Otological Congress has not had the support of his energetic and cheery presence.

Now, friends, it seems to me that at the opening of our Congress it is well that we should recall briefly the story of the birth and growth of Otological Science, and with your permission I will say a few words on this subject, dwelling more particularly on the advances made in it during the last thirty years.

Although TOYNBEE is generally acknowledged to be the father of *modern* Otology, for the date of its birth we must go back some 3,400 years to the then flourishing country of Egypt.   For Prof. Roosa, in his excellent treatise, refers to a certain ancient papyrus (called, after its discoverer, the Papyrus Ebers) on which is written a monograph on "Medicines for ears hard of hearing" and "for ears from which there is a putrid discharge."   And here, in our Museum, may be seen a confirmation of the fact that ear troubles not only existed in those days, but that they could be cured ; for we have the good fortune to possess a curious old Egyptian relic, consisting of a wooden tablet on which are portrayed, in bas relief, two effigies of the Sacred Bull, and two Auricles; this was undoubtedly a votive offering to the god Hathor from some "grateful patient."

In spite of its early birth, however, Otology, except perhaps with regard to its anatomy and physiology, did not make itself of great importance until the second half of the present century. It is true that here and there a surgeon might have been found who had turned his attention, to some extent, to this subject; and, indeed, our own Royal Ear Hospital in Dean Street, Soho, which is acknowledged to have been the first successful aural clinique in Europe,—and I believe in the world—was established in 1816. But, speaking generally, we may safely assert that aural surgery continued to be more or less in the stage of infancy until between 1840 and 1860, when the study was vigorously taken up by Sir William Wilde and Toynbee, who thus gave a fresh impetus to the study of the pathology and treatment of diseases of the ear. Even then its importance was by no means generally recognised; indeed, only thirty years ago it was a favourite saying of more than one celebrated surgeon that "Ear diseases may be divided into two classes; those which can be cured by any general practitioner, and those which, being incurable, may be relegated to the tender mercies of the Ear specialist."

Is it any wonder, therefore, that in those days Aural Surgery was not only considered to be, but actually was, very much mixed up with the name of quackery; for as scientific men refused to have anything to do with it, the door was left open for any charlatan to enter, and many strange stories gained credence as to methods of treatment which the patient was required to undergo. Indeed, one of my earliest boyish recollections of aural surgery was hearing the story of how a child, a deaf mute, had been cured by a skewer having been passed through his head from one ear to the other. Although a somewhat better knowledge of anatomy has since made me doubt the accuracy of this statement, still it is certain that strange things were both said and done in the olden times, which did not redound greatly to the honour of the specialist.

In my own student days I well remember the sarcastic manner of Prof. Partridge — Dicky, as we used to call him — when he said, "Ah, gentlemen, a little wax is a god-send to an aurist;" meaning, of course, that its removal was an easy method of earning a reputation. And, no doubt, there is a certain truth in these words, though not exactly in the sense implied by the good old professor; for which of us has not found that, by removing a plug of cerumen which has either not been diagnosed or which has resisted all the efforts of the general practitioner to dislodge, we have gained *kudos* and an appreciation which many of our more delicate operations have failed to secure.

Yes, Otology had indeed a hard battle to fight before it could be said to have won honourable recognition among men of standing in the medical profession; and I shall never forget the letter which one of these wrote to me in 1872 when he first learnt that I intended to devote myself to this branch of study. After lamenting my decision, however, he did conclude by saying, "*Now* I suppose that I must not regard *all* aural surgeons as quacks." And may I add, as a kind of commentary on this letter, that within a few years afterwards, the writer of it came to me as a patient.

Things have indeed changed since then, for, instead of a few aural surgeons scattered here and there in Great Britain, we have now at least a couple of hundred; while the number of cliniques in London alone has been increased from two or three, to near upon twenty. And in many other countries this branch of medical science is even more strongly represented.

As a natural result of the increased interest in the work, let me call attention to the unique Museum connected with this Congress, wherein is to be found the largest and most valuable collection of Otological specimens ever formed, a collection which could only have been brought together by the union of our international forces.

But in one respect there is still room for improvement. I refer to the need for the better recognition of Otology by our Universities and Colleges. I am glad, however, to be able to report that a step has lately been made in this direction, for the University of Edinburgh has now made it one of the qualifying subjects for her medical degrees, and I look forward, with hope, to the time when her example will have been generally followed.

This "new departure" will, I trust, lead to a fuller recognition of the position of teachers of aural surgery. In this respect we, in the British Isles, are sadly behind other countries, where Chairs of Otology are numerous; whereas here, among all our Universities and Colleges, —where so many able lecturers are to be found—in King's College, London, alone, is the dignity of a professorship conferred upon its teacher of aural surgery.

Let me now pass in brief review the progress of the last 30 years.

So far as the ANATOMY and PHYSIOLOGY of the auditory apparatus are concerned comparatively little has been added to the store of knowledge already gained, although a more intimate study of its parts has made that knowledge more complete and precise.

In PATHOLOGY as may be expected, there has been considerable advance.

In disease of the meatus, although aspergillus was discovered before this period by Meyer, Schwartze, and Wreden, yet the subject was not elaborated with any fulness until later. Also, the nature and classification of exostoses have been worked out within this period.

Our knowledge of the changes in chronic middle ear catarrh, and in sclerosis, has considerably advanced, although much here yet remains to be done.

The effect of pathological conditions of the nose and naso-pharynx upon the auditory apparatus, adenoid vegetations more especially, has practically been discovered.

In chronic suppurative catarrh, disease of the ossicles, the implication of the attic, the antrum and the mastoid cells have been worked out; also the intracranial complications which sometimes follow. The nature of granulations and polypi are now better understood; and although Toynbee had already called our attention to cholesteatoma, its pathological importance in connection with mastoid disease was not fully realised until quite lately.

In the pathology of labyrinthine disease there has not, perhaps, been so much advance; but Ménière's disease is now better understood; and Politzer has made known to us a disease of the bony capsule. Finally, the pathology of congenital syphilis affecting the internal ear has been partially worked out.

Our MEANS OF DIAGNOSIS have been considerably improved.

The diagnosis between affections of the conducting apparatus and the auditory nerve, which formerly was often confused, is now much more easily made out; this is chiefly due to the study of the tuning fork.

Methods of illumination have very greatly improved, to the immense advantage of the surgeon.

Bacteriology, again, has done much, and, in all probability, will do even more in the future, to help us in our diagnosis. Unfortunately, the essential apparatus is enclosed in such dense bone that the Röntgen rays have been of but little assistance.

In TREATMENT there have been immense strides.

Even in chronic middle ear catarrh and in sclerosis, those diseases which hitherto have baffled our most strenuous efforts, a distinct advance has been made indirectly, especially in prophylaxis, by treatment of the nose and naso-pharynx.

In suppurative disease there has been very great improvement in treatment. By means of boric acid, alcohol, and other suitable antiseptics, simple otorrhœa has become much more manageable; and a far larger proportion of such cases are now healed, even without operation.

In the case of its complications—caries, granulations, and polypi—the advance made is most striking, and, in consequence, the large protruding polypus is now rarely seen; and no aural surgeon at the present time would be able to show so large a collection of these as Dr. Warden, of Birmingham, was in the habit of displaying some twenty-five to thirty years ago.

Curetting of carious spots, and the removal of ossicles, so important in the treatment of many cases, has only recently been introduced.

This brings us to the wonderful stride made in the treatment of antrum and mastoid disease, for which we have chiefly to thank Profs. Schwartze and Stacke, although many others have contributed to the advancement. How much agony has been relieved, how many lives have been saved, by these operations!

And, gentlemen, this advance of surgery has carried us still further; for, by the joining hands of general surgery and otology, intracranial suppuration has been robbed of many of its victims.

But how, and why, is this? How is it that, formerly, our surgeons were unable to cope with these intracranial conditions? How is it that, now, we are able to operate on the tympanum, attic and mastoid, practically with impunity?

Gentlemen, this is due to the adoption of ANTISEPTIC SURGERY. May I beg your indulgence for proudly claiming to be pupil, colleague, and brother professor of him whom I regard as the greatest man living to-day—Lord Lister. Were it not that you would exclaim at my inconsistency, I should be tempted to add 'compatriot' also. But yes, gentlemen, I will add the word. Not, however, in the sense in which I was just about to use it, that of English nationality; but with reference to that ideal country to which I alluded at the beginning of my speech, and of which we otologists are all the naturalized subjects. Here, on the common ground of our chosen land, the land of Science, we may all proudly claim Lord Lister as our compatriot, all rejoice to serve under such a leader in the battle against disease and death. The world does not as yet understand the full benefits which he has conferred upon mankind, but we, naturally, being his compatriots, have a better opportunity for doing so; and I can only add my earnest conviction that it is by faithfully following the counsels of our superior officer that our advancing column can best secure future victories.

Such, ladies and gentlemen, is the brief, and therefore necessarily inadequate, record of the progress of Otology which I desired to lay before you.

We have seen that this nineteenth century, which has brought to the world so many wonderful blessings in other directions, has not been unmindful of our branch of medical science. For, whereas at its commencement the ear was regarded almost as a *terra incognita*, scarcely worth consideration except as the seat of one affection only—that which was generally-known as 'a deafness'—now, at its close, this organ is fully-explored ground, and has been proved well worth the exploration. Otology has been raised from the rank of pseudo-quackery to an honourable position in scientific surgery, and its importance and bearing upon the body as a whole is now fully recognised.

But while we rejoice in the progress made in the past, we must remember that much still remains to be done. For instance, we have yet to clear away that opprobrium of aural surgery, namely, chronic non-suppurative disease of the middle ear. Shall we, in the near future, be enabled to cope successfully with this hitherto invincible foe? Judging from the advance made in other directions I am bold enough, and sanguine enough, to think that we shall; and assuredly when that help comes we shall all unite in blessing the victor over this foe.

Now, it is the province of our Otological Congresses to take this and similar problems into consideration. But the real value of these gatherings is not to be measured merely by papers and discussions. This is one of their uses, it is true, for interchange of ideas is always good; still, the chief value of thus meeting together with others who are all interested in one common subject is the kindling of enthusiasm which is engendered, an enthusiasm which should serve to stimulate older and younger members alike to renewed efforts in the paths both of research and of practical treatment; and therefore, in conclusion, I desire most heartily to wish that this, our sixth Congress, may be successful in all these directions.

MR. CRESSWELL BABER, Honorary Secretary-General of the Organization Committee, then said :—

I have received letters regretting their inability to attend the Opening Meeting of the Congress from H.R.H. the Prince of Wales, and from the Lord Mayor of London.

I have also received communications from the following colleagues, who, for various reasons, are prevented from being with us to-day, viz:— Messrs. Gellé, Lubet-Barbon, and Baratoux (Paris); Noquet (Lille); Delstanche (Brussels) ; Stacke (Erfurt) ; Passow (Heidelberg) ; Rosenberg (Berlin) ; Bezold (Munich); Sachs (Hamburg); Cozzolino (Naples) ; Masip (Barcelona) ; Spencer (Haverhill, Mass.) ; Tansley (New York) ; Szenes (Budapest) ; Dadysett (Bombay).

Dr. Laurence Turnbull, of Philadelphia, in making his excuses, writes: "It would have afforded me much pleasure, as one of the oldest members of this organization to have responded to the invitation of the Society, and met you on English ground, but my health is so much impaired that I cannot be with you, nevertheless my heart is, and I send to all my many friends a hearty greeting, and wish you 'God speed' in your work."

The following members of the British Organization Committee have written expressing their regret at being unable to be present :—Messrs. Bilton Pollard (London) ; Harsant (Clifton) ; Mackenzie Booth (Aberdeen); Swanzy and Fitzgerald (Dublin); Hatch and Cursetji (Bombay), and Ferguson (New Zealand).

The following have been appointed Delegates to this Congress :—

DR. M. A. GOLDSTEIN, St. Louis, and DR. LEDERMAN, New York, Delegates from the "American Laryngological, Rhinological, and Otological Society." The former represents also the "Western

Ophthalmologic and Oto-Laryngologic Association," of which he is Vice-President.

DR. ALLEN T. HAIGHT, Chicago, Delegate from the "Chicago Ophthalmological and Otological Society," and also from the "Chicago Medical Society."

PROF. LUCAE, Berlin, President of the Society, DR. A. HARTMANN, Berlin, and PROF. STACKE, Erfurt, Delegates from the "Deutsche Otologische Gesellschaft."

The PRESIDENT next proposed a cordial vote of thanks to the Royal College of Physicians of London, and to the Royal College of Surgeons of England, for having placed at the disposal of the Congress their Examination Hall. He further expressed his thanks to the Royal College of Surgeons of England for the loan to the Congress Museum of some of its most valuable and interesting specimens, more particularly mentioning those of the Toynbee collection, and of Professor Stewart, illustrating the comparative anatomy of the ear and nose.

SIR WILLIAM MACCORMAC, BART., President of the Royal College of Surgeons of England, in the absence of the President of the Royal College of Physicians of London, acknowledged the compliment and congratulated the President of the Organization Committee on his address, and on the large numbers attracted to the Congress in the cause of Science. The Royal College of Surgeons of England, he said, had great pleasure in lending specimens from their collection to the Congress Museum. A Congress such as this did much good amongst its members, in promoting a knowledge of one another, and of the work of each other.

PROF. GRAZZI, of Florence, President of the last Congress, delivered the following address :—

As it is usual for the President of the last Congress to say a few words at the opening meeting, the honour has devolved upon me to address you after the President of the year 1899, who has just delivered such a splendid speech.

I do not consider it necessary to occupy your time with an academical discourse, but will make my remarks as short as possible, for we have come here from distant climes for the purpose of augmenting the knowledge which we have already acquired.

Before proceeding further, I must tell you what pleasure I feel in being amongst you to-day. The organization of the Fifth Congress in Florence, gave me much thought and anxiety, but I feel fully repaid for all my exertions by seeing the continued extension of my work, and the realization of the hopes I then expressed that our reunions should be held regularly every four years. I hope and trust, that in future, so long an interval may not occur again, as that which took place between the Fourth and Fifth Meetings of the International Otological Congress. It was through no fault of mine that this long interval occurred.

At the Second Meeting of the Congress held in Milan, Professor Voltolini, of Breslau, Founder of the Organization, remarked :—" Ce n'est pas pour sûr un cas fortuit que la première session du Congrès international d'Otologie *en Europe* se tienne en Italie, car, à mon avis, c'est à un Italien que nous devons la résurrection de notre spécialité, à Corti, dont les découvertes nous ont révélé un nouveau monde dans l'organe de l'ouïe ? "

To corroborate the above assertion, Voltolini referred to the opinions of Kölliker and Deiters. I must not, however, quote his discourse at any length, as it is not my desire to honour the memory, nor to extol the merits of Corti (recognized by all), but rather to recall to your recollection the Congress of Milan.

Few remain among us, unfortunately, who can remember that epoch, some twenty years ago, which marked the beginning of the progress since made in Otology.

To paraphrase the words of Voltolini :—"It is not by mere chance that London has been chosen as the seat of this Congress—two illustrious London men, Wilde and Toynbee having contributed very largely to our speciality." Of Sir William Wilde, Prof. Roosa writes:— " Sir William Wilde probably did more to place our science upon a sound basis than anything that has been done since the days of Valsalva. He led Otology out of the *terra incognita* of the ancients and brought it to a point where it could be investigated by the average practitioner, and where it was respected by all." Wilde was the first to call this branch by the name of *aural surgery*. Otologists allowed many years to elapse before putting into practice the suggestions of Wilde, nevertheless, we must give him the credit of forcing on all, the acknowledgement that our speciality is eminently surgical. I agree with those who wrote :—" Wilde deserves to be named the Father of Modern Otology."

No less useful to the progress of our speciality, are the patient, arduous studies of Toynbee. He was the first to seriously study the pathological anatomy of the ear. Even at the present time, his investigations are of the greatest value, and a subject of admiration to us.

Wilde and Toynbee must be considered as two great lights, illuminating our modern science of Otology. Tröltsch, who has himself contributed very greatly to the progress of our speciality in Germany, declares himself to be a disciple of these two British Otologists.

In conclusion, I offer to all here a hearty salutation from Florence, who remembers with pride, the honour done to her in 1895, when she was chosen as the place of meeting for the Fifth International Otological Congress. London and Florence, although differing in many ways, are united. Florence, known as the City of Flowers, is most popular with the English people, for her artistic beauty, and the selection of London for this meeting was a happy one, and has been received with universal

approbation.   Before I close, I must offer my thanks to Prof. Urban
Pritchard and to the British Organization Committee for all they have
done to render this reunion a scientific success and for the kind welcome
they have accorded to us in the metropolis of the United Kingdom,
a welcome which will be engraved for ever on the hearts of all
those who take part in this Congress.

Prof. GRAZZI proposed that the following telegram should be
addressed to H.M. the Queen :—"The Sixth International Otological
Congress, which opened in London this day, begs, on the proposition of
Prof. Grazzi, of Florence, to offer to your Majesty its respectful
congratulations on the completion of the 62nd year of your Majesty's
prosperous reign."

Prof. POLITZER (Vienna) then said :—In order to efficiently carry out
the work of our Congress, it is necessary to appoint the officials, to
whom we can with confidence, hand over the direction of the work, and
I have the honour to suggest for your approval the following list of
officers :—

I. President of the Congress.

I am quite sure the name I am about to mention will meet with
your unanimous and hearty approval.   It is that of our distinguished
and congenial colleague, Dr. Urban Pritchard.   It is unnecessary to
speak at length of his exceptional scientific merits and high qualifications for the Presidency.   The former are well known to you all, in
regard to the latter, those of us who have had the pleasure of meeting
him, either in London or abroad, are well aware that he possesses all
these attainments and gifts, which will enable him to direct this
Congress so that it may not only be a source of scientific profit to the
world, but of pleasure to the Members.

II.   Treasurer : Mr. Cumberbatch.

III.   As Secretary-General I have to propose Mr. Cresswell Baber.

It will be largely owing to his genius for organization, backed by
incessant and laborious work, that this Congress will be brought to a
successful issue.

IV.   As Secretaries :—

Dr. Barr (Glasgow); Dr. Benni (Warsaw); Dr. Bobone (San
Remo) ; Dr. Hartmann (Berlin) ; Dr. Lermoyez (Paris).

The above also to form the Editorial Committee for the Transactions
of the Congress.

The proposition was seconded by Prof. LUCÆ (Berlin), and carried.

This concluded the business of the Inaugural Meeting.

SECOND MEETING.

TUESDAY, AUGUST 8TH, AT 3 P.M.

CHAIRMAN   -   PROF. URBAN PRITCHARD.

The following telegram from Dr. Morpurgo, of Trieste, addressed to Prof Politzer, was read :—

"Bedauern fern zu bleiben. Huldigung Praesident. Grüsse Collegen. Erfolg Congress.—MORPURGO."

ON A NEW METHOD OF MEASURING
THE QUANTITATIVE HEARING POWER BY MEANS OF TUNING FORKS.
DR. E. SCHMIEGELOW, Copenhagen.

Gentlemen,—Many are the experiments made in the course of latter years in order to find a reliable method of measuring the quantitative hearing power by means of tuning-forks.

I will here only mention the methods of *Hartmann*, *Gradenigo*, and *Zwardemaker*, which, however, cannot be called satisfactory, as they do not give exact results.

In order to use the time of vibration of certain tuning forks in measuring the hearing power, it is necessary to know the curve of extinction of the vibrations of these forks (the vibration curve).

If it were possible to measure the amplitude of each tuning-fork from the moment it was set in vibration to the moment when the tone died away, the difficulty in using forks as reliable tests of quantitative hearing would be solved.

In the light of our present knowledge and with the means of experiment at our command, this is impossible in the case of most tuning-forks, the amplitudes of the deeper forks *only* being measurable.

Bezold and *Edelmann* have, by means of a very ingenious instrument, constructed the vibration-curves of the deeper forks (from D^1 to F) and from these they have constructed a standard curve.

They furthermore presumed, that this curve being almost the same in all the deeper forks, must be the same for all forks, even the *highest* ones.

It seems, however, that *Bezold* and *Edelmann* have started from wrong premises, and that the results of their experiments do not agree with the theory.

According to the theory, the amplitudes decrease in an approximately geometrical progression, that is to say, that, the logarithms of the amplitudes diminish directly with the time. This theory is no doubt correct, but only as far as the small amplitudes are concerned

(Jacobson), or, in other words the logarithmical decrement is greater and irregular at the beginning, but towards the end it becomes nearly constant. If we now examine the curve found by *Bezold* and *Edelmann* (l.c. P. 179), it will be seen, that the differences between the logarithms of the amplitudes, corresponding to the time of 0 – 10 – 20 etc.—100 sec. to begin with decrease, as they ought to do,—but afterwards increase, as they ought not to do.

Time.	Amplitude.	Logarithms of the Amplitude.	Difference.
0 Sec.	100	2.	
10 ,,	42.2	1.625	0.375
20 ,	22.6	1.354	0.271
30 ,	13.5	1.130	0.224
40 ,	9.2	· 0.964	0.166
50 ,	6.5	0.813	0.151
60 ,	4.5	0.653	0.160
70 ,	3.1	0.491	0 162
80	1.9	0.279	0.212
90 ,	0.83	0.919 ÷ 1	0.360
100 ,,	0.32	0.505 ÷ 1	0.414

According to the theory we should expect that the difference after decreasing, as it does to 0.151, ought to remain pretty nearly *constant*. The difference, however, increases again, which means that for some reason or other, the vibrations are impeded at an increasing rate and the curve therefore is not correct.

It is furthermore improbable that the curve of vibrations should be the same for all forks, on the contrary everything tends to prove that the curve of the *higher* forks is different from that of the deeper ones, and that each fork has its own special curve.

In order to find the curve of vibration for each tuning fork, *G. Forchhammer* and I propose the following method : A tuning fork is struck, and the time during which it is heard at different distances from the ear is determined.

The abscissæ of the curve represent the distances, the ordinates the duration of perception.

The correctness of this method is founded on the fact, that the amplitude (a) is proportional to the distance (A) at which the tone disappears, the intensity of the tone, $(\frac{a}{A})^2$ being constant, when the " Hörschwelle " is reached, which is the moment when the tone can no longer be heard.

The method is also practical in so far that instead of the microscopic amplitudes (a), the macroscopic distances (A) are measured ; an advantage which is all the greater because the amplitudes of the higher tuning-forks cannot be measured microscopically.

The forks examined were made by *Edelmann*, in Munich, and are as follows :—C – G – c – g – c^1 – g^1 – c^2 – g^2 – c^3 – g^3 – c^4 – g^4 – c^5 ; all of them unloaded.

The experiments were made under as good conditions as could possibly be procured in the open air at some distance from town.

If, for instance, we are going to find the curve of the C^1 fork (261 vibrations), we proceed in the following way :—

By 6 series of experiments we find that C^1, properly struck, is normally heard for 7 sec. at a distance of 160 cntm. from the ear, 14 sec. at a distance of 80 cntm., 23 sec. at 40 cntm., 37 sec. at 20 cntm., 62 sec. at 10 cntm., 88 sec. at 5 cntm., and 117 sec. when held as close to the ear as possible without touching it.

	Sec.	Difference.
160 Cntm. from the ear	7	7
80 ..	14	9
40	23	14
20	37	25
10 ..	62	26
5 ,,	88	
x (close to the ear)	117	

In order to use these figures in constructing the curve we must make a few corrections.

First of all we have to calculate the distance x.

According to the theory the differences between the time at the distances: 5 – 10 Cntm., and the distances 10 – 20 Cntm. should be the same, because close to the ear where we have to do with small amplitudes, the time increases in an *arithmetical* ratio (*i.e.*, with constant difference), if the distance diminishes in a *geometrical* ratio.

This theory is actually proved by our experiments. At the beginning of the curve (from 160 – 20 cntm. distance), we find that the differences in time are smaller at the greater distances from the ear, that they increase up to about 20 cntm. distance, and then become constant as far as the final part of the curve is concerned.

By means of the times found experimentally for the distances x – 5 – 10 and 20 cntm. we are able to calculate the distance x from the point o (the origin) of the curve, because we have the following equation :

$$\log. \; a = \log. \; a \div \beta.t$$

in which 'a' denotes a certain distance, 't' denotes the time, and a and β are constants of which a is the maximum distance at which the fork can be heard, and we have now

$$\log. \; x = \log. \; a \div \beta. \; 117$$
$$\log. \; 5 = \log. \; a \div \beta. \; 88$$
$$\log. \; 10 = \log. \; a \div \beta. \; 62$$
$$\log. \; 20 = \log. \; a \div \beta. \; 37$$

and are able to find x.

Before doing this, however, the distances, especially the smaller ones, must be corrected.

The fact is that a tuning-fork does not emit the tone from the external surface of the prongs, but the vibrations are presumed to spread out from two points which are situated between the external surfaces of the prongs. By a series of experiments we have found that the distance between "the toncentre" and the external surface of the tuning-fork is about 1 cntm. for the forks C, G, c, g, c^1, g^1, and c^2, whilst the distance is about 1.5 cntm. for the forks g^2, c^3, g^3, c^4, g^4, and c^5.

As the distances in our experiments are reckoned from that surface of the prong which faces the ear, we must therefore add to the distances 5—10 and 20 cntm. the distance of the toncentre from the external surface of the tuning-fork.

With regard to the fork c^1 the addition would be 1 cntm. and we come to the following equations :—

$$\log.\ \ x = \log.\ a \div \beta.117$$
$$\log.\ \ 6 = \log.\ a \div \beta.88$$
$$\log.\ 11 = \log.\ a \div \beta.62$$
$$\log.\ 21 = \log.\ a \div \beta.37$$

The average value of β is 0.011 and $\times$ = 1.3 Cntm.

We are now able by means of the calculated value of x and the other experimentally found data to construct the curve for c^1.

If a patient hears the fork c^1 for instance 7 sec., the fork being struck powerfully and held close to the ear, it means, that this patient's " *Minimum hearing Amplitude* " or his " Hörschwelle " is $\frac{16.9}{}$ = 123 times the normal, his hearing distance $\frac{1}{123}$ times the normal, and his hearing power $(\frac{1}{123})^2$ = $\frac{1}{15129}$ of what is normal. If the normal hearing power is equal to 1, the reduced hearing power will be equal to 0.00007.

Suppose on the contrary the patient heard the fork 62 sec., his minimum hearing amplitude would be $\frac{11}{1.3}$ = 8·5 times the normal, his *hearing distance* $\frac{1}{8·5}$ times the normal and the *hearing power* $(\frac{1}{8·5})^2 = \frac{1}{72·25}$ times the normal = 0.0138, if the normal hearing power is equal to 1.

In this way we are able to construct the curve for every tuning fork, and thereby to find how much the hearing power is diminished, if we only know the time in which the fork is heard at a certain distance from the ear.

By comparing the curves of the different forks, we now see, how greatly they differ, some of them (the deeper forks) are steep and short, others (the higher forks) are flattened and long. In other words, the assumption of *Bezold* and *Edelmann*, that the curves are always the same, is not correct, and one cannot in employing their method (l.c. P. 184) get at reliable results.

This can easily be illustrated by some examples. Take for instance the forks $C - g^1 - c^2 - g^3 - c^4$. They are, according to my experiments,

FIG. 1.

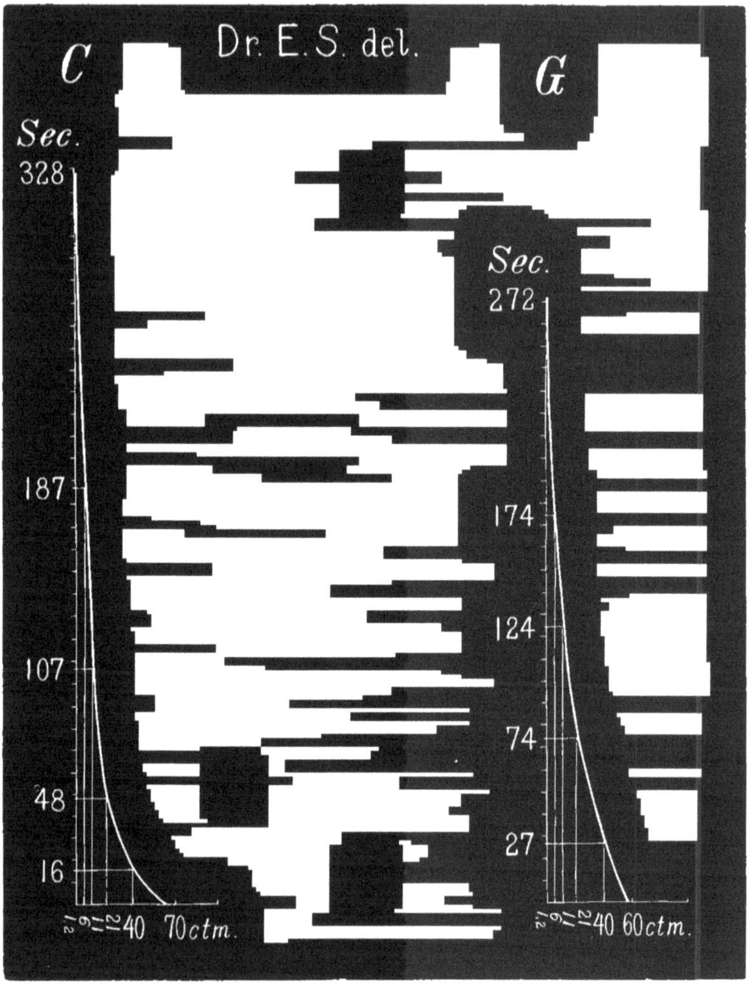

DR. E. SCHMIEGELOW.—CURVES OF TUNING FORKS.

FIG. 2.

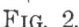

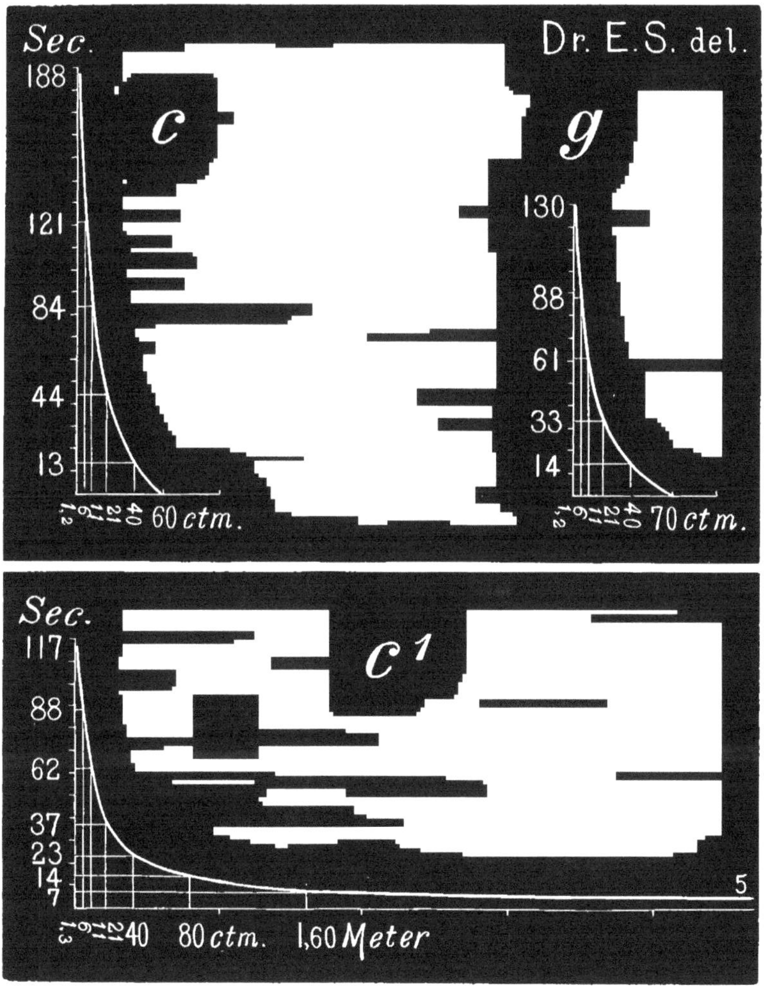

DR. E. SCHMIEGELOW.—CURVES OF TUNING FORKS.

FIG. 3.

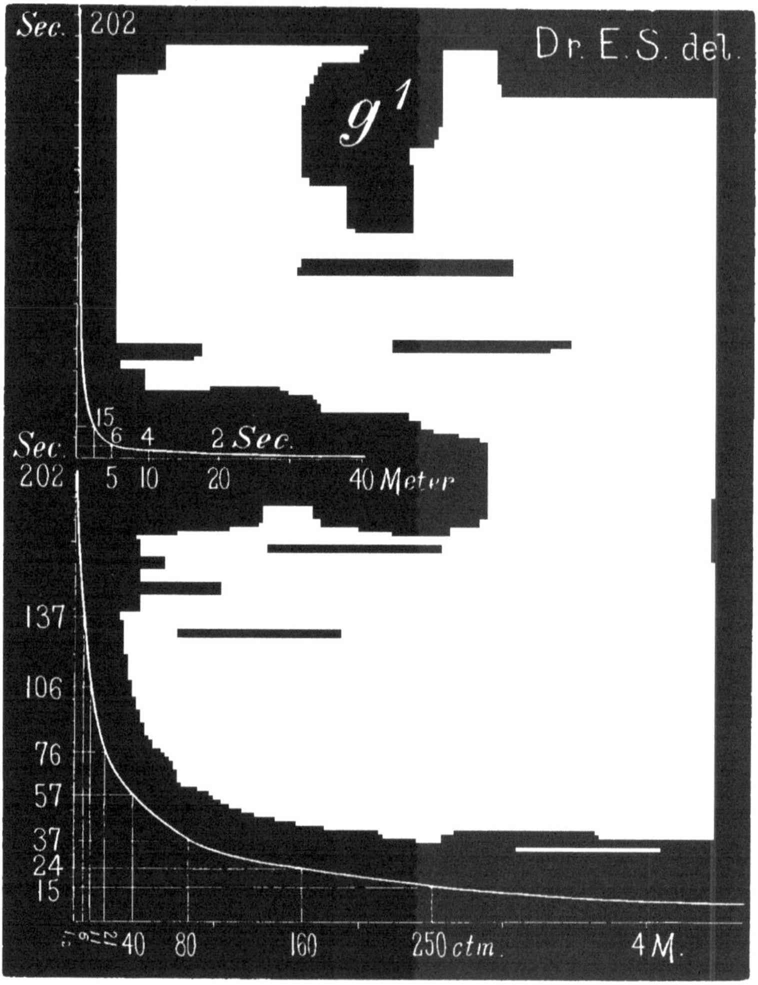

DR. E. SCHMIEGELOW.—CURVES OF TUNING FORKS.

FIG. 4.

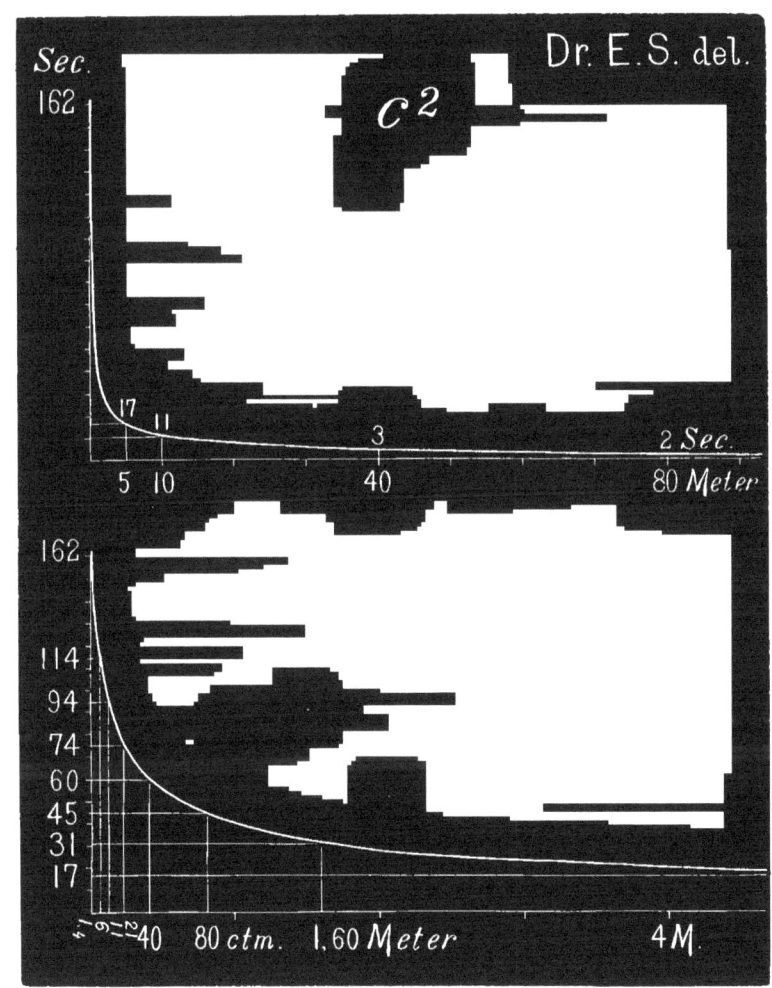

DR. E. SCHMIEGELOW.—CURVES OF TUNING FORKS.

FIG. 5.

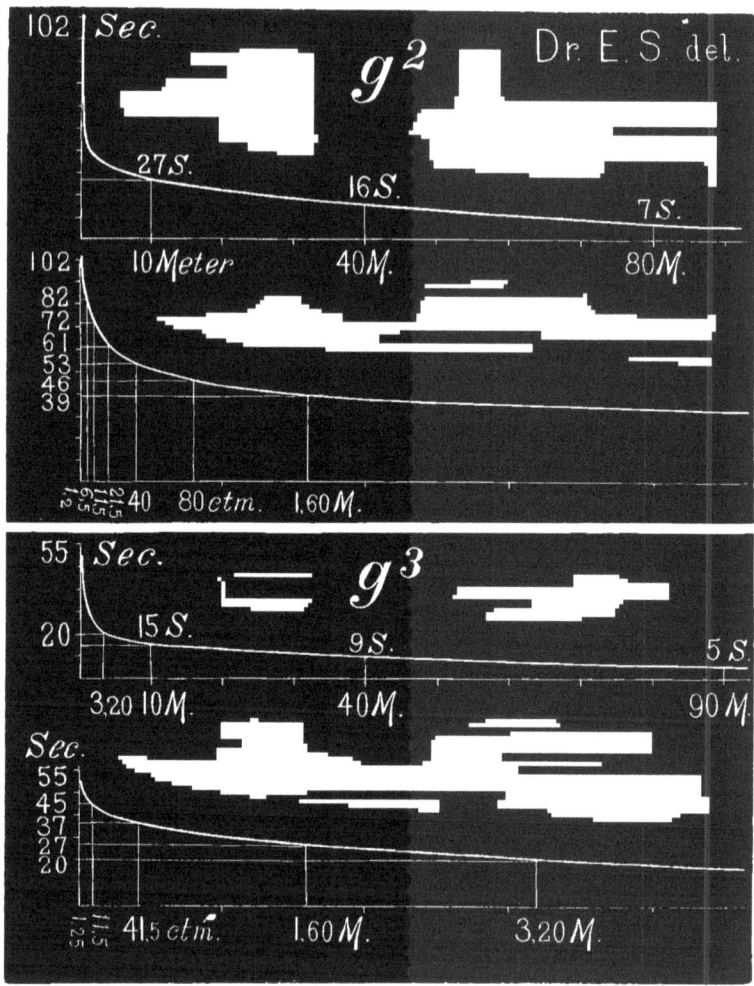

DR. E. SCHMIEGELOW.—CURVES OF TUNING FORKS.

FIG. 6..

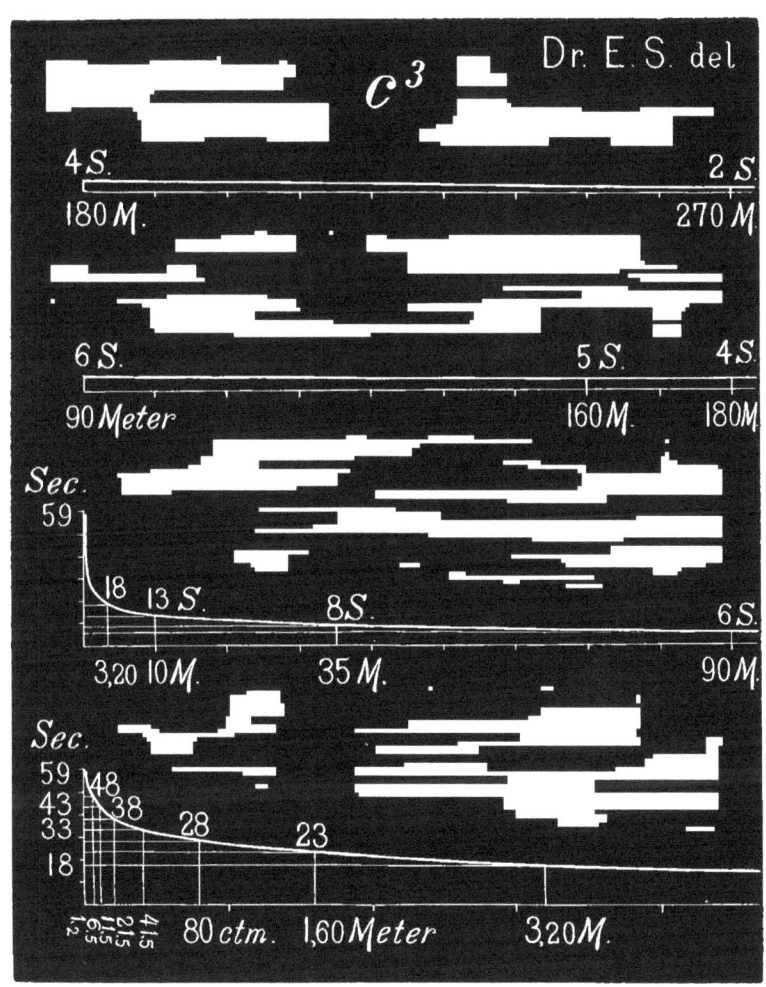

DR. E. SCHMIEGELOW.—CURVES OF TUNING FORKS.

FIG. 7.

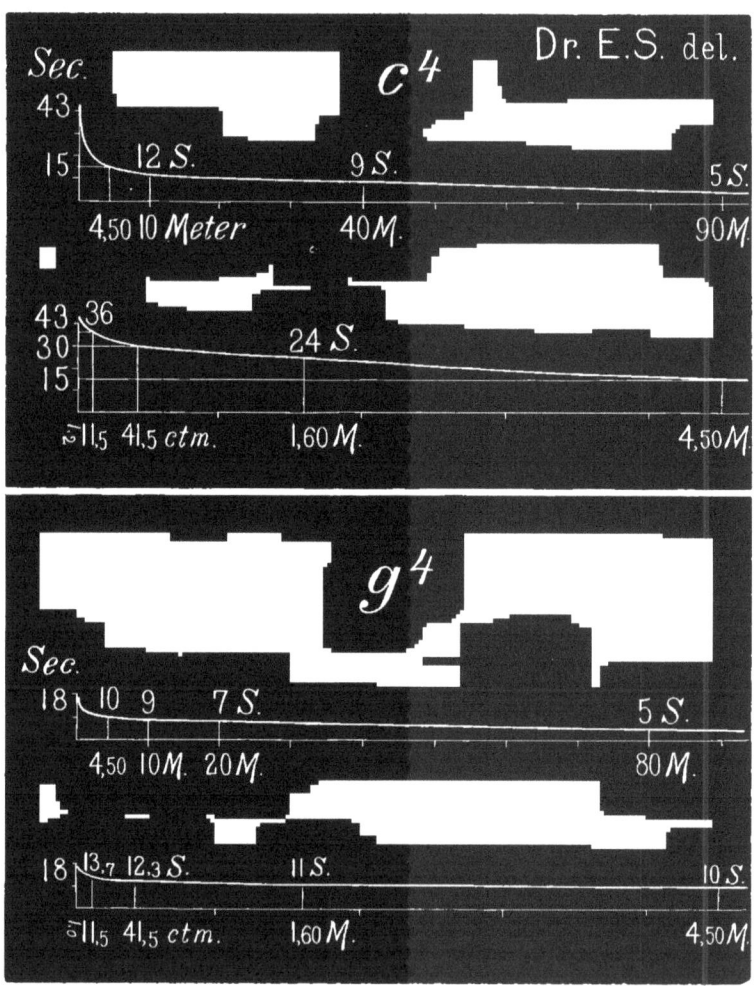

DR. E. SCHMIEGELOW.—CURVES OF TUNING FORKS.

FIG. 8.

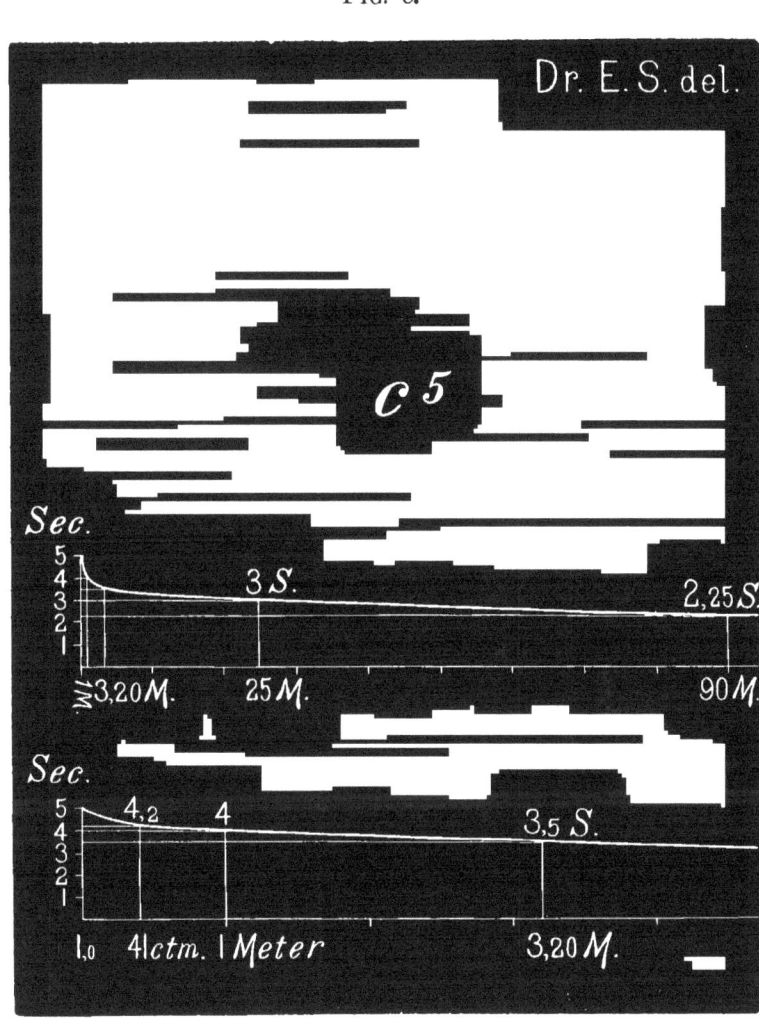

DR. E. SCHMIEGELOW.—CURVES OF TUNING FORKS.

normally heard, close to the ear, during respectively 328, 202, 162, 55, and 43 sec. Suppose now that we have a patient who hears these forks for only half the time, namely respectively during $164 - 101 - 81 - 27$ and 22 sec., the normal hearing power being equal to 1, the diminished hearing power would according to *Bezold-Edelmann* for all tuning forks be equal to $0.049 = \frac{1}{20}$.

If, on the contrary, we use the special curve of each fork, the result will be quite different, because we find that the decrease of the hearing power for C will be equal to 0.026 $= \frac{1}{39}$ of the normal hearing.

,,	g^1	,,	,,	0.012	$= \frac{1}{100}$	,,	,,	,,
,,	c^2	,,	,,	0.007	$= \frac{1}{144}$	,,	,,	,,
,,	g^3	,,	,,	0.00006	$= \frac{1}{17384}$	,,	,,	,,
,,	c^4	,,	,,	0.000025	$= \frac{1}{40000}$	,,	,,	,,

The enormous difference between the results given by this and by *Bezold-Edelmann's* method is obvious.

I believe, therefore, if one wishes to use the time in which a fork is heard to measure the quantitative hearing power, it will first of all be necessary to know the curve of the forks employed.

In order to find these curves I hope that the method given above will prove to be useful.

PROF. POLITZER asked Dr. Schmiegelow if he had found any proportion existing between the results obtained by his experiments, and those obtained by the test with the human voice (whispered or conversational), and whether we could judge from these results of the real distance at which the voice was heard.

DR. DUNDAS GRANT found Hartmann's and Gradenigo's methods of tabulating percentages of hearing power for different forks of clinical value. He asked whether Professor Schmiegelow had arrived at any means of tabulating the results as corrected by his experimental results.

DR. SCHMIEGELOW thanked Prof. Politzer and Dr. Dundas Grant for the interest they had taken in his paper. It was of the greatest value to know the relation between the quantitative hearing power when tested by the tuning fork, and by the human voice, especially when one had to do with deaf mutes, whose hearing was not quite lost. The methods of Hartmann, Bezold, and others, gave practical results, but one could not judge anything from them, because the results given were far from the reality.

A SCHEME FOR THE UNIFORM NOTATION OF THE RESULTS OF THE INVESTIGATION OF HEARING POWER.

PROF. GIUSEPPE GRADENIGO, Turin.

The method, which I propose, has already been in use for some time with good practical effects at the Clinic and the Polyclinic at Turin.

The language employed is Latin ; the various experiments are indicated by the initial letters of the names of the authors who have described them. The scheme is as follows :—

$$
\begin{array}{cc}
& \text{AD} \\
\text{S (18}'') \text{ W} & \text{R (+ 16}''), \text{ H, Hm, Ht, P, v, V,} \\
& \text{AS} \\
& \text{AD} \\
& \text{C c c}^1 \text{ c}^2 \text{ c}^3 \text{ c}^4 \text{ c}^5. \\
& \text{AS}
\end{array}
$$

Explanation.

AD, AS = Auris dextra, auris sinistra.

S = *Schwabach's* experiment (c = 128 vibr.). Duration of normal perception with my tuning fork c = 18''.

W = *Weber's* experiment (c). An arrow designates the side, to which the lateralisation takes place.

R = *Rinne's* experiment (C). Normal Perception with my tuning fork C = +16.

H, Hm, Ht = *Horologium*, watch per aër, ad mastoidem, ad tempora.

P = *Politzer's* acum.

v = vox aphona, whispering voice ; V = vox communis, conversational voice.

The results of the measuring of the hearing power for the various tuning forks are expressed in one-hundredths of the normal duration of perception.

An example will better demonstrate the method :—

	AD—9	prope	+	+	> 5	0.30—0.15	> 5
S (18) +6 W	R (+16)	H,	Hm,	Ht,	P	v.	V
	AS—15''	0.05	+	+	> 5	2.00—1.00	> 5
AD	12	42	72	95	100	95	100
	C	c	c^1	c^2	c^3	c^4	c^5
AS	50	80	87	95	100	100	100

A NEW OPTICAL METHOD OF ACOUMETRY.

PROF. GIUSEPPE GRADENIGO, Turin.

When we place at the end of one of the branches of a tuning fork, which vibrates with sufficient amplitude, a well marked drawn figure, we observe that the less ample the vibrations the more extended become the portions of the figure, whose images are superimposed, *(field of double image)*, so as to appear to the eye of the observer with distinct outlines in comparision with the rest *(field of single image)*.

If we choose a figure in the form of an inverted V (∧) black upon white ground, and mark various segments transversely with lines or steps *(see figures)* we obtain an exact index of the amplitude of vibration at every instant of the tuning fork's decrement. Since the

FIG. 1.

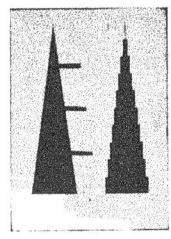

FIG. 2.

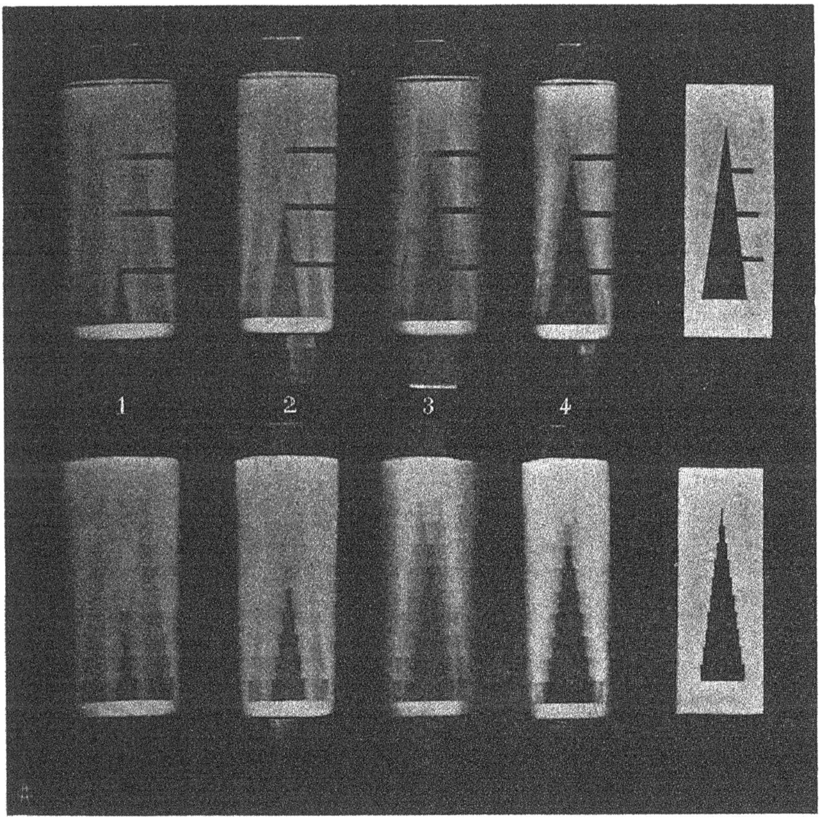

PROF. G. GRADENIGO.—A METHOD OF ACOUMETRY.

amplitude of vibration is directly proportionate to the intensity of the sound, we have thus an excellent clinical method of acoumetry.*

The best results are obtained with forks, whose branches make wide excursions (60 vibrations per minute); the method can even be used with forks up to 250 vibrations.

As the examination with low notes has a great value in the study of the affections of the sound-conducting apparatus, the method is very useful in spite of this limitation.

Of the facts, which I have been able to ascertain I will only here refer to the two following :—

(1) During the period of vibration measured by the said method, the decrease of amplitude is in direct geometrical proportion to the time.

(2) The individual mistakes in the appreciation of the duration of the sound-perception are in persons not accustomed to this kind of re-search — that is in the majority of our patients — much greater than one could believe without such direct objective control.

Experimentelle Untersuchungen ueber acustische Phaenomene in fluessigen Medien.

Dr. R. Kayser, Breslau.

Nach allgemeiner Uebereinstimmung befindet sich die Stelle, an welcher die physicalisch-mechanischen Schallvorgänge in Nerven-erregung umgesetzt werden, im Labyrinth und zwar in der Schnecke speciell in der Membrana basilaris, also in Organen die allseitig von Flüssig-keit umspült werden. Die letzten für das Gehör entscheidenden Schall-schwingungen finden also in flüssigem Medium statt. Es erscheint daher von hohem Interesse die Schallphaenomene schwingungsfähiger Körper in Flüssigkeiten zu studiren. Indess ist das bisher nur in ganz geringfügigem Masse geschehen. Das hatte seinen Grund in den grossen, bisher fast unüberwindlichen Schwierigkeiten die Schall-schwingungen irgend eines Körpers innerhalb einer Flüssigkeit objectiv zu erkennen. Es existirt nur eine einzige Beobachtung von Hensen, welcher die Hörhaare gewisser niederer Thiere im Wasser durch Schallzuführung von aussen unter dem Mikroskop in Schwingungen gerathen sah. Im vorigen Jahr hat Dennert Versuche in dieser Richtung unternommen. Es ist ihm aber nicht gelungen einen schwingungsfähigen Körper spec. eine Stimmgabel durch einen gleichgestimmten Ton von der Luft aus ohne directe Berührung des Gefässes in Mitschwingungen zu bringen.

Ich glaube nun eine Methode gefunden zu haben, durch welche Mitschwingungen eines Körpers im Wasser in bequemer und leicht

---

* I have to thank Dr. G. Ostino, Prof. G. Reymond, Dr. C. Gaudenzi, and Dr. O. Pes for their valuable help in these researches.

B

demonstrirbarer Weise hervorgerufen werden können. Dieselbe beruht
auf der Anwendung des Telephons und zwar habe ich das Telephon
derartig modificirt, dass die schwingende Platte völlig von Wasser
umspült wird. Das geschieht in folgender Weise: der ein wenig
herausgerückte Magnet ist in 2 mm. nach unten von seinem freien Ende
von einer wasserdicht abschliessenden Platte umgeben, welche das
Abfliessen des Wassers und die Benetzung der Drahtspirale verhindert.
Hierdurch entsteht unterhalb der schwingenden Platte ein 2 mm. hoher
mit Wasser zu erfüllender Raum. Die Platte selbst hat 2 seitliche
Löcher, durch welche der untere Wasserraum mit dem oberem
communicirt. Der Wasserraum über der Platte hat eine Höhe
von 5-6 mm. und ist allseitig abgeschlossen. Nur seine Decke hat in
der Mitte eine resp. 2 Oeffnungen. Ausserdem besteht noch eine
seitliche abschliessbare Eingussöffnung. Ueber die beiden Oeffnungen
ist ein 15 mm. hohes Ansatzrohr geschraubt. Ist der Raum über
und unter der Platte mit Wasser gefüllt—wozu beiläufig 50 ccm.
ausreichen — so entspricht derselbe einigermassen der Schnecke
während die Telephonplatte ein Analagon zur Membrana basilaris
bildet. Setzt man nun dieses Wassertelephon mit einem 2ten
gewöhnlichen Telephon in grösserer Entfernung in leitende Verbindung, so kann man in diesem 2ten Telephon hören, sobald die
Platte des Wassertelephons durch irgend eine Schallwirkung in
Schwingungen versetzt wird. Zu dem Zwecke spricht man einzelne
Laute gegen das Ansatzrohr oder man hält eine schwingende Stimmgabel in seiner Nähe—aber ohne jede directe Berührung—dann muss
eine andere Person am 2ten Telephon die betreffenden Schalleinwirkungen
wahrnehmen. Man kann die Sache noch einfacher machen, wenn man
die Decke des oberen Wasserraumes weglässt und das Telephon mit
freier Platte in ein grosses Gefäss mit Wasser stellt, so dass die Platte
sich unter Wasser befindet. Schliesslich kann man die Anordnung
auch umkehren, indem man in das 2te gewöhnliche Telephon spricht
oder eine schwingende Stimmgabel vorhält und das Wassertelephon zum
Hören benutzt, wobei natürlich dessen Platte gleichfalls im Wasser
schwingen muss. Um eine weitergehende Uebereinstimmung mit dem
menschlichen Gehörorgan zu erzielen ist die Decke des Wassertelephons
nicht bloss von einem, sondern, wie erwähnt, von 2 Löchern durchbohrt,
die den beiden Labyrinthfenstern entsprechen. In diese Löcher lassen sich
leicht Membranen oder auch eine feste Platte anbringen. Man kann
noch weiter gehen und über die äussere Oeffnung des Ansatzrohrs eine
Membran—analog dem Trommelfell—spannen und diese durch einen
knöchernen Stab—analog der Columella—mit einer Fenstermembran in
Verbindung bringen. Kurz, es lassen sich wenn einmal die Methode
gegeben ist, die verschiedensten Variationen ausführen. Ich will mich
nun darauf beschränken die wichtigsten Resultate mitzutheilen, die
ich bisher mit dieser Methode erlangt habe.

(1.) Spricht man in das Wassertelephon einige Laute oder hält eine ganze Reihe Stimmgabeln davor, so ist die Wahrnehmung am 2ten Telephon *schwächer* als wenn unter gleichen Verhältnissen *ohne* Wasser experimentirt wird. Das wird besonders deutlich bei den Stimmgabeln. Ohne Wasser kann man auch tiefe und sehr hohe Stimmgabeln hören, mit Wasser fallen die höheren und tieferen aus, man hört dann nur noch die Stimmgabeln im Bereiche von c^3 (1027 Schw.) und c^2 (562 Schw.) und die zwischen liegenden Töne, also g^1 und a^1, während c^1 und c^4 nicht mehr gehört werden. Dasselbe tritt bei umgekehrter Anordnung ein. Die Abschwächung ist um so grösser, je dicker die Wasserschicht ist, die über die Telephonplatte lagert, sie nimmt ferner zu, wenn man statt Wasser eine zähere Flüssigkeit, z. B. Glycerin oder Milch, anwendet. Der Grund dieser Abschwächung der Schallschwingungen liegt wohl in dem Uebergang von einem Medium in das andere. Diese Abschwächung wird nicht nachweislich vermindert, wenn der Uebergang ins Wasser durch eine Membran vermittelt wird. Man kann über die beiden oberen Löcher des Wassertelephons Membrane spannen, man kann weiter die eine Membran durch ein Knochenstäbchen—columella— mit einer über das Ansatzrohr gespannter Membran—Trommelfell—in Verbindung bringen ohne nachweisbaren Erfolg. Die Einrichtung des Gehörorgans, dass sein akustischer Endapparat in Flüssigkeit suspendirt ist, bewirkt also an sich eine Verminderung der Schallintensität. Es ist natürlich nicht ausgeschlossen, dass diese Verminderung durch compensatorische Einrichtungen ausgeglichen ist.

(2.) Bekanntlich haben Helmholtz und Andere der Lehre zum Siege verholfen, dass die Gehörknöchelchen als Masse schwingen, dass also der eindringenden Steigbügelplatte eine Ausbuchtung der runden Fenstermembran entsprechen muss. Demnach wird durch Starrheit dieser Membran oder Verschluss des runden Fensters das Gehör aufgehoben resp. sehr bedeutend herabgesetzt. Diese Anschauung ist allerdings wiederholt bis in die jüngste Zeit angefochten worden. Aber alle diese Angriffe blieben erfolglos, weil sie sich nur auf unsichere theoretische Deductionen stützten. Mit dem Wassertelephon ist es aber zum ersten Male möglich die Sache experimentell zu untersuchen. Man kann die eine der beiden Schallzuleitungsöffnungen des Telephons dicht verschliessen, also dem Wasser jede Massenausweichung versperren und den Einfluss dieser Veränderung auf die Function des Apparats feststellen. Es ergiebt sich nun, dass durch eine solche Versperrung des Ausweichens der Wassermasse auch mit columella und Trommelfell die Tonwahrnehmung im Telephon nicht merklich beeinflusst wird speciell nicht geringer ist als ohne Versperrung. Es reichen demnach die Molecularschwingungen für die Gehörwahrnehmung volkommen aus. Allerdings zeigt sich, dass bei 2 offnen Zuleitungsöffnungen die Schallintensität immer stärker ist als bei einer. Hierbei ist es aber völlig gleichgültig, ob die Oeffnungen ganz frei sind oder durch eine Membran geschlossen oder ob eine Oeffnung mit columella und Trommelfell in Verbindung steht oder nicht. Ich bin mir wohl bewusst, dass es der Vorsicht bedarf wenn man die Telephonexperimente auf das Gehörorgan übertragen will. Indessen ist durch die beschriebene Methode meines Wissens zum ersten Male Gelegenheit gegeben die physicalischen Vorgänge des bisher ganz unzugänglichen akustischen Endapparats einer experimentellen Untersuchung zu unterziehen.

PROF. LUCAE findet, dass die Abschwächung des Tones durch das "Wassertelephon" sehr natürlich ist. Interessanter ist das Factum dass die hohen Töne der viergestrichenen Octave nicht mehr durch den Apparat fortgepflanzt wurden. Er möchte daher fragen ob denn nicht die menschliche Stimme sehr erheblich *tiefer* wahrgenommen wurde. Es würde dies mit dem bereits von *Chladni* am Anfang dieses Jahrhunderts nachgewiesener Thatsache übereinstimmen, dass Stimmgabeln, welche nach dem Anschlagen mit ihren Zinken in Wasser getaucht werden, sehr vertieft werden. Er habe selbst gefunden, das der Ton der Stimmgabel c⁴ im Wasser um eine None tiefer wurde.

DR. KAYSER.—Ich habe gleichfalls die Erniedrigung des Stimmgabeltones in Wasser constatirt. Hierbei ist der Telephonapparat sehr brauchbar indem man in einem mit Wasser gefüllten Gefäss das Telephon ohne Platte bringt und statt der Platte eine Stimmgabel in Wasser anschlägt und kann dann am zweiten gewöhnlichen Telephon den viel tieferen Ton der Stimmgabel gut erkennen. Allerdings habe ich eine so starke Vertiefung auf 1 Octave nicht gefunden, sondern nur um circa 2 Töne.

Ob beim Wassertelephon der Timbre der menschlichen Stimme geändert wird, etwa durch Ausfall der höheren und tieferen Töne habe ich gleichfalls beachtet. Indess habe ich eine solche Veränderung nicht gefunden.

UEBER TUBERCULOSE DES MITTELHORS.

DR. O. BRIEGER, Breslau.

Die Anschauungen über das Vorkommen tuberculöser Erkrankungen des Gehörorgans haben innerhalb weniger Jahre mehrfache Wandlungen erfahren. War man früher, vor der Entdeckung des Erregers der Tuberculose, geneigt, auf Grund klinischer Vorstellungen Caries und Tuberculose ohne Weiteres zu identificieren, und solche Processe im Bereich des Mittelohrs, welche wegen destructiver Veränderungen an der knöchernen Wand oder dem knöchernen Inhalt der Mittelohrräume zur "Caries" gerechnet wurden, als tuberculös zu bezeichnen, so ist man andererseits in der Bekämpfung dieser allerdings in solcher Form unhaltbaren Auffassung vielfach über das Ziel hinausgeschossen. Die Tuberculose localiert sich viel häufiger, als man gelten lassen wollte, und in mannigfaltiger Form am Gehörorgan. Der Schwierigkeit, Tuberkelbacillen im Ohrsecret nachzuweisen, ist es wol hauptsächlich zuzuschreiben, dass dem bekannten klinischen Bilde der symptomlos einsetzenden, fast latent verlaufenden Mittelohreiterung Tuberculöser andere neue Typen der Verlaufsform bei Tuberculose des Gehörorgans noch nicht an die Seite gestellt, oder wenigstens nur unvollkommen durch Mitteilung vereinzelter Fälle belegt worden sind. Die anatomische Untersuchung der durch die Section gewonnenen Gehörorgane kann die Kenntnis des *klinischen* Verlaufs der Mittelohrtuberculose nur bedingt fördern. Denn es ist natürlich, dass zur Zeit des Todes Tuberculöser sich gewöhnlich, wie auch der Verlauf des Processes sich klinisch gestaltet haben mag, ziemlich einheitliche, nur graduell, hinsichtlich der Ausdehnung des Processes, verschiedene Befunde am Trommelfell ergeben. Der hohe Wert der anatomischen Untersuchungen an sich wird dadurch nicht im mindesten verringert. Nur gewinnt gerade die *Klinik* der Mittelohrtuberculose mehr dadurch, dass durch einwandsfreie Beweismittel, durch den Nachweis der specifischen Erreger oder, wo dieser misslingt, durch die Feststellung der für die Tuberculose characteristischen Gewebsveränderungen in excidierten Stücken, die Zugehörigkeit zur Tuberculose auch für solche Processe nachgewiesen wird, welche vom Standpunkt unserer bisherigen klinischen Anschauungen zwar als gelegentliche Begleiterscheinungen der Lungentuberculose gekannt, aber nicht als charakteristische Formen wirklich tuberculöser Processe gewürdigt sind. Denn mit dem Krankheitsbilde, wie es die Lehrbücher meist als typisch für die Tuberculose des Mittelohrs darstellen, wird das Wesen der Erkrankung bei Weitem nicht erschöpft. Auch unter scheinbar unverdächtigen Bildern, unter den Symptomen einer gewöhnlichen chronischen Mittelohreiterung, kann sich eine Tuberculose des Mittelohrs verbergen. Klinisch statistische Angaben, bei denen das Vorhandensein einer Mittelohrtuberculose lediglich aus dem als charakteristisch angesehenen Ohrbefund bei gleichzeitiger Gegenwart anderweitiger tuberculöser Processe erschlossen wird, können daher nur ein Bild von der Häufigkeit, in welcher Erkrankungen des Mittelohrs überhaupt bei Tuberculose auftreten, nicht aber von der Frequenz, mit welcher das Gehörorgan von specifischen, tuberculösen Processen ergriffen wird, gewähren.

Ueberraschender Weise ergeben die bisher vorliegenden klinisch-statistischen Ermittelungen, trotzdem man dabei eigentlich naturgemäss einen weit höheren Prozentsatz erwarten sollte, niedrigere Ziffern für das Häufigkeitsverhältniss der Beteiligung des Mittelohrs bei Tuberculose, als die anatomischen Untersuchungen, bei denen doch niedrigere Ziffern resultieren müssten, weil dabei die zur Tuberculose gehörigen Processe mit grösserer Sicherheit von den accidentellen, durch andersartige Infectionen bedingten Eiterungen getrennt werden können. Normale Befunde findet man bei der anatomischen Untersuchung von Schläfenbeinen Tuberculöser allerdings relativ selten. Freilich steht die grosse Mehrzahl dieser Veränderungen ausser Beziehung zur Natur der Grundkrankheit. So sieht man gerade hier, wie überhaupt bei Obductionen solcher Individuen, welche an langdauernden chronischen Krankheitsprocessen zu Grunde gegangen sind, relativ oft Befunde, wie sie fast regelmässig bei Sectionen von Kindern aus den ersten Lebensjahren sich ergeben : Ansammlung von Secret in der Pauke bei intacter Beschaffenheit des Trommelfells. Derartige Befunde, welche als finale Erscheinungen anzusehen, wenn auch in ihrer Genese sonst vorläufig noch unklar sind, scheiden natürlich ohne Weiteres von vorn herein aus. Von ihnen sind leicht die seltenen Fälle zu unterscheiden, in denen eine Mittelohrtuberculose in einem Stadium zur Obduction kommt, in welchem bei ausgedehnter Infiltration der Paukenschleimhaut doch das Trommelfell in seiner Continuität erhalten ist, wenn auch das Stratum mucosum selbst schon von dem tuberculösen Process ergriffen gefunden wird. Auch wenn man solche Befunde, bei denen ein Zusammenhang mit Tuberculose von vornherein bestimmt ausgeschlossen ist, ausscheidet, bleibt noch immer ein erheblich grösserer Prozentsatz für die Beteiligung des Mittelohrs mit Tuberculose übrig, als in klinischen Beobachtungen ermittelt wurde.

Alle bisherigen anatomischen Untersuchungen stellen die Thatsache des häufigen Vorkommens tuberculöser Processe in den Mittelohrräumen übereinstimmend fest. Als practisch verwertbare Unterlagen für eine procentuale Berechnung sind aber auch sie deshalb nicht recht zu verwerten, weil die Ergebnisse der einzelnen Autoren nicht unerheblich differieren. Man kann im Allgemeinen in etwa dem vierten Teile aller obducierten Fälle von Tuberculose Veränderungen im Gehörorgan erwarten. *Unter 141 Fällen von Tuberculose*, deren Gehörorgane innerhalb der beiden, letzten Jahre von mir, bezw. meinen Assistenten anatomisch untersucht wurden, ergab sich 37 Mal der Befund chronisch entzündlicher Processe in den Mittelohrräumen; in 18 von diesen Fällen wurde die tuberculöse Natur des Processes sicher festgestellt. Aber auch für die übrigen Fälle, welche nicht alle gleich vollständig untersucht worden waren, ist nach dem Verlauf der Untersuchung die Möglichkeit, dass, trotz scheinbar unverdächtiger Bilder, doch Tuberculose zu Grunde lag, nicht durchweg mit Sicherheit auszuschliessen. Gelegenheit zur tuberculösen Infection der Paukenhöhle ist bei tuberculösen Individuen so reichlich gegeben, dass diese Häufigkeit tuberculöser Processe im Mittelohr nicht im mindesten überraschen kann. Der Infectionsweg ist, wie die Untersuchungen HABERMANN'S zuerst gelehrt haben, hierbei der gleiche, wie bei fast allen andersartigen Infectionen der Paukenhöhle. Die Tuberkelbacillen gelangen meist im Lumen der Tube, unter Umständen aber auch in der Continuität der Tubenwand vom Nasenrachenraum zum Mittelohr. Infectionsfähiges Material ist im Nasenrachenraum Tuberculöser, zum mindesten zeitweise, wol in jedem Falle vorhanden. Es ist nicht notwendig, dass Tuberkelbacillen sich primär im Nasenrachenraum ansiedeln, und erst hier die characteristischen Veränderungen auslösen, um dann von der Oberfläche tuberculöser Geschwüre des Nasenrachenraums in die Paukenhöhle einzuwandern. Die Häufigkeit des Vorkommens tuberculöser Ulcerationen im Nasenrachenraum ist auch nach meinen Erfahrungen wesentlich geringer, als bisher auf Grundlage früherer Untersuchungen angenommen wird. Uebrigens sind hier klinische Untersuchungen tuberculöser Individuen oft zuverlässiger, als der anatomische Befund erodierter Schleimhautstellen, wenn dieser nicht durch histologische Untersuchung der ulceriert gefundenen Partieen ergänzt worden ist. Bei klinischer Beobachtung aber stellt sich das tuberculöse Geschwür des Nasenrachenraums als eine sehr seltene Localisation der Tuberculose dar. Man kann, wie sich mir bei Untersuchungen, welche auf die Feststellung der Frequenz tuberculöser Ulcerationen im Nasenrachenraum hinzielten, ergab, eine sehr grosse Zahl von Phtisikern untersuchen, ehe man einmal einer Ulceration begegnet, welche man, nach ihrem klinischen Aussehen oder nach dem Ergebniss der histologischen Untersuchung eines excidierten Gewebsstücks, sicher als tuberculös ansprechen dürfte. Insbesondere habe ich bei Kranken mit tuberculösen Mittelohrprocessen gleichartige Zustände im Nasenrachenraum fast regelmässig vermisst, oder gelegentlich auch erst secundär entstehen sehen, indem anscheinend das aus der Paukenhöhle durch die Tube abfliessende Secret den Nasenrachenraum inficierte. Ebenso schienen mir, um das hier gleich einzuschalten, die oft tiefgreifenden Veränderungen im knöchernen Abschnitt der Tube meist nicht auf primäre Ansiedlung von Tuberkelbacillen oberhalb des Isthmus zu beruhen, sondern eher secundär, durch Ausbreitung des tuberculösen Processes in der Pauke gegen das Ostium tympanicum hin, bedingt zu sein.

Für die Mittelohrtuberculose der Kinder besonders, kommt die Möglichkeit der Fortleitung von einer *latenten Tuberculose der Rachenmandel* in Betracht. Die Coincidenz latenter Rachenmandeltuberculose mit Tuberculose der Paukenhöhle habe ich wenigstens wiederholt direct nachweisen können. Ein derartiger Zusammenhang war auch schon durch die Untersuchungen von SCHUETZ wahrscheinlich gemacht, welcher als Ursache der bei Schweinen ausserordentlich häufigen Mittelohrtuberculose die Fortleitung "lymphatischer Nasenrachenkatarrhe" nach der Paukenhöhle beschrieben hat.

Auch specifische Mittelohrerkrankungen bei *Lupus der Nase* werden, anscheinend nicht selten, durch die continuierliche Fortsetzung tuberculöser Processe vom Nasenrachenraum, dessen Beteiligung bei Lupus ausserordentlich häufig ist und anscheinend relativ frühzeitig erfolgt, vermittelt. Allerdings kann auch hier das Bindeglied zwischen dem lupösen Process an Nase und Gesicht und dem secundären Ergriffenwerden des Mittelohrs eine latente Tuberculose der Rachenmandel, nicht ausschliesslich solche Processe darstellen, welche mit dieser anatomisch zwar identisch sind, klinisch aber so different sich verhalten, dass man sie, eben dieser klinischen Differenz wegen, als lupöse Veränderungen der Mandel, anzusprechen pflegt. Man findet bei Lupus mit Beteiligung des Mittelohrs das Eine, wie das Andere: sowohl die "latente" Tuberculose mit dem klinischen Bilde der einfachen Hyperplasie der Rachenmandel, als ulceröse oder narbige Processe, welche zum Schleimhautlupus gerechnet werden müssen.

Neben der Infection durch die Tube kommen andere Infectionsmodi praktisch kaum in Betracht. Die Möglichkeit der Entwickelung tuberculöser Herde im Mittelohr im Verlauf miliarer Aussaat von Tuberkelbacillen ist, besonders durch BARNICK, sicher erwiesen, aber für diejenigen Mittelohreiterungen Tuberculöser, welche zur *klinischen* Beobachtung gelangen, relativ unerheblich. *Die Infection auf dem Wege des Gehörgangs* ist sicher nur ein ganz ausnahmsweises Vorkommniss. Es ist wenig wahrscheinlich, dass, insbesondere bei chronischen Mittelohreiterungen mit epidermisierter Paukenschleimhaut, eine Invasion der durch eine Trommelfelllücke eingewanderten Tuberkelbacillen durch die resistente, neugebildete Auskleidung der Mittelohrräume häufig zu Stande kommen wird. Die Gelegenheit dazu ist relativ leichter im Gehörgang gegeben, wo eine Begünstigung der Infection durch mechanische Momente leichter möglich ist. Trotzdem sind auch Tuberculosen des Gehörgangs, besonders in den tieferen Abschnitten desselben, ausserordentlich selten. Der Beobachtung v. TROELTSCH'S, welcher ein wahrscheinlich tuberculöses Geschwür im knöchernen Gehörgang beschrieben hat, kann ich einen gleichartigen Befund an die Seite stellen: bei einem Kranken mit linksseitiger Mittelohrtuberculose bestand in der Tiefe des rechten Gehörgangs ein ausgedehntes, den Knochen arrodierendes tuberculöses Geschwür, welches bis unmittelbar an das intacte Trommelfell heranreichte. Wenn aber derartige Infectionen in den periphersten Abschnitten des Gehörorgans schon zu den Seltenheiten gehören, wird man zugestehen müssen, dass dieser Infectionsmodus überhaupt, erst recht also für die Tuberculose des Mittelohrs, kaum ins Gewicht fallen kann.

Die Tuberculose des Mittelohrs verläuft am häufigsten unter dem als typisch beschriebenen Bilde, dessen characteristische Eigentümlichkeit die lange Latenz des Processes und die schmerzlose Entstehung der Eiterung darstellt. Diese *Schmerzlosigkeit* bleibt gewöhnlich im ganzen Verlauf der in dieser Weise entstandenen Mittelohreiterung bestehen. Selbst in solchen Fällen, in denen ausgedehnte Einschmelzungen des Knochens zu Stande gekommen waren, in denen die Tuberculose auf die Wand des äusseren Gehörgangs übergegriffen, und selbst das Kiefergelenk erreicht hatte, blieben die Beschwerden, bei dieser Form dauernd gering. Man sieht solche eigentümlich latent verlaufenden Tuberculosen, nicht bloss bei vorgeschrittenen Lungenprocessen, sondern unter Umständen sogar als erstes manifestes Symptom der Tuberculose, bei langsamer schleichender Entwickelung der Lungenerkrankung, die dann nach Entwickelung des Processes im Ohr, zuweilen in zeitlichem Anschluss an die Infection der Paukenhöhle, gewissermassen durch diese eingeleitet, sich zuweilen rasch ausbreitet.

Aber nicht alle in dieser Weise entstehenden Processe bei Tuberculose sind durch Infection mit Tuberkelbacillen bedingt. Diese werden vielmehr auch in Fällen mit typischem klinischen Verlauf doch im Secret dauernd vermisst. Dank der geringen Resistenz der Gewebe bei vorgeschrittener Tuberculose, können auch gewöhnliche pyogene Infectionen zu rapidem und ausgedehntem Zerfall führen, ohne dass erhebliche Reactionserscheinungen zu constatieren wären. Diese Beeinflussung des Verlaufs accidenteller Infectionen ist aber nicht eine ausschliessliche Eigentümlichkeit der Tuberculose, sondern ebenso gelegentlich bei allen, die Widerstandskraft der Gewebe schädigenden Allgemeinkrankheiten zu beobachten. Jedenfalls darf man danach der klinischen Diagnose aus dem als typisch angesehenen Trommelfellbild nur bedingten Wert beimessen. Deshalb sind z.B. auch nicht alle in der Literatur niedergelegten Heilungen solcher Mittelohrprocesse bei progredienter Lungentuberculose, welche lediglich wegen der klinischen Uebereinstimmung mit dem 'typischen' Bilde, auch genetisch identificiert worden sind, nicht ohne Weiteres zuzugeben. Für die Anerkennung der tuberculösen Natur eines Processes bedarf es stringenterer Beweise, als solcher rein klinischer Befunde. Dabei soll nicht bestritten werden, dass das Trommelfellbild bei der Tuberculose des Mittelohrs für praktisch diagnostische Zwecke unzweifelhafte Bedeutung besitzt. *Die Multiplicität der Perforation,* die hier dem Zerfall multipler tuberculöser Infiltrate entspricht, wird zwar gelegentlich auch bei anderartigen entzündlichen Processen der Pauke, hier aber immerhin so selten beobachtet, dass ihr Nachweis zweifellos als ein wesentliches diagnostisches Moment für die klinische Erkennung tuberculöser Processe anerkannt werden kann. Sie stellt aber natürlich nur ein Stadium in der Entwickelung des tuberculösen Processes dar und wird oft rasch durch die Confluenz der Perforationen, durch die Entwickelung totaler Defecte des Trommelfells abgelöst, so dass sie der klinischen Beobachtung vollständig entgehen kann. So ist auch bei Obductionen tuberculöser Schläfenbeine der Nachweis multipler Trommelfellperforationen meist nicht mehr möglich.

Nicht selten dauert das Stadium der tuberculösen Infiltration sehr lange an. Meist ist in diesem Falle die Functionsstörung, bedingt

durch Infiltration der Schleimhaut, besonders auch in den Fenster-
nischen, das einzige für den Kranken auffällige Symptom.   Man sieht
in solchen Fällen das Trommelfell entweder in toto infiltriert, oder von
der Oberfläche, an welcher sonst meist Niveauunterschiede und
Details nicht mehr zu differenzieren sind, einzelne gröbere Prominenzen
sich abheben.   Derartige Bilder habe ich wiederholt bei Lupösen gesehen.
Wurden bei diesen dann Tuberculininjectionen vorgenommen, so
entwickelten sich als Ausdruck localer Reaction, nach Ablauf der diffusen
entzündlichen Schwellung erst deutlich erkennbar, eigentümliche
Veränderungen welche an dem Vorhandensein tuberculöser Infiltrate an
diesen Stellen keinen Zweifel lassen.   Es kam im Bereich der vorher
vorhanden gewesenen Prominenzen zum Zerfall mit vorübergehend
ziemlich starker Secretion ; im Secret waren nunmehr auch Tuberkelbacillen nachweisbar.   In einigen Fällen entwickelten sich allmählich
grössere, multiple Defecte ; das Bild unterschied sich dann kaum noch
von dem der gewöhnlichen Mittelohrtuberculose.   In einem Falle kam
es auf diesem Wege nach wiederholten Tuberculininjectionen zu
vollständiger Exfoliation der tuberculösen Herde, und zur Heilung des
Processes mit Verschluss der im Verlauf der Injectionen entstandenen
drei Perforationen.   Solche umschriebenen Infiltrate werden oft—
zu Unrecht—als Miliartuberkel bezeichnet.   Ob man otoskopisch
überhaupt Gebilde, welche dem anatomischen Begriff des Miliar-
tuberkels entsprechen, würde differenzieren können, ist mehr als
zweifelhaft.   Die Infiltrate entsprechen vielmehr, wie man leicht
feststellen kann, Conglomeraten von Tuberkeln, grösseren Granulations-
knoten.   Eine solche scheinbar isolierte Tuberculose des Trommelfells
konnte ich durch histologische Untersuchung der dem Kranken excidierten Membran feststellen.   In einem Falle von initialer Lungentuberculose bestand, bei mässiger Herabsetzung der Hörfähigkeit, eine um-
schriebene gelbrötliche Infiltration der hinteren Trommelfelhälfte.   Das
Trommelfell wurde zum grössten Teile excidiert.   Die histologische
Untersuchung ergab, dass die beschriebene Partie einen Granulations-
knoten darstellte, welcher mehrere Tuberkel mit den characteristischen
Elementen und den der Tuberculose eigentümlichen Producten
regressiver Metamorphose enthielt.   Der Process kam aber mit der
Excision nicht zum Stillstand ; vielmehr lehrte die weitere Beobachtung,
dass wahrscheinlich schon zur Zeit der Erkrankung des Trommelfells
latent gleichartige Processe an den andern Abschnitten der Paukenhöhle
bestanden hatten.   Diese Beobachtung bestätigt gleichzeitig die
klinischen Befunde anderer Autoren, welche nach dem Vorgang
SCHWARTZE'S, solche tuberculösen Infiltrate des Trommelfells beschrieben
haben.   Sie ergänzt diese Befunde insofern, als die klinisch vermutete
tuberculöse Natur dieser Veränderungen hier durch Excision der
betreffenden Partie des Trommelfells, und histologische Untersuchung
des excidierten Stücks vervollständigt werden konnte.   Praktisch that

man in solchen Fällen allerdings vielleicht besser, sich aller Eingriffe, welche eine Communication mit dem Gehörgang herbeiführen können, zu enthalten. Bei dieser Form besteht meist eine relativ geringe Tendenz zum Zerfall. Kommt es aber durch Vermittelung einer Trommelfelllücke zur Mischinfection, dann kann eine überraschend schnelle Destruction des Trommelfells eingeleitet werden. Incisionen des Trommelfells mögen nach dieser Richtung meist belanglos sein. Ich habe aber in einem Falle, in welchem ich den langen Bestand der Trommelfellinfiltrate selbst controlliert hatte, nachdem von anderer Seite das Trommelfell incidiert, und durch wiederholte Spülungen wahrscheinlich der Transport von Mikroorganismen aus dem Gehörgang in die Paukenhöhle begünstigt worden war, innerhalb kurzer Frist eine ausgedehnte Zerstörung sich entwickeln sehen. Die *Mischinfection* spielt bei der Entwickelung des Bildes der Mittelohrtuberculose eine nicht minder grosse Rolle, als bei tuberculösen Processen in andern Körperregionen, wo ebenfalls wie in der Paukenhöhle die Gelegenheit zu secundärer Invasion anderer Bacterienarten reichlich gegeben ist.

Vielleicht verdankt *die acute Form der Mittelohrtuberculose*, welche bisher nur in vereinzelten Fällen beschrieben worden ist, die eigentümliche Gestaltung ihres Verlaufs ebenfalls einer Mischinfection. Tuberculosen der Paukenschleimhaut manifestieren sich in seltenen Fällen unter dem Bilde einer gewöhnlichen acuten Mittelohrentzündung. In den Fällen, welche ich beobachtet habe, zeigte das Bild anfangs keinerlei von den Symptomen der acuten Otitis media abweichenden Eigentümlichkeiten. Nach Incision des Trommelfells kam es, im Gegensatz zu der sonst bei Tuberculose relativ beschränkten Granulationsbildung, neben rascher Destruction des Trommelfells zu so üppiger Wucherung der Paukenschleimhaut, dass bereits in den ersten Tagen der Erkrankung grosse polypenartige Granulationstumoren in den Gehörgang vorgedrungen waren. Die Untersuchung solcher durch Excision gewonnenen Gewebsstücke ergab das Vorhandensein von Tuberculose. Die excidierten Polypen bestanden aus Granulationsgewebe mit zahlreichen eingestreuten Tuberkeln. Dabei waren im Secret Tuberkelbacillen nicht immer nachweisbar. Die von mir beobachteten Fälle dieser Art zeichneten sich übrigens fast durchweg durch rasche Progredienz des Processes, frühe Destruction der Knochenwände,—in einem Falle schon nach 10 Tagen Durchbruch der hinteren Gehörgangswand durch die aus dem Antrum vordringenden Granulationsmassen,—und schnelle Entwickelung labyrinthärer Symptome aus. Man kann sich natürlich vorstellen, dass in solchen Fällen bereits eine Zeit lang latent eine Tuberculose der Mittelohrschleimhaut bestanden hat, welche erst durch eine accidentelle Infection der Paukenhöhle mit pyogenen Erregern manifest geworden ist. Dagegen spricht allerdings die in meinen Beobachtungen durchweg constatierte vollständige

Abwesenheit aller solcher Erscheinungen, welche auf eine dem acuten Stadium etwa voraufgegangene Erkrankung der Paukenhöhle hindeuten könnten, ebenso wol auch die Structur der excidierten Gewebsstücke, welche dem Bild tuberculöser Granulationen vollständig entsprach. Man wird daher die Möglichkeit des Vorkommens acut verlaufender Tuberculosen des Mittelohrs, welche ich übrigens, vielleicht entsprechend der auch im Verlauf des Ohrprocesses zu Tage tretenden hochgradigen Virulenz der Tuberkelbacillen, bei rasch progredienten Lungentuberculosen jugendlicher Individuen beobachtet habe, zugeben müssen.

Ebenso, wie unter dem Bilde acuter·Mittelohrentzündung, kann die Tuberculose unter den Erscheinungen einer gewöhnlichen *chronischen Mittelohreiterung* verlaufen. Es ist bereits oben erwähnt, dass die characteristischen Erscheinungen der Trommelfelltuberculose im weiteren Verlauf verloren gehen, wenn die Einschmelzung fortschreitet und schliesslich zur Entstehung eines Totaldefects des Trommelfells geführt hat. Man findet bei Sectionen solcher tuberculöser Individuen welche scheinbar gewöhnliche chronische Eiterungen klinisch gezeigt hatten, Befunde, welche dann doch an der Entstehung des Ohrprocesses durch tuberculöse Infection nicht zweifeln lassen.

Besonders bei solchen Kranken, welche an Lupus des Gesichts und der Nase litten, war die grosse Häufigkeit gleichzeitiger chronischer Mittelohreiterungen auffällig. Freilich sind natürlich bei Weitem nicht alle derartigen Processe im Ohr, welche den Lupus begleiten, tuberculöser Natur. Ich habe bereits früher darauf hingewiesen, wie gerade auch beim Lupus die Gelegenheit zur gewöhnlichen eitrigen Infection der Paukenhöhle ausserordentlich gross ist. Aber dass hier auch unter ganz unverdächtigen Erscheinungen, d.h. unter den Symptomen einer chronischen Eiterung der Paukenhöhle sich Tuberculose verbergen kann, lehrte mich die Beobachtung eines Falls, in welchem die Reaction auf Tuberculin-Injection, welche des Lupus der Gesichtshaut wegen erfolgt war, das Bild vollständig veränderte. Unter dem Einfluss der reactiven Schwellung entwickelte sich sofort eine Facialislähmung. Die blossliegende Paukenschleimhaut bedeckte sich mit einem festhaftenden grauweissen Belage, welcher der von SCHEIBE bei Mittelohrtuberculose beschriebenen fibrinoiden Auflagerung glich. Im Secret waren, während der Befund in dieser Richtung früher negativ war, nunmehr reichlich Bacillen nachzuweisen. Die acuten Erscheinungen gingen allmählich zurück; auch die Facialislähmung, welche wahrscheinlich dadurch entstanden war, dass der Nerv in Folge tuberculöser Zerstörung seiner Knochenwand freilag und durch die acute Gewebsschwellung comprimiert wurde, wich nach einiger Zeit ebenfalls. Die Menge der Tuberkelbacillen im Ohrsecret nahm allmählich wieder ab. Das Bild gestaltete sich im weiteren Verlaufe also wieder so, wie es vor der

Tuberculin-Injection gewesen war; es fehlten im weiteren Verlauf wieder alle, auf Tuberculose hindeutenden, characteristischen Momente, obwohl nunmehr an der tuberculösen Natur des Processes kein Zweifel sein konnte.

Ebenso wie in diesen Fällen, wurden auch in andern Beobachtungen sehr häufig ausgedehnte Zerstörungen an den Wänden der Mittelohr-räume nachgewiesen, ohne dass während des Lebens erhebliche Stö-rungen und deutliche Anzeichen vorgelegen hatten. Die symptomlose Entwickelung ausgedehnter cariöser Defecte am Tegmen oder am Sulcus sigmoideus bei relativ geringfügigem Paukenprocess ist bei Tuberculose ja vielfach beobachtet worden, und unzweifelhaft ziemlich häufig. Man findet dann Bilder, welche vollständig den Vorgängen bei der perforir-enden Tuberculose im Schädel entsprechen. Es liegt indessen, wie ich im Gegensatz zu KOERNER hervorheben möchte, keine Veranlassung vor, selbst bei scheinbar von den erkrankten Bezirken abgelegenen cariösen Destructionen die tubare Infection auszuschliessen, und für diese Fälle eine Infection auf dem Wege der Gefässbahn anzunehmen. Eine solche Discontinuität des tuberculösen Processes im Bereich des Schlä-fenbeins ist ebenso wenig eine ungewöhnliche Erscheinung, wie die Perforation nach dem Schädelinnern bei scheinbar geringfügigen Pro-cessen in der Paukenhöhle.

Die Erkrankung der Gehörknöchelchen bei Tuberculose ist in den Arbeiten von HABERMANN, SCHWABACH, BARNICK u.A. eingehend gewürdigt. Es handelt sich ebenso, wie bei den auf andere Weise entstandenen, ebenfalls als Caries bezeichneten destructiven Processen an den Gehörknöchelchen gewöhnlich um Uebergreifen der Erkrankung vom Periost auf den Knochen, in den die tuber-culösen Granulationen hereinwachsen. Auffällig ist, wie bereits SCHWABACH betont hat, hier das frühe Ergriffenwerden der Steig-bügelschenkel. Man findet zuweilen die beiden äusseren Gehörknöchelchen in ihrer Form noch relativ erhalten, durch den Bandapparat oder pathologische Adhäsionen fixiert, während vom Steigbügel nichts mehr zu entdecken, und das ovale Fenster bereits perforiert ist.

Die Häufigkeit des *Durchbruchs der Labyrinthfenster* bei der Tuber-culose ist bekannt. In meinen Obductionsprotokollen sind 7 derartige Befunde verzeichnet. Bei 3 Kranken war das runde Fenster, bei 2 das ovale, bei den beiden übrigen beide Fenster gleichzeitig perforiert. Weit häufiger sind mir, sowohl bei Sectionen, als auch bei Operationen Arrosionen der medialen Adituswand und am Facialkanal begegnet. Auch hier bestätigt sich übrigens die von anderen Labyrintheiterungen bekannte Erfahrung, dass die Gefahren, welche aus der Communication des perilymphatischen Raumes mit dem Subarachnoidalräume resultieren könnten, bei weitem nicht in dem Masse vorhanden sind, wie man erwarten sollte. Auch bei den tuberculösen Processen, welche auf das Labyrinth übergreifen, macht sich die Tendenz zu reparativen Vorgängen, zur

Bindegewebs = und selbst Knochen = Neubildung innerhalb des perilymphatischen Raums so wirksam geltend, dass es gewöhnlich zu frühem Abschluss des von der Tuberculose erreichten Bezirks und damit zu einem Schutz gegen die Infection der Meningen kommt. Meningeale Tuberculose kann sich natürlich auch gelegentlich auch durch Fortleitung im Labyrinth und Acusticus-Stamm entwickeln, kommt aber auf diesem Wege anscheinend seltener zu Stande, als z.B. bei Arrosion des carotischen Canals durch Entwickelung von Tuberkeln in der Adventitia der Carotis, deren Verzweigungen an der Hirnbasis sich dann die Entwickelung miliarer Tuberkel der Pia direct anschliesst.

Eine Sonderstellung nimmt die *Tuberculose des Warzenfortsatzes* ein. Die Auffassung KUESTER'S, dass primäre Tuberculose des Warzenfortsatzes häufig sei, und oft secundär erst die Veränderungen der Schleimhaut herbeiführe, ist unbewiesen geblieben. Nur wenige Fälle, in denen man berechtigt war, primär ossale Processe deswegen anzunehmen, weil die Paukenhöhle garnicht, oder relativ unerheblich beteiligt war, sind bis heute bekannt geworden. Vielleicht sind aber auch diese häufiger, als man bis jetzt anzunehmen geneigt ist. Vielleicht erschwert in manchen Fällen nur die rasche Ausbreitung des Processes die richtige Deutung der Fälle im Sinne der KUESTER', schen Auffassung. Ich will hier nur kurz zwei Fälle erwähnen in denen bei Kindern im ersten Lebensjahr unter Bildung eines subperiostalen Abscesses bei normaler Paukenhöhle sich eine durch Untersuchung der ausgeschabten Granulationsmassen als solche sicher festgestellte, bis in das Occiput reichende Tuberculose des Warzenfortsatzes zeigte. In beiden Fällen führte die Entfernung des tuberculösen Herdes zu dauernder Heilung. Auch hier darf man aber klinischen Thatsachen nicht zu grosse Beweiskraft für die Annahme der Tuberculose einräumen. Es kommen vielmehr im diploetischen Warzenfortsatz des Kindes, sehr selten allerdings, Ostitiden vor, welche ebenfalls auf den Warzenfortsatz beschränkt sind, die Paukenhöhle dauernd freilassen, und doch, trotz voller Uebereinstimmung des Befundes bei der Operation, histologisch als tuberculös nicht agnosciert werden können.

Die klinische Diagnose der Tuberculose begegnet hier, wie überhaupt, deswegen grossen Schwierigkeiten, weil der Nachweis der specifischen Erreger meist sehr schwer ist. Die Zahl der Tuberkelbacillen im Ohreiter ist bei Mittelohrtuberculose im Allgemeinen gering. Man erlangt positive Befunde oft erst dann, wenn man, wie ich es bereits früher empfohlen habe, das bröcklige, käsige Secret aus der Pauke und ihren Nebenräumen mittels Paukenröhrchens direct ausspült, und dann die Spülflüssigkeit sedimentieren lässt oder noch besser centrifugiert. Aber auch positive Befunde besitzen nur unter gewissen Voraussetzungen volle Beweiskraft. Nicht bloss im Cerumen, sondern auch im Secret chronischer Mittelohreiterungen, besonders bei cholesteatomatösen Processen, finden sich Bacillen, welche tinctoriell sich ähnlich den *Smegmabacillen* verhalten. Man muss deshalb bei Untersuchungen von Ohreiter auf Tuberkelbacillen diese Fehlerquelle durch Combination der Säure-Entfärbung mit Einwirkung von absolutem Alcohol und durch entsprechende Dauer der ganzen Entfärbung zu vermeiden suchen.

Dort, wo Granulationen ohne Schwierigkeiten zu erreichen, oder operativ zu entfernen sind, wird die Diagnose am besten durch histologische Untersuchung solcher durch Excision gewonnener Massen gestützt. Auch hier ist allerdings eine reiche Quelle für Irrtümer durch die Häufigkeit der sogenannten Fremdkörpertuberculose, gerade in Granulationswucherungen im Ohr, gegeben. Es bedarf hier nur eines kurzen Hinweises auf die besonders durch MANASSE gewürdigte Thatsache, dass, wie auch aus den demonstrierten Zeichnungen meiner Präparate hervorgeht, solche Granulationsherde mit Riesenzellen sich im Mittelohr sowohl um von aussen eingedrungene Fremdkörper, als auch um Producte der Eiterung selbst, besonders bei cholesteatomatösen Processen bilden können. Der Nachweis der Tuberkelbacillen in excidierten Gewebsstücken ist nicht minder schwierig und misslingt nicht minder häufig, als bei der Untersuchung des Eiters. Man muss sich deshalb für diagnostische Zwecke meist mit dem Nachweis der characteristischen tuberculösen Structur und besonders der für die Tuberculose characteristischen Degenerationsvorgänge begnügen. HAUG und WANTSCHER haben auf die diagnostische Bedeutung *mastoidealer Lymphdrüsenschwellung* für die Erkennung centraler, tuberculöser Ostitis hingewiesen. Klinisch beweist natürlich die Anwesenheit einer geschwollenen Drüse nicht das Mindeste für das Vorhandensein eines Processes im Innern des Warzenfortsatzes, ja nicht einmal für die Anwesenheit einer Erkrankung des Ohrs überhaupt, wie man ja solchen Lymphadenitiden auch im Verlauf von Retronasalkatarrhen bei acut entzündlicher Infiltration der Seitenstränge begegnet. Andererseits aber hat sich wiederholt dort, wo operativ tuberculöse Caries im Bereich des Warzenfortsatzes aufgedeckt wurde, die Thatsache bestätigt, dass, wenn in den aus den Knochenräumen entfernten verkästen Granulationsmassen die characteristischen Elemente der Tuberculose nicht mehr nachweisbar waren, in der bei der Operation excidierten Drüse, vielleicht weil die Veränderungen hier frischer waren, typische tuberculöse Structur noch gefunden wurde. Die Excision dieser dem Warzenfortsatz aufliegenden Drüse ist also dort, wo sie geschwellt ist, schon deswegen ratsam, weil man auf diesem Wege am einfachsten Gelegenheit findet, die Natur des Processes im Knochen zu erkennen. Negative Befunde bei Untersuchung der Drüse entbehren natürlich jeder Beweiskraft. Es ist selbstverständlich nicht unmöglich, dass bei Tuberculosen des Warzenfortsatzes einfach entzündliche Processe in dieser Drüsengruppe sich abspielen.

SIEBENMANN und MILLIGAN haben ebenso, wie auch ich schon, die *Verimpfung excidierter Granulationen* auf empfängliche Tiere für diagnostische Zwecke empfohlen. Nach meinen Erfahrungen führt indessen subcutane Uebertragung, wahrscheinlich wegen relativer Spärlichkeit der Bacillen im Gewebe, meist nicht zu positiven Resultaten. Intraperitoneale Impfung aber bedingt, entsprechend der Regelmässigkeit der Mischinfection bei tuberculösen Mittelohreiterungen, so sehr die gleichzeitige Uebertragung pyogener Bacterien, dass der frühe Eintritt eitriger Peritonitis meist die Beobachtung des Impfergebnisses hinsichtlich der Tuberculose verhindert.

Die *Therapie der Mittelohrtuberculose* kann nur eine operative sein. Zweifelhaft ist nur, welche Fälle operativer Behandlung noch zugänglich sind. Die Möglichkeit, dass eine primäre Tuberculose des Warzenfortsatzes durch operative Eliminierung des ganzen Herdes definitiv heilen kann, wird durch unsere Beobachtungen auf's Neue belegt und wol kaum bestritten. Aber auch an der Heilbarkeit secundärer, von der Schleimhaut aus entstandener Mittelohrtuberculosen ist meines Erachtens nicht zu zweifeln. Auch das Vorhandensein einer Tuberculose der Lunge kann, vorausgesetzt, dass sie nicht so ausgedehnt ist, dass die Chancen für Erhaltung des Lebens, zum mindesten auf längere Zeit hinaus, von vornherein ungünstig sind, eine absolute Contraindication gegen operative Behandlung nicht darstellen. Ebenso wie andere tuberculöse Localerkrankungen operativer Behandlung zugänglich sind, ist dies auch bei der Mittelohrtuberculose, unter gewissen Vorausset, zungen, der Fall. Bei den Fällen, bei welchen sich die als typisch bezeichnete Hauptform der Tuberculose symptomlos entwickelt und, fast latent, um sich greift, kann natürlich eine Operation schon deswegen kaum einen Erfolg haben, weil es sich dabei, wenn auch nicht immer, so doch meist, um Kranke mit vorgeschrittenen Lungenprocessen handelt. Man würde in solchen Fällen mit einem Versuche operativer Ausschaltung der Localtuberculose im Ohr nichts erreichen. Wird man in solchen Fällen durch irgend welche äussere Gründe,—Eintritt cerebraler Symptome, Abscesse an der Aussenfläche des Warzenfortsatzes, etc.,—ausnahmsweise zu einem Eingriff gezwungen, so erreicht man meist nichts weiter, als dass der Process in den nunmehr freiliegenden Mittelohrräumen, jetzt nur besser übersehbar, fortdauert.

Allerdings ist selbst in solchen Fällen mit ausgedehnter Einschmelzung an den knöchernen Wänden der Mittelohrräume ein Erfolg nicht absolut ausgeschlossen. Als Beleg führe ich nur eine Beobachtung an : Ein Knabe mit tuberculöser Coxitis und initialer Lungenerkrankung trat mit einer tuberculösen Mittelohreiterung zu einer Zeit in meine Beobachtung, als schon eine totale Perforation bestand, und ein tuberculöser Herd im Warzenfortsatz durch die Corticalis unter das Periost durchgebrochen war. Nach Freilegung der Mittelohrräume und möglichster Ausschaltung der tuberculösen Partieen kam es hier zu

vollständiger Heilung. Der Knabe starb etwa drei Jahre nach der
Operation an seiner Lungentuberculose. Bei der Obduction zeigte sich
der Process auf der operierten Seite vollständig ausgeheilt, während am
anderen Ohr, auf welchem zur Zeit der Operation ebenfalls eine
chronische Mittelohreiterung bestanden hatte, ausgedehnte, destructive
Processe mit Ansammlung reichlicher käsiger Massen in allen Räumen
vorlagen. Errinert man sich der alten Erfahrung v. TROELTSCH'S,
welcher lange vor der Entdeckung des Tuberkelbacillus, auf die
Bedeutung der Ansammlung solcher käsiger Massen in den Mittelohrräumen für den Allgemeinzustand des betreffenden Kranken hinwies,
so wird man es kaum principiell ablehnen dürfen, Fälle, in denen die
Tuberculose des Mittelohrs den am weitesten fortgeschrittenen tuberculösen Process bei einem Individuum darstellt, doch, trotz der
gleichzeitigen Erkrankung der Lungen, operativ in Angriff zu nehmen.

Thatsächlich habe ich denn auch in mehreren Fällen, in denen ich
trotz gleichzeitiger, relativ geringfügiger Erkrankung der Lunge die
Radicaloperation vornahm, nicht nur vollständige Heilung des localen
Processes im Ohr, sondern selbst eine ganz augenfällige Besserung des
Allgemeinbefindens folgen sehen. Drei von diesen Fällen sind seit Jahren
controliert. Bei zwei dieser Fälle ist von dem Lungenprocess
gegenwärtig überhaupt nichts mehr nachzuweisen. In diesen Fällen
wurde allerdings die tuberculöse Natur der Ohrerkrankung nicht
durchweg erwiesen. Es handelte sich also auch um gewöhnliche
chronische Eiterungen, deren operative Behandlung von den gewöhnlich dafür massgebenden, " prophylaktischen " Gesichtspunkten aus
indiciert war. Die Indication für die Einleitung operativer Therapie
hängt in solchen Fällen von der Körperbeschaffenheit und dem Lungen-
befund ab. Wenn Jemand voraussichtlich nur noch kurze Zeit zu leben
hat, wird man ihn nicht operieren, um ihn vor den möglicher Weise in
Jahren auftretenden Consequenzen seiner Ohreiterung zu schützen.
Ebenso wäre es aber auch verkehrt, angesichts der unbestreitbaren
Heilbarkeit initialer Lungentuberculosen den Nutzen frühzeitiger
Ausschaltung solcher Eiterheerde besonders bei jugendlichen Individuen
leugnen zu wollen. Einen schädlichen Effect habe ich von der Operation
selbst dort nie gesehen, wo ich, aus vitaler Indication oder aus der
Tendenz symptomatischer Therapie heraus, bei schon sehr herabgekom-
menen Individuen operierte. Auch *endocranielle Complicationen* einer
Mittelohrtuberculose können operativ zur Heilung gelangen. In einem
Falle ausgedehnter tuberculöser Caries mit Thrombophlebitis des Sinus
transversus gelang es, die Sinusthrombose so vollständig zur Heilung
zu bringen, dass bei dem mehrere Monate danach wegen Lungen-
tuberculose erfolgten Tode die vollständige Obliteration des Sinus als
Effect der Operation nachgewiesen werden konnte. Hat in diesem
Falle der Operierte, bei dem wegen Indicatio vitalis die sofortige
Vornahme der Operation unabweisbar war, einen bleibenden Vorteil

davon auch nicht gehabt, so ist doch mindestens die Heilbarkeit der Sinusthrombose auch bei ausgedehnter tuberculöser Ostitis und allgemeiner Tuberculose damit sicher bewiesen. Wiederholt boten die Kranken, welche an einer auf das Labyrinth übergreifenden Tuberculose der Paukenhöhle litten, Erscheinungen dar, welche dem Symptombild der sogenannten Meningitis serosa entsprachen. In einem derartigen Falle, in welchem eine Lähmung des Facialis bestand, die Functionsstörung ausserordentlich hochgradig und dabei der Lungenprozess sehr weit vorgeschritten war, waren die cerebralen Störungen so hochgradig, dass, trotz der Unmöglichkeit den Process dauernd zur Heilung zu bringen, doch die Eröffnung der Mittelohrräume vorgenommen werden musste. Die Entfernung der diese ausfüllenden Käsemassen, die Extraction der Sequester, die Sicherung des Eiterabflusses aus den vorher durch Granulationen verschlossenen Labyrinthfenstern, führte zu einem so raschen und subjectiv wohlthätigem Rückgang der meningealen Erscheinungen, dass die Frage, ob man selbst in solchen Fällen, in Sinne symptomatischer Therapie, operieren darf, jedenfalls nicht ohne Weiteres von der Hand zu weisen ist. Es liegt mir fern, etwa auf Grund meiner eigenen günstigen Erfahrungen, die operative Behandlung chronischer Mittelohreiterungen bei tuberculösen Individuen durchwegs principiell zu empfehlen. Man wird sich für operatives Vorgehen um so eher entscheiden müssen, je mehr Anhaltspunkte sich im speciellen Falle dafür ergeben, dass sich unter dem Bilde der gewöhnlichen chronischen Mittelohreiterung eine Tuberculose verbirgt. Es kommen dabei die gleichen Gesichtspunkte in Betracht, die für die Behandlung tuberculöser Localerkrankungen überhaupt massgebend sind. Wenn man aber diesen Gesichtspunkten folgt, wird man zugeben müssen, dass die Anschauung, welche in dem Vorhandensein einer Lungentuberculose schlechthin eine Contraindication gegen die operative Behandlung sonst nicht heilbarer chronischer Mittelohreiterungen erblickt, absolute Geltung nicht mehr beanspruchen kann.

TUBERCULOUS DISEASE OF THE MIDDLE EAR.

DR. MILLIGAN, Manchester.

Frequency of the disease.

Predisposing causes.

Paths of infection.

Clinical features : Condition of middle ear; of facial nerve; of glandular structures around the ear.

Diagnosis : Bacteriological ; by inoculation experiments.

Course of the disease : Complications ; prognosis ; treatment, non-operative, operative.

The widespread interest which has of late been manifested in this and other countries in the endeavour to check the ravages of tubercular disease in its numerous forms, has an interest to the Otologist not only on account of the general merits of the case, but more especially on account of the frequency with which tubercular lesions are met with in and around the middle ear.

The factors which come into play in producing tubercular lesions of the middle ear and its adnexa are but imperfectly understood, and their investigation opens up a wide field for research and experiment.

Does the bacillus gain entrance to the middle ear by way of the Eustachian tube, or is it conveyed along vascular or lymphatic channels ? What also is the relation between tubercular naso-pharyngeal adenoid vegetations and tubercular middle ear disease ?

Questions such as these are not easily answered, and yet their solution must appeal to all as being of much importance.

For some years past I have been particularly interested in this subject, and as opportunity has presented itself, have endeavoured to investigate these questions both in their practical·and in their scientific aspects.

That a large proportion of the cases of suppurative middle ear disease with accompanying bone lesions met with in practice are of a tubercular nature will, I think, be admitted by all, and that the prognosis in such cases is not very favourable will, I believe, be conceded by those who have had large clinical experience.

The characteristic features of tubercular middle ear disease may be somewhat masked on account of an accompanying pathogenic infection, and an accurate diagnosis may be impossible if one relies upon finding the bacillus of tubercle in the secretion from the middle ear.

Time after time it has been my experience to examine cover glass preparations of pus from the middle ear for bacilli, and with negative results, although the tubercular nature of the lesion has been proved beyond all doubt by means of inoculation experiments, and by the subsequent clinical history of the case. In my experience, primary tubercular lesions of the middle ear and adjoining mastoid cells are comparatively common, especially amongst the children of the poorer classes, and I believe also, that secondary tubercular infection from such a primary focus is by no means of infrequent occurrence.

Amongst causes which may be considered predisposing, are the following :—

(1) Hereditary tendency.
(2) Unhealthy environment.
(3) Unsuitable feeding.
(4) Exposure to infection from tuberculous relatives.
(5) The presence of tuberculous naso-pharyngeal adenoids.

The relation of nasal obstruction to tubercular middle ear disease deserves special consideration. In many of my cases postnasal adenoids have been present, and in a small proportion have themselves been tuberculous. The almost constant degree of Eustachian catarrh, which their presence implies, produces a soil which is favourable to the growth of the tubercle bacillus, and once it has found a footing in the middle ear the conditions favourable to its development are present, viz.: a suitable soil and a more or less uniform temperature, &c. In the early stages these tubercular foci appear as slightly elevated yellowish points in the mucosa, after a time coalescing and breaking down to form superficial tubercular ulcers.

Should the deposit occur upon the inner aspect of the membrane, perforation ensues. Such perforations may be multiple and the destruction of tissue is usually quite painless. The edges of such perforations have a pale indolent looking appearance, and the accompanying discharge from the middle ear is usually thin, ichorous, and frequently fœtid.

Within the mastoid cells such deposits are also frequent, and I am inclined to think that in some cases at least the disease begins first of all within the mastoid and subsequently spreads to the middle ear. At a very early stage the bone becomes affected and undergoes an amount of destruction which is almost inconceivable, considering the comparatively slight external indications present. In some cases which have come under my observation, practically the entire cancellous tissue of the mastoid — occasionally of both mastoids — has been eaten away, leaving merely a bony shell upon which the middle fossa is poised. Owing to this early and extensive destruction of bone, the facial nerve in part of its course is exposed with resulting facial paralysis. In fact, early facial paralysis in a case in which sthenic symptoms have been absent should I hold be looked upon with suspicion, and as a possible, if not probable, manifestation of an underlying tubercular lesion. Early implication and enlargement of the glandular structures around the ear is also a most important symptom, and when masses of enlarged glands occur around the ear any discharge from the tympanic cavity should be microscopically examined for bacilli.

To definitely establish the fact that the aural lesion is of a tubercular nature the characteristic bacillus must be found. This may be an exceedingly difficult task, but in all cases it is worth while staining and examining the secretion from the middle ear. Should no evidence of its presence be found in this way, small pieces of granulation tissue may be removed by forceps, pressed between two cover glasses and stained in a suitable manner. Occasionally bacilli will be found in such preparations. The method which I believe gives the most reliable results however is the inoculation of guinea-pigs with small fragments of tissue removed from the middle ear or adjoining mastoid cells, and I believe it is advisable to inoculate with fragments of bone and mucous membrane from an area where the disease is seen to be advancing. In many such cases where the mastoid process has been opened for the purposes of treatment a pultaceous looking mass will be found filling up the cavity, but this material is practically valueless for experimental purposes, consisting as it does of broken down tissue, inspissated purulent débris and epithelial cells. When, however, it has been removed by means of a spoon and the underlying bone exposed, it will then be seen where the disease is making progress and from where a scraping of bone should be taken. In my experiments I have inserted a fragment of tissue, obtained as above described, into a guinea-pig's hind leg just above the knee joint, all hair having previously been removed by singeing with a platinum knife. A small pocket is now made with a sterilised needle and the tissue carefully inserted. In a few weeks' time, should the tissue inoculated be tuberculous, the inguinal glands will be found enlarged, and as time goes on the tubercular virus will be found to have spread over the animal's body, the glands and the viscera being attacked in the following order, according to the results obtained by Prof. Delepine. (B.M.J., Sept. 23rd, 1893):—

During the Second Week after inoculation the lymphatic ganglia upon the same side of the body below the diaphragm and the spleen will be found enlarged.

During the Third Week, the liver, the mediastinal, and the bronchial ganglia.

During the Fourth Week, the lungs, the cervical, and the axillary ganglia.

After the Fourth Week, some of the lymphatic ganglia of the opposite side of the body below the diaphragm become affected, but this takes place extremely slowly, and the sublumbar and popliteal glands escape for a considerable time.

Microscopic sections made from these glands and stained for bacilli will frequently be found to reveal their presence.

In this way a definite diagnosis of the actual character of the underlying lesion can be made, and the value of the knowledge thus obtained is naturally immense, as regards both prognosis and treatment.

The course of such tubercular lesions is only too often a downward one despite the most elaborate and painstaking treatment. The practical difficulties encountered in removing tubercular deposits within bone are immense, and in no region of the body are these difficulties greater than when tubercle attacks the temporal bone, for reasons which must be obvious to all here.

The complications which have to be feared are

(1) Meningitis.
(2) Tubercular enteritis.
(3) General marasmus.

The treatment of such cases must be considered from two points of view, according as it is non-operative or operative. Cases will be met with, especially in infants, where any operative interference will from the first be seen to be hopeless.   Such are the cases where marked debility and emaciation are present, where advanced facial paralysis and masses of enlarged glands have been early symptoms, and where the discharge is abundant, fœtid and frequently blood-stained.   In such cases palliative measures, antiseptic treatment, and, if possible, residence at the seaside are indicated, but I am bound to say that in the majority of such patients whose cases I have followed, an early death has been the usual history.   The prognosis I believe to be essentially bad.

In other cases, however, where the general condition of the patient is good (and often enough it is so), and where the tubercular lesion may be regarded as primary and local, much can be done by suitable operative interference.   It is almost superfluous to say that the first and main essential is to provide free drainage.   This implies opening and cleansing the mastoid cells, and it is a remarkable fact how often in such cases without any external and objective sign or indication, the mastoid cortex will be found extensively perforated, and a pultaceous mass immediately exposed to view.   Under good illumination, a very careful toilet of the part should be affected, and this can generally best be done by means of a sharp spoon.   All softened and carious bone must be scraped away, and as smooth a cavity left as possible even if this necessitates laying bare the dura and walls of the lateral sinus.   The cavity thus obtained should be allowed to granulate from the bottom, and care must be taken to stimulate any sluggish area by means of applications of chloride of zinc, nitrate of silver, etc.   Frequently more than one scraping is necessary, as fresh foci of disease appear.   In one particular case which came under my treatment some years ago, and when the cause was proved to have been feeding with milk from a tubercular cow, four operations had to be undertaken before the disease within the mastoid process was eradicated, which however it finally was, and the child has now grown up to a healthy and sturdy boy.   In very many of the cases the middle ear has been so extensively destroyed, that its function as a sense organ may be disregarded.   Under such circumstances its contents should be freely curetted, and middle ear, antrum and mastoid cells thrown into one cavity, and allowed to become obliterated by means of healthy granulation tissue.   Where, however, a fair degree of hearing is present, efforts should be made to preserve the function of the organ so far as is possible.

An important point arises in connection with the treatment of the accompanying enlarged glands.   Some of the glands may be enlarged purely as the result of septic absorption, and if the morbid cause be removed this enlargement will gradually subside, especially if aided by suitable treatment.   But many of the glands are of a tubercular nature and are prone to undergo caseous degeneration, while at the same time they are a source of possible systemic infection. Hence I hold that after the mastoid area and the cavity of the middle ear have been attended to, and as soon as the condition of the patient admits of it, another operation should be undertaken with the object of removing these enlarged and tuberculous structures.

The facial paralysis which so often accompanies tubercular disease of the middle ear is unfortunately frequently permanent. Something, however, may be done by facial massage and the internal administration of strychnine to assist in maintaining the tonus of the facial muscles.

General treatment, such as the administration of cod liver oil, iodide of iron, syrup of iodine, etc., is useful, as also is change of air and liberal diet.

The general conclusions from a study of a number of cases may be summarised as follows :—

(1). That primary tuberculous disease in and around the middle ear is of fairly frequent occurrence, and that it most usually attacks the children of the poor, especially the poor of our larger cities.

(2). That a generalized tubercular infection may arise from a primary focus within or around the middle ear.

(3). That the prognosis of such cases is not very favourable, at least 40-50 per cent. of the cases succumbing even after operative treatment has been undertaken.

(4). That in many of the cases operative interference is contra-indicated owing to the extent of the existing disease and the asthenic condition of the patient.

(5). That when operative interference is feasible, the main object should be to scrape away all foci of disease and to provide efficient drainage.

(6). That the best and most reliable means of establishing the tubercular nature of the disease is by means of properly conducted inoculation experiments.

PROF. KUEMMEL hat gerade solche acute tuberkulöse Mittelohreiterungen wie Brieger auch gesehen und stimmt mit ihm überein, dass solche Fälle ganz wie gewöhnliche acute Mittelohreiterungen verlaufen können, auch die massenhafte Granulationsbildung konnte Kümmel beobachten. Für die Diagnose hält er die bei seinen Fällen auffallende Labyrintherkrankung für wichtig. Dagegen darf, nach seiner Meinung, Nachweis einer tuberculösen Erkrankung der Drüse auf dem Warzenfortsatz nicht ohne Weiteres als Beweis für tuberkulöse Natur der Otitis angesehen werden. Zuweilen gelingt der Nachweis der Tuberkulose besser als in Granulationen und Drüsen im erkrankten Knochen.

PROF. POLITZER said : Dr. Brieger had favourable results from operation in chronic tuberculous suppuration of the middle ear, even with extensive destruction in the temporal bone. He agreed with Dr.

Brieger that a tuberculous process in the temporal bone was no contra-indication for operative interference.   He only operated if there were symptoms of beginning tuberculosis ; but he never operated in phthisical individuals, as according to his experience the operation only accelerated death.

DR. MCBRIDE asked a question as to the diagnosis without resorting to inoculation, which was difficult to carry out in this country.

DR. BRIEGER hat Spontanheilungen bei den acuten Formen der Mittelohrtuberculose nie gesehen.   Sie zeichneten sich durch sehr schweren Verlauf aus, und führten meist bald zum Tode.   Labyrinth-erscheinungen waren in diesen—übrigens sehr seltenen Fällen—bald vorhanden, bald fehlend.

Zur Diagnose gelangte Brieger durch histologische Untersuchung excidierter Granulationen.   Der Impfversuch eignete sich für diese Zwecke nicht; subcutane Impfung war bei diesen—meist bacillenarmen—Gewebsstücken meist zwecklos, die intraperitonale Uebertragung bedenklich, weil gleichzeitige Uebertragung pyogener Mikroorganismen Peritonitis und zu frühen Tod des Versuchstieres oft herbeiführte.

Tuberculose der über dem Warzenfortsatz gelegenen Lymphdrüsen war bei Weitem nicht immer, aber gelegentlich geeignet, die Erkennung eines Prozesses im Warzenfortsatz als Tuberculose zu erleichtern.   Man fand mikroskopisch diese Drüsen charakteristisch verändert zu einer Zeit, zu der im mastoidealen Heerde die Elemente der Tuberculose nicht mehr nachzuweisen waren.

ANGEBORENES FEHLEN DES AEUSSEREN GEHOERGANGES UND ERWORBENER VERSCHLUSS DESSELBEN.

DR. ARTHUR HARTMANN, Berlin.

Die Sektionsberichte über angeborenes Fehlen des äusseren Gehör-ganges, wofür in der Literatur in der Regel die nicht entsprechende Bezeichnung Atresia auris congenita gebraucht wird, sind nicht sehr zahlreich.   Es wurden von Joel 12 Fälle zusammengestellt, welche von Bezold auf 16 ergänzt wurden.   Ruedi bringt in einer kürzlich erschienenen Arbeit die Zahl auf 46, wobei allerdings Fälle mitgezählt sind, die nur am Lebenden beobachtet wurden.   Ich selbst habe vor 6 Jahren die Präparate von einem Neugeborenen demonstrirt.   Bei dem-selben fanden sich beiderseits die Ohrmuscheln nur rudimentär ent-wickelt und keine Spur eines äusseren Gehörganges.   Bei der Präpara-tion zeigte es sich, dass der Annulus tympanicus und das Trommelfell vollständig fehlten.   In der Paukenhöhle, die ebenso wie das Antrum mastoideum gut entwickelt ist, sind die Gehörknöchelchen wenn auch rudimentär entwickelt.

Neuerdings kam ich in der Besitz eines Präparates vom Erwachsenen, auch hier war das äussere Ohr wie das Gypsmodell zeigt rudimentär entwickelt, von dem äusseren Gehörgange und vom Trommelfell ist keine Spur vorhanden. Das Unterkiefergelenk artikulirt auf der vorderen Fläche des Warzentheiles des Schläfenbeins. Auch hier ist wie an dem vorgelegten Präparate zu ersehen — Paukenhöhle und Antrum vorhanden, ebenso die Gehörknöchelchen, in einer von der normalen nur wenig abweichenden Form.

Ich glaubte Ihnen die Präparate vorlegen zu dürfen da sie in praktischer Beziehung für die Beurteilung der Versuche bei der sog. Atresia auris congenita einen neuen Gehörgang herzustellen von Wert sind. Aus der Literatur konnte ich nur in den Besitz einer italienischen Veröffentlichung gelangen von Vannoni aus dem vorigen Jahrhundert. Vannoni beschreibt wie er an der Stelle des äusseren Gehörganges eine Incision machte in die Tiefe drang, einen mit Flüssigkeit gefüllten Gehörgang fand. Es gelang ihm die Oeffnung dauernd herzustellen. Er schildert nun wie sich bei dem Patienten der vorher vollständig taub war, allmälig das Gehör wieder zum normalen entwickelte. Da bei allen sonst beobachteten Fällen das Gehör bei erhaltenem Labyrinthe so weit vorhanden ist, dass die Patienten laute Sprache verstehen, und nicht taubstumm werden, und die Schilderung der Erlernung der Sprache bei dem operirten Patienten etwas abenteuerlich klingt, möchte ich diesen Fall nicht als feststehend betrachten.

In den älteren Lehrbüchern der Ohrenheilkunde finden sich die Methoden angegeben auf operativem Wege bei Fehlen des äusseren Gehörganges einen solchen herzustellen. Bevor ich die Verhältnisse kannte, habe ich vor 8 Jahren einen solchen Versuch gemacht und den betreffenden Patienten bei der zweiten Versammlung norddeutscher Ohrenärzte vorgestellt. Bei dem Patienten war die Ohrmuschel wenn auch etwas verkleinert gut entwickelt, die Auskultation auf dem Warzenfortsatz bei Katheterismus ergab kräftiges Eindringen des Luftstromes in das Mittelohr, das Gehör für Sprache und Stimmgabel wies auf normales Funktioniren des Labyrinthes. Der Operationsversuch wurde nicht wie in den Lehrbüchern empfohlen an der Stelle der Gehörgangsmündung gemacht, die Ohrmuschel wurde von hinten abgelöst und entlang der vorderen Fläche des Warzenfortsatzes eingedrungen. An Stelle des äusseren Gehörganges fand sich der Gelenksfortsatz des Unterkiefers. Nach Vernähung der Wunde, trat Heilung per primam intentionem ein.

Erfolglose Operationsversuche wurden trotz meiner Mitteilung später von Kiesselbach und neuerdings von Mahr gemacht. Ich glaube wenn man einzelne Präparate gesehen hat, wird man von solchen Operationsversuchen Abstand nehmen.

Ueber das Hörvermögen bei der sog. Atresia auris congenita hat vor Kürzem Ruedi eingehende Untersuchungen angestellt. Es konnte von ihm bestätigt werden, dass bei beiderseitigem Fehlen des äusseren Gehörganges, Conversationssprache gut, Flüstersprache nur in nächster Nähe des Ohres vernommen wird. Die Stimmgabelprüfung ergibt das für Schallleitungshinderniss bei intaktem Labyrinthe charakteristische Schema.*

Während wir über die Verhältisse bei angeborenem Fehlen des äusseren Gehörganges eine beträchtliche Anzahl von Mitteilungen besitzen, sind diejenigen über erworbenen knöchernen Verschluss weniger zahlreich. Ich erlaube mir desshalb über einen von mir beobachteten und mit Erfolg operirten Fall einige Bermerkungen zu machen.

Der Patient hatte in der Kindheit durch Scharlachdiptherie beiderseitige eiterige Mittelohrentzündung bekommen, mit Verlust der Gehörknöchelchen und Meningitis. Dieselbe verursachte linksseitige Lähmung. Es blieb zurück Atrophie des linken Armes und Beines, und nicht vollständige Lähmung des Gesichtsnerven. Auf beiden Seiten war der Verschluss des Gehörganges ein vollständiger. An Stelle der Oeffnung befand sich beiderseits eine glatte Oberfläche mit knöcherner Unterlage. Flüsterstimme wurde beiderseits nur in einer Entfernung von 10 cm gehört. Tiefe Stimmgabeln wurden nicht durch Luft, gut durch Knochenleitung gehört. Beim Valsalva'schen Versuch dringt die Luft in beide Ohren.

Ich führte auf der linken Seite die Operation in der Weise aus,dass die Ohrmuschel von hinten abgelöst wurde. Die Knochenneubildung am Eingang des Gehörganges wird mit dem Meissel entfernt und ebenso die hintere Gehörgangswand in der bei der Radikaloperation üblichen Weise abgetragen und die Mittelohrräume freigelegt. Aus der Ohrmuschel bildete ich einen Lappen nach der Körner'schen Methode. Der Lappen wurde nach hinten angenäht und die hintere Wunde durch die Naht geschlossen. Auf diese Weise entstand eine sehr weite Oeffnung an der Stelle des Gehörganges. Die Nachbehandlung erforderte zahlreiche Aetzungen mit Chromsäure und die Anwendung des Galvanokauters. Trotz der anfänglich sehr beträchtlichen Grösse des neugebildeten Gehörganges wurde derselbe immer enger, so dass schliesslich zum Offenhalten ein Zinnrohr eingelegt werden musste, welches die Oeffnung dauernd erhielt. Das Hörvermögen wurde so beträchtlich gebessert, dass Flüstersprache in 2 Meter Entfernung gehört wird.

Dr. Holinger said he was personally very much obliged to Dr. Hartmann, because he was just at present confronted by the question whether or not to operate in a case of double-sided absence of the auditory meatus. In examining 510 deaf and dumb children at the State Institution of Illinois, he had met with a girl of fifteen years. She had had scarlatina at the age of two years. which broke through the mastoid process behind each auricle. The hearing was pretty good in

*Arch. f. Ohrenheilk, Bd. 19, S 127. Annales des Malad, de l'oreille, etc., No. 6, 1899.

the beginning, but during the last few years had been getting very bad. At the present time there was an opening behind each ear, and from time to time the suppuration recurred. This case, he thought, answered the question whether to operate or not. We could create a perpetual opening if we opened the middle ear through the mastoid—high enough not to get into the joint—removed the malleus and incus, allowed the wound to granulate, and finally covered, according to Siebenmann, with Thiersch's grafts.

MR. CRESSWELL BABER said that he had seen the case last referred to by Dr. Hartmann. It was a very interesting one, and from the patient's own account, his hearing had much improved. The wearing of a metal tube was necessary to prevent contraction. He said that in a case recently under his care of acquired occlusion of both meatuses, in which the tuning fork was perfectly heard, he operated on one ear, and at first drilled with a bur, but without penetrating the obstruction in the meatus. He afterwards performed a Stacke's operation, but little or no improvement in hearing had resulted.

DR. HARTMANN.—In Fällen von angeborenem Fehlen des äusseren Gehörganges ohne Entzündung ist die Herstellung einer dauernden Oeffnung im Warzenfortsatze nicht zu empfehlen, da es sehr fraglich ist ob eine Verbesserung des Gehörs dadurch erreicht werden kann. In einem Falle von Exostosenbildung, in welchem eine Oeffnung von ihm nach dem Antrum hergestellt wurde, trat keine Hörverbesserung ein.

UEBER BLAUE DIAPHANITAET AM TROMMELFELL UND UEBER VARIXBILDUNG AN DEMSELBEN.

DR. F. ROHRER, Zurich.

Die Farbe des Trommelfelles ist eine Combinationsfarbe, die sich aus der Eigenfarbe der Membran, der angewendeten Lichtart und der Menge und Farbe der von der Innenwand der Trommelhöhle zurückgeworfenen Strahlen zusammensetzt (Politzer, Atlas der Beleuchtungsbilder des Trommelfelles 1896 IV. S. 43.)

Ausser der normalen neutralgrauen oder perlgrauen Farbe des Trommelfells bei Erwachsenen haben wir das blassgraue oder grauröthliche noch glanzlose Trommelfell des Neugeborenen und Säuglings und die leicht grau getrübte oft matte Membran des Kindesalters. Im Greisenalter beobachten wir die typische Veränderung der Verdickung, Opacität, Verfettung, Verkalkung, und Narbenbildung. Nicht selten nimmt das opake Trommelfell einen bläulichen oder blaugrünen Ton an, und bei genauem Zusehen, finden wir, wenn auch nur ausnahmsweise, Trommelfelle mit ziemlich reinen, blauen Farbentönen. Doch handelt es sich in diesen Fällen wohl ausnahmslos um die Eigenfarbe der Membran.   Sehr selten nur kommt eine eigentliche blaue Diaphanität des Trommelfells zur Beobachtung.   In dieser Beziehung finden wir die erste Andeutung in dem von Dr. Ludewig in der Halle'schen Ohrenklinik beobachteten, und im Arch. f. O. Bd. XXIX. S. 234/37 beschriebenen Fall von "lebensgefährlicher Blutung bei Paracentese des Trommelfells durch Verletzung des Bulbus venae jugularis." Ausdrücklich meldet Ludewig: "Auffällig war uns wohl die blaue Färbung des hinteren unteren Quadranten oder richtiger-gesagt ein durchscheinendes Blau an dieser Stelle!" Bekanntlich erfolgte in diesem Fall 25 XI. 88 bei Erweiterung der Paracentese durch Dilatation des Einstiches mit der Paracentesennadel eine colossale Blutung, wobei circa 1 Liter Blut in ganz kurzer Zeit aus dem Gehörgang in weiten Bogen herausschoss.   Der 5 jährige Knabe genas trotz des grossen Blutverlustes, unter Tamponade des Meatus auditorius externus mit Iodoformgaze.   Bei Besprechung dieses Falles hat L. die einschlägige Literatur, soweit sie sich auf Lücken in der knöchernen Wand der Paukenhöhle, insbesondere auf Dehiscenz-bildungen am Bulbus V. jugularis bezieht zusammengestellt. V. Tröltsch hat zuerst auf die eminent praktische Bedeutung dieser Dehiscenzen für pathologische Processe in der Trommelhöhle und für operative Eingriffe hingewiesen (4 Aufl. S. 133. 7 Aufl. S. 165) während Toynbee in seinem berühmten und seltenen "Descriptive Catalogue" (1857 S. 44) eine Reihe von anatomischen Präparaten anführt No. 453-482 unter dem Titel N. "The inferior osseous wall deficient, the mucous membrane of the tympanum being more or less in contact with the outer surface of the jugular vein!" Gerade für den von mir selbst seit einigen Jahren beobachteten Fall von blauer Diaphanität des Trommelfells und Varixbildung in beiden oberen Quadranten desselben ist von besonderer Wichtigkeit die weitere Anführung von Präparaten aus Toynbee's "Descriptive Catalogue" und zwar sub. L. "Superior osseous wall expanded!" "No 411. The tympanic cavity is so expanded that its superior and posterior walls are so thin as to be translucent," und M. "Superior wall partly deficient, the mucous membrane of the tympanum being more or less in contact with the dura mater."

Eine besonders genaue Würdigung der Dehiscenzen der knöchernen Wandungen der Paukenhöhle verdanken wir Zuckerkandl, (M. f. O. VIII. No 7 II. "Beitrag zur Anatomie des Schläfenbeins"), während Friedlowsky in der M. f. O. 1867 auf Dehiscenzen am Boden der Paukenhöhle aufmerksam machte.   Zuckerkandl sagt: "Durch die beschriebenen anatomischen Veränderungen der Fossa V. jugularis sehen wir die *Venae jugulares* mit dem Inhalte der Paukenhöhlen, mit der Dura mater, mit den Gesichtsnerven, Hörnerven, und mit den oberen Felsenbeinblutleitern in Berührung treten" (vergl. Hessler "Otogene Pyaemie"). In Bd. XXX. des A. f. O. bringt Körner einen sehr bemerkenswerthen Artikel : "Ueber die Fossa jugularis, und die Knochenlücken im Boden der Paukenhöhle." Körner betont mit v. Tröltsch die Möglichkeit der Entstehung einer Sinusphlebitis, ausgehend vom Bulbus V. jugularis und wiederholt die Thatsache, wie sie Zuckerkandl und V. Tröltsch bereits erwähnten, dass die Fossa jugularis links und rechts am gleichen Schädel oft verschieden gross sei und verschieden tief in den Knochen eindringt. Diese Unterschiede sind durch die verschiedene Stärke der beiden Venae jugulares bedingt. Nach Bezold, Rüdinger, H. v. Meyer, und Körner ist der Sinus transversus rechts stärker als links, dasselbe bemerkt Rüdinger auch für die Fossa jugularis, die rechts durchschnittlich grösser und tiefer ist als links. Daher auch die entsprechende Knochenwand, welche sie von der Paukenhöhle trennt, dünner sein und häufigere Lücken zeigen muss. Körner hat diese Verhältnisse an 449 Schädeln studirt. Das Ergebniss dieser Studien bestätigt das vorher gesagte.

Schädel-
zahl

76 — Fossae jugulares waren beiderseits gleich weit und gleich tief in 16, 9%

264 — „ „ „ rechts weiter und tiefer als links 58, 8%

109 — „ „ „ links weiter und tiefer als rechts 24, 3%

bei 30 Schädeln fanden sich Lücken und zwar 22 mal rechts, 8 mal links. Mehrmals fand sich siebartige Durchlöcherung dieser Stelle und zwar bei 23 Schädeln : 12 mal rechts, 7 mal links, 4 mal beiderseitig. Ebenso fand K. pneumatische Räume in der trennenden Knochenwand. An der 66 Versammlung deutscher Naturförscher und Aerzte in WIEN hielt Dozent f. O. Dr. B. Gomperz in der Section f. O. am 26. IX. 94, einen Vortrag über : "Die Erkennung der Vorwölbung des Bulbus Venæ jugularis in die Paukenhöhle am Lebenden." Gomperz besprach den Fall Ludewig's und führt zwei analoge Beobachtungen an, den einen aus der Gruber'schen Klinik 1888, den andern aus der Trautmann'schen Klinik A. f. O. XXX. S. 183 von Hildebrandt veröffentlicht. In allen 3 Fällen handelt es sich um das rechte Ohr. In den beiden letzten Fällen fanden sich nach der Operation im hinteren unteren Quadrante ein livider bläulich rother Fleck, und bei Hildebrandt's Fall eine gelblich rothe Vorwölbung, die bei Compression der Vena jugularis sich änderte—Dehiscenz ! Ein 4ᵉʳ Fall von Brieger endete durch Pyaemie letal, nachdem der Bulbus V. jugularis mit dem Galvanocauter eröffnet worden war. Fall 5 von Seligmann, publicirt A. f. O. XXXV. S. 134, rechtes Ohr, Heilung. Gomperz sah gar nicht selten im hinteren unteren Quadranten "blaue Verfärbungen, welche nach Sitz, Ausdehnung und Farbe nichts mit dem Schatten der runden Fensternische gemeinhatten, der an zarten Trommelfellen öft wahr zu nehmen ist. Man findet diese blauen Flecke meist kreisabschnittförmig oder biconvex oder mit wellig verlaufender oberer Grenzlinie sich der unteren Trommelfellperipherie anschliessend, die Convexität nach oben und vorne wendend,—meist einseitig, manchmal auch doppelseitig, dann aber auf einer Seite stärker ausgeprägt."

Gomperz beschreibt nun drei beobachtete Fälle mit besonders stark ausgeprägter blauer Diaphanität. Im ersten Fall zeigte das linke Ohr in nahezu der ganzen unteren Hälfte des Trommelfells die blaue Verfärbung. Bei Anwendung des Siegle'schen pneumatischen Trichters zeigte es sich, dass die blaue Farbe nicht im Trommelfell selbst, sondern hinter demselben ihren Ursprung nahm. Im 2ten Fall handelte es sich um Zerstörung des rechten Trommelfells und der Ossicula—narbige Degeneration der Paukenhöhle, " von deren Boden ein tief dunkelblauer Buckel von 5 mm Länge und 3mm Querdurchmesser sich emporwölbte." Der 3te Fall betraf einen 13 jährigen Knaben, dessen rechtes Ohr in der ganzen unteren Hälfte und einem Teil des hinteren oberen Quadranten ein tief dunkles Blau zeigte, das nahe der unteren Trommelfellperipherie in ein DUNKLES VIOLETT UEBERGEHT. Siegle's Trichter zeigt, dass es sich um Diaphanität handelt. Nonengeräusche sind hörbar, was übrigens bereits v. Tröltsch beobachtete. Praktisch von hoher Bedeutung ist in solchen Fällen die Frage der Paracentese. Gomperz besitzt Präparate, wo das vorgewölbte Dach des Bulbus stark in die Nische des runden Fensters hinein ragt. Besonders gefährlich sind in solchen Fällen von Dehiscenz die acute und chronische eitrige Entzündung. Der von mir beobachtete Fall von "Blauer Diaphanität des Trommelfells" und Auftreten von "Varixknoten im Trommelfell" ist seit Februar 1894, in meiner Beobachtung. Es betrifft einen Knaben, "Johann Gamp," geboren 1887, der am 21. II. 94. wegen leichter Gehörstörung hervorgerufen durch Tubencatarrh und Ansammlung von Ohrfett in den Gehörgängen in meine Behandlung trat. Flüstersprache wurde damals links auf 3 M, rechts auf 2 M. Distanz gehört, die Kopfknochenleitung war gut erhalten, hohe und tiefe Töne wurden gut percipirt. Der Knabe zeigte Erscheinungen von Scrophulose und abgelaufener Rachitis und hatte in früher Kindheit Anfälle von Eclampsie gehabt. Nasen-Rachenraum belastet, Adenoide Vegetationen und Aprosexia sind nachweisbar. Linkes Trommelfell ist in der Membrana propria blau durchschimmernd, Hammer retrahirt; am hinteren Rand des rechten Trommelfells ein dunkelblaurothes Gebilde das prima vista den Eindruck einer Blutblase machte. Der sichtbare Rest des rechten Trommelfells war tiefblau. Im Laufe der Beobachtung überzeugte ich mich, dass es sich um einen reellen Varix in der hinteren oberen Hälfte des Trommelfells handelte. Im Laufe der Jahre von 1894—1899 ist dieser Varix mehrmals verschwunden, wobei an seine Stelle eine mit radiär angeordneten Falten versehene Narbe tràt und alternirend eine Varixbildung am linken Trommelfell auftrat.

Der Varix links nimmt die ganze obere Hälfte des Trommelfells ein, und reicht erbsengross in das Lumen des knöchernen Gehörganges herein. Gegenwärtig entwickelt sich am rechten Trommelfell neuerdings ein grosser, tief dunkelblauer Varix in der hinteren Hälfte der Membran, während in dem vorderen Quadranten eine dunkelblaue Diaphanität besonders schön sichtbar ist. Der Fall wird demnächst in einer Inaugural-Dissertation in extenso publicirt werden.

L'INVOLUTION PRÉCOCE DU TISSU ADENOÏDIEN SUR LA RIVIERA.

DR. T. BOBONE, San Remo.

MESSIEURS,

J'ai publié, en 1885, dans le " Bollettino per le malattie dell 'Orecchio, Naso, e Gola," un petit Travail, dans lequel, me basant sur les observations que j'avais instituées pendant une saison de bains, je faisais ressortir la fâcheuse influence que sous certaines conditions les bains de mer peuvent exercer sur l'oreille saine et sur l'oreille malade, influence que je mettais toute sur le compte du bain, de l'eau, et pas de l'air maritime.

Dans une des séances du 4ᵐᵉ Congrès International d 'Otologie à Bruxelles, M. Moure de Bordeaux relata les résultats d'observations personnelles, d'après lesquelles l'air de la mer serait, plus encore que l'eau, nuisible aux oreilles car il favoriserait les dermatoses, rendrait plus grave la surdité et les bourdonnements et *provoquerait l'accroissement momentané des végétations adenoïdes.*

Si je vous rappelle aujourd'hui cette communication de notre très estimé confrère, que vous n'avez certainement pas oubliée, c'est pour vous dire que, ayant renouvelé, depuis cette époque, mes observations, j'ai non seulement gardé, mais fortifié davantage mon ancienne opinion, à savoir que l'air maritime, sur notre littoral, plus que nuisible peut être, au contraire, utile aux oreilles.

J'ai cru pouvoir m'expliquer cette différence de vues par le fait, sur lequel je vous entretiendrais tout à l'heure, que l'air maritime n'est pas égal partout, et que notamment entre l'air maritime de ce morceau de littoral qui est universellement connu sous le nom de "Riviera," et l'air maritime de Bordeaux la diversité est si grande, qu'il est aisé de comprendre comment ces deux airs puissent agir sur notre organisme d'une façon toute différente, et parfois diamétralement opposée.

Au cours de mes recherches je suis venu, un peu spontanément, un peu guidé par le hasard, à porter mon attention sur la façon dont se comportent, dans notre climat, les végétations adenoïdes, dont l'extrême rareté, chez les indigènes, n'avait pas été sans me frapper depuis très longtemps. En effet, je puis dire que les indigènes, affectés de végétations adénoïdes, qui sont tombés sous mon observation pendant l'espace de presque vingt ans, je pourrais les compter sur les bouts des doigts. La très grande majorité des enfants que j'eus à traiter, appartenait à des familles venues du Nord de l'Europe ou de l'Italie pour passer l'hiver à San Remo, ou s'y fixer définitivement. Une partie parmi eux, envoyés chez nous par leurs médecins à cause de leur constitution faible, de leur tendence aux migraines, aux rhumes de cerveau, aux maux de gorge, aux bronchites, n'étaient, au fond que des adenoïdiens, et il m'arriva bien souvent d'être le premier à poser le diagnostique de végétations adenoïdes qui n'avait pas été fait jusque là, et de parler à leurs parents de la nécessité d'une opération que, avec la suffisance que donne la conviction, je mettais devant leurs yeux comme un *aut-aut*, comme le seul moyen pour redonner aux petits malades la santé ou de les débarasser de leurs bobos.

L'on comprend aisément que non obstant toutes les affirmations sur le danger qui accompagnait la vraie cause de la maladie, et la nécessité de l'extirper au plus vite, l'intervention sanglante était la plupart des fois refusée par des parents qui se trouvaient loin de leur residence habituelle, ou à l'étranger, et qui répondaient, presque invariablement, que si l'opération était vraiment nécessaire, ils désiraient la laisser faire une fois rentrés chez eux.

Eh bien, en dépit de mes prophéties, d'après lesquelles il n'y aurait dû avoir, hors de l'opération, point de salut, il m'est arrivé de voir bien souvent des adenoïdiens laissés sans traitement, ou traités avec des moyens qui, presqu'à l'uninamité, sont déclarés comme absolument inutiles par les otologistes, s'améliorer peu à peu, soit dans l'état local que général, changer de physionomie et d'expression, retrouver leur réspiration nasale, perdre leur tendance à s'enrhumer et tousser pour un rien, et se développer rapidement comme ils n'avaient pas fait jusque là : de sorte qu 'après une ou deux saisons il aurait été impossible de persuader leurs parents que leur restait encore quelque chose dans l'arrière-gorge. En effet, les granulations, très réduites, comme volume et comme quantité, ne les gênaient plus. Quoique les observations de végétations adenoïdes chez les adultes, et même chez les vieillards (Putrzeck en trouva chez un homme de 78 ans) soient loins d'être rares, les auteurs s'accordent, cependant, en admettant que, à l'âge de la puberté, c'est-à-dire à partir de 15 ans, les végétations subissent un processus d'involution, qui serait complet à 25. J'ai dit : involution. Mais d'après Arslan, Gradenigo et d'autres ce terme serait mal choisi, car il indiquerait une chose qui n'est pas. En effet, Arslan parle de regression, et Gradenigo de cicatrisation. Cela pour indiquer qu'il ne s'agit d'une guérison vraie, si bien d'une cicatrisation, qui laisse derrière elle des altérations anatomiques et fonctionnelles de la muqueuse, telles que irrégularité, sillonnements, stagnation des sécrétions, catarrhe etc. Delavan n'est pas moins explicite lorsqu'il admet que l'involution pure et simple des végétations adenoïdes, c'est à dire la regression de l'hypertrophie en laissant la muqueuse du rhino-pharynx dans un état normal, ou à peu-près, ne se fait pas; mais qu'il reste toujours un certain degré d'hypertrophie, ou bien l'atrophie complète de la muqueuse de la voute du pharynx très difficile à guérir, ou bien encore la maladie de Torn-waldt.

Je ne suis pas toujours si heureux pour pouvoir suivre tous mes malades pendant le temps nécessaire pour constater le résultat final d'un séjour prolongé sur notre littoral, car j'ai à faire, très souvent, avec des étrangers que l'on perd trop facilement de vue, mais d'après les amélio-rations si rapides que j'ai si souvent constatées soit dans leur état général que dans le local, et d'après ce que j'ai pu observer chez quelques malades que j'ai pu suivre assez longtemps, je me suis persuadé que l'involution pure et simple est possible, et que sur la Riviera, et encore dans d'autres localitées qui jouissent des mêmes conditions climatolo-giques que la Riviera, cette involution se fait en réalité, et, de plus, se fait précocement, c'est à dire même avant la puberté.

Cela, Messieurs, est dû, sans aucune doute, à la même cause qui fait que sur la Riviera les végétations adénoïdes sont, d'après mes observa-tions, si rares. Cette cause je la trouve dans le climat chaud et surtout sec de la Riviera et dans la grande luminosité de son atmosphère. Et si d'une part ces facteurs empêchent les indigènes de devenir adénoïdiens rien ne s'oppose à admettre aussi qu'ils doivent favoriser l'involution des végétations chez les adénoïdiens importés.

Il m'est nécessaire ici de rappeler les opinions les plus courantes sur l'étiologie des végétations adénoïdes et sur leur distribution géogra-phique.

Vous savez que les opinions à propos des moments étiologiques qui produisent ou favorisent l'éclosion des végétations adénoïdes sont très disparates. A côté de W. Meyer, De Roaldès, Morell Mackenzie, qui croient que les végétations sont plus fréquentes dans les climats froids que dans les chauds, on trouve d'autres, comme Trautmann, Arslan, Gradenigo, Fraenkel, Cuvillier, pour qui le climat n'entrerait nullement en ligne de compte. Ils reconnaissent respectivement comme causes des végétations soit la suppuration nasale, soit l'hérédité, la tuberculose, la syphilis; soit les infections, telles que la diphtérie, la scarlatine, la coqueluche, la rougéole; soit la scrophule, soit encore qu'ils les considèrent comme congénitales.

D'autres enfin, et parmi eux Delavan, dont l'opinion est partagée aussi par Mm. de Roaldès, et M. Mackenzie réconnaissent dans l'humi-dité du climat le facteur le plus important des végétations adénoïdes.

Je crois que cette dernière interprétation est encore la plus juste; et je le crois d'autant plus que, en analysant le peu de données que nous possédons sur la distribution géographique des végétations adénoïdes, j'ai remarqué que les pays où on les a signalées ont des climats humides par suite des conditions du sol, ou bien doivent leur humidité au voisinage et à l'influence du grand courant équatorial et du courant du Golfe, qui en est la continuation. L'humidité, plus encore que le froid, joue un rôle important dans l'étiologie des végétations adénoïdes, lesquelles dans un climat simplement froid, ou chaud et sec, se comportent bien autrement que dans un climat chaud et humide. Une autre preuve de ce que j'avance, je la trouve dans la distribution géographique des végétations adénoïdes en Italie. En effet, tandis qu'à San Remo, je les trouve très rares, Massei et Cozzolino les trouvent aussi également rares à Naples (0.01—0.5% sur les malades de la spécialité) ; De Rossi ne les trouve pas trop fréquentes à Rome (0, 8%), tandis que Poli, Corradi, Kruck, Gradenigo, Arslan, Ficano les ont trouvées très fréquentes, c'est à dire dans une proportion qui varie entre 5 et 8%, respectivement à Gênes, Verone, Milan, Turin, Padoue, Palerme.

On voit, donc, qu'aussi en Italie les V. A. sont distribuées d'une façon aussi différente que l'est la climatologie. Les pays de l'Italie, où les V. A. sont absolument rares, ou très peu fréquentes, jouissent d'un climat chaud et sec, tandis que les autres où elles abondent, ont un climat humide. En effet, d'après des données dont l'exactitude est garantie, à San Remo et sur la Riviera di Ponente l'humidité rélative atteint le maximum de 60 à 65° ; à Rome de 65° à 68°, tandis qu'à Venise elle varie entre 80°-84°, à Padoue entre 68°-70°. Nous avons donc en Italie des climats chauds et secs, comme celui de San Remo et de toute la Riviera di Levante, Naples etc. ; des climats chauds et peu secs, exemple Rome et Pise ; des climats décidemment humides, comme celui de Milan, de Venise, de Padoue, de la plaine du Po en général, de Catane, de Palerme etc. A chacun de ces climats corréspond une distribution différente des végétations adénoïdes. D'après cela, on comprend aisément que dans les pays où les V. A. pullulent on n'observe pas leur involution pure et simple, mais ces processus de cicatrisation qui sont aussi ennuyeux que la maladie même. Cela explique aussi pourquoi dans quelques endroits, où l'humidité rélative est, selon toute vraisemblance très élevée, on observe un si grand nombre d'adénoïdiens aussi parmi les adultes.

Pour comprendre l'influence que peut avoir le climat sur l'involution des V. A., il faut d'abord se poser la question, à savoir si les V. A. sont de leur nature, susceptibles de subir une involution pure et simple, après laquelle la muqueuse reste dans un état qui, s'il n'est pas tout à fait normal, il s'y avoisine de beaucoup, sans être, de toutes façons, si piteux comme beaucoup de nos confrères l'ont décrit, et comme ils l'ont observé à la suite de la regression des V. A. par la force de l'âge ? A cette question je crois pouvoir répondre affirmativement.

Je dois dire, d'abord, que je ne sais pas concevoir les V. A. que sous une seule et unique forme, laquelle, d'après les données anatomo-pathologiques que nous possédons la dessus, est très simple et n'admet pas,

par conséquence, des variétés. La classification des V. A. en scrophul-
euses, lymphadeniques, syphilitiques, tuberculeuses (Dansac et
Lermoyez), je la trouve bien artificielle. Dans ces cas il me parait bien
plus simple de parler de syphilis, de tuberculose pharyngienne, localisée
dans les follicules closes du rhino-pharynx, et d'appeler pseudo-
végétations la forme qui en résulte. Il est évident que pour ces formes
la question de climatologie reste tout-à-fait hors de cause.

En vous parlant de végétations adénoïdes je n'ai donc en vue que
cette unité clinique décrite par W. Meyer à laquelle, contrairement à
l'avis de M. Lermoyez je ne crois pas qu'il soit déjà nécessaire de faire
subir de révision.

L'anatomie pathologique des V. A. ainsi comprises, est des plus
simples : le nom en dit assez plus que la chose ne le mérite. Ici, comme
Mm. Gradenigo et Ménière l'ont proposé, un peu de revision serait
nécessaire, laquelle en faisant justice du terme de végétations adénoïdes,
et de l'autre, plus hyperbolique, de tumeurs adénoïdes, désignait le mal
avec une dénomination plus conforme à son essence. Au fond, il ne
s'agit d'autre chose que d'un tissu normal qui subit une hyperplasie.
Réduisons encore ce fait à sa dernière expression, et nous arriverons à
pouvoir dire que toute la question des V. A. se réduit à un déplacement
de leucocites.

Eh bien, Messieurs, qu'est-ce-qui s'oppose à admettre qu'un tissu
simplement hyperplastique puisse, sous des circonstances favorables,
après suppression de sa cause, reprendre son état normal ? Et
pourtant ça ne s'observe pas dans les pays où les végétations
abondent. Et pourquoi ? Parceque chez tous les adénoïdiens,
surtout sous l'influence du froid, de l'humidité, des brumes, des
brouillards, des refroidissements, et des maladies infectieuses qui
retentissent sur la gorge et sur les diathèses, il ne tarde à arriver
quelque chose qui vient gàter, compliquer, la constitution si simple des
V. A : j'ai nommé les *poussées d'adénoïdite*. L'hypertrophie du tissu
interfolliculaire (Hynitzsch), les petits foyers purulents (Hynitzsch,
Trautmann), les petits kystes, les épaississements de l'épithélium, l'inflammation active permanente de la muqueuse . . . toutes ces altérations
que beaucoup d'entre vous ont, tour au tour, signalées, sont, plus que la
suite nécessaire de l'hyperplasie du tissu adénoïdien normal, la conséquence de l'adénoïdite qui s'y jete, de temps à autre, dessus. Depuis
l'âge où les végétations commencent, jusqu'à l'âge de 20 ans, l'adénoïdite
a assez de temps pour accomplir ses ravages. Alors on comprend que
l'on n'observe pas d'involution, si bien cette regression ou cicatrisation
dont ci-dessus, avec ses conséquences.

Le climat de la Riviera, comme celui des autres localitées de l'Italie
où mes confrères voyent aussi peu d'adénoïdiens que moi, outre à ne
pas être favorable au développement de l'hyperplasie adénoïde, il ne
l'est pas non plus au développement de ces attaques répétées d'adénoï-

dite, qui doivent être si fréquentes dans le Nord. Par conséquent, les adénoïdiens sur la Riviera échappent presque constamment à l'adénoïdite: d'où une probabilité de plus que leurs végétations puissent y subir l'involution dans le sens strict du mot.

Il nous reste à voir de quelle façon ce climat peut agir sur les V. A J'ai déjà dit plus haut, qu'il agit par deux facteurs principales : sa sécheresse et sa luminosité, auxquelles il faut ajouter la température élevée et la pureté de l'air : ce qui forme un ensemble qui donne à ce climat sa physionomie toute caractéristique.

On comprend que dans les pays froids et humides, on reste trop exposé aux refroidissements, catarrhes, rhumes de cerveaux, tonsillites, bronchites, etc., et que les adénoïdites soient là aussi très fréquentes chez les adénoïdiens.

Mais aussi les pays où l'air est humide et chaud, ceux surtout qui doivent cet air au courant du Golfe (en Europe : pays côtiers du Golfe de Gascogne, du Nord-ouest de la France, des îles de la Grande Bretagne, et de la Norvége) ne sont pas mieux situés au point de vue des adénoïdiens. L'air chauffé et saturé de vapeurs du courant du Golfe rencontre, en arrivant à la côte, des courants d'air froid, s'y mêle, en donnant naissances aux pluies et aux brouillards. Ici l'air chaud et humide rend atoniques les muqueuses, diminue les forces digestives et nerveuses, d'où une sorte d'énervement et un manque de résistance aux causes nocives externes. Dans ces climats les adénoïdites sont aussi fréquentes comme le sont les végétations. J'ajouterai que dans les climats chauds et humides, l'excrétion de l'eau soit à travers la peau que les poumons est diminuée, ce qui fait que lorsque, chez des adénoïdiens arrivent de ces insuffisances rénales, même transitoires, dont la fréquence est signalée de jour en jour de plus, en résultent des états oedemateux de la muqueuse du rhino-pharynx, qui sont plus faits pour augmenter les V. A. existantes que pour en favoriser l'involution. Bien autrement se passent les choses dans les climats chauds et secs. Le séjour dans un air sec produit une augmentation dans l'excrétion cutanée et bronco-pulmonaire, et, par conséquent, une diminution dans les secrétions de la muqueuse du tractus respiratoire : ce qui établit déjà dans le rhino-pharynx une condition peu favorable pour l'hyperplasie adénoïde. Sous ce climat l'échange matériel est augmenté, l'activité des tissus stimulée, le dynamisme nerveux accru. Les enfants, porteurs de V. A., faibles, scrophuleux, s'y rélèvent physiquement.

La lumière s'ajoute à compléter les bienfaits de la chaleur et de la sécheresse de l'air. L'air, qui y est, pour cette raison, d'une grande limpidité, permet aux rayons ultra violets d'exercer toute leur action chimique sur notre organisme. La limpidité de l'air, laisse passer un très grand nombre de celles qu'on appela radiations *actiniques.* C'est cette puissance actinique qui, d'après Duclaux est la base des manifestations eutrophiques que la lumière exerce sur l'organisme vivant ; c'est elle qui favorise les échanges moléculaires à la surface du corps, et la régénération des ematies de la nappe sanguine énorme contenue dans les vaisseaux du derme (Guimbail). On comprend comment tout cela doit exercer une action extraordinairement favorable sur les organismes qui sont encore en train de se développer.—Messieurs, c'est la connaissance de ces faits qui peut nous permettre de comprendre aussi comment, les pays qui jouissent d'un climat si bienfaisant, ne sont pas des pays où les V. A. peuvent alligner. Le tout est contre elles. Pas de merveille, donc, qu'on y observe, chez les adénoïdiens importés cette involution pure et simple de l'hyperplasie adénoïde, sans residus facheux ; involution niée par presque tous les otologistes, pour la simple raison qu'ils ne sont pas ordinairement placés dans des conditions favorables pour l'observer.

Messieurs, l'opération des V.A. est, sans contredit, surtout lorsqu'on opère sous l'anéstésie générale, la plus simple de notre specialité, et la moins risqueuse. Cependant on a eu après cette opération, quelquefois des désagréments et des accidents, tels que hémorragies, angine lacunaire, processus infectieux accompagnés de fièvre, douleurs de tête, delire, etc. quelquefois, même, l'issue fatale. Avec tout ça, l'opération s'impose et tous sont d'accord sur la nécessité de l'imposer aux parents des petits malades, car, médicalement, il parait qu'il n'y a rien à faire. Les guérisons que Marage dit d'avoir obtenu en badigeonnant le tissu adénoïdien avec des solutions de resorcine au 50 et au 100%, n'ont pas été, malheureusement, confirmées par d'autres observateurs. Moi même j'ai commencé des essais de traitement par les badigeonnages avec la solution aqueuse-alcoolique d'acide arsénieux que Czerny proposa, il n'y a pas longtemps, contre le cancer epithélial. Les résultats ne me déplaisent pas, mais je ne vous en parle, pour ne pas me hâter à avancer des conclusions qui seraient encore trop hasardées. Au demeurant, l'opinion générale est, comme M. Chatellier la résume, qu'il faut se garder des traitements purement médicaux quels qu'ils soient, car ils font perdre un temps précieux sans aucun profit pour le malade.

Mais nous trouvons, trop souvent encore et surtout lorsqu'il s'agi, de malades qui viennent à notre consultation privée, des parents qui refusent net toute intervention sanglante sur leurs petits, ou qui, avant de l'accepter, ils veulent avoir de nous un tel tas d'assurances et de promesses que nous ne pouvons pas leur donner sans trop charger notre responsabilité.

Dans ces circonstances je me prends garde maintenant, d'avancer des prophéties qui peuvent être démenties par les faits, car je ne peux plus affirmer, d'une façon si absolue qu'autrefois, que hors de l'opération il n'y a point de salut. Moi je ne veux plus me prendre la responsabilité d'opérer ces malades presque par force, du moment que je sais que dans mon pays, ils peuvent guérir même sans opération. Ces malades là, je ne les abandonne plus " à leur triste sort," en disant aux parents qu'ils sont responsables des malheurs que l'avenir réserve à leurs enfants, mais je les soigne maintenant médicalement, avec l'un ou l'autre de ces remèdes déclarés absoluments inutiles, et j'obtiens, aidé par l'influence du climat ou, si vous voulez mieux, par le climat seul, quelques guérisons que l'on ne saurait pas espérer.

NASO-PHARYNGEAL ADENOIDS AS A CAUSATIVE FACTOR IN EAR DISEASES.

DR. ALLEN T. HAIGHT, Chicago.

Among the most interesting cases that come before the Otologist are those pertaining to post-nasal vegetations affecting the hearing, and there are few patients to whom more satisfaction can be rendered than to those so affected. Adenoid vegetations seem not to be restricted to countries, to climates, to sex, to colour, or race of man. Dr. William Meyer gives the results of his collected evidence of the existence of affections of adenoid growths in various parts of the world, and in various races of man. He says in Greenland in 60 Esquimaux children, between six and fourteen years of age, Helms only found 16 free from adenoid vegetations. In North Dakota of the United States, Quarry found adenoid vegetations frequently among the native tribes of Indians, but the growths were very little developed in adults. Cantley, of Hong Kong, reported that native Chinese of the Mongolian race, as also those belonging to the mixed Chinese-Portugese race, frequently suffered from them. While in Bangkok, Denietzer rarely found the disease among the native Siamese. Meyer concludes that adenoid vegetations are often to be found in varying degrees of frequency in at least three parts of the world, namely : Europe, America, and Asia. The Mongolian race is almost as much prejudiced as the Aryan. A cold climate seems more favourable to their development than a warm one. Arslan, of Padua, commenting upon the frequency of adenoid vegetations in Italy, states that of 300 children examined in the schools of Padua, he had found the growths present in two-thirds. He attributes the preponderating role to heredity, a number of his patients showing that their antecedents presented exactly the same symptoms. Balme, who collected statistics on the subject of adenoid growths, considered as a sign of degeneracy, in examining for adenoid vegetations backward and degenerate children at the Van Cluse Colony, found that of 113 children examined, 56 suffered from adenoid vegetations or enlarged tonsils, or most frequently from both lesions simultaneously. I agree with Meyer, Professor Stoker, Lennox Browne, and others, that post-nasal growths are just as common among the best classes of society as among the poorer.

Let us consider first what naso-pharyngeal vegetations are. They are an hypertrophy of the lymphoid tissue forming a mass situated in the vault of the pharynx bounded on either side by the orifice of the Eustachian tube, and presenting on its surface several vertical furrows which partially subdivide it. The structure covers the roof of the naso-pharynx back of the septum, and extends backward on the posterior wall, while prolongations are often met with in the fossæ of Rosenmüller and even in the orifices of the Eustachian tubes. Many writers have impressed me by the frequency with which they have found various forms of middle ear disease to depend upon morbid conditions of the naso-pharyngeal mucosa, and it is my opinion, based on several years' experience in the Illinois Charitable Eye and Ear Infirmary, and in private practice, that the main factor in producing both suppurative and non-suppurative inflammatory conditions of the tympanic and Eustachian mucous membranes, is the presence of naso-pharyngeal adenoids, or the condition of the post-nares subsequent to their removal or absorption. The naso-pharynx is an important cavity to the ear, by its relation from the nose through the Eustachian tube, and morbid conditions there readily exert an injurious influence upon the ear. Adenoid vegetations may produce inflammation of the middle ear (1) by constant irritation on account of the obstruction to the circulation of the blood by pressure; (2) by blocking the orifices of the Eustachian tubes partially or completely; (3) by their injurious effect upon the general economy of the child and particularly upon the nerves of special sense; (4) by leaving as a sequela a post-nasal catarrh which sooner or later establishes some form of middle ear disease.

Blake advocates the theory that the first stage of inflammation, hyperemia, is produced in the middle ear by an interference with the return circulation, owing to the pressure exercised by the adenoid mass upon the pharyngeal veins and those of the deep-seated tissue.

In children who suffer from adenoid vegetations the hearing is generally very sensibly impaired, and it is the common thing for a child so affected to have questions repeated often and in a louder tone of voice, to say nothing of earaches and discharge from the ears. In many cases the Eustachian tube is completely blocked by dry secretions in the posterior nares. I have observed diminution of power of hearing on the side where the adenoids existed. On the opposite side where the post-nasal space was clear the hearing was normal. I have seen cases where the hearing was seriously impaired, and the drum membranes normal in appearance, yet with safety I assume the faulty hearing to be dependent upon the growths in the naso-pharynx. Mr. Bosworth, I believe, agrees with me in this statement.

Mouth-breathing, the most prominent objective symptom of children affected with adenoids, I believe has an important etiological bearing on the subject. In this form of respiration the upper parts of the lungs are never normally expanded, a fact which can be readily demonstrated by observing a child with normal respiration, and one with the sucking respiration of mouth-breathers. The mouth-breather is usually found shallow through the upper part of the chest, and with very small lung capacity. The mouth-breather does not inhale sufficient air, the blood therefore is not sufficiently oxygenized, and is surcharged with carbonic acid. This excess of carbonic acid retained in the blood causes the lassitude, headache, stupidity, and sleepiness commonly met with in mouth-breathers, and gradually renders the nerves of special sense less active and responsive to stimuli. This excess of carbonic acid and lack of oxygen, I also believe to be the cause of the loss of appetite, malnutrition, and general cachexia, so often found accompanying mouth-breathing. We frequently meet with children affected with adenoids who are not mouth-breathers, and these children are plump, well-developed, and of healthy appearance, although they usually have some ear complication.

Lennox Browne found that not only were these growths present where the tonsils were not enlarged, but that in most cases of deafness, formerly considered due to enlarged tonsils, there was co-existence of adenoids, and that failure to cure deafness after tonsillotomy would be less frequent if the vault of the pharynx were always explored and cleared of additional lymphoid overgrowth. It was also probable that adenoids did not always disappear at an early age, and several cases are quoted in which they were present, and were the cause of deafness in patients over twenty-one years of age.

Alderton believes that disease of the naso-pharynx is directly causative of middle ear disease in from 35 to 88 per cent. of all cases. White states that out of 565 cases treated for naso-pharyngeal affections, he found disease of the middle ear in 197. Of the whole number, 134 had hypertrophy of the third tonsil, and of these 62, or 20 per cent., had impaired hearing. Bronner, before the British Medical Association, stated that upon examination of 250 school children, he found 8 per cent. suffering from adenoid vegetations. Eighty-five per cent. of 125 cases carefully examined showed symptoms of past and present affections of the middle ear. Laveand calls attention to cases in which adenoid vegetations produce total deafness in children. He considers that a cause of deaf-mutism, and says the removal of the vegetations may act as a cure.

A number of cases of post-nasal growths in the new-born have been reported, and Sendziak believes that many children develop adenoids in the first year of their lives, and frequently become deaf from this cause, and are not able to learn to speak, or forget what they know.

According to many authors it has been shown that adenoids are much more frequent among deaf-mutes than among other children. In my examination of 26 children for deaf-mutism, I found only 4 free from post-nasal adenoids ; 16 of those examined showed marked facial defor-mity from mouth breathing.

Frankenberger cites many authors who have investigated the frequency of adenoid vegetations in normal children : Meyer, 1 per cent. in 2,000 cases ; Schmiegelow, 5 per cent. in 581 examinations ; Wroblewski, 7 per cent. in 650 children ; Kafemann, 9 per cent.   This does not show a very large percentage, but when we arrive at the deaf-mutes, we find Lemcke reports 58 per cent.; Wroblewski, 57½ per cent.; Peissen, 58 per cent. ; Frankenberger, 59 per cent. ; Albrich, 73 per cent.

The principal function of the Eustachian tube is to supply air to the middle ear.   This equalizes the atmospheric pressure on the outer and the inner sides of the drumhead.   If the post-nasal cavity is blocked with the presence of adenoids, and we have a mechanical obstruction of the orifices of the Eustachian tube, either from the dried secretion or proliferation from the adenoids, the air supply to the middle ear is partially or completely cut off.   This inequality of atmospheric pressure causes a contraction of the drumhead, and such a condition will cause deafness to some extent, which will increase as the further pathological process develops ankylosis of the ossicles and atrophy of the tympanic membrane.

Wright Wilson reports 235 cases which he had treated for post-nasal vegetations.   He found the proportion of sex about equal.   Ten cases presented deafness as the only symptom.   Wilson points out the importance of exploring the naso-pharynx in every case of deafness.

Halbies found adenoids to be the cause of inflammatory process in the middle ear in 33 per cent. ; Meyer, 78.8 per cent. ; Hartmann, 74⅓ per cent. ; Ingals, 34 per cent.; Braislin, 58 per cent.   Max Schaeffer, of Bremen, reports a series of 1,000 cases of adenoid growths of the pharynx treated by himself.   Of these, 768 were treated surgically, 99 with the galvanic cautery, 81 by local applications, 52 were merely observed.   In 467 cases there was deafness, in 107 otorrhea ; 20 were improved, and 331 were cured.

I coincide with Harrison Allen, and Sisson, who hold the opinion that there are many children in homes for the feeble-minded and idiots all over the world who are affected with this disease, and who by a comparatively trifling operation could possibly be restored to use-fulness and their families.   Interference with the condition may or may not complicate the case.   Much depends on the relation of the Eustachian orifice to the vault of the pharynx.   If the orifice be situated high up, a comparatively small amount of growth will block it, and cause an auditory trouble ; but if it be low down, there may be extensive vegetations without the Eustachian tube being implicated. It would be superfluous to mention every analogous case reported of deaf-mutes who, after the removal of adenoid vegetations, gave evidence of hearing and began to speak some words.

The general belief that adenoid vegetations are never present after the thirteenth year is contradicted by Conetoux of Nantes who operated upon a man of sixty-five to cure a marked unilateral deafness. Adenoids are apt to become smaller and more dense as age advances, yet I have found vegetations in ages above sixty, and frequently between the ages of thirty and forty. They do not differ histologically from adenoids in children. It is not uncommon to observe these formations in the aged who are hard of hearing.

Notwithstanding all the writings of the last ten years, I cannot say that the pathological enlargement of the lymphoid tissue of the naso-pharynx has received sufficient attention in the world's medical text-books.

If the symptoms of these growths were more generally recognized by the family physician and their removal accomplished, we would not find so many chronic suppurative and non-suppurative inflammations of the middle ear with the history dating back to an attack of diphtheria, scarlet fever, measles, or other fevers.

I believe that these obnoxious growths are of great importance to the health of the child, not only in the present, but also the future development of all its faculties.

As to treatment, I would say, it is never too early nor is it too late. At the first recognition of existing growths, the operation should be performed at once, by whatever method is best suited to the case in hand. I do not believe in chemical cauterization or caustics, nor even the thermal cautery, especially in children as they require so many séances to accomplish a cure. I find that curetting is the only true basis of treatment, and worthy of consideration.   It may be done with Trautmann's, Hartmann's or Gottstein's curette; Meyer's ring knife, Löwenberg's forceps and various other modifications.   Such operations are recommended by Messrs. Hovell, Field, Lennox Browne, Politzer, Löwenberg, Trautmann, Bronner, Goldstein, Rousseaux, and many others. I am not a believer in general anæsthetics in children over the age of twelve years, as local anæsthesia after the age of twelve makes such an operation absolutely free from danger ; but there are some cases where a general anæsthetic must be administered, especially in refractory children and nervous adults. In children it is advisable to anæsthetize in a sitting posture. I prefer bromide of ethyl to any other of the numerous anæsthetics. It is easily administered, anæsthesia is quickly produced, and is of sufficient duration for the expert operator to remove both tonsils and adenoid vegetations, if necessary. The child recovers from the anæsthetic quickly enough to clear its throat and prevent strangulation from hæmorrhage. As it is common to find children suffering from adenoid vegetations to . be constitutionally affected, restorative tonics, nutritious food, and plenty of outdoor fresh air are indicated after the operation.

BIBLIOGRAPHY.

Meyer, Hospitals-tidende, Copenhagen, No. 3, 6, 7, 1895.

Bahne, Regis, Thèse de Bordeaux, 1895.

Arslan, La Médecine, 1895.

Laveand, La Semaine Médicale, 1890.

von Klein, Transactions of the International Medical Congress, Rome, 1894.

Bronner, British Medical Journal, 1889.

Lennox Browne, British Medical Journal, 1889.

Wright Wilson, Medical Press and Circular, 1890.

Ingals, Journal American Medical Association, vol. 23, 1894.

Alderton, Archives of Otology, vol. 20., 1894.

Kafemann, Revue mensuelle des Maladies de l' Enfance, 1892.

Max Schaeffer, Deutsche Mediz. Wochenschrift, 1892.

Coulloux, Revue Générale de clinique et de Thérapeutique, 1888.

O. Toole, Journal American Medical Association, vol. 30, 1898.

PROF. GRAZZI : Bobone ha detto nel principio della sua comunicazione che i bagni di mare sono dannosi per gli orecchi : ed è vero, come ha dimostrato con alcuni esperimenti Masini di Genova, ed un suo assistente, il Dott. Ugo Mariani, che pubblica un articolo intitolato "Influenza dei bagni di mare sulla funzione uditiva" nel mio Bollettino delle Malattie dell 'Orecchio (Gennaio, 1899). Ma non solo i bagni marini sono nocivi certe volte, ma anche i bagni caldi sono dannosi per l'orecchio come mi resulta da esperimenti che feci l'anno scorso e sto ripetendo quest'anno allo stabilimento climatico delle Prese. Dice le ragioni per le quali egli crede che il bagno caldo prolungato, anchè nei sani, spesso produce diminuzione dell' udito.

PROF. EEMAN recommande vivement l'anésthésie *générale* pour l'opération des végétations adénoïdes chez les enfants. Il y a recours dans tous les cas, et il ne se sert jamais que du Bromure d'Ethyle. Il estime que, si cette méthode n'est pas encore employée par tout le monde, c'est qu'on lui attribue des dangers. Ceux-ci peuvent être absolument écartés, si au lieu d'employer la dose de 8 à 10 grammes et plus, on ne donne jamais plus de 6 grammes, chez des enfants jusqu 'à l'àge de 10 à 12 ans. Chez des enfants plus jeunes, 3, 4 grammes suffisent. Il est nécessaire d'employer un produit absolument pur ; le Dr. Eeman emploie du Bromure d'Ethyle fourni par la maison Merck de Darmstadt dans des tubes scellés renfermant chacun 6 grammes.

DR. H. KNAPP uses ether in refractory children, but produces only an initial anæsthesia. When this is obtained, the operation can be begun and finished, however long it may last. It is not the pain but the fright that makes the child struggle, and this fright is over when the beginning of the operation is done without hurting the child.

PROF. GRADENIGO. Devo dire qualche parola intorno alla distri-
buzione geografica delle vegetazioni adenoidi.   Io non credo che si debba
attribuire grande valore alle statistiche su questo punto ; se tale
affezione è in genere segnalata raramente nella parte meridionale
d'Italia, lo è perche si tratta per lo più di forme non molto pronunciate,
che restano latenti se non si ricercano metodicamente.   Per mio conto
trovo in Torino una proporzione assai elevata di adenoidei : più che il 50%
dei malati di orecchio al dissotto dell'età di 15 anni.—Del resto Ficano,
Faraci e Garbini hanno segnalato anche in Sicilia il grande numero di
vegetazioni adenoidi.   Sono dispiacente di non esser d'accordo col
collega Bobone anche sull'influenza favorevole, per la involuzione della
tonsilla faringea ipertrofica, del clima della Riviera.   Per mia parte ho
visto l'affezione resistere alle cure generali e climatiche di tutti i generi ;
alla fine i malati, se hanno voluto guarire, hanno dovuto farsi operare.

THIRD MEETING.

CHAIRMAN   -   PROF. URBAN PRITCHARD.

The following reply from Sir Arthur Bigge to the telegram sent to H.M. the Queen, was read by the President :—

"To President, Otological Congress, Examination Hall, Victoria Embankment. The Queen desires me to convey to the Sixth International Otological Congress the thanks of Her Majesty for its congratulatory message received yesterday.—BIGGE."

GENERAL DISCUSSION ON INDICATIONS FOR OPENING THE MASTOID IN CHRONIC SUPPURATIVE OTITIS MEDIA.

OPENING ADDRESS BY
PROF. A. POLITZER, Vienna.

It was a good idea of the Committee of Organization of our Congress to put the present theme on the programme for our discussion. Indeed, no question of modern Otology has acquired an actual interest of such practical importance as the free opening of the middle ear in chronic suppuration.

For experience has definitely shown, that the free opening of the middle ear is of the most vital importance, and that by it we are often able to save the life of the patient, and to prevent other consequences of middle ear suppuration hurtful to the organism.

Some years ago the result of such a discussion would have been very doubtful; to-day, our experience of the result has been so much enlarged, that we are able to state with much more precision the indications for this operation.

The indications for the radical operation are generally acknowledged and in most of the well marked cases surgeons are likely to be in perfect agreement. Consequently there will be but little new to say in reference to the indications which are founded on marked objective and subjective symptoms.

The chief point in the present discussion will be to decide, whether in cases of chronic suppuration of the middle ear, without well marked symptoms it is justifiable to operate as frequently as has been maintained by some operators.

In order to gain a view of the object of the present discussion it is advisable to enumerate shortly the indications for the radical operation hitherto recognized, and I shall take the liberty of making some remarks based upon my own clinical experience.

As you know these indications are founded on the clinical picture which the objective and subjective symptoms taken together give us.

We shall see later, that certain objective symptoms alone, or certain subjective symptoms alone, are sufficient in themselves to call for the radical operation.   But generally in practice there is a combination of both which assists us in coming to a definite conclusion.

The objective symptoms which, according to my experience, indicate the radical operation, are the following :—

1.   Well marked caries of the walls of the tympanic cavity.

2.   Extensive proliferation of polypi and granulations in the tympanic cavity growing from the antrum and attic and recurring even after repeated removal.

3.   Carious fistulæ situated either in the posterior superior wall of the external auditory canal, or on the outer surface of the mastoid process.   In such cases there is usually caries of both the mastoid process and tympanic cavity, and sequestra and cholesteatoma are also frequently associated with this condition.

The fact, that such fistulæ may heal up spontaneously with or without exfoliation of a sequestrum must never influence the indication for the operation, because such carious and necrotic processes in the temporal bone, particularly in children and lasting for years, are not only deleterious to the general health, but may also be the cause of death by extending to vital organs.

4.   A pathological change, which I have found in nearly 50 per cent. of my operation cases, is the occurrence of cholesteatoma.

Cholesteatoma, as is well-known, may last for years latent, without any symptoms, till from some cause, for instance, water penetrating into the ear, or the use of a vapour-bath, the pathological micro-organisms contained in it become active, and provoke an inflammation in the temporal bone.   This not unfrequently leads to death from cerebral abscess, meningitis, or phlebitis of the sinus, as is shown by post-mortem examination.   According to my experience the prognosis in cases of cholesteatoma, in which the radical operation is performed on account of pyæmic symptoms is very unfavourable.

I would here remark, that there are cases in which the suppuration apparently ceases spontaneously or after treatment, and suddenly after an interval of weeks or months, headache and vertigo may occur with or without pain in the mastoid region.

In these cases, in which the radical operation is clearly indicated, cholesteatoma in the antrum and attic is often found to be the cause of the serious symptoms.

5.   The fifth indication is a hyperostotic stricture, or complete atresia of the external auditory canal, leading to retention of pus and formation of cholesteatomatous or cheeselike greasy deposits.

6.   Facial paresis or paralysis.   Although this is not always to be

considered as a symptom of caries of the Fallopian canal, still its occurrence is always to be looked upon as a very serious symptom, especially if combined with headache, vertigo, or other brain symptoms, it being not unfrequently the precursor of a carious necrotic process, passing over to the labyrinth and the cranial cavity, ending in death.

The indication for the radical operation is in such cases so much the stronger, as we know by experience, that after operative interference facial paresis or paralysis, if not of too long duration, may entirely disappear.

7. The seventh indication is a painful swelling over the mastoid process or the formation of an abscess. This may be due either to a complication of the chronic process with acute mastoiditis and fistulous perforation of the cortical surface of the mastoid process or to the presence of a cholesteatoma or sequestrum in the mastoid cells.

8th Indication. When there is an obstinate, long continued, septic, bad smelling discharge, which has resisted all forms of treatment, especially when the perforation of the drum is situated in the posterior superior quadrant, and the rest of the drum is adherent to the inner wall of the tympanic cavity. If in such cases a large quantity of purulent matter can be aspirated through the perforation by means of Siegle's speculum, there is probably a focus of suppuration in the attic or antrum, especially if there are crumby particles of epithelium, which no treatment except radical operation will cure.

9th Indication. If symptoms of commencing tuberculosis appear in cases of chronic suppuration, the operation has not only a favourable influence on the local affection, but also on the general health, as I have seen in several of my cases. On the other hand, if the suppuration begins in those who are already affected by phthisis, it is a strong contra-indication for the operation, which only—as far as my experience goes—tends to accelerate the fatal termination.

Among the objective symptoms, which indicate the necessity for the radical operation, must be mentioned fever with a high temperature preceded by shivering and rigor, or fever marked by sudden rising or falling of the temperature, which usually indicates septicæmia. This may be due to a phlebitis taking place in the sinus, or to an immediate absorption of septic material into the blood. Another important symptom, especially when combined with headache and other brain symptoms, is vomiting. These symptoms, although strong indications for the radical operation, must nevertheless be regarded as most serious for the prognosis.

Another objective symptom, which must never be overlooked, is the *state of the fundus of the eye.* Ernest Delstanche has shown, that in 50 per cent. of serious cases there were changes in the fundus of the eye, consisting in papillitis, retinitis optica, and congestion of the blood-vessels. I have also observed hemorrhages, thrombosis, and new formation of blood-vessels in the fundus oculi in cases, which have recovered after the operation.

The subjective symptoms, which accompany the suppurative processes in the temporal bone, and which, by their appearance, indicate the radical operation, are the following :—

1. Persistent or frequently recurring pains in the ear and in the mastoid region, headache, which may be either constant or recurring at short intervals. Particularly important is persistent and fixed pain in the parietal or occipital regions, which is increased by percussion, as this frequently points to temporal or cerebellar abscess.

2. Intermittent or permanent attacks of vertigo, which indicate sometimes an erosion of the horizontal semi-circular canal or an extension of the suppurative process to the labyrinth. The latter is probable, if there is total deafness in the affected ear, bone conduction is abolished, and Weber's experiment is localized in the opposite ear. Such cases demand the immediate performance of the radical operation, which should include the removal of the labyrinth, as recommended by Jansen, in order that the suppurative process should not extend through the meatus internus to the cranial cavity.

3. Well-marked brain symptoms such as headache, heaviness, and pressure in the head, drowsiness, torpor, loss of consciousness, etc.

Although any one of the above-mentioned symptoms under certain circumstances may necessitate the performance of the operation, so much the more will it be called for, if the objective signs be accompanied by any of the already mentioned serious subjective symptoms.

I may be here permitted to remark, that urgent symptoms of serious brain complications, such as extradural abscess, abscess of the brain, even after loss of consciousness, do not contra-indicate, but rather call for the immediate performance of the radical opening of the skull. I will not enter into a description of this important part of our discussion, considering that the distinguished pioneer of brain-surgery, Prof. Macewen, of Glasgow, will give us his very valuable experience on this subject.

I only wish to remark that cases with well marked symptoms of meningitis, which as you are aware, offer the least chances of a successful result of an operation, are not entirely hopeless. The operation should only be carried out, if the cerebrospinal fluid aspirated by means of the lumbar puncture does not show any signs of purulent infection. Quite recently I have had a favourable result after operation in a case of meningitis serosa, in which the symptoms of purulent meningitis were distinctly pathognomonic, but the previous lumbar puncture had shown the cerebrospinal fluid to be normal. Lucae has lately reported a similar successful case.

To sum up I wish to accentuate my opinion on the question under discussion, as to whether in chronic middle ear suppuration without marked symptoms it is right to have recourse so often to the radical operation in order to cure the discharge.

Experience teaches us that the clinical symptoms do not always correspond to the pathological changes found during the operation in the temporal bone. Sometimes only insignificant changes, such as a small quantity of granulation tissue in the attic or antrum, are found in cases where we have performed the operation on account of dangerous symptoms.

On the other hand we may find grave changes, cholesteatoma or sequestrum, where before the operation we should not have expected them.

These circumstances render it more difficult to draw strict lines in regard to the indications, and there will always be cases in which some surgeons, on account of the impossibility of predicting exactly the pathological changes in the temporal bone, will hold the opinion that it is not advisable to await the appearance of well marked symptoms, and will decide to operate at once, while other surgeons will advocate more conservative methods, from the fact, that in numerous cases they have succeeded in healing the discharge without operative interference.

That many cases of chronic suppuration of the middle ear can be healed by vigorous antiseptic treatment, by the removal of granulations or cholesteatoma in the tympanic cavity and the attic, by curetting and partial removal of the rough wall of the attic, has been shown by the daily experience of those surgeons who cure such cases by conservative methods.

Now although I am a strong advocate for the radical operation in suitable cases, I cannot agree with those surgeons who not only perform it when the above mentioned indications are present, but also often for the *mere purpose of curing the discharge*, at least until strenuous efforts have been made to stop it by other means.

I think, that in these cases it is not justifiable to have recourse to an operation, which although not necessarily dangerous in the hands of a skilled operator, is still a serious one, especially when we consider :—

1.   The many important structures in the vicinity which may be injured.

2.   The possible permanent impairment of hearing in those who before the operation could hear fairly well.

3.   The protracted healing process after the operation, which very often renders the patient "hors de combat" for many months.

4.   That in a considerable number of cases, in spite of the radical operation, the middle ear suppuration continues.

It is my firm belief that these views will in course of time receive general assent, when further anatomical researches and more extended clinical observations have cleared up those points, about which at present our judgment is still in doubt.

E

OPENING ADDRESS BY
PROF. MACEWEN, Glasgow.

MR. PRESIDENT AND GENTLEMEN,

I have to thank you for the honour you have conferred upon me by asking me to open a discussion on "The indications for opening the mastoid in Suppurative Otitis Media."

Instead of enumerating the individual indications for opening the mastoid, which may be found in more or less detail, in most recent Otological works, and which may require to be supplemented or reduced as our experience ripens, it is thought desirable to regard the subject from a broader basis, and one which may be found more generally applicable. The following forms a useful practical rule :—

When a pyogenic lesion exists in the middle ear, or in its adnexa, which is either not accessible, or which cannot be effectually eradicated through the external ear, the mastoid antrum and cells ought to be opened.

As there are many ways of opening the mastoid, some more, and many less complete, the observations made in this note cannot be equally applicable to all of them.

Some operators content themselves in "opening the mastoid" by sinking a narrow shaft into the antrum, through which they can inject fluid, and others perform a typical operation, irrespective of the pathological condition revealed.

The author does not follow the classical operations of Küster, Stacke, or Schwartze, but operates, by first opening the mastoid at the base of the supra-meatal triangle. From that point he follows the pathological lesions anteriorly into the middle ear, especially exposing and carefully scrutinizing in all cases the attic of the antrum and tympanum, when, if found eroded, these plates are removed, along with the morbid contents of the middle ear. He then passes backwards and downwards, through the mastoid cells toward the sigmoid sinus, following the pyogenic erosions wherever they may lead in that direction, and when necessary, exposing the knee of the sigmoid sinus. After opening the mastoid antrum and cells, the further procedure has a purely pathological basis : if the disease revealed be extensive, so must be the operation. The greater part of this operative procedure is performed by means of the rotatory bur, which is the safest instrument for such a purpose. One of the first objects of the operation is to secure the patient against subsequent pyogenic extension to the brain on the one hand, and the cerebellum and sinus on the other ; and this may be done with a probable certainty, as far as the two most frequent localities for brain and sigmoid sinus invasion are concerned. It is to such an operation (with its pathological basis), for "opening the mastoid" that the following remarks apply :—

The ablation of the mastoid, while at once eradicating a suppurative process, chiefly located in the mastoid antrum and cells, affords at the same time ready access to the attic and inner wall of the tympanic cavity, and to the auricular extremity of the Eustachian tube. Immediately following the operation, one can initiate the formation of a vascular tissue and thus create an efficient barrier against pyogenic extension to the otherwise most accessible and most vulnerable parts of the brain, the cerebellum and the sigmoid sinus.

In persistent otitis media purulenta, the mastoid operation has at least three advantages over that of the treatment by way of the external auditory meatus. First, by exposing to ocular inspection all the affected area, and by thus enabling the operator to follow and eradicate all the recesses in the bone made by pyogenic invasion. In this way, one does not act in the dark, as the whole pathological field is open to inspection. Secondly, by being able to secure asepsis, and Thirdly, by raising an efficient barrier against pyogenic extension between the most vulnerable parts of the brain and the sinus.

INDICATIONS FOR OPENING THE MASTOID IN PURULENT OTITIS MEDIA.

1. There are many cases of purulent discharge from the middle ear, of such long standing, and so intractable to all remedies administrable through the external auditory meatus, that most surgeons would agree that in such the mastoid ought to be opened. When the symptoms are obtrusive, the pain severe, the discomfort great, the discharge profuse, and possibly foul smelling, the patients themselves will demand relief, which the Otologist will readily grant. It is not, however, to such pronounced cases that special attention is here directed. It is rather to those in which the decision is much more difficult, especially in the presence of very slight discharge, continuous, though apparently subdued by treatment. Many believe that very slight, though persistent otorrhœa, can lead to no untoward result, the patient living a considerable number of years, possibly even a long life, with the discharge never properly away, and yet not sufficient to arrest attention. Its long duration causes the bearer of it to pay little attention to it, and by and by it may be disregarded and even forgotten.

The pyogenic process may however proceed inwards, giving rise to symptoms often misunderstood or attributed to other causes, and may eventually either prove fatal or, by undermining the constitution, thereby pave the way for the advent of other lesions. Many patients thus affected, though able to pursue their usual avocations, are yet subject to periods of malaise, with occasional recurrent slight febrile attacks:—irritability and nervous hypersensitiveness, exhibited in unevenness and irrascibility of temper, which attacks last from a few days to a week or more,—leaving the patient slightly weaker, though relieved from the depression, and fit to enjoy life. These attacks are so frequent, and the patient becomes so used to them, that he comes to regard them as part of his ordinary habit, and often attributes them, with considerable plausibility, and sometimes with point, to colds, chills, biliousness, indigestion, &c.

When they occur however in the presence of pyogenic otorrhœa of old standing, they may bear a different interpretation, and in the absence of other definitely assignable causes, they may be considered as the result of slight absorptions. In some cases the cause and effect are a little more evident, as when patients have pyogenic pulmonary catarrh, with organisms in the lung secretion similar to those found in the slight purulent otitis media, and when these pulmonary attacks are mainly coincident with the recrudescence of the otorrhœa. In some such slight cases, after every other assignable cause was exhausted, and after treatment in other directions had failed, the mastoid was opened, when, in the midst of eburnation and sclerosis of the bone, marked osseous erosions, containing small quantities of secretion filled with pyogenic organisms were found, and generally these led more or less directly to the sigmoid sinus, the coats of which bore evidence of long-standing irritation, and through which, no doubt, the pyogenic absorptions had taken place.

After the operation, these patients greatly improved in health, all their old general symptoms having disappeared along with the cessation of the otorrhœa.

Cases with a history of an initial period, somewhat similar to the above, have been seen at a later stage by the Author, coming under observation in a moribund condition from pneumonia, due to septic infarctions from thrombosis of the sigmoid sinus, originating in a purulent otitis media of old standing ; the passage between the cells and the sigmoid sinus being in some instances very small and tortuous, and not unlike those apertures seen in the cases with slight symptoms just referred to.

When it is recollected that in many instances the otitis media purulenta is obscure and overlooked, and that the symptoms of the purulent absorption may be of a "typhoid" as well as of a "pulmonary type," one can easily understand that death may be attributed to pneumonia or to enteric fever.

It is quite true, that with chronic otitis media purulenta, a fatal issue ensues only in a limited number of cases,—a proportion, however, perhaps greater than is generally believed—but as one cannot, with any data obtainable at present, foretell which of these apparently slightly affected patients are to become the victims of a fatal issue, ordinary prudence dictates its removal even while it is slight.

It cannot be too often recalled that the virulence of the otorrhœa cannot be measured by the quantity of the secretion, its odour, or the slightness of its initial symptoms, and that the pyogenic process may proceed insidiously until some slight exciting cause or accidental circumstance precipitates a dangerous or fatal crisis.

2. Another question arises, whether there be lesions in the middle ear, which, though it may be mechanically possible to remove them through the external auditory meatus, could yet be removed with greater safety through the mastoid. This must be answered affirmatively, while the middle ear and its adnexa are in a septic condition, and when by applications through the external auditory meatus, they cannot be made aseptic prior to the performance of an operation entailing the exposure of a fresh surface to the action of pyogenic organisms and their products. To operate through the external ear, under such conditions, is to court disaster. By opening the mastoid, one can efficiently remove therefrom the suppuration and can eradicate its cause, after which any operation involving exposure of a fresh surface can be proceeded with in safety.

In numerous instances, cases of intracranial pyogenic extension have occurred in immediate sequence to the removal by way of the external auditory meatus of granulation tissue masses—so called "aural polypi"—which were protruding into the middle ear. Some of these granulation masses protrude through the bone from the dura mater which they serve to protect, *as long as they remain intact*, but when they are removed, a fresh surface with open mouths of vessels is exposed and absorption through the softened brain membranes is apt to occur.

Besides rendering the operation safe by asepsis, the opening through the mastoid enables one to demonstrate the exact locality from which these granulation masses spring. This is difficult and sometimes impossible to do, by operating through the external auditory meatus. One must recollect that many of these granulation masses presenting at the upper and back part of the middle ear, protrude through eroded bone, and that their presence is to be regarded as indicative of a diseased process which has attacked the osseous tissues as well as the soft parts, and therefore to an extent these granulation masses are symptomatic, and by removing them alone, the disease is not removed, but only *one* of its indications.

As long as these masses are left *intact*, they may secrete, but they do not readily absorb, as they are destitute of lymphatics, and therefore in the midst of certain pyogenic organisms, not only may the granulation masses be left with safety, but they afford for the tissues from which they spring, a definite protection from the invasion of certain pyogenic organisms. They are a provision thrown out by Nature in an attempt at repair.

In the presence of such granulation masses, one does not devise an operation merely for their removal, but for the eradication of the disease, which has occasioned them. In removing them one has also to make provision that absorption will not take place through the wounded surface left thereby.

3.   In many, if not all of these persistent pyogenic otorrhœas the osseous tissue is involved, and it is very difficult, by means of treatment through the external auditory meatus, to eradicate the organisms that have housed themselves in the recesses of a minute particle of necrotic bone.   In the interior of such harbours of refuge, situated in the mastoid, the pyogenic and other organisms are safe from any antiseptic wave or blast introduced through the external ear, and wait—and they have endless patience, even beyond that of the aurist—until the antiseptic has exhausted its energies, when they again sally forth, in the tide of a catarrhal effusion, disseminating themselves and affecting fresh areas.   Erosion often steadily progresses within the mastoid cells, even when the middle ear has been rendered sweet.   In such cases the surgeon would be deceived were he to form an opinion on the asepticity of the mastoid cells, from the condition of the discharge issuing through an external ear which he has rendered aseptic by chemicals, as a slight pyogenic discharge issuing through such chemicals would probably be rendered aseptic in transit.

In other parts of the body where a necrotic bone filled with pyogenic organisms is even exposed to view and of easy access, it is extremely difficult, sometimes it is impossible, to entirely destroy these organisms by direct applications of antiseptics of such strengths as the neighbouring tissues would withstand without themselves being destroyed.   If this be so under such conditions, how much more difficult must it be by way of the external ear, to eradicate pyogenic organisms through hidden, narrow, tortuous, and sometimes almost inaccessible passages, which are often found in the mastoid process and cells.

4.   In recurrent cases of purulent otitis media, one cannot pronounce the patient safe, even when the otorrhœa ceases temporarily.

In one such instance, treated through the middle ear on the most approved principles, with great care, by an aurist of undoubted ability and experience, the patient who had had a slight pyogenic otorrhœa was pronounced cured by the aurist, the discharge having disappeared and the condition of the middle ear appearing to him in every way satisfactory.   Within about three weeks of this time the patient came under my observation, suffering from pronounced symptoms of cerebellar abscess, and was plunged in profound coma, accompanied with great respiratory difficulty.   He was operated on, two ounces of pus being removed from the cerebellum, after which he made a rapid recovery.

The middle ear contained only a few drops of pus, the mastoid antrum and cells contained more, and an erosion in the mastoid exposed the sigmoid sinus which was thickened, the disease having spread to the cerebellum by continuity of tissue.

With the data at the disposal of the aurist in this case, it would have been difficult for him to have acted otherwise than he did, and had he done so, it would have been at variance with the teaching of the day. This case, however, demonstrates that the information obtainable by inspection of the middle ear, is not sufficient to reveal the pyogenic invasion of the recesses of the mastoid region.

Had the case been treated by opening the mastoid in the way described, the formation of the abscess in the cerebellum would have been prevented.

5. Cholesteatoma and tubercular processes with secondary pyogenic involvement are also conditions for which the mastoid requires to be opened, as it is only in this way that these diseases can be efficiently removed.

6. The problems connected with the question of operation upon recurrent attacks of purulent otorrhœa are somewhat similar to those which arise in connection with appendicitis. Purulent otitis media and appendicitis have many analogies. They are both pyogenic, but while the latter is the result of the action of a well-known bacillus, whose course is definite, the former may be the result of one or other of a variety of organisms of greater or less virulency, and producing different pathological effects. Both are apt to invade neighbouring structures, the one the peritoneum, the other the intracranial tissues. Both are insidious in their action, and as long as they exist, they are apt to undermine the health, and reduce the vigour of the individual, both tending to precipitate a sudden, serious illness, and one which is often fatal. In both, an early and complete operation, not only at once relieves the patient from the depressing effects of the disease, but at once removes the possibility of a sudden and fatal termination. In both, many lulled into a sense of security by the apparent passivity of the disease and its long duration, and arguing from the fact that as the patients have recovered from one attack, they are equally likely to recover from another, postpone operation until the peritoneum in the the one case and the brain in the other become involved, and a fatal termination is imminent, and then it may be too late to save the patient.

7. With regard to the flora occurring in that perfect incubating chamber—the middle ear and its adnexa—and their relative pathological significance, the time at disposal prevents us dwelling at present further than to state that valuable indications may be derived from the identification of the particular form or forms of organism which may be present in such cases.

8. After what the author has elsewhere written, he presumes that it may be understood that the opening of the mastoid must always be undertaken as a preliminary step to operating upon those intracranial lesions originating in purulent otitis media—abscess of the brain, cerebellum and sigmoid sinus thrombosis. To operate upon the several

complications and to leave uneradicated the paths by which pyogenic organisms enter, is to render the patient's recovery doubtful, and to expose him to fresh attacks.

9. Syme is credited with saying that diseases of the ear were of two kinds, the one which is curable and is treated by the surgeon, the other which is incurable and is treated by the aurist. Whatever be the special province of the present day aurist or surgeon, let us hope that we relegate to neither, many cases of incurable disease.   The anatomy and pathology of the mastoid region were not understood in Syme's day, and the operation of opening the mastoid in its present conception was unknown.   As the subject which you, Mr. President, have arranged for this discussion is the indications for opening the mastoid in purulent otitis media, we are precluded from entering into the consideration of the results attending that operation.   The personal experience of the author leads him however to state that he regards the operation of opening the mastoid as the safest and most efficient way of eradicating otherwise persistent purulent otitis media.   In conclusion, he adds that the more the pathology of purulent otitis media is studied, the more frequent the complete ablation of the mastoid recesses is undertaken, the fewer will become the so-called incurable cases of "*ear disease.*"   He regards the operation of opening the mastoid as substantially contributing to the well-being of human comfort and happiness, and as materially lengthening life.

OPENING ADDRESS BY

DR. LUC, Paris.

Les indications pour l'ouverture de l'apophyse mastoïde, assez simples quand il s'agit d'une suppuration aiguë de l'oreille, puisqu'elles se résument alors dans l'ensemble des signes caractéristiques de la rétention purulente dans l'antre ou dans les cellules mastoïdiennes, sont au contraire nombreuses et variées, en cas d'otorrhée chronique. Ici également des phénomènes de rétention peuvent éclater, à un moment donné, après des mois et des années d'une suppuration, dont rien jusque là n'avait contrarié l'écoulement et qui, ne causant aucune douleur au malade, avait été plus ou moins négligée par lui. Mais ce n'est là qu'un point tout-à-fait limité de la question, et à cette première indication, qui était la seule connue, aux débuts de la chirurgie auriculaire, d'autres sont venues s'ajouter, depuis que les progrès de nos méthodes de diagnostic nous ont appris que, dans la majorité des cas, le caractère rebelle de bien des otorrhées résulte de lésions localisées dans les régions de l'oreille moyenne inaccessibles à nos moyens d'action par les voies naturelles : l'attique et l'antre. Et c'est ainsi que nous avons appris à ouvrir l'apophyse, non plus seulement pour assurer l'écoulement de pus retenu dans cette cavité, mais pour y atteindre les limites extrêmes du foyer suppuratif et tarir ainsi d'une façon radicale une suppuration autrement incurable. Nous tenons à rappeler ici que Schwartze (de Halle) Zaufal (de Prague) et Stacke (d'Erfurt) ont été les principaux promoteurs de ce mouvement qui s'est si largement généralisé depuis. Voilà donc un second ordre d'indications tout-à-fait distinct du premier, pour l'ouverture mastoïdienne.

Il en est un troisième. Les nombreuses tentatives d'ouverture crânienne faites dans ces dernières années pour enrayer les accidents d'infection intracrânienne si fréquents dans le cours des otorrhées ont effectivement conduit la plupart des chirurgiens auristes à la conviction, que l'antre représente la voie la plus sûre pour atteindre les foyers initiaux, soit de méningite, soit d'encéphalite, soit de thrombophlébite, d'origine otique, et que, par conséquent, son ouverture mérite d'être considérée comme le prélude ou la première étape devant précéder la recherche de l'un des foyers en question. Notre sujet se trouve donc de la sorte tout naturellement divisé en trois chapitres que nous allons aborder successivement.

I.—INDICATIONS DE L'OUVERTURE MASTOÏDIENNE DANS L'OTORRHÉE CHRONIQUE, EN CAS DE RÉTENTION PURULENTE.

Notre intention n'est pas de nous étendre longuement sur ce sujet, les indications de l'opération apparaissant ici avec une physionomie à peu près identique à celle qu'elles présentent dans les suppurations aiguës de l'oreille.

Il s'agit en somme d'un accident intercurrent, survenant le plus souvent inopinément, dans le cours d'une vieille otorrhée plus ou moins négligée jusque là. Généralement par le fait du développement exubérant de fongosités dans la caisse, et particulièrement au niveau de *l'aditus ad antrum*, le pus, qui s'était toujours facilement écoulé de l'antre dans la caisse et dans le conduit, éprouve un obstacle à son évacuation régulière, et le malade ressent pour la première fois dans l'oreille une douleur qu'il localise généralement à la base de l'apophyse. En même temps, la fièvre peut s'allumer, tandis que l'état général s'altère.

L'exploration de l'apophyse y révèle une sensibilité marquée à la pression, prédominant ou limitée le plus souvent à sa base, sauf dans les cas où son système lacunaire s'étend jusqu'à sa pointe, cette dernière région pouvant alors correspondre au siège du maximum d'endolorissement.

Lorsque l'antre est étroit, profond, et séparé de l'extérieur par une épaisse couche de tissu éburné, la rétention purulente dont il est le siège pourra n'avoir d'autre expression clinique que la coïncidence d'une otalgie plus ou moins intense, généralement accompagnée de sensibilité à la pression de la base de l'apophyse et d'un état fébrile persistant, avec un arrêt ou une diminution de l'otorrhée. Par conséquent la persistance et surtout l'accentuation de cet ensemble symptomatique, constituent une indication formelle à intervenir, après toutefois que l'on aura fait le nécessaire pour rétablir l'écoulement du pus, en procédant par exemple à l'extraction des polypes fongueux qui obstruent si souvent en pareil cas, soit le conduit, soit la profondeur de la caisse, dans la région de l'aditus.

La douleur, à elle seule, mérite, à notre sens, de décider l'intervention quand elle atteint un certain degré d'intensité, privant par exemple, le malade de tout sommeil. Différer en pareil cas l'opération dans l'attente d'autres symptômes tels que gonflement mastoïdien, œdème. . . . c'est s'exposer à voir apparaître à leur place, les signes de la transmission de l'infection à l'intérieur du crâne.

La symptomatologie de la rétention purulente intra-mastoïdienne, dans le cours de l'otorrhée chronique, n'est heureusement pas toujours aussi obscure ; bien souvent en effet la douleur et la sensibilité de la région apophysaire ne tardent pas à être suivies de l'apparition des signes locaux classiques de la "mastoïdite" disons plutôt: de la rétention mastoïdienne ; car il est bien établi aujourd'hui que la mastoïdite suppurée accompagne toute suppuration de l'oreille, et que les signes locaux en question (gonflement, œdème, rougeur de la peau) indiquent non la simple suppuration de l'antre, mais *l'emprisonnement du pus à son intérieur.* Toujours est-il que ces signes, révélant la marche naturelle du pus vers les parties molles extérieures, doivent être considérés comme favorables, et bienfaisants: favorables, en ce sens qu'ils impliquent habituellement des cavités mastoïdiennes superficiellement placées et écartent par là même la menace de l'irruption du pus vers l'endo-crâne ; bienfaisants, en ce sens qu'ils lèvent toute espèce de doute dans l'esprit des médecins les plus hésitants et les plus temporisateurs, à l'égard de la nécessité d'opérer sans retard.

Quelle doit être en pareil cas, la nature, ou plutôt quelle doit être l'étendue de l'intervention ?

Nous croyons pouvoir ériger en principe que, toutes les fois qu'il y a indication à ouvrir l'apophyse dans le cours d'une otorrhée chronique, qu'il s'agisse de phénomènes de rétention purulente, ou que l'on se propose d'y découvrir et d'y détruire les lésions entretenant la suppuration, l'ouverture opératoire et le curettage consécutifs doivent porter sur la totalité des cavités de l'oreille moyenne. Peu importe que l'on commence par l'antre pour atteindre de là l'attique, le long de l'aditus, à la façon de Zaufal, ou que, suivant la méthode de Stacke, l'on aille de l'attique à l'antre : encore une fois : toutes les cavités, tous les prolongements de l'oreille moyenne doivent être ouverts et curettés. Procéder autrement et se borner à l'ouverture de l'antre et des cellules mastoïdiennes, notamment dans le cas de rétention mastoïdienne, ce serait évidemment

courir au danger le plus pressant, mais ce serait exposer le malade à
la persistance de son otorrhée et à la reproduction, dans l'avenir, des
accidents que l'on vient de combattre.

II.—Indications de l'ouverture mastoïdienne visant à la cure radicale de l'otorrhée chronique.

Nous croyons pouvoir émettre ce principe, que *tout foyer suppuratif,
quelque invétéré qu'il soit, ne résiste pas au traitement chirurgical qui
réalise le triple résultat de découvrir puis de nettoyer et de drainer la
totalité de sa surface suppurante.*

Ce qui a longtemps justifié l'expression *d'otorrhée rebelle,* c'est que,
jusqu'à une époque encore peu éloignée, en dehors des accidents de
rétention purulente mastoïdienne, créant une indication urgente
d'ouvrir l'antre, toute la thérapeutique des suppurations auriculaires se
limitait à la région de la caisse accessible par le conduit. Or ce n'est là
qu'une minime partie des cavités de l'oreille moyenne. Au-dessus d'elle
est la logette des osselets, ou attique, dérobée à nos regards par le rebord
osseux qui résulte de la différence de niveau entre sa paroi supérieure et
celle du conduit auditif. En arrière d'elle, et sur un niveau un peu
supérieur à elle, est l'antre pétreux communiquant avec elle par un canal
étroit, l'aditus, et s'étendant plus ou moins loin vers la base de l'apophyse
mastoïde.

Prolongements, en haut et en arrière, de la caisse du tympan,
l'attique et l'antre sont le plus souvent solidaires de ses processus
pathologiques et notamment de ses suppurations. En outre, certains
détails de leur disposition anatomique les rendent tout particulièrement
favorables à la rétention purulente et à l'éternisation de la suppuration
à leur niveau.

Pour toutes deux cette particularité s'explique par leur situation,
qui les rend inaccessibles, par les voies naturelles, à nos regards et à nos
moyens d'action. Ajoutons, pour l'antre pétreux, que, descendant plus
ou moins bas dans l'apophyse, au dessous du niveau de l'aditus, qui est
son déversoir naturel, et se confondant même souvent, dans les cas
d'ostéite ancienne, avec les cellules mastoïdiennes en une vaste caverne
suppurante, qui s'étend jusqu'à la pointe de l'apophyse, il ne peut
évacuer son pus vers la caisse que par trop plein, circonstance favorable
au développement de lésions fongueuses, qui à leur tour, entretiendront
la suppuration, et ne disparaîtront que sous l'action de la curette. Pour
ce qui est de l'attique, il semblerait, au premier abord, que sa situation,
immédiatement au dessus de la caisse, se prête, on ne peut mieux, à
l'écoulement, vers cette dernière, du pus sécrété à son intérieur ; mais ici
le mécanisme de la rétention purulente est d'une nature spéciale : il se
trouve réalisé par la présence, au beau milieu de la cavité en question,
de la plus grande partie des osselets, maintenus dans leur position

respective par un appareil ligamenteux, compliqué, dont les mailles ne laissent circuler le pus qu'avec la plus grande difficulté ; à quoi il faut ajouter que, atteints, le plus souvent eux-mêmes, par le processus de l'ostéite fongueuse ambiante, les osselets contribuent activement à entretenir l'otorrhée.

Les considérations précédentes n'avaient pas échappé aux chirurgiens de cette école de Halle où, nous devons le reconnaître, a pris naissance la chirurgie auriculaire moderne, devenue si féconde, depuis, dans ses résultats.   Schwartze, le premier, tenta d'obtenir la guérison de certaines otorrhées rebelles, en pratiquant l'ouverture de l'antre, dans le but d'obtenir un contre-orifice pour l'écoulement des lavages pratiqués par le conduit.

D'autre part, un de ses élèves, Ludewig obtenait la guérison d'autres otorrhées chroniques par l'extraction du marteau et de l'enclume cariés. La route se trouvait ainsi ouverte dans la direction du traitement véritablement rationnel des formes les plus rebelles de l'otorrhée ; mais il était réservé à Stacke (d'Erfurt) de donner la solution complète du problème, en proposant une nouvelle méthode opératoire qui permettait de découvrir et de nettoyer, d'un seul coup, la totalité des cavités de l'oreille moyenne.

Stacke limita pourtant ses premières interventions à l'attique, mais bientôt l'expérience lui montra que l'intervention ainsi limitée échouait le plus souvent, les lésions rencontrées dans cette cavité existant presque toujours simultanément dans l'antre, et il arriva à cette conclusion, à laquelle nous avions été nous même conduit par notre propre expérience et que nous ne saurions trop élever ici en principe : que *l'antre mastoïdien, véritable prolongement postérieur de l'attique, dans la base du rocher, participe, dans la grande majorité des cas aux lésions suppuratives de ce dernier, et doit par conséquent être ouvert et curetté en même temps que lui, lorsqu'une tentative suffisamment prolongée de traitement local de l'otorrhée par le conduit auditif, a échoué.*

Nous nous trouvons donc naturellement amené à étudier l'ensemble des signes qui, dans le cours d'une otorrhée chronique, indiqueront que la cavité attico-antrale participe à la suppuration, si même elle n'en constitue la source unique ou principale, et que par conséquent une intervention chirurgicale s'impose, répondant au but précis de rendre accessible à l'action de la curette, puis au drainage une région qui naturellement échappe à nos moyens d'action, par le fait de sa situation anatomique.

Cliniquement l'otorrhée chronique, d'origine antro-mastoïdienne se présente sous deux aspects distincts, suivant qu'elle s'accompagne ou non d'une fistule.   Nous allons aborder successivement l'étude symptomatique de ces deux formes.

Dans la majorité des cas, la fistule mastoïdienne occupe la face externe de l'apophyse et, de préférence, sa base, mais on peut la rencontrer plus en arrière, ou au voisinage de sa pointe. Dans ces conditions rien n'est plus facile et en même temps plus instructif que l'exploration du trajet pathologique, à l'aide d'un stylet. On est, pour ainsi dire, alors, amené directement en contact de la lésion osseuse, et lorsque, l'instrument a pénétré dans la cavité antro-mastoïdienne, il fournit souvent des renseignements précieux sur sa situation et ses dimensions.

Mais la fistule mastoïdienne n'occupe pas toujours la face externe de l'apophyse. Elle peut affecter d'autres sièges, qu'il est d'autant plus important de connaître qu'ils sont plus insolites.

Mentionnons d'abord les cas, non précisément rares, où elle siège au niveau de la paroi postérieure du conduit auditif. Nous venons précisément d'en observer, cette année même, un remarquable exemple chez une dame diabétique, de notre clientèle, âgée d'une cinquantaine d'années, qui nous avait été adressée comme atteinte d'une otorrhée simple. Une première particularité frappa notre attention : l'insufflation d'air dans la caisse ne s'accompagnait pas de bruit de perforation ; d'autre part le fond du conduit était obstrué par une grosse fongosité implantée sur sa paroi postérieure. Après avoir extrait cette granulation, au moyen d'une curette, nous notâmes la parfaite intégrité du tympan, et, à la place de la fongosité, un orifice fistuleux d'où nous vîmes du pus s'échapper en abondance. Nous soupçonnâmes aussitôt une fistule mastoïdienne antérieure.

Dans ce cas, nous ne pûmes, en raison de l'étroitesse et de la direction oblique du trajet osseux, confirmer notre diagnostic par l'emploi du stylet, ni par le lavage explorateur au moyen de la canule de Hartmann, mais la lésion observée nous ayant paru suffisamment caractéristique pour nous permettre de proposer à la malade l'ouverture chirurgicale des cavités mastoïdiennes, nous eûmes, quelques jours après, l'occasion de vérifier l'exactitude de notre diagnostic. L'ouverture de l'apophyse nous la montra effectivement convertie en une vaste caverne suppurante d'où le pus ne s'échappait que par trop plein, à travers l'étroite perforation de sa paroi antérieure.

Déjà délicat, quand la perforation osseuse occupe cette situation, le diagnostic de la mastoïdite chronique devient tout à fait difficile, lorsque, consécutivement à une mastoïdite de Bézold devenue chronique, elle siège au niveau de la paroi interne de l'apophyse, le pus s'écoulant de là le long d'un trajet profond, sous-jacent au muscle sterno-cleido-mastoïdien, pour aboutir à un orifice cutané souvent fort éloigné de la région mastoïdienne, en sorte que la première idée que cette lésion éveille dans l'esprit est, qu'il s'agit là de l'orifice fistuleux d'un abcès froid cervical ganglionnaire.

Nous avons publié, au commencement de cette année dans les *Archives internationales d'otologie*, un remarquable et, croyons nous, un unique exemple de cette forme clinique observée par nous chez un jeune homme de vingt ans, qui était venu nous demander de le guérir d'un orifice fistuleux cervical, siégeant sur le côté droit, du cou, immédiatement en arrière du bord postérieur du muscle sterno-cleido-mastoïdien, à plus de six centimètres au dessous de la pointe mastoïdienne. Cette fistule persistait depuis quatre ans et était le seul vestige d'un phlegmon diffus du cou qui s'était developpé à la suite d'une suppuration aiguë de l'oreille. Lors de notre premier examen, nous constatâmes que le tympan était détruit, et que l'oreille suppurait encore faiblement. Cette coexistence d'une fistule cervicale avec une otorrhée ancienne nous mit sur la voie diagnostic, et notre soupçon se confirma à la suite de l'exploration du trajet à l'aide d'une sonde que nous pûmes faire pénétrer, de bas en haut, d'abord sous la masse charnue du muscle sterno-cleido-mastoïdien, puis jusqu'en dedans de l'apophyse. Le jeune homme guérit à la suite d'une longue et laborieuse intervention qui consista, d'une part, à ouvrir et à curetter la totalité des cavités de l'oreille moyenne, d'autre part, à ouvrir, sur toute sa longueur, le trajet fistuleux, de façon à la transformer en une gouttière profonde, enfin à réséquer la plus grande partie de l'apophyse mastoïde, de façon à atteindre les fongosités qui s'étaient développées en dedans de sa pointe, autour de la perforation de sa paroi interne.

Il nous reste à aborder maintenant l'étude des signes auxquels on pourra reconnaitre la deuxiéme catégorie des cas de mastoïdite chronique, ceux dans lesquels il n' existe pas de trajet fistuleux faisant communiquer plus ou moins directement le foyer mastoïdien avec l'extérieur.

C'est ici, qu'en dehors de tout accident de rétention, le diagnostic offre son maximum de difficultés. Aussi le terme de *mastoïdite latente* nous parait il convenir essentiellement à cette forme clinique.

Ici en effet, l'inspection et la palpation de la région mastoïdienne n'y révèlent absolument aucune particularité anormale: il n'y a ni fistule, ni rougeur de la peau, ni gonflement, ni sensibilité à la pression. Toute l'expression symtomatique de l'affection se borne à une otorrhée rebelle, dans le sens habituel du mot, c'est-à-dire résistant aux moyens thérapeutiques les plus variés appliqués par la voie du conduit auditif, y compris l'extraction des osselets.

Que nous apprend en pareil cas l'examen de la membrane tympanique? Nous la trouvons toujours perforée, cela va sans dire, mais ses perforations peuvent être généralement ramenées, à 3 types distincts, faciles à schématiser.

1° Il y a d'abord le type *perforation de Schrapnell* siégeant au dessus de la petite apophyse martellaire ;

2° puis le type *perforation circum-martellaire*, caractérisée par une vaste destruction tympanique, s'étendant tout autour du manche du marteau, qui pend au milieu d'elle. Souvent des végétations fongueuses occupant la région postérieure de la perforation, c'est à dire le voisinage de l'aditus, indiquent que c'est de ce côté que vient le pus, et les lavages pratiqués, dans cette direction, au moyen de la canule de Hartmann, confirment cette présomption, en provoquant l'expulsion de pus grumeleux et fétide.

3° Enfin le type *perforation postéro-supérieure*, caractérisé par une petite perte de substance de la membrane, siégeant dans la région de l'aditus. Cette perforation, de même que les précédentes, livre fréquemment aussi passage à de petites masses polypeuses, récidivant invariablement après toutes les tentatives d'extraction, et les lavages pratiqués à travers d'elle, au moyen de la canule de Hartmann, donnent les mêmes résultats que dans les cas précédents.

Indépendamment de ces végétations polypeuses, les divers types de perforation que nous venons de passer en revue permettent parfois d'apercevoir des masses blanchâtres, nacrées, qui ne sont autre chose que des agglomérations cholestéatomateuses, occupant la région attico-antrale. En pareil cas, la canule de Hartmann joue encore son rôle merveilleux, comme moyen de diagnostic, en expulsant ces produits pathologiques, si caractéristiques, et en les mettant directement sous les yeux de l'observateur.

Les diverses constatations otoscopiques que nous venons d'énumérer établissent donc une forte présomption en faveur du siège du foyer suppuratif, dans la région attico-antrale, surtout, si, en cas de vaste perforation tympanique, l'examen de la région inférieure de la caisse n'y révèle aucune lésion susceptible d'entretenir la suppuration.

Ce diagnostic entraîne-t-il d'emblée l'indication d'ouvrir l'apophyse et l'attique ? Ce n'est pas là notre pensée. Dans le cas, que nous avons supposé, d'une otorrhée chronique rebelle, mais non accompagnée de phénomènes de rétention, ni de menace de complication intra-crânienne, il n'existe aucune urgence à intervenir ; c'est donc un devoir rigoureux de ne recourir à la grande ouverture chirurgicale en question, qu'après avoir épuisé les moyens locaux rationnels, applicables par le conduit.

Au nombre de ces moyens, nous placerons en première ligne les lavages pratiqués à travers la perforation, dans la direction de l'attique et de l'aditus, au moyen de la canule de Hartmann, cet instrument si simple et qu'il nous faut vanter maintenant, comme moyen curatif, de même que nous l'avons loué tout à l'heure comme moyen de diagnostic. Effectivement ces lavages pratiqués régulièrement et suivis d'insufflation de poudres antiseptiques diverses, et de tamponnements pratiqués, aussi à fond que possible, donnent bien souvent la guérison, dans des cas que l'on serait tenté, au premier abord, de considérer comme n'étant justiciables que de l'ouverture chirurgicale.

Si ces moyens employés avec méthode et régularité pendant quelques semaines viennent à échouer, avant de recourir à la grande ouverture en question il est encore une tentative à laquelle il sera indiqué de recourir : nous voulons parler de l'extraction des osselets par les voies naturelles, surtout lorsqu'il s'agit d'une perforation de

Shrapnell, ou quand les osselets paraissent manifestement atteints par l'ostéite.

Cette opération devra être suivie d'un curettage aussi complet que possible de l'attique, au moyen de petites curettes recourbées en divers sens, puis la caisse sera tamponnée au moyen de mèches de gaze, que l'on s'appliquera à faire pénétrer jusque dans son étage supérieur.

Après quelques semaines de ce traitement consécutif, on sera fixé sur ses résultats : si la suppuration persiste, intarissable, avec ou sans reproduction de fongosités dans la région de l'aditus, si les injections pratiquées au moyen de la canule de Hartmann, en haut et en arrière, dans la direction de l'antre, continuent de provoquer l'expulsion de nouvelles quantités de pus, si surtout ce pus est fétide, chargé de grumeaux et de lamelles nacrées, il n'y a plus à hésiter : l'extraction des osselets n'a permis d'atteindre qu'une partie des lésions, et il reste un autre foyer à ouvrir et à nettoyer, mais celui-là ne peut être atteint qu'au prix d'une brèche opératoire, nécessitant une plaie extérieure : dès lors l'ouverture chirurgicale attico-mastoïdienne s'impose d'une façon absolue.

III.—INDICATIONS DE L'OUVERTURE MASTOÏDIENNE DANS L'OTORRHÉE CHRONIQUE, EN CAS DE MENACE DE COMPLICATION INTRA-CRÂNIENNE.

Nous venons de passer en revue deux catégories de faits, dans lesquels l'ouverture mastoïdienne se présentait comme une nécessité, mais avec un caractère très différemment pressant : pour les premiers, en effet, il s'agissait d'intervenir sans retard pour assurer l'écoulement du pus supposé retenu dans les cavités mastoïdiennes et du même coup, par la même occasion, de tarir le foyer suppuratif, en l'ouvrant et en le nettoyant dans toute son étendue : pour les seconds au contraire cette dernière tàche était la seule que l'on avait à remplir : on était en présence d'une otorrhée qui s'était montrée rebelle à tous les modes de traitement dirigés contre elle, par les voies naturelles : d'où la conclusion, que le foyer entretenant la suppuration était inabordable par ces voies et qu'il fallait l'attaquer par une voie artificielle. Mais là, nulle urgence à intervenir, l'opérateur pouvait prendre son temps et ne se décider à intervenir qu'après s'être assuré de l'inefficacité des autres moyens.

Nous avons maintenant à aborder une troisième catégorie de faits, dans laquelle l'urgence de l'intervention se présente plus impérieuse encore que dans la première ; car il ne s'agit plus seulement de rétablir un écoulement purulent qui se fait mal, et par là de mettre un terme à des douleurs plus ou moins vives, en même temps que l'on prémunit le malade contre le danger possible, d'une irruption du pus vers l'endo-cràne, il s'agit de combattre sans retard le danger réel d'un commence-ment d'infection méningo-encéphalique.

Avant d'entrer dans ce sujet, il est un symptôme se rapportant à une complication bien connue de l'évolution de l'otite moyenne suppurée chronique, dont nous croyons devoir nous occuper ici, au point de vue spécial des indications de l'ouverture mastoïdienne. Nous voulons parler de l'apparition d'une hémiplégie faciale, du côté de l'oreille malade. Il nous semble que nous sommes tous d'accord pour accorder à cette éventualité, dans les circonstances supposées, une gravité spéciale. Elle marque en effet une progression dans la marche du travail de-structeur de l'ostéite et il n'est pas rare de la voir suivie, de plus ou moins près, par l'explosion d'accidents d'infection intra-crânienne. Dans tous les cas, cet accident pouvant être la conséquence de la compression du nerf, soit par un séquestre, soit par des fongosités entassées dans la région de l'aditus, il est indiqué d'aller au secours du nerf en péril et de remédier à temps au danger d'une paralysie faciale définitive. Pour toutes ces raisons nous croyons devoir considérer l'apparition d'une hémiplégie faciale périphérique, du côté de l'oreille malade, dans le cours d'une otorrhée chronique, sinon comme une indication assez décisive pour déterminer à elle seule l'intervention, au moins comme un argument de nature à lever toute hésitation à l'égard de la nécessité d'opérer sans retard, dans le cas où l'ensemble des signes présentés par le malade paraîtrait déjà légitimer l'ouverture chirurgicale de l'oreille.

Simplement relative, en cas d'apparition de l'hémiplégie faciale, d'origine otique, dans le cours d'une otorrhée rebelle, l'urgence de l'ouverture mastoïdienne devient absolue, en présence de toute manifes-tation symptomatique, trahissant un commencement d'infection intra-crânienne, avec ou sans rétention purulente concomitante, l'écoulement régulier du pus antral par la caisse et le conduit n'empêchant aucunement l'ostéite fongueuse de poursuivre sa marche destructive et de mettre, à un moment donné, la face externe de la dure-mère en contact avec les germes infectieux du foyer auriculaire.

Nous ne croyons pas avoir à tracer ici un tableau symptomatique complet de l'infection intra-crânienne, d'origine auriculaire, qu'il s'agisse d'un début de méningite, d'encéphalite ou de thrombo-phlébite du sinus latéral. Il est de toute évidence que, lorsque l'ensemble symptomatique classique de l'une de ces complications se trouve réalisé, l'ouverture du crâne et la recherche du foyer intracrânien s'imposent sans retard, comme la seule ressource susceptible de sauver le malade.

Or, en pareille circonstance, même dans le cas de l'existence de certains symptômes, dits *symptômes de foyer*, tendant à faire admettre l'existence d'un foyer d'encéphalite plus ou moins éloigné du rocher, notre opinion (que nous savons d'ailleurs être aussi celle de la plupart de nos collègues en chirurgie auriculaire) est, qu'au lieu de baser le choix du siège de l'ouverture crânienne sur des considérations de localisation cérébrale, le plus sage est de précéder tout d'abord à l'ouverture antro-mastoïdienne, en poussant la résection osseuse jusqu'à la dénudation de la dure-mère de l'étage moyen du crâne, si l'on a plutôt des raisons de soupçonner une lésion du lobe sphénoïdal, tandis qu'on découvrira la dure-mère de l'étage postérieur et le sinus latéral, si les symptômes observés font plutôt songer à une lésion cérébelleuse ou à des accidents de phlébite du sinus.

Nous venons de supposer le cas d'une infection intra-crânienne confirmée ; mais, avant d'en arriver là, les malades passent souvent par une sorte de phase prémonitoire, dont il importe de bien connaître la signification, car, en procédant dès ce moment à l'ouverture mastoïdienne, l'on a grande chance d'enrayer les accidents par une désinfection limitée au foyer osseux, ou du moins ne dépassant pas la barrière représentée par la dure-mère.

Nous ne saurions donc trop insister sur la symptomatologie de cette période où le danger peut encore être conjuré par une opération simple et n'entraînant pas les conséquences graves de toutes celles qui dépassent les limites de la dure-mère.

Au premier rang de cette énumération symptomatique, nous placerons la douleur de tête, non plus localisée à profondeur de l'oreille, ni à la région mastoïdienne, mais se diffusant vers le front ou le vertex et affectant le caractère gravatif de la céphalée.   Souvent cette céphalée s'accompagne d'un certain degré de photophobie et le visage prend l'expression contractée, si particulière à la méningite initiale. D'autres symptômes peuvent s'ajouter aux précédents et en accentuer la signification, alors qu'il n'existe pourtant pas encore de méningo-encéphalite constituée, ainsi que le prouvera le résultat de l'ouverture mastoïdienne pratiquée dès cette période : c'est un état vertigineux empêchant le malade de se tenir debout et accompagné souvent de nausées ; ce sont des vomissements bilieux absolument analogues à ceux de la méningite confirmée ; c'est parfois une nuance d'inégalité pupillaire.   Enfin la température ne reste pas toujours normale à cette période, surtout si les accidents en question s'accompagnent de rétention purulente, ou s'il s'agit d'un commencement d'infection du sinus latéral, auquel cas la fièvre peut déjà présenter ses grandes oscillations thermiques si caractéristiques.

Encore une fois nous ne saurions trop insister sur l'urgence que crée, à l'égard de l'ouverture mastoïdenne, non pas l'apparition simultanée de tous les symptômes précédents, mais la constatation nette d'un seul d'entre eux.

En pareille circonstance, nous érigeons en principe, que *l'ouverture osseuse doit non seulement, comme dans tous les cas d'otorrhée chronique, porter sur toutes les cavités de l'oreille moyenne, mais qu'elle doit être poussée jusqu'à la dénudation de la dure-mère.*   Au reste, cette peine est le plus souvent épargnée à l'opérateur et, dans bien des cas, où il aura été déterminé à une intervention prompte par l'apparition de quelques unes des manifestations *méningitiformes* que nous venons d'énumérer, il trouvera l'explication des symptômes en question dans la constatation d'une perforation de l'une des parois profondes de la cavité attico-antrale, laissant la dure-mère dénudée et en contact direct avec le pus du foyer.

Le devoir de l'opérateur, dans les cas de ce genre est de pratiquer une désinfection minutieuse de la totalité des parois du foyer et notamment du territoire dénudé de la dure-mère, et de laisser la plaie opératoire suffisamment ouverte pour permettre une surveillance ultérieure des cavités osseuses opérées : mais, d'autre part, notre opinion ferme est *qu'il ne doit pas, dans cette première intervention, ouvrir la dure-mère :* car la simple désinfection extra-durale peut suffire et suffit souvent pour amener l'arrêt complet des accidents méningitiformes les plus inquiétants. Or ceux d'entre nous qui ont quelque expérience des interventions crâniennes savent assez combien varie le prognostic post-opératoire suivant que la dure-mère a été ouverte ou respectée !

Elle ne devra donc être ouverte que dans une seconde séance opératoire à laquelle on se décidera d'ailleurs sans hésitation et sans retard, si une surveillance de 24 heures, à la suite de la première opération, révèle une persistance et surtout une accentuation des symptômes d'infection intra-crânienne.

Si cette nécessité d'une opération plus profonde s'impose, elle se trouve singulièrement facilitée par la première qui a eu pour effet de mettre à découvert la région de la dure-mère, derrière laquelle se trouve le plus souvent, soit immédiatement à la surface de la pie-mère, soit à une très faible profondeur du tissu cérébral, le foyer cherché.

Dans ces conditions l'ouverture mastoïdienne aura donc marqué la première étape rationnelle de l'intervention intracrânienne ; elle aura servi à en justifier, puis à en simplifier l'exécution.

CONCLUSIONS.

A.—*L'ouverture mastoïdienne est indiquée dans le cours de l'otorrhée chronique dans trois circonstances distinctes :—*

1° dans le but de donner issue au pus, en cas de rétention purulente.

2° dans le but d'enrayer des accidents menaçants ou initiaux d'infection intracrânienne, d'origine auriculaire.

3° dans le but de tarir l'otorrhée, après qu'il a été reconnu que celle-ci s'est montrée rebelle aux divers modes de traitement local appliqués par le conduit auditif, y compris l'extraction des osselets et le curettage des fongosités accessibles par cette voie.

B.—*L'opération n'a caractère d'urgence que dans les deux premiers cas.*

C.—*Dans tous les cas d'otorrhée chronique, l'ouverture osseuse doit être étendue de l'antre à l'attique, ou de l'attique à l'antre et être suivie d'un curettage et d'une désinfection complets de la totalité des cavités de l'oreille moyenne.*

D.—*En cas de menace de complications intra-crâniennes, la brèche osseuse doit être poussée d'emblée jusqu'à la région suspecte de la dure-*

mère, qui ne sera franchie elle même, que dans une séance suivante, après un délai d'expectation armée aussi court que possible, si l'on voit persister et surtout s'accentuer la menace en question.

OPENING ADDRESS BY
DR. HERMAN KNAPP, New York.

MR. PRESIDENT AND GENTLEMEN,

When along with three others, I was asked to introduce by some remarks the discussion on the above subject, I hesitated to accept the honour, in the full conviction that, besides the gentlemen who shared it with me, there were many in this Convention that were much more competent than myself. Only the great, I may say enthusiastic, interest I take in the subject emboldened me to recommend to your consideration, some fragments of knowledge gleaned from reading, travel, and a limited personal experience.

In the presentation of the subject, I shall dwell less on the symptomatology of a given disease than on its pathogenesis, as determined by structural and etiological differences. I think it is in order not to consider the indications only at a certain period of the difficulty, but to point out how they change in its course, I mean we do not only want to be informed that under such conditions the mastoid should be opened, but also when, where, and how, in particular, how extensively it should be opened, the description of the mere technique of the operation however, lying outside the question.

Omitting the discussion of the generally known symptoms, such as pain becoming more acute on stoppage of the discharge, tenderness on pressure on the post-meatal pit and other parts of the mastoid, bulging of the posterior-upper portion of the drum-head, swelling, abscess, fistula of the mastoid, etc., I beg to call attention to the following four propositions :—

A.—*When acute purulent otitis media is on the border line of becoming chronic, or has just become chronic, opening of the mastoid is indicated both as a curative and a prophylactic measure.* I do not mean that every case of acute purulent otitis media, if the discharge does not stop in six weeks, should be operated on, but I would watch and treat those protracted cases carefully, for they are the ones that relapse readily, and come to be operated on later in life, after the infliction of a good deal of suffering and irreparable damage to hearing. *This applies particularly to children.* The indication for opening the mastoid is strengthened if tuberculosis, diabetes, syphilis or some other constitutional disease is present. Why do children contract otitis so readily, why is their recovery so much slower, and why are relapses in them so much more frequent than in adults? The first and second propositions may be explained by the frequency and virulence of the cause, the exanthemata, especially scarlet fever, but this does not account for the frequency of relapses. The latter, I think, is owing to the *structural conditions of the infantile mastoid*. The tympanum of the child is nearly the size of that of the adult, whereas the mastoid is diminutive, consisting of a small antrum cavity, surrounded by very little bony substance, which has the peculiarity of never being pneumatic, but cancellous (diploïc), almost compact, though soft and vascular. The discharge from the tympanic cavity readily drains off; the antrum and bone yield but little discharge, as there is but little mucous tissue to produce it. This *simulates* recovery, and the child is dismissed "cured." In the diminutive and very vascular interstices of the cancellous bone, germs and decaying material of diminished virulence may lie in small quantity quasi dormant without causing distress for months or years, but wake to life again when a new irritation, "a fresh cold," sets in. This need not lead to larger accumulations of pus (abscess), but is apt to produce molecular disintegration (Einschmelzung) of the bone.

I have noticed this condition typically in the compact mastoid of a man of about 48 years. He acquired an acute purulent otitis media, pain, bulging of posterior part of drum membrane, tenderness over the whole mastoid, increase of temperature. On paracentesis of drum membrane, discharge, improvement, simulating recovery in two or three weeks. Then relapse, tenderness less over antrum pit, more over tip and posterior border, discharge. I opened the mastoid at once. The bone was compact, no pus in the antrum, but a bead of pus here and there in the hard bone. Removing the beads did not lead to the discovery of fistulæ. The trace of the suppuration simply was lost. I chiselled away a considerable quantity of bone substance, but stopped when I found that the walls of the wound cavity though congested were otherwise normal. The patient soon recovered, but only temporarily. Subsequently he developed a post-occipital abscess under the deep cervical fascia which was split and drained by a counter-opening. He recovered permanently and with perfect hearing, only after the tip of the mastoid had been resected. The posterior cranial fossa having been exposed was found healthy.

This case demonstrated that the suppuration may leave the tympanic cavity, attic, and antrum, but extend into and beyond the tip of the mastoid. The pus cells in this case travelled through the condensed bone in passages so small that they could not be followed with the naked eye.

As to treatment of these conditions I am sure to speak the sense of the Congress in declaring that *the indications for operation in advanced cases of destructive, sub-acute, or chronic mastoiditis are absolute, and in the relapses of suppurative mastoiditis almost absolute.*

The prognosis in both cases is favourable. I have seen children recover that had a whole mastoid and a good deal of the adjacent temporal bone converted into gelatinous and lardaceous masses, and the dura extensively covered with soft, discoloured granulations.

What special indications may be derived from the well-known fact that in children mastoid operations are slowly recovered from and readily followed by relapses ?

First, let us try to find the reason for the slowness of healing in infants. When we operate on children, unless the vital indication be paramount, we endeavour to cause as little impairment of hearing as possible. I, for one, have been in the habit of cleaning out the interior of the mastoid of all the morbid, or even suspicious material that I could discover, but with a tendency not to interfere with the conductive and perceptive parts, avoiding especially damage to the intratympanic structures. As in most operations the wounds were rather deep, I did not immediately close, but tamponed them so as to be able to watch the course of healing. In most of them there was no particular disturbance, the wounds looked clean and filled up nicely, but there was *a small fistula at the bottom* into which a probe could be introduced one or two centimetres. Some of the cases required repeated scraping of the granulations, and also of bone which in the course of weeks or months had become brittle and soft. All cases, however, were cured. In some, the last period of the recovery was abridged by perforated silver-tubes introduced into the fistula, which were replaced by shorter and thinner ones, according as the fistulæ closed from the bottom. In the last cases I have tried to ascertain during the operation *where the fistula originated.* By cautious examination of the walls of the wound with the probe, I found that the yielding point was the antro-tympanic passage (the aditus ad antrum). With a delicate sharp spoon I enlarged the latter forward and upwards, carefully avoiding interference with the anvil on the one hand and the Fallopian canal on the other. The last case (in the Spring of this year), is still well in my memory. I succeeded in widening the aditus to 3 or 4 mm, without disturbing the anvil or the facial nerve. The recovery, by loose plugging, was smooth and shorter than in the previous cases.

The same treatment, as long as a radical tympano - mastoid operation is not indicated, refers to acute cases as well as chronic. In fact the best treatment of cases *which from the beginning show a predisposition to long duration,* for instance, otitis purulenta in tuberculous persons, is to perform the first opening of the mastoid, and conduct the subsequent local and constitutional treatment with the utmost care and perseverance, so as to *prevent the affection from becoming chronic.*

As particular requirements in such cases I would lay stress on :

1, *large, deep, and angular incision* of the drum head and the adjacent part of the posterior wall of the ear canal as soon as there is bulging; 2, *opening the mastoid and thorough removal of all diseased tissue;* 3, *enlarging the antral canal by cautious scooping;* 4, *watching the course of recovery, using dry treatment rather than syringing* ; *loose tamponing.*

B.—*In chronic suppurative otitis media, without symptoms of mastoid involvement, that has resisted topical treatment and intratympanic operations, attic-antrectomy is indicated.* In many cases it is difficult to determine the time when this should be done. During the last years intratympanic operations steadily have lost ground. Formerly they were extensively practised in non-suppurative otitis media to improve hearing and relieve distressing tinnitus. At present, as far as I have noticed, they are not completely abandoned, but waning, in chronic ear catarrh. In the same way the indications for their use in suppurative middle-ear disease have been curtailed in favour of tympano-mastoid operations. Many aural surgeons report good results from removal of the ossicles and cleansing the attic in cases of chronic otorrhœa with or without cerebral symptoms. I myself have witnessed a number of successful intratympanic operations in the practice of others, and have had some in my own, but unfortunately the good results in most of them have not proved permanent. Finding it difficult in many cases to remove the incus, and cleanse the attic thoroughly through the external ear canal, I have detached the integument from the posterior and upper walls of the meatus, and operated according to Stacke, which made the removal of the ossicles and the various portions of the walls of the attic easier and more efficient. The patients felt better, the discharge soon lost its odour and almost disappeared, but it was difficult in some cases to control the reappearance of small granulations and the swelling at the end of the detached skin.

In support of my standpoint, I may allude to a patient who had been treated long by intratympanic procedures, namely, scraping, and the use of the tympanal syringe, but received only temporary relief.

It was a lady, now 27 years old, who had had otorrhœa from her tenth year, when she came to me in 1893, with attic caries, showing the usual local and general symptoms. Local medical treatment, the tympanic syringe, removal of granulations and polypi improved her condition considerably, but failed to prevent occasional relapses. In October, 1896, intratympanic operation under ether :—enlarging a nipple-shaped perforation in Shrapnell's membrane, removal of a piece of carious anvil (no malleus found), and thorough scraping of the attic. She felt tolerably well the whole winter, but still had occasional headache and dizziness. In the fall of 1897, after a pretty good winter, she came again. The discharge, which had never completely stopped, was offensive, and she had had several attacks of intense occipital headache, and great dizziness. I made a *radical operation, penetrating from the mastoid into the tympanic cavity.* The lateral wall of the attic was removed, and the walls of attic and antrum thoroughly scraped. The ossicles were absent. No fistula or discoloured bone pointed toward extension of the suppuration into the cranial cavity. Perfect recovery. No relapse of inflammation. I saw the patient in June, 1899. The tympanic cavity was clean and evenly cutisized.*

Similar cases have determined me not to lose much time with intratympanic operations, though I would not go so far as an excellent otologist whose operations I had the privilege of witnessing lately, and who told me that he had practically abandoned them altogether. He said the removal of the anvil was a difficult and unsatisfactory task. Where the anvil was carious, the aditus and antrum always were so too. This is also the opinion of Stacke, who, if the probe detects caries at the anvil or in the aditus, at once makes a radical operation which he begins at the antrum, not as he did before from the aditus.

C.—*In chronic otitis media with evident symptoms of mastoid involvement, opening of the mastoid is indicated unquestionably and its extent is to be determined by the conditions ascertained before and during the operation.*

1. *Simple attic and mastoid caries.*

If the tympanic membrane is defective in its lower part, the handle of the malleus bare, the anterior part of Shrapnell's membrane thickened, the posterior part bulging, perhaps pouting, the probe discovers rough bone in the epitympanic recess and antral canal, may the antrum region be or not be painful to the touch, attic-antrectomy should be made without first trying other modes of treatment. If during the operation nothing but caries is found, all diseased bone should be removed by thorough scraping, and the wound may be plugged for a week or two, or closed immediately.

2. *Advanced caries with limited deposition of cheesy and cholesteatomatous masses.*

There is more pronounced tenderness and slight redness and swelling in the mastoid region. The posterior part of the attic and the adjacent part of the posterior wall are swollen, rough, uneven, and tender to the touch of the probe. Besides caries of the ossicles and the antral walls we frequently find cheesy and membranous masses in the epitympanic recess, the antrum and adjacent anterior wall of the mastoid, and the posterior wall of the ear canal. In these cases the removal of bone should be extensive, the lateral (outer) wall of the attic chiselled or broken off, and the osseous walls of the wound cavity evened and smoothed with a burr, the wound according to its extent may be entirely or partially closed with sutures, or healed with a permanent opening by a plastic

---

* Compare an article on Radical Tympano-Mastoid Operations, in Arch. of Otol., 1898. No. 2. p. 145.

operation, so as easily to detect and cure relapses. The latter are frequent in these cases.

3. *If the disintegration of bone goes beyond the antrum, attic-antrectomy and the removal of the anterior wall and the contents of the whole mastoid are indicated.*

The inner table, if intact, may be left as a protection of the dura mater. In these cases if there is only disintegration of the parts the wound may be partially closed with sutures, and if the healing be smooth, *i.e.*, without granulations and discharge, it may be allowed to close entirely. But if besides the disintegration of tissue there is degeneration—cholesteatoma—present, it is better to leave a permanent opening.

D.—IF THE DISEASE EXTENDS BEYOND THE MASTOID PROCESS, THE RADICAL TYMPANO-MASTOID OPERATION HAS TO BE FOLLOWED BY OPERATIONS ON THE AFFECTED PARTS OUTSIDE THE EAR.

1. *If the outer wall of the mastoid is perforated and an abscess or a fistula present* it is indicated to evacuate the abscess, seek the perforation, and, guided by it or the fistula, open the mastoid freely and remove all morbid material. This is better than to let the patient take the uncertain chances of a spontaneous recovery which rarely is complete and permanent.

2. If the medial wall of the tip of the mastoid is perforated (the so-called Bezold mastoiditis), and an *abscess* forms *on the side of the neck,* either *before* the sterno-cleido-mastoid muscle, or *behind it under the deep cervical fascia, the anterior table and the whole tip should be resected,* and all diseased bone on the inner table and the tegmen removed. The abscess cavity on the neck should be probed, and either *split* in its whole length *and plugged,* or *incised* at the deepest point, syringed *and drained.* I have seen good cures either way, the former leaving a deformity, the latter none.

W. MACEWEN* reports a good case :—a large abscess, under the deep cervical fascia, pointing in the upper third of the posterior cervical triangle, ten ounces of pus evacuated. The large cavity rapidly filled with granulation tissue and soon cicatrized.

If the pus burrows still deeper, for instance into the mediastinum, the assistance of a general surgeon is indicated.

3. *If in chronic purulent otitis media the anterior wall of the mastoid bulges*—which means a suppuration in the cells adjacent to the posterior wall of the ear canal—a *free incision down to the bone is indicated.* We then should explore the wall with a probe. or—as the skin is swollen and painful—wait a few days and see whether the mastoid should be opened from the outer surface or from the anterior. In two marked cases of this kind, I have had a permanent recovery from enlarging the perforation in the posterior wall of the bony meatus, and scraping the adjacent cells with a sharp spoon.

*Pyogenic Infective Diseases of the Brain Spinal Cord. 1893. Cas., LX., p. 287.

4. *If in chronic purulent otitis media pus extends from the ear into
the pharynx, forming a retropharyngeal abscess*, I would open the
mastoid, and expose the tympanic cavity and attic clear to the tympanic
orifice of the tube, and free it as far as possible from pus and disin-
tegrated tissue. Little is known about retropharyngeal abscess.
L. JACOBSON* says, "Retropharyngeal abscesses are infrequently
produced by suppuration of the middle ear with caries of the
temporal bone." W. MACEWEN† writes, "Purulent inflammation
in the tympanic cavity may extend into the Eustachian tube, in the
walls of which pus may form and ultimately produce gravitation
abscess in the naso-pharynx." O. KÖRNER‡ says : "Pharyngeal
lymphatic glands, in the course of mastoiditis, may suppurate, and
produce at the lateral wall of the pharynx, abscesses which have been
mistaken for gravitation abscesses from the ear along the tube." The
rule I expressed above, is derived from the condition of a fatal case from
my own practice.§ "The upper part of the tympanic cavity was full of
pus which collected along the semi-canalis pro tensore tympani, in the
tissues surrounding the tube, and formed a prominence in the upper
pharyngeal cavity. A probe, passed from the attic through the
collection of pus, could be felt with the finger introduced into the mouth.
I cut through the soft palate to the adjacent superior wall of the
pharynx, evacuating the collection of pus—an otitic retropharyngeal
abscess, connecting with the middle ear. Then I removed the tube with
its surroundings and could ascertain that the pus had not passed
through the tube itself, but through the tissue surrounding it, chiefly
the tensor canal."

5. *If the infection invades the posterior cranial fossa, the opening of
the mastoid and removal of its posterior wall is indicated.* This extension
of the disease is so important and so frequent that the removal of the
posterior wall, in particular that part of it which forms the sulcus of
the sigmoid sinus, has been recommended and practised by some
competent aurists in all cases. They support their opinion by the
experience that in a number of cases in which the outer aspect of the
posterior wall of the mastoid showed no trace of disease and the patient
had no symptom of intra-cranial trouble, nevertheless, epidural
abscess, perisinuitis, and thrombosis have been found when the posterior
cranial fossa was opened. If the posterior wall shows no flaw on the
closest search and the suppuration is limited, I have left the wall alone,
but when the contents of the mastoid have undergone extensive
molecular disintegration, I consider the exploratory partial exposure of
the sigmoid sinus and dura mater correct practice. That symptoms of
epidural or cerebellar abscess, perisinuitis, thrombosis, and pyemia,

---

*Text book. 2nd edition, 1898, p. 474.   †Pyogenic Infective Diseases, 1893, p. 84.
‡Die eitrigen Erkrankungen des Schläfenbeins, J. F. Bergmann, Wiesbaden, 1899, p. 30.
§Arch. of Otol., vol. xxiv., p. 128.

indicate the opening of the mastoid as the initial step to further procedures is self-evident.

6. *Similar indications result from the extension of the suppuration into the middle cranial fossa,* an occurrence less frequent than its extension into the posterior fossa. The symptoms are : offensive discharge, roughness and defects of bone felt with the probe, ossicles exposed or absent, dark spots and fistulæ in the tegmen, headache, vomiting, dizziness, rise of temperature, slow pulse in cerebral abscess, accelerated pulse in epidural abscess or meningitis. Sensory aphasia, optic neuritis and hemianopia are important symptoms in certain cases of abscess. A radical tympano-mastoid operation, with clean removal of the lateral wall, should be made as the initial step, then the upper wall of the tympanum carefully searched for black specks and defects in the bone, and if these are present, the roof of the tympanum should be removed, the dura mater exposed and examined the same way. It is the merit of KOERNER to have emphatically pronounced the fact that abscesses of the brain are situated near the perforation in the bone and dura. We know now where to seek and attack them.

7. *Extension of the suppuration in the petrous bone may indicate opening of the mastoid as an initial step for removing carious and necrosed portions of the petrous, or evacuating pus,* which passes *from the middle ear through the petrous bone*—fenestræ, vestibule, labyrinth, internal auditory meatus—*into the posterior cranial fossa,* producing epidural abscess on the posterior surface of the petrous bone. The symptoms are, besides those of purulent otitis media, caries in the medial wall of the tympanic cavity, complete deafness, headache, vomiting, dizziness, weakness of equilibration, fever, facial paralysis, etc. The beginning of meningitis is accompanied by aggravation of these symptoms, and stupor, excitement, convulsions. Meningitis in the first stage may be recovered from by opening of the mastoid, and middle and posterior cranial fossæ, exposing boldly the posterior surface of the petrous, and liberating the pus.

8 *Necrosis of different portions of the temporal bone indicates the opening of the mastoid in most cases.* It is rare that sequestra of the petrous or other portions of the temporal bone exfoliate spontaneously, and even then it will be judicious to open the mastoid and cleanse its interior from other dead or decaying masses.

From this long array of indications which the discussion no doubt will rather increase than diminish, it is evident that the opening of the mastoid in its recent development by the combined efforts of general and aural surgeons takes rank among the most important operations.

ZUR RADICALOPERATION
BEI CHRONISCHER PURULENTER MITTELOHRENTZÜNDUNG.
Paper by
PROF. LUCAE, Berlin.

MEINE HERREN,

Als Einleitung zu meinem Vortrage kann ich nicht genug hervorheben, dass ich auf die genannte Operation als ein ausserordentliches Heilmittel bei chronischen Mittelohreiterungen einen hohen Werth lege, zumal ich nur mit Hülfe der Operation bei einer grossen Zahl von Fällen die Heilung gesehen habe. Die folgenden Beobachtungen sollen nur dazu dienen, den *Missbrauch* der Operation möglichst einzuschränken.

In der unter meiner Direction stehenden Universitäts-Ohrenklinik in Berlin, sind vom April, 1881 (Gründung der stationären Klinik), bis August, 1899, *1935 operative Eröffnungen des proc. mastoideus* vorgenommen worden, 852 bei der acuten, und 1083 bei der chronischen Form der Eiterung. Bei oberflächlicher Betrachtung dieser Zahlen könnten diese, selbst was die chronischen Fälle betrifft, gross erscheinen, während der erfahrene Sachverständige mir zugeben wird, dass die Zahl der chronischen operirten Fälle im Verhältniss zu den acuten eine keineswegs grosse ist.

Es ist selbstverständlich, dass nur ein Bruchtheil aller operirten chronischen Fälle die sog. Radical-operation (Eröffnung aller Mittelohrräume) betrifft, welche allgemeiner überhaupt erst in den letzten Jahren ausgeübt worden ist. Um nun die Zahl der Radical-Operationen in den chronischen Fällen genauer zu würdigen, habe ich das procentualische Verhältniss der Operationen zur Summe der Ohreiterungen berechnet, und hierzu die letzten 4 Jahre ausgewählt. Es sind hierbei die in Preussen üblichen sog. Etats-Jahre von April bis April gemeint. Es geschah dies hauptsächlich darum, weil in diese Periode die seit 1895 von mir angewandte Behandlung mit Ausspritzungen von Formalin-Lösung fällt. Dieselbe hatte einen doppelten Vortheil, indem es mir gelang eine grössere Zahl von Fällen auch ohne Operationen zu heilen resp. zu bessern, andererseits wo das Mittel einen negativen Erfolg hatte, die Indication zur Operation genauer festzustellen. Es ergeben sich in dieser Zeit nun (von April bis April) :—

1. $18^{95}/_{96}$ in Summa 2061 Eiterungen des Mittelohrs, davon
   648 acute mit 86 Operationen = 11,72%.
   1413 chronische mit 118 Operationen = 8,35%.
2. $18^{96}/_{97}$ in Summa 1736, davon
   528 acute mit 66 Operationen = 12,5%.
   1208 chronische mit 85 Operationen = 7,03%.
3. $18^{97}/_{98}$ in Summa 1700, davon
   581 acute mit 69 Operationen = 11,87%.
   1119 chronische mit 69 Operationen = 6,16%.

4. $18^{98}/_{99}$ in Summa 1661, davon
    530 acute mit 61 Operationen = 11,51%.
    1131 chronische mit 90 Operationen = 7,95%.

In diesen Ergebnissen sei zunächst hervorgehoben, dass dabei die
Zahl aller neuen Ohrenkranken keineswegs abgenommen hat, sondern in
der Zeit von 1895-99 eine Zunahme von 6536 auf 6704 ergiebt.

Die Zahlen der Procente sprechen wohl für sich selbst laut genug
und zeigen, dass die Zahl der Operationen in den chronischen Fällen
gegenüber den acuten eine weit geringere ist; im Jahre $18^{97}/_{98}$ beträgt sie
sogar nur die Hälfte der Operationen in den acuten Fällen.

Ausserdem ist es von Interesse, wie klein der absolute Procentsatz
der Operationen in den chronischen Fällen überhaupt ist, und dass auch
die acuten Fälle verhältnissmässig wenig Operationen erforderten. Ein
statistischer Vergleich dieser vierjähriger Formalin-Periode mit den
früheren Jahrgängen würde keine sicheren Resultate ergeben, weil die
meisten chronischen Eiterungen in der Poliklinik (als " Out-patients ")
und nur wenige auf der stationären Klinik behandelt wurden, und, wie
es leider in jeder Poliklinik vorkommt, nicht regelmässig wiederkehrten.
Wir hatten jedoch den allgemeinen Eindruck, dass der Erfolg der
Formalinbehandlung ein grösserer war als die mit andern Mitteln
erzielten Resultate.

Ganz besonders hat sich die Formalin-Behandlung bewährt in allen
"kalten" ohne alle drohenden Symptome verlaufenden Fällen, wo nur
wegen foetider Beschaffenheit des Secretes der Verdacht auf ein tieferes
Ohrenleiden vorlag.

Die allgemeine Regel war, dass wo die durch 4-6 Wochen täglich
mehrmals sorgfältig vorgenommene Behandlung absolut keine Veränderung des Foetors bewirkte, die nachfolgende Operation stets schwerere
Erkrankung des Felsenbeins (Empyem, Caries, Cholesteatom) ergab.

Das Formalin hat den doppelten Vortheil, dass es nicht nur ausserordentlich desinficirend wirkt, sondern auch sehr billig ist. Die Stärke
der zu den Einspritzungen von mir angewandten Lösung ist 15-20
Tropfen auf 1 Liter abgekochten Wasser. Besondere und namentlich
andauernde Reizerscheinungen habe ich dabei niemals beobachtet.
Das einzig Unangenehme, namentlich bei furchtsamen Kindern ist,
dass das Mittel durch Abfliessen durch die Tuba Eustachii mitunter
vorübergehende Schmerzen im Pharynx hervorbringt, was sich jedoch
durch Gurgeln mit Wasser leicht beseitigen lässt. Eventuell kann man
in solchen Fällen bei der grossen Wirksamkeit des Formalins eine
schwächere Lösung wählen.

Gentlemen,—As I think in German, I have spoken in my native
tongue. But I now wish to say just a few words for those of our
British friends who do not understand German. I am of opinion that
the opening of the mastoid and of the tympanic cavity is a very important help in the treatment of chronic otorrhœa. But one may also

succeed in many cases without operating. I beg to add, that instead of being proud of saying, "I have operated on so many patients," one should be prouder of saying, "I have cured so. many patients without operating."

DISCUSSION.

PROF. GUYE said:—I had no intention of speaking on this question, but being asked to express my opinion by the President, as well as by Prof. Politzer, I will not refrain from giving it. I join in the opinion expressed by Profs. Lucae and Politzer, that one may often be proud of having cured a patient of chronic otorrhœa, without, as well as by operation. For my part I do not find in chronic otorrhœa, without any dangerous symptoms, sufficient indication for the mastoid operation. I will simply say, what in my opinion are three important points in the cure of chronic otorrhœa: (1) Keeping clean the meatus and tympanum by injections. (2) The application of antiseptics. The formaline recommended by Prof. Lucae, I have not yet used. I use the Carbolglycerine, introduced into aural practice by our regretted friend Bendelack Hewetson some ten or fifteen years ago. (3) I lay great stress on the care to be taken that air be freely blown through the tympanum. When the patient is not able to blow air through freely by the experiment of Valsalva, I make him Politzerise himself. I make him take a menthol insufflator and teach him to Politzerise himself by means of this instrument. After the air has passed through the tympanum, I make a second injection into the meatus to remove matter which has been blown through the tympanum—for this I generally use sublimate 1 in 1,000—and after all I introduce a long cotton wool tampon dipped in carbolglycerine. With this treatment I have seen patients for years keep in a very satisfactory state, and not present any indication for other treatment

DR. MOURE remarqua:—Les spécialistes sont en général assez divisés au point de vue des interventions à faire sur l'apophyse mastoïde, dans les cas aigus. Les uns veulent presque toujours appliquer le traitement médical, les autres au contraire le traitement chirurgical. Pour ma part je me rallie complètement à l'opinion des opérateurs, car j'estime que la mastoïdite aiguë peut être tout à fait comparée à l'ostéomyélite ; nous ne savons jamais dans quels cas l'affection guérira par les soins médicaux, et ceux au contraire dans lesquels surviendront une série d'accidents graves, capables d'emporter le malade. La raison en est dans la structure variable de l'apophyse, dont la corticale externe peut être épaisse et éburnée ou, au contraire, poreuse et facile à perforer. Dans le 1er cas, le pus a des tendances à perforer la table interne et à fuser dans la cavité crânienne. Dans la 2e il peut se faire jour à l'extérieur. L'opération bien réglée, étant sans aucun doute bénigne, il

y a des inconvénients graves, à s'abstenir lorsqu'elle est indiquée.—
J'estime que la persistance d'une suppuration abondante, et l'existence
de douleurs spontanées violentes, empêchant le sommeil sont des indications suffisantes pour ouvrir. Dans les cas chroniques, en dehors des
indications formulées par MM. les rapporteurs j'ajouterai qu'il faut
opérer les suppurations qui *semblent* guérir, mais qui reapparaissent peu
de jours après que l'on a cessé le traitement.

En résumé, j'estime que plus on intervient, plus on devient inter-
ventionniste.

DR. MCBRIDE understood Prof. Macewen to recommend
operations in cases of chronic middle ear suppuration with persistent
discharge, which continued to some extent in spite of treatment. He
desired to associate himself with the more conservative views of Profs.
Politzer, Lucae, and Guye. He submitted that even if Prof. Macewen's
proposals were right they were impracticable, because of the frequency
of chronic middle ear suppuration. He, however, excepting in special
cases, objected to so-called prophylactic operations. Time did not
permit him to give more reasons than the one which seemed most
cogent, viz., that we can never in chronic cases promise a cure. On the
other hand Dr. McBride was much in favour of operation in acute cases
which were just beginning to become chronic, because thus hearing was
generally saved and discharge stopped.

DR. JANSEN remarked :—There remains very little to be said
after the exhaustive publications of Politzer. There will be differences
of opinion in the difficult relations which are here under discussion that
cannot be set aside. In general we are on a firm basis. Naturally we
must operate if we have symptoms of threatening intracranial complications, and I believe I can prove that meningitis serosa was not
mentioned by the preceding speakers, furthermore, we must operate if
retention symptoms exist in the antrum or mastoid process, or both. I
missed the complete discussion of the same by Luc. These symptoms
are, however, of great practical value, associated with them are headache, profuse suppuration, depression of the posterior superior wall of
the auditory canal—labyrinthine symptoms. The depression or bulging
downward of the posterior superior wall of the auditory canal is
regarded as of great importance in this direction.

The differential diagnosis between suppuration in the antrum and
in the mastoid process is only of any value in cases without symptoms
of retention of pus.

One should not cling to the term, or name, "chronic middle-ear
suppuration" in speaking of the indications for radical operation.

We should locate the pus as nearly as possible, then we shall have
more definite indications. An empyema of the Eustachian tube
demands the radical operation ; a suppuration limited to the drum
cavity, on the contrary does not. Those limited to the region of the

drum of the ear or to the posterior part of the drum cavity require, even if of long duration, no other treatment than that *per vias naturales.*

Suppuration in the mastoid process is curable only by operation, and must be operated on for the reason that suppuration here always shows a tendency to increase, although the increase is sometimes slow. Suppuration limited to the antrum may occasionally heal spontaneously, especially where the antrum is small and lies high. Where the antrum lies deep and is of large capacity a cure will usually only be obtained by operation.

If the case is one in which the discharge of pus is small in amount and escapes easily, with sclerosis of the mastoid and but little swelling of the mucous membrane in the antrum, it is probably one unattended with danger and an operation is not necessary.

It is, therefore, necessary to have important guides to determine if the suppuration is only in the antrum or also in the mastoid process, or if it comes from a large antrum. I have here only in view those cases without visible signs of pus retention.

A suppuration, small in amount, but of constant flow without fetor, mucous in character, coming from above, without subjective symptoms, speaks for suppuration limited to the antrum with an unimpeded passage for the escape of the discharge. On the contrary, a discharge in which the flow is irregular or very offensive, points to suppuration in the mastoid.

If there is a feeling of pressure and fulness of the region behind the ear, of the occipital region, or of the top of the head, or if headache is added, the probability is greater that the location of the pus is in the mastoid process, and this too even in the absence of local tenderness, or it points at least to an increased distension within the antrum. We may be still more certain that the pus is located here if it is thick and lumpy in character, or is quite free from mucus, or very offensive.

At times it is certainly difficult, and occasionally impossible, to differentiate between the two.

The expression to operate early or late does not solve the difficulties of this question.

PROF. GRADENIGO.—Sono ancora io del parere che si esageri coll'operare nelle forme croniche semplici, e che molte volte un opportuno intervento dalla via del condotto è sufficiente per portare la guarigione.

Io ho avuto buoni risultati colla pinza osteotoma, che ora presento, di Faraci, colla quale, dopo estratti gli ossicini, si può aprire l'attico dalla via del condotto anche senza narcosi generale. Riguardo alla diagnosi, non ho avuto buoni risultati dalla transilluminazione nè dalla radioscopia, invece il metodo di ascoltazione binauricolare, metodo di Okuneff modificato da Ostino (Annales des maladies de l oreille etc. mars 1899) ha dato nella mia Clinica buoni risultati nelle endomastoiditi centrali. Con questo metodo si può confrontare contemporaneamente la transmissione del suono di un diapason vibrante al vertice dal lato leso e dal lato sano.

Desidero ancora accennare all'aggravamento che talvolta segue l'atto operativo sulla mastoide e sulla cavità timpanica per improvvisa l'esplosione di processi infettivi latenti; tali casi hanno grande importanza nella pratica privata.

Riguardo al significato della puntura lombare, io ho recentemente potuto conseguire con un atto operativo sull'osso temporale e su una raccolta ascessuale estradurale, la guarigione di due casi, nei quali la diagnosi di meningite purulenta potè esser confermata dai risultati della puntura lombare. (Archiv für Ohrenheilkunde, xlvii. 155.)

DR. NOYES remarked that for certain cases of chronic suppurative otitis media, a non-operative treatment will bring most satisfactory results. These cases may ensue after acute otitis media catarrhalis, or may result from scarlet fever, measles, etc; the method is the so-called dry treatment. To make it applicable we must exclude caries of bone, either of the ossicula or of the walls, also granulation tissue, tuberculosis, also syphilis, and perhaps some other cases in which the general health is much depreciated by anæmia, bad hygiene, etc. It is the so-called dry treatment, which some years ago was greatly in vogue, but which of late, since the days of antisepsis, has fallen into disrepute, for fear of propagating a simple middle ear suppuration into the antrum and the mastoid. I do not in any sense disparage the value in some cases of operative methods. But to employ this method is far more easy among patients of a public clinic than with those whom we have in private practice. It certainly is always a good rule to try first the mild methods before resorting to those of a more formidable character. Again, the character of the population among which one exercises his functions, must be borne in mind. For myself, I know that in private practice in New York City, measures will not be accepted which are employed in a public clinic there— and still more easily in a public clinic of Europe—as I know to my chagrin. Patients will quietly but steadfastly refuse operative measures, when local measures of another sort will meet with no objection. I therefore have come back with no little hesitation, after an interval of many years, to the old proceeding of packing the external auditory canal with powdered boric acid. Naturally there must not be any considerable secretion—no caries. The *modus operandi* is not to blow in a small quantity of powder, but to pack the canal two-thirds full. Use a common goose quill, squared at each end, dip it into a bottle of the powder and take up about half an inch, push this into the canal with a proper stick as one would load a gun from the muzzle. Pack the powder down firmly. If there be much secretion the fluid will dissolve the powder, and within two or three days it may need

G

renewal. But if the case has been happily chosen, a week will elapse with no discharge, and finally the mass of powder will come out in dry pellets. Should this treatment be of no avail within three weeks then one may insist on operative measures and will enjoy the advantage of having convinced the patient that nothing less serious will avail. This treatment is essentially antiseptic, because the tight packing excludes air and germs, and it has the great advantage of not demanding frequent syringing. I must protect myself against a possible accusation of being careless as to antisepsis, by noting that should there be any tenderness over the mastoid or its tip I would not resort to what I have recommended. But I put in a plea for a real antiseptic method by *packing* with boric acid as a prelude to the more important surgical methods. I do not hesitate about the latter in my own mind, but we have also to take into account the necessity of convincing the patient, and the avoidance of external scar. I make these remarks without premeditation, and have not gone into many details which would naturally suggest themselves as to diagnosis, irrigations and various kinds of local remedies.

PROF. KUEMMEL. In den gehaltenen Vorträgen ist kein Hinweis geschehen auf die hysterischen Phänomene, die intracranielle oder labyrinthäre Complicationen vortäuschen. Hysterische Personen können sogar Fieber, selbst Facialislähmung neben den genannten Symptomen simuliren, und Kümmel kennt eine Patientin, bei der vor mehreren Jahren die " Radicaloperation " bei chronischer Mittelohreiterung wegen solcher Symptome gemacht wurde, und bei der seither viermal Trepanationen des Schädels, zahllose Probepunctionen ins Gehirn, etc., gemacht sind, weil die Patientin immer wieder andere Aerzte aufsuchte und mit ihren Künsten hinter das Licht führte. Man soll deshalb auch bei den "Indications d'urgence " vorsichtig sein.

PROF. EEMAN est partisan enthousiaste de l'intervention opératoire large, mais il faut, pour qu'elle soit justifiée, que l'on ait épuisé d'abord les autres ressources ; il en est une qui parait un peu discréditée c'est l'extraction du marteau.

A la clinique de Gand, cette opération appliquée aux cas d'otite moyenne purulente chronique avec perforation de la membrane de Shrapnell, a donné 15% de guérisons, avec amélioration ou conservation de l'ouïe. Parmi ces cas, il s'en est trouvé qui pour d'autres observateurs auraient relevé immédiatement de l'opération radicale: rétrécissement du conduit, retention du pus, douleur, fièvre, symptômes cérébraux.   Un traitement palliatif a eu raison de ces accidents aïgus et ultérieurement l'extraction du marteau a amené une guérison radicale.

M. Eeman fait remarquer à ce propos que les résultats de son expérience clinique ne concordent pas avec les assertions de l'école de Halle. Il a trouvé très souvent la carie limitée à la tête du marteau, sans aucune lésion de l'enclume.

Dr. Brieger : Unter den Indicationen für die Radical-operation ist die Erfolglosigkeit früherer arzneilicher Localtherapie angeführt worden. Nach dem gegenwärtigen Stande unserer Kenntnisse wird man diese Indication auch bis zu einem gewissen Punkte anerkennen müssen. Indessen wäre es irrig, wenn man daraus den Schluss zöge, die Operation mache jede weitere Behandlung überflüssig. Im Gegentheil: bei der operativen Freilegung der Mittelohrräume können solche Alterationen der Schleimhaut, welche neben den operativ angegriffenen Knochenheerden bestehen, weitere Localtherapie nothwendig machen. Man kann durch deren Combination mit der postoperativen Behandlung hie und da die Nachbehandlung abkürzen. So empfiehlt sich z. B., besonders bei Prozessen, die sich durch lang dauernde Maceration der neugebildeten oder implantierten Epidermis auszeichnen, Tamponade mit Alkohol-getränkter Gaze. Auch Formalin eignet sich für diese Zwecke, ebenso wie die anderen Medicamenten, z. B. schwache alkoholische Silbernitratlösung—je nach der Natur der im speciellen Fall vorliegenden Processe.

Luc empfahl principiell die Ausräumung der Mittelohrräume. Wenn damit auch der Rat, bei der Radicaloperation regelmässig die Gehörknöchelchen zu entfernen, gegeben ist, so muss dem entgegengehalten werden, dass von anderer Seite im Interesse der Erhaltung der Function empfohlen worden ist, die Ossicula stehen zu lassen. Im Allgemeinen ist dieser Rat gegenstandslos, weil in solchen Fällen gewöhnlich die Continuität der Columella, insbesonders durch Destruction des langen Ambosschenkels, unterbrochen ist. Richtig ist, dass gelegentlich durch diese—technisch meist complicierte—Methodik die Function sich auffällig gut gestaltet. Anderseits aber kommt es vor, dass—nach völliger Ueberhäutung der Mittelohrräume—von cariösen Stellen des stehen gebliebenen Hammers fötide Secretion fortbesteht, die schon deswegen der Behandlung weniger zugänglich und damit zugleich auch bedenklicher ist, weil durch Verwachsungen etc. die räumlichen Verhältnisse in unberechenbarer Weise verändert werden. Jedenfalls müssen die Fälle, in denen man die Ossicula stehen lassen darf, sorgfältig ausgewählt werden.

Was die Contra-Indicationen gegen die Operation anbelangt, so möchte Dr. Brieger die Meningitis ausscheiden. Es giebt Fälle, in denen ausgeprägte meningeale Erscheinungen vorliegen, und doch nur eine circumscripte eitrige Exsudation besteht, die heilen kann, wenn der Nachschub neuer Infectionserreger von den Mittelohrräumen aus durch die Operation verhütet wird. Aber auch bei diffuser durch Lumbalpunction sicher gestellter eitriger Meningitis kann Heilung erreicht werden, wenn man einerseits durch die Radicaloperation den primären, infectiöses Material liefernden Heerd im Ohr ausschaltet, und anderseits durch die Lumbalpunction, in Folge der Abfuhr der im Cerebrospinalsack angesammelten Erreger, vielleicht auch in Folge der damit angeregten Production neu transsudierender, vielleicht bactericid wirksamer Lymphe günstige Bedingungen für die Heilung des meningitischen Processes schafft. Naturgemäss sind solche Erfolge bei ausgebreiteter Meningitis selten, aber doch immerhin so sicher, dass man angesichts der Unschädlichkeit der Operation in diesen verzweifelten Fällen, ihr Bestehen als absolute Contraindication gegen die Operation keineswegs anerkennen kann.

DR. BARR regretted that this discussion did not include the methods of operation and the results, especially the latter. The most interesting and important class of cases was that in which there was no symptom demanding immediate operation, but where there had been simple discharge for years, which it had not been possible to arrest by ordinary methods. Prof. Macewen's words of warning as to the danger of continuing the simple treatment too long, and postponing operation indefinitely, were calculated to be very useful in a Congress of Otologists. Dr. Barr placed great value on the treatment of the attic before the mastoid operation. The attic syringe, however, should be wide enough, not the thin bored tube which sends a stream of no mechanical force. To use these tubes efficiently it was often necessary to remove the malleus and incus, so as to allow of a wide clear opening, into which the tube of the syringe might be introduced, and a proper syringe attached. Dr. Barr had experienced excellent results from this mode of treatment, and generally carried it out as preliminary to the radical operation through the mastoid.

PROF. GUISEPPE FARACI: A quanto il Prof. Gradenigo ebbe la compiacenza di dire a proposito dell'utilità della mia pinza osteotoma aggiungo le seguenti considerazioni frutto della mia personale esperienza: Io ho trovato che nella maggior parte dei casi è bastata la rimozione dei grandi ossicini e la resezione della parete esterna dell'attico timpanico e dell'antro mastoideo, per guarire completamente la malattia; io credo quindi poco giustificato in questo caso aggredire la mastoide in tutti casi di suppurazione cronica dell'orecchio senza prima tentare l'operazione per il condotto uditivo. Nei casi di minaccia di complicazione endocranica, bisogna distinguere due casi;

1°. La complicazione è avvenuta? allora la natura del trattamento chirurgico dev'essere subordinato a quello della complicazione endocranica, in questi casi l'apertura della mastoide non rappresenta lo scopo principale dell'operazione ma una semplice parte di quest'ultima.

2°. Si tratta di semplice minaccia di complicazione endocranica? In questi casi basta la sola operazione dal condotto. Sul proposito cito il caso di una giovanetta che dopo un mese di suppurazione nell'orecchio destro fu presa da una meningite basilare con sintomi manifesti, specialmente nella sfera oculare. Ebbene, in questo caso è bastato la sola rimozione del martello e dell'incudine per arrestare la malattia e conseguire la guarigione.

Io vengo quindi alle seguenti conclusioni :

1°. Bisogna aprire la mastoide quando questa in tutta o in parte è invasa dal processo morboso.

2°. Quando tutti gli altri metodi di cura, compresa l'ablazione dei grandi ossicini, e la resezione della parete esterna dell'attico timpanico e dell'antro mastoideo sono riusciti infruttuosi.

3°. Nei casi manifesti di complicazioni endocraniche ed in questo caso bisogna far seguire quegli atti operativi che la complicazione endocranica richiede.

DR. SUAREZ DE MENDOZA : Dans son excellent rapport dont j'admets volontiers presque toutes les conclusions, notre savant confrère le Dr. Luc nous dit (chapitre 1er, par. 5). " La douleur à elle seule, mérite, à notre sens, de décider l'intervention quand elle atteint un certain degré d'intensité "—et plus loin dans le même chapitre, paragrafe 8, il dit : " Nous pouvons ériger en principe que, toutes les fois qu'il y a indication à ouvrir l'apophyse dans le cours d'une otorrhée chronique, qu'il s'agisse de phénomènes de retenfion purulente, ou que l'on se propose de détruire les lésions entretenant la suppuration, l'ouverture opératoire doit porter sur la totalité des cavités de l'oreille moyenne." " Peu importe," ajoute t'il, " qu'on aille de l'attique à l'antre, ou de l'antre à l'attique." Je crois, Messieurs, qu'en étant aussi exclusif, on s'exposera à faire quelquefois des délabrements inutils. Car dans un nombre de cas obscurs dans ceux où comme dit mon savant confrère, la douleur seulement fait décider l'intervention, et où la suppuration de la caisse est devenue nulle, ou presque nulle il arrive quelquefois de trouver la mastoïde saine ou presque saine, et que la douleur est produite par l'ébournement des cellules mastoïdiennes. Dans ces cas une simple trépanation (faite à la gouge ou mieux encore, à l'aide de la fraise des dentistes, mue par le moteur électrique, ou à son défaut par la machine de White, comme je l'ai conseillé il y a déjà 15 ans) suffit à faire cesser les accidents, et la guérison se fait alors en quelques semaines, au lieu de trainer quelques mois.

Je crois donc, que dans ces cas obscurs, où l'indication est née de l'élément de douleur, il faut être éclectique et commencer toujours par la trépanation classique pour pouvoir s'arrêter si la condensation du tissu osseux et le manque de suppuration et de bourgeonnements nous permet d'attribuer la douleur à la condensation du tissu osseux.

A propos de l'emploi des fraises dans la chirurgie de l'apophyse, et du sinus frontal et maxillaire, dont je ne saurais trop me louer, je vous demande la permission de vous faire connaître une petite pièce que j'ai fait ajouter à l'arbre flexible du moteur électrique que le commerce nous fournit. Cette petite pièce nous permet de mettre à contribution à très bon compte, les inombrables modèles de fraises, burins, brosses, dont disposent les dentistes, et qui deviennent extrêmement chers si on les fait fabriquer expressement pour notre usage.

DR. MILLIGAN said that in those cases of chronic suppurative middle ear disease which had resisted a prolonged and careful local treatment, and in which a definite focus of bone disease could be made out, operative interference was not only advisable, but was called for. By local treatment he meant the use of antiseptics, the removal of granulations and polypi, the removal of ossicles, and at times the removal of the outer attic wall. If under those circumstances purulency persisted, he thought that, in the light of our knowledge regarding its risks, a radical mastoid operation was the proper thing to do. In cases such as described, a perfectly fair inference, was that a focus of disease existed which the previous treatment had failed to reach. The opening up of the the mastoid in such cases he regarded as affording the only means of ascertaining the exact nature of the septic focus and the paths of pathogenic infection, and the importance of the information thus obtained could, he thought, not be overestimated. He wished to associate his views with the views of Prof. Macewen, that in cases of old standing suppuration which resisted the ordinary methods of local treatment, operative treatment should be undertaken.

In addition he would like to call attention to the great improvement which took place in the general health of the patient after operative interference and after the obliteration of the focus of sepsis.

MR. T. MARK HOVELL thought that the mastoid process should always be opened in cases of chronic suppurative inflammation of the middle ear, after a fair trial had been given to treatment by the meatus, but that the mere existence of a discharge for a long period was not a justification for the operation being immediately performed. In the case of a lady who came for an affection of the throat about ten years ago, her husband remarked that she had a discharge from one ear, which had existed for forty-three years. The discharge was treated in the usual manner with an antiseptic lotion and dry powdered boric acid, with the result that the discharge ceased in six weeks, and had not since returned. In the event of an operation being undertaken, it was best in all cases to open the mastoid antrum, for if the ossicula only were removed, another operation might have to be undertaken to remove septic matter lodged in that cavity.

DR. HOLMES said:—I take it, that in chronic suppurative otitis media, the surgeon will not operate until other means of treatment have been faithfully tried; unless the symptoms are such as to demand prompt operative interference.

As for the indications for opening the mastoid in chronic suppurative otitis media, I have in the past, and expect to continue, to practice along the lines indicated in the classical work of Prof. Wm. Macewen, which aside from some variation in technique is practically the same as I was taught by my honoured teacher, Prof. Schwartze, that is, *a radical operation*, which means removal of every particle of diseased tissue if possible. If this is done and the after treatment is carefully carried out then I fail to understand why Dr. McBride should take such an unfavourable view of the results following this operation.

When the attic is extensively diseased I believe that the antrum is always involved, and therefore, *in such cases* prefer to make the radical operation with positive results, in preference to obtaining uncertain results by removal of the hammer and anvil and curetting *by touch only*, such a delicate and irregular space as the tympanic cavity. By this I do not mean that the radical operation should be performed in all cases with attic disease, for where the symptoms point only towards a chronic inflammation of the mucous membrane or at most slight involvement of the ossicles, there I would operate through the external canal only; after explaining to the patient that the radical operation may have to follow should the disease be more extensive than existing symptoms indicate.

PROF. DENCH remarked that each case must be treated according to the local condition present. In certain cases ossiculectomy and thorough curettement of the tympanic vault will effect a perfect cure. When the mastoid is involved, a *complete mastoid operation* is imperative. If during the operation the surgeon finds that infection of the lateral sinus has taken place, or that there is either an extradural or cerebral abscess, he must not hesitate to deal with these conditions, so as to remove every source of infection.

In one of the speaker's cases, a second operation was necessary, owing to jugular involvement. The internal jugular with its branches was resected from a point just below the bulb to a point just below the clavicle. All vessels excised were divided between two ligatures. The patient made an excellent recovery.

In a second case of jugular involvement, the mastoid cells were healthy; resection of about two and a half inches of the vessel and its branches in the manner above described was followed by a perfect cure.

In certain cases of chronic suppuration of the middle ear, the "Stacke-Schwartze" operation is the best procedure. The speaker had operated on seventeen cases by this method. Of these cases, twelve had been entirely cured, while the remaining five had been greatly improved.

MR. CRESSWELL BABER thought that we were most of us agreed, that in chronic suppuration of the middle ear, accompanied by mastoid symptoms, the bone should be opened. The interesting point to consider, was whether the mastoid should be opened in cases of chronic suppurative otitis media without any symptoms, except the discharge. In those cases he thought, as a general rule, that first of all every means of arresting the discharge through the meatus (such as careful cleansing, curetting, removal of ossicles, etc.) should be tried, and if the purulent discharge from the tympanum still continued, the risks of pyogenic infection from this focus should be put before the patient or his friends, and the chances of an operation on the mastoid placing him in a safer position explained, although, of course, no certainty of a cure could be promised until the parts had been exposed by operation, and the full extent of the disease ascertained.

DR. HOLINGER said that while as a rule Otologists were all more or less conservative about mastoid operations, conservatism was absolutely out of place in cases where, in the course of a chronic suppuration, an acute attack on the base of influenza set in. Under these circumstances we should have to operate right away, and not lose time.

MR. DE SANTI remarked that as a general surgeon as well as an aural surgeon, he had had great opportunities of dealing with chronic suppurative otitis media.

He had taken special interest in the operation on the mastoid for chronic intractable otorrhœa, and was reading before the Congress a paper based on the results obtained by him in 1896-1897.

First of all, he would say that he entirely agreed with all that had been said by Prof. Macewen, who, in every sense, was a type of the highest form of scientific surgeon. Mr. de Santi could not understand those who advocated non-operative treatment in suitable cases. As a general surgeon it struck him as being against all principles of good surgery to let a discharge go on for an indefinite period from cavities so adjacent to the brain and big sinuses, as the tympanum and its adnexa.

In no other part of the body would a surgeon countenance such a course of neglect. It was obvious that *all* cases of chronic otorrhœa did not require operative treatment of the mastoid, but in selected cases operation gave in his hands excellent results.

In his paper he gave the history, etc., of eighteen patients suffering from otorrhœa of durations varying from six months to fifteen years. In all cases skilled treatment had been tried first, by the external meatus and Eustachian tubes. On these eighteen patients, twenty-six operations had been performed (some being operated on on both sides), and in only one case, out of eighteen patients, had the operation proved a failure. In all the others the cure was permanent, and in every way satisfactory. In no operation on the mastoid itself had he had a fatal result.

The conditions which he considered justified the operation were :—

1. Simple chronic purulent inflammation of the middle ear which has resisted prolonged treatment through the external meatus and Eustachian tubes.

2. The same condition when accompanied by the formation of granulations and polypi which recur after removal and in which carious bone is diagnosed.

3. Attic suppuration in which carious ossicles if present have been

removed and counter-drainage in the membrane made, and intra-tympanic syringing carried out but without success.

4. Cholesteatomata in the tympanum and mastoid antrum.

5. Constant pain in the mastoid pointing to sclerosis.

6. Great narrowing or closure of the external meatus from chronic inflammation, etc.

7. In cases with a sinus leading from the mastoid or deep external meatus.

MR. FAULDER WHITE thought that it would be a subject for regret if an impression were created that Otologists were against any treatment but operative. The object of the surgeon should be to arouse tissue vitality, and this could best be done by hot antiseptic irrigation; considering the size of the cavites concerned and the communicating spaces the external auditory meatus makes a fair means of entry. Treatment should be carried out by skilled hands, and good results would generally be obtained.

DR. LEDERMAN observed that after listening to the remarks of the previous speakers he had arrived at the conclusion that a conservative stand was a proper one to assume. A number of the gentlemen had stated that they attacked the mastoids of these cases in a radical manner, after treating the disease through the auditory canal for a certain length of time without stopping the discharge. Would the gentlemen who followed him be good enough to state more concisely what they presumed to be a reasonable length of time. He did not feel justified in opening every mastoid in which the suppuration did not cease immediately upon the application of local treatment.

They were all agreed that *prolonged* conservatism would prove disastrous in some of the more advanced cases, but this fact did not warrant the assumption that every case of running ear should be operated upon in a radical manner.

PROF. URBAN PRITCHARD said he was very sorry that the very valuable papers of Profs. Politzer and Macewen were not received in time to be printed, so that they could have been studied. On the subject of the discussion, he thoroughly agreed with Dr. Barr of Glasgow. In spite of the very great difference of opinion expressed, he should not be surprised if in an individual case, those apparently most opposed agreed.

DR. MACEWEN in reply, thanked the members of the Congress for the kindly reception and consideration they had given his paper. He had no intention of replying to all the points discussed, but would confine attention to two points. It had been said by one gentleman, that Dr. Macewen advocated opening the mastoid in every case of "simple otorrhœa." He (Dr. Macewen) did not use the term "simple otorrhœa," as he did not know what it meant. It had no pathological significance, but if it assumed that Dr. Macewen advocated opening the mastoid in every case of non-pyogenic otorrhœa, he had to say that such was not the case. Not even in pyogenic otorrhœa did he propose to open the mastoid "in every case." The statement was quite at variance with his practice, and he had never spoken or written to that effect. Reference to his paper would show his precise meaning. It was however, not only necessary to write carefully, it was equally necessary to read carefully what had been written.

It had been said that the mastoid operation was not followed by a cure of the purulent discharge. This depended on the particular part of the ear affected, and on the special kind and thoroughness of the operation adopted. If the disease were situated in the mastoid antrum and cells and these were ablated, one failed to understand how the disease could possibly longer exist. On the other hand, when disease existed in the inner ear or in the inner wall of the tympanic cavity, the mere removal of the mastoid antrum and cells would, of course, not remove the discharge, though the free access to the parts would aid in keeping it in check. In the latter kind of cases the ablation of the inner ear—a much more serious operation, and one requiring to be performed in two stages, the latter after the parts had been rendered aseptic—might be required. It was by this route that pyogenic meningitis so often gained entrance and therefore it required to be very thoroughly looked to.

DR. LUC, in replying, protested against Prof. Guye's opinion that simple otorrhœa, not connected with serious symptoms, was no sufficient reason for opening the antrum, as the first appearance of a *serious symptom* might prove fatal to the patient.

DR. KNAPP replied as follows:—I wanted to say a word on your own remarks, Mr. President. The operation which we call radical, means to stamp out all disease in the temporal bone that we can discover at the time. We have, of course, to depend on our senses, and may not be able to detect all foci of disease. The result will be a relapse, which has to be dealt with later. With the earnest endeavour to be thorough (radical), we must preserve all tissue that appears sound to our means of diagnosis. This refers particularly to cases of cholesteatoma, which feel well some years after the first operation, the same after a second and third operation, but they will ultimately be cured permanently. We do the best we can with such almost desperate cases. We have of two evils to choose the least, which in the present case is to operate, if necessary several times—to ward off death.

FOURTH MEETING.

WEDNESDAY, AUGUST 9TH, AT 3 P.M.

CHAIRMAN   -   -   -   -   PROF. A. POLITZER.

DIE ANATOMIE DES SINUS FRONTALIS, UND DER VORDEREN
SIEBBEINZELLEN. MIT PROJEKTION.

DR. ARTHUR HARTMANN, Berlin.

Indem ich suchte die sehr verwickelten Formen des Sinus frontalis,
und der vorderen Siebbeinzellen in Einklang zu bringen mit den
Resultaten der embryologischen Forschung, gelang es mir ein sehr
klares und einfaches Bild der verschiedenen Formen zu gewinnen.
Beim Embryo beginnt die Gliederung der Oberfläche der äusseren
Wand der Nasenhöhle mit dem Auftreten verschiedener Furchen der
späteren Nasengänge, welche Wülste zwischen sich lassen, die späteren
Nasenmuscheln. Nach Zuckerkandl sind es 4 solche Furchen, während
nach Killian, dessen Darstellung ich hauptsächlich folge, 6 von ihm
sogenannte Hauptfurchen bestehen. Einzelne der Hauptfurchen versch-
melzen mit einander, so dass in der Regel später nur 3 zur Beobachtung
kommen. Die unteren Hauptfurchen haben im vorderen und hinteren
Teil eine knieförmige Biegung—Ramus ascendens und Ramus descendens.
An dem oberen Ende des Ramus ascendens bildet sich eine sackartige
Bucht der Recessus frontalis,—die Stirnbucht. Aus dieser entwickelt
sich die Stirnhöhle, indem sich die Ausbuchtung zwischen die Tafeln des
Stirnbeins vorschiebt. Auf der lateralen Fläche der Stirnbucht treten
3 kleinere Furchen auf—Nebenfurchen, gleichfalls mit zwischenliegenden
Wülsten. Aus diesen entstehen die vorderen Siebbeinzellen, die Cellulæ
frontales, so dass wir in der Regel 3 solche Zellen finden.

Die Stirnhöhle kann entstehen, nicht nur durch die Ausbuchtung
und das Vorschieben des Recessus frontalis zwischen die Tafeln des
Stirnbeins, sondern auch durch das Vorschieben einer Frontalzelle, was
Killian als indirekte Bildung der Stirnhöhle bezeichnet.

An einer grösseren Anzahl von photographischen Aufnahmen
anatomischer Präparate erlaube ich mir Ihnen die verschiedenen Formen
der Anordnung der Zellen und der Stirnhöhle zu zeigen.

1. Präparate von Stirnhöhle ohne Frontalzellen.

a). Mit freier Oeffnung der Stirnhöhle nach dem mittleren Nasengange.

b). Mit einer Oeffnung welche durch eine Bulla ethmoidalis verengt ist.

Bei der Operation des Stirnhöhlenempyems, muss in diesen Fällen die Communikation nach der Nasenhöhle in der Höhe des Ansatzes der mittleren Muschel hergestellt werden.

2. Präparate bei welchen durch 3 Frontalzellen ein Ductus nasofrontalis gebildet ist.

a). Regelmässige Anordnung der Zellen.

b). Unregelmässige Anordnung der Zellen.

3. Herniöse Entwickelung der Stirnhöhle. Eine Frontalzelle hat an ihrer oberen Wand eine zweite Oeffnung, welche die einzige Verbindung der Stirnhöhle durch die Zelle mit der Nase bildet.

4. Indirekte Bildung der Stirnhöhle.

5. Fehlen der Stirnhöhle.

6. Frontalschnitte durch die Stirnhöhlen an welchen die verschiedene Ausdehnung derselben und das Vorspringen der Frontalzellen zu sehen ist.

In Fällen bei welchen Frontalzellen vorhanden sind, genügt es nicht nach Eröffnung der Stirnhöhle beim Empyem derselben den Boden nach der Nase zu abzutragen, es muss auch der Boden der Frontalzellen abgetragen werden. Dies wird in der Weise gemacht, dass ausser der Oeffnung auf der vorderen Fläche der Stirne, eine zweite Oeffnung angelegt wird von der inneren Orbitalwand aus. Die Wandungen der Zellen, werden mit einer Knochenzange von dieser Oeffnung aus entfernt. Vorauszuschicken ist die Abtragung des vorderen Endes der mittleren Muschel.

DR. ALDREN TURNER, London, gave a lantern-slide demonstration on the course and connections of the Central Auditory Tract.

THE TOPOGRAPHY OF THE FACIAL NERVE IN ITS RELATION TO MASTOID OPERATIONS.

MR. ROBERT DWYER JOYCE, Dublin.

In two papers on the applied anatomy of the mastoid region published in the Transactions of the Royal Academy of Medicine, Ireland, 1890-1891, Professor Birmingham recorded the examination of 100 temporal bones, in which he had investigated the chief relations of the mastoid antrum and the anatomy of the operations for opening that cavity. In these papers the relations of the facial nerve were but briefly referred to, and, at Dr. Birmingham's suggestion, I have carried out in his laboratory, a systematic examination of 30 temporal bones, with the object of determining the precise relations of this nerve to the exterior of the skull in the adult, its depth, as well as that of the external semi-circular canal, from the surface, and the relations of both these structures to the operations for exposing the mastoid antrum and to "the radical operation."

For the material upon which the investigation was carried out, and for much help and many valuable suggestions, I am greatly indebted to Professor Birmingham, of Dublin.

Method: Each bone was cut from before backwards, beginning near the angle between the squamous and petrous portion, so as to expose the Aqueduct of Fallopius in its entire length; the external semi-circular canal was also cut across by the same section in every case.

Then I projected the facial canal on the surface by a method devised by Professor Birmingham in his investigations, namely, the method of drilling from the exposed canal outwards. In order to utilize this method, it was necessary to make the holes accurately at right angles to the sagittal plane, and of course thus parallel to one another. To do this I constructed the following simple contrivance.

An accurately made wheel drill was fastened down on a sliding bed, so that the drill was capable of backward and forward movement only, without any lateral wobbling. To the end of the baseboard, in which the sliding drill-bed moved, I fastened an end-board at right angles to the line in which the drill worked, in such a way that it could be shifted about in a vertical plane perpendicular to the line of the drill. Each temporal bone was now accurately fastened in correct position to this end-board, with the exposed facial canal towards the drill, by embedding it in dentists' "modelling composition." This material, which becomes soft in hot water and hard again in cold, is very suitable for such a purpose. Thus the drill always working in the same direction, and the bone being capable of adjustment, while remaining in the plane at right angles to the drill (i.e., Sagittal, as the bone was in correct position) I was enabled to get on the outer surface a perfectly true projection of the facial canal.

Next I measured, with the aid of a fine sliding callipers graduated to $\frac{1}{2}$ millimetres, the distance of the facial canal from three points on the surface (see figure), viz. (a) a point immediately behind the external auditory meatus on a horizontal line passing through its centre; (b) a point immediately behind the upper part of the meatus and immediately below a horizontal line passing through its upper margin; (c) a point high up above the middle of the meatus on the posterior root of the zygoma.

The measurements from (a) and (b) were taken horizontally inwards and parallel to the posterior wall of the meatus; that from (c) straight in and slightly downwards to the horizontal part of the facial canal which lies on the inner wall of the attic. I have not used the suprameatal spine in any of my measurements, first, because it is very frequently absent, and second, because when it is present, it varies considerably in length. The points *(a)* and *(b)* are taken as representing the anterior edge or lip of the cavity made in the bone by the drill or chisel, when the mastoid is opened below or above respectively. Also the point *(b)* is the point from which, as Birmingham has shown, the antrum may in every case be tapped, without any danger to either the lateral sinus or the cranial cavity, by a small drill sent straight in, *i.e.*, perpendicular to the sagittal plane. The distance of the facial canal from the point *(c)* will come into consideration in removing the outer wall of the attic from the external meatus.

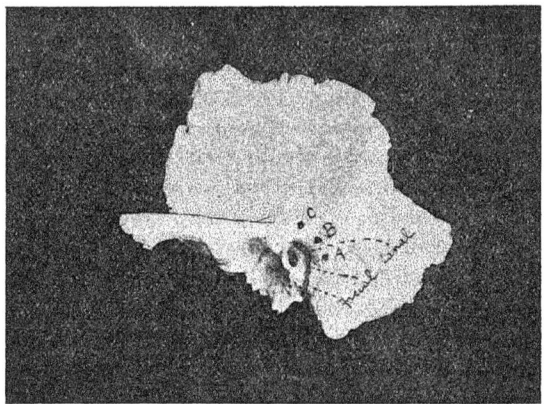

Outer surface of temporal bone, showing points (*a*), (*b*), and (*c*), and also line of projection of facial canal.

Results : The line of projection of the facial canal on the surface is very constant in position. It lies on the posterior and superior walls of the external auditory meatus, about midway between the sulcus tympanicus and the outer margin of the bony meatus, its position between these two points varying however with the obliquity of the meatus. The lower part of the canal runs perpendicularly downwards, or has a slight inclination forwards, and its upper part beyond the bend runs almost horizontally forwards, with a slight inclination upwards. As Politzer shows in his "Lehrbuch der Ohrenheilkunde" in its whole. course from above downwards, the facial canal slopes out, being thus farther from the surface above than from the surface below. In a. coronal section exposing the canal, it will be seen, however, that its inclination outwards is not regular and gradual when traced from above downwards, but that at the genu it frequently makes a bend either outwards or inwards, both directions being about equally common. As regards its relations to the surface of the mastoid, a straight drill hole 3 to 4 mm. behind the posterior wall of the meatus and parallel to it, will in every case strike it. This last holds true from the level of the floor of the meatus to within 4 mm. of the roof.

I have found the distance of the facial canal from the surface to vary very considerably. From the first point (*a*) (immediately behind the meatus, on a horizontal line passing through its centre), its average distance was about 16.75 mm. ; the maximum being 22 mm., and the minimum 13.25 mm. In the case where it measured 22 mm. the surface of the mastoid at the measuring point was considerably bulged out.

DISTANCE OF FACIAL CANAL FROM POINT (*a*) WAS

in 1 case 22 mm.
 ,, 2 cases 19.5 ,,
 ,, 2 ,, 18.75 ,,
 ,, 4 ,, 18 ,,
 ,, 1 case 17.75 ,,
 ,, 2 cases 17.25 ,,
 ,, 5 ,, 17 ,,
 ,, 5 ,, 16 ,,
 ,, 2 ,, 15.25 ,,
 ,, 2 ,, 14.5 ,,
 ,, 3 ,, 14 ,,
 ,, 1 case 13.25 ,,

From the second point (*b*) (immediately behind the upper part of the meatus and immediately below a horizontal line passing through its upper margin), the average distance was about 18.5 mm.; the maximum being 22.75 mm., and the minimum 14.75 mm., this last being in a case of solid mastoid. The first (22.75 mm.) was in the same case as gave the maximum distance from the point (*a*).

DISTANCE OF THE FACIAL CANAL FROM POINT (*b*) WAS

in 1 case 22.75 mm.
 ,, 4 cases 21.25 ,,
 ,, 1 case 20.5 ,,
 ,, 3 cases 20 ,,
 ,, 2 ,, 19.25 ,,
 ,, 4 ,, 19 ,,
 ,, 5 ,, 18.5 ,,
 ,, 2 ,, 17.75 ,,
 ,, 1 case 16.75 ,,

in 2 cases 16 mm.
,, 1 case 15.75 ,,
,, 3 cases 15 ,,
,, 1 case 14.75 ,,

From the third point (c) (above the middle of the meatus on the posterior root of the zygoma) the average distance was about 19.4 mm., the maximum being 21.75 mm., and the minimum 17 mm.

DISTANCE OF FACIAL NERVE FROM POINT (c) WAS

in 1 case 21.75 mm.
,, 2 cases 21.25 ,,
,, 2 ,, 21 ,,
,, 4 ,, 20.75 ,,
,, 6 ,, 20 ,,
,, 5 ,, 19 ,,
,, 4 ,, 18.5 ,,
,, 2 ,, 18 ,,
,, 1 case 17.75 ,,
,, 2 cases 17.25 ,,
,, 1 case 17 ,,

As mentioned above, the external semi-circular canal was always exposed by the same cut as opened up the facial canal. Its outer sweep lies about 1.5 mm. above the horizontal part of the facial canal and parallel to it. Its depth from the surface was measured from the points (b) and (c).

From (b) the average distance was about 18.56 mm. ; the maximum being 22 mm., and the minimum 13.75 mm. (this last in a solid mastoid).

DISTANCE OF THE EXTERNAL SEMI-CIRCULAR CANAL FROM POINT (b) was

in 1 case 22 mm.
,, 1 ,, 21.25 ,,
,, 3 cases 20.75 ,,
,, 4 ,, 20 ,,
,, 2 ,, 19.75 ,,
,, 4 ,, 19.25 ,,
,, 2 ,, 18.5 ,,
,, 1 case 17.75 ,,
,, 5 cases 17.5 ,,
,, 2 ,, 15.5 ,,
,, 2 ,, 14.75 ,,
,, 2 ,, 14.5 ,,
,, 1 case 13.75 ,,

From the point (c) the average distance was about 18.5 mm. ; the maximum being 20.5 mm., and the minimum 16.25 mm.

DISTANCE OF THE EXTERNAL SEMI-CIRCULAR CANAL FROM POINT (c) was

in	1 case	20.5	mm.
,,	1 ,,	20.25	,,
,,	5 cases	20	,,
,,	3 ,,	19.5	,,
,,	4 ,,	19	,,
,,	3 ,,	18.25	,,
,,	5 ,,	18	,,
,,	5 ,,	17.25	,,
,,	2 ,,	17	,,
,,	1 case	16.25	,,

Summary: 1. The facial canal lies altogether in front of the anterior border of the mastoid process ; and a drill sent *straight in* from the surface of the mastoid (point *b*) to open the antrum, cannot injure the nerve.

2. Measured from the point (*b*) and slightly more forwards than the direction of the posterior wall of the meatus, and also slightly upwards, the facial canal in 43.3 per cent. of cases was *more* superficial than the external semi-circular canal; in the same percentage of cases this was just reversed, and in the remaining 13.4 per cent., they were the same distance from the surface (at *b*). Thus the external semi-circular canal cannot be taken as a guide to the depth of the facial nerve. The distance between the facial and the semi-circular canals, measured in the same way (*i.e.* from the point (*b*) slightly upwards and in a direction more forwards than the posterior wall of the meatus) was never more than 1.5 mm., except in one case where the latter was 4.25 mm. more superficial than the former.

3. The average distance of the facial canal from the point (*b*) is slightly *less* than that of the semi-circular canal when the measurements are made to corresponding points on both (*i.e.*, points on the same perpendicular line).

4. In order to avoid the facial canal in every case while drilling the mastoid from the point (*a*) the drill-hole must never be more than 13 mm. deep, if it is horizontal and parallel to the posterior wall of the meatus.

5. From the point (*b*) 14.5 mm. must be the maximum depth of the hole, if it is horizontal and parallel to the posterior wall of the meatus ; but if the drill or chisel be sent in with a stronger inclination forwards, and also slightly upwards the greatest safe depth would be 13.5 mm., as in one of the specimens, the external semi-circular canal was only 13.75 mm. from this point.

H

6. The anterior lip of the bone wound (as above) is the point from which these measurements are to be taken.

7. It has been stated that the points (*a*) and (*b*) are immediately behind the meatus. But on account of the gradual way in which the surface of the mastoid slopes into the meatus, and as the drill has to be kept parallel to the posterior wall of the meatus, it is not possible to make a drill hole nearer the posterior wall than about 3 mm. In other words, a line drawn inwards from either (*a*) or (*b*) parallel to the posterior wall of the meatus, will be about 3 mm., distant from the meatus, the measurement being taken, of course, at a point in the canal sufficiently far in, to be beyond the gradual slope leading from the mastoid into the meatus.

8. In removing the outer wall of the attic, it should be remembered that the external semi-circular canal is almost always (91 per cent.) nearer the surface of the skull at the point (*c*) than the facial nerve ; but as it is about 1.5 mm. higher than the latter it is almost out of danger ; besides it has a thicker covering of compact bone in this situation than the facial nerve. From the meatus, the chisel or scoop ought not to go in more than 16.5 mm., or if sent in very high 16 mm. measured from the point (*c*).

PROF. EEMAN fait remarquer à propos de la 3ième préparation montrée par le Dr. Joyce, qu'il n'est point exact d'affirmer d'une manière absolue que l'on peut, sans danger de blesser le sinus transverse pénétrer dans l'antre en partant du point *b* (situé immédiatement derrière le bord postérieur du conduit auditif externe à la hauteur du milieu de ce bord). Le Prof. Eeman a montré à une réunion de la Société d'Otologie Belge, une préparation où le tissu osseux situé entre la paroi postérieure du conduit auditif externe et le sinus transverse, avait à peine une épaisseur de 2 millimètres. Dans ce cas il eut été absolument impossible d'arriver à l'antre sans blesser le sinus. Le Dr. Eeman regrette de ne pas avoir apporté cette préparation au Congrès, mais fait remarquer que le Dr. Moure a exposé au superbe Musée du Congrès, deux préparations absolument démonstratives à cet égard.

DR. L. KATZ, Berlin, demonstrirte eine Reihe macroscopischer und microscopischer Præparate des Gehörorgans sowie mehrere chirurgische Instrumente für Ohr und Nase.

1. Stereoscopische Ansichten der complicierten anatomischen Verhältnisse der Gegend des foramen rotundum und speciell der Membran des runden Fensters. Es unterliegt keinem Zweifel, dass man durch eine derartige stereoscopische Betrachtung viel besser als durch anatomische Zeichnungen dem Studierenden die Verhältnisse klar machen kann. Es handelt sich in den vorgelegten Præparaten um Ansichten von Aussen und Innen. Bei letzteren sieht man auch das Verhältniss der convex gekrümmten nierenförmigen Membran zum

Eingang in den aquæductus cochleæ sowie zum Anfang der lamina spiral. ossea, und des im Bogen von Aussen nach Innen verlaufenden ligam. spirale. Bei der Betrachtung der Stereogramms von Aussen tritt der von Katz früher beschriebene recessus sub fenestra rotunda, welcher durch einen mehr oder weniger deutlich hervortretenden Knochenwall von der eigentlichen fenestra rotunda getrennt ist, deutlich in die Erscheinung. Dieser Recessus ist hier ausserordentlich lang (c. 1 cm) und erstreckt sich in horizontaler Richtung von hinten nach vorn unter der Schnecke an der Grenze zwischen medialer Labyrinthwand und Boden der Paukenhöhle.

2. Eine Anzahl von stereoscopischen Ansichten des gesammten, *durchsichtig* gemachten Labyrinths, der Paukenhöhle, des Trommelfells, etc., welche dem Beschauer ein sehr instructives Bild dieses so verwickelten Gebietes gewähren. Die Methode des Durchsichtigmachens des Knochens hat Katz im 37ten Band des Archivs für Ohrenheilkunde beschrieben.

3. Microscopische Præparate besonders des-Cortischen Organs, welche bis in die kleinsten Details uns Aufschluss über die Epithelgebilde der papilla spiralis und der feinen dazu gehörenden Nerven gewähren. Katz bespricht die Methode der histologischen Conservierung. Zunächst müssen die Objecte in $\frac{1}{4}$-$\frac{1}{2}\%$ Osmiumsäure für 5-10 Stunden gehärtet werden, dann werden sie in eine Lösung von $\frac{1}{2}\%$ Chromsäure + $\frac{1}{2}\%$ Essigsäure gebracht und zwar für 4-8 Tage, sodann werden sie für 8-14 Tage in 5-10% Salpetersäure oder 2-6% Salzsäure zum Entkalken gelegt. Es kommt bei der Concentration der Säure auf die Grösse und Härte des betreffenden Felsenbeins selbstredend sehr an. Uebrigens muss die Entkalkungs Flüssigkeit öfter gewechselt werden.

4. Macroscopische Præparate spec. die Labyrinthwand, welche mit dem Zeiss'schen binocularen Præparier-Microscop in plastischer Weise zur Ansicht gelangen.

5. Instrumente zu Operationen in der Nase und im Ohr, die von Katz früher beschrieben worden sind. (Siehe Berl. Klin. Wochenschrift 1899, No. 5).

(a). Curette für adenoide Vegetationen im Nasenrachenraum. *(b).* Verstellbare und fixierbare Curette für Nasenoperationen, spec. das hintere Ende der unteren Nasenmuschel. *(c)* Sonde mit goldenem, kronenformigem Ansatz zum Anschmelzen von Chromsäure und Argentum nitricum für Nase und Ohr. *(d)* Verstellbarer Aetzmittel-träger (kleiner Teller) für die Nase. *(e)* Sicherheits Meissel für die Radical-Operation an der lateralen Atticus-Wand. (Zu erhalten bei Pfau, Berlin, Dorotheenstrasse).

THE OPERATION OF THE REMOVAL OF ADENOID GROWTHS
WITH THE HEAD HANGING OVER THE TABLE WHILE THE PATIENT IS
UNDER THE INFLUENCE OF CHLOROFORM.

DR. P. RUDLOFF, Wiesbaden.

In an address delivered before the third Congress of the German
Society of Surgery, in 1874, Rose[1] introduced his method of performing
operations on the hanging head in cases in which there is danger of
blood suction. This method excludes the dangers arising from the
aspiration of blood and particles of tissue, and on that account it has
been generally adopted in the larger operations on the head and throat,
such as uranoplasty, staphylorrhaphy and laryngotomy, and also in
the operation at present under consideration, which has a particular
interest for aurists. It was a surgical friend who first drew my
attention to this method, and having made use of it during a period of
eleven years, my experience justifies my bringing the subject before
you. Adopting Rose's method I perform the operation of the removal
of adenoid vegetations in the following manner : The patient is placed
upon the operation table, chloroform is administered in drops until
complete unconsciousness is induced and voluntary muscular motion is in
abeyance; then the body of the patient is lifted beyond the edge of the
table until the edge is on a line with the shoulders and the head hangs
downwards. The head is supported in an oblique line by an assistant,
stationed on the left side of the patient, and I pass my left
index finger, which is protected by von Langenbeck's thimble,
into the left side of the mouth, while the tongue is drawn
out by a second assistant, stationed on the right side. Having
on a former occasion diagnosed the growths either by digital
examination or by posterior rhinoscopy, I am now in a position to
ascertain by means of the right index finger their extent and consistency.
In examining the growths I am as careful as possible to avoid separating
a part from the entire mass and thus to cause hæmorrhage. Then I
introduce Boecker's curette into the naso-pharynx and place it so that
the ring of the instrument catches the middle part of the growths at
the end facing towards the choanæ, I pass the instrument with moderate
pressure over the fornix and the posterior wall of the pharynx as far as
the vegetations extend, and lastly out of the pharynx and mouth,
bringing the separated mass with me. A second and third stroke on
the right and left sides of the first then follow, and having disposed of
the instrument I re-examine the naso-pharynx. Generally it is found that
the principal part of the mass has been removed, but that remnants are to
be met with in the fornix and at the entrances to Rosenmüller's fossæ.
Occasionally these remnants are not only confined to these points, but
they extend deeper into Rosenmüller's fossæ, or they are to be found

on the anterior walls of Rosenmüller's fossae, extending to the pharyngeal orifice of the Eustachian tubes, also downwards into the furrows descending from these recesses. If larger remnants are to be found— say of the size of a pea—then Boecker's curette is again brought into play; should however only smaller remnants remain, I employ Hartmann's curette, passing it from the entrance of the one Rosenmüller's fossa—or if necessary from a deeper part of the recess—over the fornix to the other fossa and I then repeat the stroke in a reverse direction. If remnants are to be found either at the pharyngeal orifice of the tube or extending downwards from the fossæ, then I remove them with a gentle sweep carrying Hartmann's curette round the plica salpingopharyngea, holding the instrument somewhat obliquely. Should the naso-pharynx be small, as is the case in early childhood, I use smaller instruments, such as these. *

I am very careful in removing all the remnants; they can be felt by the index finger as small eminences projecting above the level of the mucous membrane. Sometimes one cannot tell whether it is a remnant of soft tissue or a clot of coagulated blood; if the latter, it is easily removed without pressure by means of the curette. I should like to lay special emphasis upon the fact, that in performing the operation the exertion of all strong pressure is unnecessary, because it is apt to be injurious and even hard masses can be removed without it. Special care must be exercised in handling the instrument in Rosenmüller's fossa and carrying it round the plica salpingopharyngea. I shall return to this subject later on.

Being convinced that there are no further remnants, I put the curette aside. In the course of the operation I pass the posterior ends of the turbinated bones under digital examination; should thickening exist it is easily ascertained. Formerly I sometimes removed the hypertrophied mucous membrane from these parts, introducing Hartmann's curette from the naso-pharynx; but as there is danger of injuring the sphenopalatine artery and thus causing free hæmorrhage to ensue, and as it cannot always be ascertained beforehand whether the existing thickening will disappear after the removal of the adenoid vegetations, it is now my habit to delay a few weeks, and if necessary to apply the galvanic cautery.

If the tonsils are much enlarged, it is advisable to remove them some time before hand. This is safer, as where much tonsillar hypertrophy exists in conjunction with adenoid vegetations and a receding tongue, the air passages become considerably obstructed, and there is danger of asphyxia supervening. Technical difficulties in the employment of the instruments are of less importance, if the entrance to the pharynx is unobstructed.

During the operation the blood flows through the choanae and

* H. Pfau, Fabrik Chirurg. Instrumente, Berlin, N.W., Dorotheenstrasse 67.

escapes by the nostrils into a pail standing on the floor. In case it should happen that the blood ascends into the mouth, as the head does not hang in a vertical line but somewhat obliquely, the assistant who is holding the tongue, must have sponges in readiness. When the bleeding stops, the patient is placed in a natural position on one side with the head bent a little forward, so that the oozing blood may escape through the nostrils.

Having described the method of operation, I wish to point out two elements of risk in connection with carrying it into effect. In clearing Rosenmüller's fossa great care requires to be exercised in order to avoid injury to the pharyngeal orifice of the Eustachian tube. In following this method and using Hartmann's curette as described, this danger is reduced to a minimum. Should it, however, happen, that a small portion of cartilage is removed together with the growth as shown by this specimen, the defect involved, which will disappear to a certain extent by healing, will not interfere with the physiological function of the tube nor with the passing of the catheter. Casts, which are exhibited in the museum, show the relation between the orifice of the Eustachian tube and Rosenmüller's fossa (negatives). Of much greater importance is the risk of injuring the lateral wall of Rosenmüller's fossa. One must bear in mind, that the relation existing between this wall and the connective tissue surrounding the carotid artery, is so close, that according to Merkel[2] it is quite impossible to distinguish where the line of boundary lies. This close connection assumes importance with the sixth year of life, when the development of Rosenmüller's fossæ is nearly complete (Symington, Disse[3]), it does not exist in early childhood as long as Rosenmüller's fossæ are undeveloped. But the majority of cases which present themselves for operation, as proved by my own* and other statistics[4] are above that age. There is a specimen in the museum illustrating this relationship. So it is seen, that damage to the lateral wall might involve serious consequences to the carotid artery. How necessary this warning is, is proved by the case recorded by Schmiegelow.[5] In performing the operation as described injury to the carotid artery is rendered impossible.

I attach great importance to the necessity of thoroughness in performing the operation, because with regard to recurrence it has been observed, that in the majority of cases it takes place after an incomplete removal of the growths. At the same time I should mention, that it is not only the remnants of the growths, which produce recurrence, but that vegetations can also develop in parts of the pharynx, in which at the time of operation the adenoid tissue was in a normal condition. Then the necessity of a thorough removal becomes more apparent, when it is borne in mind, as already mentioned by Drs. McBride[6] and Delavan,[7] that a certain percentage of cases is tuber-

---

*Rudloff: 564 cases; of them 122 were 1-5 years old ; 442 older.

cular. Possibly future researches may reveal, that, if recurrence takes place after complete removal, in many cases tuberculosis of the vegetations may have been the cause of the mischief.

With regard to the results, my 'experience has verified the truth of the statistics reported by Dr. Gleitsmann[8] as being generally accepted in America and of those of Prof. Moritz Schmidt,[9] of Frankfort. I have found that out of 254 cases it was necessary to operate again on nine ; out of these nine cases the second operations were performed by other specialists in two, in four by myself under anæsthesia and in three without it, in these seven cases I found a few remnants shortly after the operation, and in performing the second operation these remnants had neither decreased nor increased, though in two cases a considerable interval had elapsed. It is not in my power to include in these statistics about 450 cases more, operated upon after this method, partly because they are not under my present control, and partly because a sufficient interval has not yet elapsed to test the result. Perhaps it is worth while mentioning, that the oldest individual was a person of fifty years, and the youngest a baby of fifteen months.

Before concluding I must add that I do not entirely confine myself to the method described, but I employ other methods as well, without anæsthesia. I consider the special circumstances in connection with each case generally in consultation with the family doctor before deciding which method to use ; but I invariably employ the method described under anæsthesia in cases of children, who have undergone a former operation without a narcotic, and who have become nervous in consequence, and in cases of their relations and friends, who have not had a glowing account of their treatment, and in all cases of inherited nervous predisposition, among whom are a certain number of patients suffering from special nervous diseases.   Further, I employ this method in cases of anatomical anomaly, occasionally to be met with, first, when the anterior arch of the atlas projects too far into the naso-pharynx, and secondly, when the junction of the posterior wall, and the roof of the naso-pharynx presents rather an angular than a circular form. These anomalies are described by Merkel ;[10] Zuckerkandl,[11] Hopmann,[12] Seifert, T. Heymann, and others also draw attention to the projection of the atlas in some cases. I first observed these peculiarities in cases originally operated on by others, in which, thorough removal had been impossible owing to the inaccessibility of the recess by the instruments employed ; for example, one of my patients, a lady fifty years of age, who had failed to get rid of the growths after having undergone many operations at the hands of operators of undoubted skill during a number of years, found permanent relief by means of the method in question.

With regard to these and other peculiarities of structure, Merkel[13] remarks in describing the anatomy of the naso-pharynx : " As there are many varieties of form it is evident, that surgical instruments, which it is necessary to introduce from the mouth into the naso-pharynx, must not be confined to one form, but must be adapted to the individual case." I must add, that not only are a variety of instruments and skilful manipulation necessary in performing the operation, but several methods ought to be made use of, if thorough removal of the adenoid vegetations is to be attained in every case.

LITERATURE.

1. Archiv für Klinische Chirurgie, Band xvii. und xxiv.
2. Merkel, Handbuch der topographischen Anatomie, Band i., Seite, 417.
3. Disse, ii. Band des Handbuches der Laryngologie und Rhinologie von Dr. P. Heymann.
4. Wex, Zeitschrift für Ohrenheilkunde, Band xxxiv., S. 207.
5. Monatsschrift für Ohrenheilkunde, Band xxxi., 1897, S. 115.
6. Sixty-sixth Annual Meeting of the British Medical Association, Edinburgh, 1898. "British Medical Journal," October 22nd, 1898.
7. Bryson Delavan, "New York Medical Journal," October 29th, 1898, pag. 620.
8. Gleitsmann, "New York Medical Journal," October 29th, 1898, pag. 638.
9. M. Schmidt, Die Krankheiten der obëren Luftwege, ii. Auflage, Berlin, 1897, S. 275.
10. Merkel, Handbuch der topographischen Anatomie, Band i., S. 411 und S. 419.
11. Zuckerkandl, Normale und pathologische Anatomie der Nasenhöhle, Wien 1892.
12. Hopmann, Die adenoiden Tumoren als Theilerscheinung der Hyperplasie des lymphatischen Rachenringes und in ihren Beziehungen zum übrigen Körper, Halle a/S. 1895.
13. Merkel, Handbuch der topographischen Anatomie, Band i., S. 411.

———

Dr. KNAPP: I would wish to get an opportunity of demonstrating a modification of Schütz's guillotine instrument by Prof Passow. He has sent it to the Museum of this Congress. It acts swiftly, thoroughly, and safely as far as I have witnessed it. I have seen the operation with reclined head performed by one of my former assistants, who was a very well-trained operator. The piece which had been removed with the curette, contained a fine slice of cartilage.

Dr. LEDERMANN: One of the disadvantages of the adenoid operation is the severe hæmorrhage which is met with at times. For this reason we should not put our patient in any condition which might predispose to this unpleasantness. For the same reason the method of operating with the head hanging over the end of the table, to my mind, is not a desirable one. We never know when we may meet with a hæmophilic disposition, and the "hanging head" would certainly increase the flow of blood from the lacerated surface.

I have operated in a large number of cases in the upright position, and am very well satisfied with the good results which can be accomplished in the following manner:—

A large post-nasal forceps is first introduced, and a considerable mass of the vegetation is removed. The second step is the application of a modified Gottstein curette, and finally the finger is introduced and all remnants are removed.

RHEUMATIC DISEASES OF THE EAR.

PROF. UCHERMANN, Christiana.

Rheumatic diseases of the ear are but little known, and seem to be rare. The symptoms are not sufficiently distinct, nor the etiology so clear, as to establish a safe conclusion with regard to cause and effect. Still, I am of opinion that a closer investigation of the matter will enable us to recognise certain common features, symptomatical and pathological, by which a clinical diagnosis of the special case can be made or rectified. To attempt this, and at the same time to draw the attention of my colleagues to an interesting group of ear diseases, as yet little known, is the aim of this paper.

At the outset we are met with the old difficulty. What is rheumatism? The usually accepted answer, from an etiological point of view, appears to be more unsatisfactory than ever. Infection admitted; is it a specific infectious disease, or is it only a kind of pyæmia dependent upon one or more pathogenic bacteria? Whatever the case may be, we have the clinical picture which cannot be mistaken. As we are well aware, the characteristics of the disease are its tendency to attack the connective tissue (fibrous or muscular), and its endothelium-lined cavities, and to form fibrinous exudations and infiltrations. In this way it appears in the joints, muscles, heart, skin, etc. In addition to this, there is its painfulness in certain localities, also its being acted upon by salicylic acid in acute forms, by atmospheric changes in chronic forms. It is necessary to set aside all cases whose only claim to being rheumatic is that they appear to have arisen after a rheuma, that is a cold or catarrh. To this class belong, for instance, many of the so-called rheumatic cases mentioned by Gradenigo in his description of labyrinthine diseases (Schwartze's Handbook). It is also necessary to differentiate between acute and chronic forms. Among the former, the best known are polyarthritis acuta (rheumatic fever), acute muscular rheumatism and erythema nodosum, among the latter the chronic rheumatic muscular and joint diseases.   All the rheumatic ear affections that have up to the present been described belong to the acute forms of rheumatism appearing as complications of rheumatic fever.   Ménière (Revue Mens. d'Otologie et de Laryngologie, Nov. 1883) mentions a case where otalgia in the form of severe intermittent pain preceded by four days the attack of ordinary acute polyarthritis.   A similar case is given by Wolff (Verhandlungen der otiatrischen Section der Wiesbadener Naturförscher Versammlung, 1887), who also adds that the joints of the ossicles can be affected by this.   The clinical or pathological proof, however, is not given.   In both cases the appearance of the drum does not seem to have been altered. Moos has observed a case of apoplectiform (Ménière's) deafness during the period of convalescence after acute rheumatic fever, complicated with endocarditis (perhaps embolic).   In a second case various cerebral hyperaesthetic symptoms appeared with attacks of pain and hyperacusis, in the eighth and ninth weeks hardness of hearing, ending in total deafness (Schwartze's Handbook, Vol. 1, p. 544).   Among the deaf-mutes in Norway is a case where an examination of the ear points to the existence of a combined middle ear and labyrinth affection, caused by this disease (Uchermann, "Deaf-Mutes in Norway," Vol. 1, p. 446).

I have seen two cases where ear affection preceded ordinary rheumatic fever.   Both cases were in adults, one a lady, 25 years of age, who had had rheumatic fever several times before, the other a gentleman of 35, of very rheumatic disposition.   In both cases there was an acute inflammation of the middle ear, with strong injection of the drum, abundant secretion of serous or sero-fibrinous fluid, together with quite an unusual amount of pain, both spontaneous and when touched, which continued even after the opening of the drum.   In the case of the lady, during the seventeen days before the beginning of the fever, an infiltration formed on the posterior wall of the bony meatus, involving the adjacent part of the drum, of the size of half a pea, red and very sensitive.

In the man's case there was a swelling of the posterior part of the drum, also a more diffuse swelling and sensitiveness of the septum cartilagineum nasi on the same side, with superficial (catarrhal) erosions. In both cases, with the beginning of rheumatic fever, the ear affections healed after eight days, possibly the result of paracentesis and salicylic acid, though the swelling of the septum did not disappear for several months and caused considerable impediment to nasal respiration.

But there are also other cases where the rheumatism from which the ear affection arises is of a chronic character, and where the ear disease runs a course less acute and violent, but sometimes more fatal for the organ itself.   In the case of a young man about 30, with a marked rheumatic history, I have seen, without any apparent cause, and

alternating with rheumatic affections of the throat, a double-sided
what is generally called otitis media serosa, that is to say a collection
of serous or sero-fibrinous yellowish fluid in the tympanic cavity with
the slightest inflammatory signs. The case ran a slow course, but finally
yielded to repeated incisions of the drum.

I venture the hypothesis that many of the cases of serous middle
ear affections, especially those marked by yellowish or amber coloured
exudation are rheumatic in origin or foundation, and that treatment
with salicylic acid should be tried before any surgical intervention is
resorted to. In another case, that of a young plethoric man, of about
34, the symptoms, when I first saw him, February 1895, were the
following : He complained that for a year he had suffered from tinnitus
aurium and deafness of progressive character, which latterly had greatly
increased. He experienced no dizziness, and hitherto he had enjoyed
good hearing and freedom from ear troubles. Occasionally he
had felt rheumatic pains, but otherwise had never had a disease
of any consequence. On examination, the right drum revealed
a small round cicatrix (as big as a shot) in the upper and hinder-
most quadrant, there was a little dulness but no retraction, the
left drum being also dull and not retracted. Both the drums
were moveable by Delstanche. By auscultation the left ostium
tubae Eustachii was found narrower than the right, otherwise there was
nothing abnormal. From the left ear the hearing of speech was gone.
He could hear neither No. 64 of Appiens set of tuning forks (64 double
vibrations per second) nor Galton's whistle ; Rinne – 5''', Schwabach
much shortened (–). Right ear Rinne + 5''', Schwabach – ; the
deeper tuning forks were heard more distinctly than the higher, Galton
not at all. On this side he heard words spoken in a loud voice at a
distance of from three to four inches. In spite of internal treatment
with salicylic acid and iodide of potassium, together with local treatment—leeches, injections of iodide of potassium and pilocarpine, massage,
(Lucæ, Delstanche)—after a couple of months he was completely deaf.
At his repeated request at last I tried a stapedectomy on the left ear.
On probing, the stapes at first gave the impression of immobility, but
by traction became loosened, and was then immediately replaced. The
only result was considerable giddiness for a month, during which time
he had to lie quite still on his back. At the same time he had rheumatic
pains in the right shoulder. About a year later, there appeared a
reddish fluctuating swelling of the left eyebrow and upper eyelid, with
its seat in the periosteal tissue. By incision, I removed about a tea-
spoonful of sero-fibrinous fluid, upon which the swelling disappeared. A
year after, however, it reappeared in nearly the same place, and yielded
to the same treatment. On this occasion there was also a swelling over
the left tuberositas frontalis. Last year he called on me for a nose
affection. There was a dry catarrh of the anterior part with a forma-

tion of crusts and a dry perforation of the cartilaginous septum of considerable size. It had developed since the last time I had seen him and proved very stubborn under ordinary treatment. [I might mention two similar affections of the nose that have come under my notice. One, the case of an elderly man, very rheumatic, who eventually died of rheumatism (articular, etc.) owing to general exhaustion. The other, a case now under my treatment, where there is no perforation, but the pale swollen mucous membrane is specked with white fibrous (sclerotic) spots.] It is then, a case of what is commonly called secondary sclerosis with involvement of both the labyrinthine bony capsule and the nervous elements. The history of the case and its accompanying symptoms make it fairly certain, that it is of rheumatic nature and, like these affections elsewhere, bound to the connective tissue. For instance, a swelling of the lining of the canaliculi for the N. Cochlearis and the lining of the vestibulum, with the result of more or less fixation of the stapes will easily account for the acoustic phenomena. While with regard to the bone (labyrinthine capsule) the result may be an eburnation (though with the preservation of the greater cavities—vestibulum, scala, etc.), or may be in some cases the apparent reverse, a rarification (Spongiosirung. Siebenmann). To sum up :—

1. Rheumatic fever is sometimes preceded (sometimes accompanied) by otalgia, alone or together with an acute swelling and injection of the drum and the adjacent bony meatus, followed by a serous or sero-fibrinous secretion in the middle ear (otalgia, myringitis, otitis externa, otitis media rheumatica) ; or it may be complicated during its progress with affections of the middle ear and the internal ear (labyrinth, perhaps the auditory nerve).

2. There are other, more independent rheumatic ear diseases in persons of a rheumatic constitution or tendency (previous rheumatic fever, &c.) The ear affection appears as an otitis media "serosa" with yellowish half fibrinous exudations, or as a (secondary) sclerosis of progressive character.

3. The characteristics of the different forms are : in the acute forms, painfulness, excessive injection, and the tendency to the formation of infiltrations and exudations ; in the chronic forms, the tendency to the formation of fibrinous exudations and the tendency to affect the bony capsule, with strong tinnitus, and slow, but steady progression. Salicylic acid seems to influence the acute forms but not the chronic. These latter, judging from the experience of a case at present under my treatment, are perhaps more influenced by a general rheumatic treatment.

DR. HARTMANN beobachtete plötzliche Taubheit bei einem Manne der eine Nacht bei starker Kälte im Freien geschlafen hatte und morgens vollständig taub aufgewacht war. Das Gehör kehrte nicht wieder zurück. Der Fall dürfte als reine rheumatische Taubheit zu betrachten sein.

PROF. UCHERMANN : I have seen several such cases in deaf-mutes. But I think it quite necessary, as I have already said, to discriminate between the pure rheumatic cases, where you have the different clinical features, as infiltration, exudation, 'etc., and cases, whose etiology only points to cold or catarrh, otherwise there will be confusion.

FIFTH MEETING.

THURSDAY, AUGUST 10TH, AT 10 A.M.

CHAIRMAN   -   PROF. GRAZZI.

TRAITEMENT DES SUPPURATIONS CHRONIQUES DE L'ATTIQUE.

DR. E. MÉNIÈRE, Paris.

La thérapeutique des perforations de la membrane de Shrapnell, avec suppuration chronique de la coupole, et carie de tout ou partie des osselets, est entrée dans une voie nouvelle depuis un certain nombre d'années.

Je ne veux pas faire ici l'historique des divers procédés opératoires mis en avant, pour arriver à tarir cette suppuration localisée dans l'attique.

A mon sens, les indications sont formelles, et en face d'un état chronique persistant, il est reconnu par les Otologistes que l'intervention opératoire donne des succès plus complets et plus rapides, que toute autre méthode.

Dans les hôpitaux, et dans les cliniques spéciales, il est assez facile de faire comprendre aux malades affectés de carie des osselets et de suppuration de l'attique, avec perforation de la membrane de Shrapnell, l'utilité, ou plutôt la nécessité d'une intervention qui, seule, peut les guérir à tout jamais, dans la majorité des cas.

Il n'en est plus de même pour les malades de la clientèle particulière. Ceux-ci, ne ressentant aucune douleur, aucune gêne, et ne pouvant même pas constater un écoulement dans le conduit, sont réfractaires, généralement, à toute intervention opératoire. Ils la regardent comme hors de proportion avec leur état de maladie, et la mettent sur le compte de la *manie opératoire* tant reprochée.

Dans ces conditions, il est urgent d'essayer un traitement actif. Je n'énumérerai pas tous les médicaments employés, toutes les méthodes mises en œuvre. Un caustique énergique, le chlorure de Zinc à saturation, est celui qui m'a donné les meilleurs résultats, toutefois bien aléatoires.

Dans ces derniers temps le hasard m'a fait employer une médication nouvelle. Au mois d'Avril dernier, j'ai communiqué à la Société d'Otologie de Paris l'observation d'un cas de périostite chronique du conduit auditif externe, guérie en 4 séances par les pulvérisations d'Ipsilène iodoformé.

Il m'est venu à l'idée d'employer ces pulvérisations dans les suppurations chroniques de l'attique, en me servant de la canule de Hartmann.

L'Ipsilène iodoformé est un chlorure d'Ethyle obtenu par un procédé spécial, et tenant en suspension de l'Iodoforme.

J'ai soumis à cette médication deux malades, un jeune homme de 22 ans, cachectique, de mauvaise santé ; affecté de carie des osselets et de suppuration de l'attique depuis 7 ans ; puis, un homme de 35 ans affecté de même maladie remontant à plus de 5 ans. Tous deux ont été soignés longtemps par divers procédés, sans effets.

Le premier malade a éprouvé une amélioration très nette après 4 pulvérisations, et je suis convaincu qu'il guérira.

Le deuxième a été soumis à 5 pulvérisations, et son état est excellent. La coupole autrefois remplie de pus s'écoulant par la perforation, est presque complètement sèche. Sa guérison est prochaine.

J'attribue ces bons résultats à l'imprégnation très vive des tissus malades par ce petit jet d'Ipsilène iodoformé, s'introduisant dans les moindres anfractuosités et favorisant la cicatrisation.

L'appareil pulvérisateur permet de modérer à volonté la force de projection.

Je signale un léger inconvénient, c'est un petit sentiment de vertige qui suit la première et la deuxième pulvérisation, mais qui disparaît vite. Il est bon, du reste, de tâter la susceptibilité particulière des malades.

Me basant sur les deux faits observés, je crois que cette médication pourra rendre de réels services aux sujets atteints d'affection chronique de l'attique, lorsqu'ils sont absolument réfractaires à toute intervention chirurgicale.

LA CONTAGION DES OTITES MOYENNES AIGUËS.

Dr. MARCEL LERMOYEZ, Paris.

Un certain nombre d'observations, que j'ai faites depuis plusieurs années, m'ont peu à peu amené à cette conviction, d'abord hésitante, aujourd'hui solide, que l'otite moyenne aiguë est contagieuse. Ce n'est certes pas une contagion patente et inéluctable comme celle des fièvres éruptives ; dans ce cas il y a longtemps qu'elle eut été reconnue. C'est, au contraire, une transmission contingente, souvent évitable, et qui, par sa variété et son insidiosité, échappe facilement à l'observation.

Il en est de l'otite, ce me semble, comme de la pneumonie. Dans l'un et l'autre cas, le refroidissement en ont accaparé l'étiologie ; cependant, pour ce qui est de la pneumonie, ce vieux type de maladie a *frigore*, une observation patiente et tenace est parvenue à démontrer sa contagiosité. Je voudrais en faire de même aujourd'hui pour l'otite moyenne aiguë, non pas que je veuille avancer que toutes les otites aiguës se prennent par contagion, loin de là ; mais je crois fermement que quelquefois l'inflammation de l'oreille moyenne ne reconnaît pas d'autre cause.

Encore une fois je n'apporte pas à la défense de mon hypothèse ces preuves dites scientifiques que réclame la nosologie actuelle. D'ailleurs ni le microscope ni l'expérimentation ne prouveraient grand'chose en l'espèce : il me faut m'en tenir au terrain clinique, toujours un peu incertain.

La communication préliminaire que je fais aujourd'hui n'a donc d'autre prétention que d'attirer l'attention sur un point de nosologie auriculaire dont des travaux ultérieurs auront à rechercher le bienfait.

———

Voici d'abord les faits que j'ai recueillis. Je ne rapporte que ceux qui m'ont paru les plus probants.

I. Un premier cas, très simple, est celui d'une femme soignant son mari atteint d'*otite moyenne aiguë catarrhale légère* au cours d'une grippe ; et qui, sans aucune prédisposition antérieure locale, sans s'être exposée au froid, puisqu'elle ne quittait pas l'appartement, est prise d'une poussée d'otite moyenne aiguë catarrhale légère.

Ces deux otites furent semblables et évoluèrent de même.

OBS. I et I *bis.* — M. L…, 40 ans.

Le 8 *octobre* 1898 est pris d'une attaque légère de grippe à forme catarrhale. Température 38°5 rectale maxima. Coryza léger catarrhal puis muco-purulent.

Le 12 *octobre*, en se réveillant, le malade ressent une douleur modérée dans l'oreille droite avec diminution légère de l'ouïe. Marteau et cadre très rouges, presque hémorrhagiques : le tympan présente une coloration un peu sombre sur laquelle tranchent des vaisseaux dilatés ; pas d'exsudat dans la caisse.

Le 13 *octobre* toute douleur a cessé. Le 14 *octobre* le tympan a repris son aspect normal.

———

La femme du malade qui jamais n'avait eu d'affection auriculaire et qui passait la journée dans la chambre de son mari, est brusquement prise, le 15 octobre, d'une douleur modérée dans l'oreille droite. Le spéculum montre, comme chez son mari, une très légère otite aiguë catarrhale, avec injection du marteau, rougeur du fond de caisse par transparence à travers le tympan sans exsudat. Guérison en quarante-huit heures.

II. Un second fait intéressant est celui de deux sœurs, demeurant ensemble. Toutes deux sont atteintes, à un degré d'intensité divers, il est vrai, *d'angine herpétique*, d'herpès vrai du pharynx.

Dans l'un et l'autre cas éclate une *otite purulente aiguë :* et dans les deux cas l'otite a le même caractère, d'être torpide, presque sans douleur, avec distension énorme du tympan qui n'arrive pas à se perforer spontanément et cependant en donnant lieu à une suppuration abondante.

OBS. II et II *bis*. — Mlle Char.... (Madeleine), 10 ans.

Au commencement de mai : mal de gorge, fièvre. Depuis cette époque traîne et garde la chambre.

Le 18 *mai* 1897 est prise d'un élancement douloureux dans l'oreille droite, très passager. Dès le lendemain surdité double, mais *sans douleurs*. Température atteinte jusqu'à 39°8 sous l'aisselle.

Je vois la malade le 24 *mai*. — Etat général mauvais : teint pâle d'une infection latente. Surdité manifeste : voix basse entendue : O. D. = 0,10 cent. et O. G. = 0,20 cent. Mais pas de douleurs ni d'écoulement d'oreilles.

Le spéculum montre à droite un tympan rouge, présentant à sa partie postéro-supérieure une poche saillante, presque prolabée, non perforée. A gauche, aspect analogue, le tympan est plat, grisâtre avec vaisseaux voilés apparents : en avant et en arrière de la courte apophyse du marteau deux poches saillantes, rouges, centrées d'un point jaune.

Le 25 *mai*. — Incision profonde et large de ces poches sous le chloroforme. Flot de pus. L'air passe ensuite largement à travers ces ouvertures.

26 *mai*. — Suppuration abondante. Toute douleur a cessé. Les poches ont disparu : les perforations sont bien béantes.

1er *juin* — Bon état général. Suppuration abondante. Ce jour-là, la malade se plaint de *souffrir de la gorge*, de la même façon, dit-elle, que les jours qui ont précédé son otite. Je constate une *plaque d'herpès* sur le pilier antérieur gauche.

2 *juin*. — De nouvelles vésicules d'herpès apparaissent sur le voile.

6 *juin*. — Suppuration d'oreille abondante. Je prescris des bains de nitrate d'argent à 1%. Le mal de gorge augmente.

Tout le pharynx (luette, piliers, épiglotte) sont le siège d'une poussée influente d'herpès.

10 *juin*.—L'éruption pharyngée diminue : en même temps la suppuration auriculaire se réduit considérablement.

25 *juin*.—Guérison.

Mlle Char. (Jeanne), 5 ans.

Cette malade est la sœur de la précédente : elle couche dans une chambre voisine : mais elle passe la journée dans la chambre de sa grande sœur et joue sur son lit.

Vers le 20 *mai*, étant légèrement grippée depuis quelque temps, elle est atteinte d'une angine herpétique typique diffuse. Quelques jours plus tard, elle se plaint de souffrir de l'oreille droite, très légèrement.

Le 1er *juin*, pas de fièvre, mais état général mauvais ; teint pâle ; anorexie.

Le spéculum montre une otite aiguë gauche, datant seulement de deux à trois jours. Le tympan, plat dans sa partie antérieure, forme en haut et en arrière une poche extrêmement saillante, presque prolabée : un point jaune au centre.

10 *juin*.—Même aspect du tympan. Ecoulement muco-purulent seulement dupuis hier ; fait une paracentèse.

24 *juin*.—Guérison.

III. L'observation suivante relate une coïncidence tout au moins curieuse. Deux sœurs, partageant la même vie, prennent ensemble la rougeole. Ensemble elles prennent une otite purulente aiguë intense et toutes deux ont, au cours de leur maladie, une même poussée d'adénoïdite. Rougeole, otite, adénoïde concordent chronologiquement : pourquoi admettre la contagion pour la première et la nier pour les deux autres ?

OBS. III et III *bis*.—Mlle Tet... (Jeanne), 6 ans.

Le 22 *mars* 1897, au douzième jour d'une rougeole normale, cette enfant est prise d'une violente douleur d'oreille. Pas de traitement spécial. Cinq jours après le début de ces accidents, sensation d'éclatement dans l'oreille gauche : écoulement de pus, sédation momentanée de douleurs.

Le 28 *mars*, je suis appelé à voir cette enfant. Conduit gauche plein de muco-pus, ayant amené une légère otite externe avec retentissement ganglionnaire péri-auriculaire. Le tympan est rouge vif, bombé : perforation insuffisante. Paracentèse. Glycérine phéniquée.

Le 3 *avril*.—Retour de douleur dû à la fermeture rapide de la perforation que j'agrandis de nouveau.

Le 9 *avril*.—L'enfant présente un peu d'enchifrènement. Légère fièvre, 38° 1 dans le rectum. Cependant la suppuration d'oreille diminue : la perforation demeure insuffisante ; le tympan se rétracte et le marteau commence à se dessiner.

Le 10 *avril*.—La température atteint 40° 2 ; il n'y a pour expliquer cette hyperthermie ni recrudescence de douleurs d'oreilles, ni augmentation de l'otorrhée ; la perforation tympanique est large, il n'y a pas de rétention. Mais l'enfant a la respiration nasale complètement entravée et le badigeonnage de la gorge ramène du naso-pharynx d'abondants masses de muco-pus. Cette poussée hyperthermique est due à une *adénoïdite* intercurrente.

Le 12 *avril*.—Température normale, suppuration auriculaire presque nulle, l'adénoïdite semble avoir agi vis-à-vis de l'otite à la façon d'un puissant dérivatif.

Le 22 *avril*.—Guérison.

———

Mlle Tet... (Madeleine), 8 ans.

Sœur de la malade précédente, demeurant dans la même chambre, est prise de rougeole en même temps qu'elle.

Deux jours après le début de l'otite de sa sœur, elle commence à souffrir surtout de l'oreille droite. Jamais d'otite antérieure ; mais adénoïdisme déjà ancien.

Je la vois le 21 *mars* 1897, en même temps que sa sœur. Mauvais état général, maux de tête ; vomissements, douleur d'oreille très vive. Pas encore d'écoulement ; à droite, le tympan est rouge vif et fortement bombé. Paracentèse d'urgence. Glycérine phéniquée. La famille se refuse à donner la douche d'air.

Le 30 *mars* l'enfant se réveille ayant mal à la tête et parfois nausées : la suppuration d'oreille continue. TR : 38°5. A midi la température atteint 39°5. L'enfant est amenée d'urgence à Paris.—A deux heures, 40°5 : maux de tête violents, prostration : l'apophyse est excessivement douloureuse au moindre frôle-ment. Le Dr. Egger, appelé à ce moment, constate une perforation tympanique très suffisante : mais la douche d'air, qui n'a pas été encore donnée, administrée vigoureusement, fait sortir une grande quantité de muco-pus accumulé dans la caisse. Le soir même les accidents cessent.

Le 1er *avril* l'enfant a bien dormi.—TR : 37°5. Toute douleur de tête a disparu. Mastoïde normale. Large perforation tympanique donnant issue à beaucoup de muco-pus.

Le 9 *avril* l'écoulement d'oreilles, très réduit les jours précédents, devient excessivement abondant.

Le 12 *avril*.—*Pousée d'adénoïdite* : TR : 39°2. Toux quinteuse, nez un peu bouché : muco-pus descendant du cerveau dans le pharynx.

20 *avril*.—Guérison.

Il faut remarquer que pendant toute la durée de leur otite les deux sœurs ont occupé deux lits jumeaux.

IV. Encore une observation du même genre.

Deux enfants, deux sœurs, prennent une grippe légère, et toutes deux font une otite aiguë à marche analogue, otite légère et courte, de type congestif avec ecchymoses tympanales.

OBS. IV et IV *bis.*—Mlle Germaine de Dal..., 5 ans.

Aurait eu, il y a deux ans, une otite aiguë gauche.

Je la vois le 9 *janvier* 1899.—Depuis cinq jours, grippe légère à forme catarrhale. Fièvre, otalgie violente.

Ce matin, après une bonne nuit, il n'y a ni fièvre, ni douleur d'oreille spontanée ou provoquée.

L'oreille gauche est seule atteinte. Le tympan est transparent, non bombé et laisse voir un fond de caisse rouge vineux, ecchymotique. Le manche du marteau a une couleur rouge sombre.

Le lendemain, le tympan a repris son aspect grisâtre : mais il y a une ligne d'ecchymoses punctiformes en arrière du manche du marteau et parallèle à lui.

Le 13 *janvier.*—Ces ecchymoses pâlissent légèrement.

Mlle Suzanne de Dal..., 8 ans.

Sœur de la précédente, soignée par moi l'année précédente pour une otite moyenne aiguë purulente gauche.

Cette enfant, couchant dans la même chambre que sa sœur, prend d'elle une grippe légère vers le 10 janvier, avec poussée d'adénoïdite.

Le 16 *janvier.*—Je suis appelé près d'elle. Depuis la veille elle souffre de l'oreille gauche ; cependant la nuit a amené une sédation. De ce côté le tympan est grisâtre et montre un fond de caisse très foncé, le manche du marteau a une teinte rouge vineuse. Pas d'écoulement.

Le 20 *janvier.*—Je constate un piqueté ecchymotique en arrière et tout le long du manche du marteau.

V. Suit un cas du même genre mais plus net. Chez un frère et une sœur, sans infection rubéolique ou grippale qui prépare le terrain, éclate une otite aiguë à forme hémorrhagique, débutant par un épanchement de sang dans la caisse avec bulle sanguine tympanale. Puis suppuration secondaire et évolution sans peine ni douleur. Il est vrai que les deux enfants lavaient leur nez au siphon de Weber : mais cette imprudence ne saurait, ce me semble, être incriminée en l'espèce, attendu que dans le cas actuel, les otites n'avaient aucunement le caractère des suppurations banales de la caisse consécutives aux lavages du nez.

OBS. V et V *bis.* — Fernand S. T.. , 6 ans.

A la fin d'un coryza subaigu, traité par des lavages divers au siphon de Weber, cet enfant est pris d'une violente douleur d'oreille gauche, sans fièvre, ni état général. Un spécialiste appelé à ce moment, porte le diagnostic de *myringite hémorrhagique phlycténulaire.* Quelques jours après, sans autre traitement que des bains locaux, l'oreille gauche se met à suppurer.

Le 1er *juin* 1897, je suis appelé pour voir cet enfant. Je constate, à gauche, une membrane tympanique rouge très tendue, avec une fistulette insuffisante, laissant échapper du pus sous pression. Mastoïdite douloureuse au frôlement. Large paracentèse : glycérine phéniquée.

3 *juin.*—Pas de douleurs, la caisse se vide bien et abondamment.

10 *juin.*—L'écoulement devient beaucoup plus filant.. Il s'écoule avec peine ; tympan rouge et très bombé.   La famille s'oppose à une nouvelle paracentèse.

20 *juin.*—Guérison.

———

Renée S. T..., 5 ans.

Pas de passé auriculaire, malgré un coryza purulent chronique très ancien. Depuis quelques jours, fait des lavages du nez très prudents, à l'aide d'une seringue anglaise.   Passe, d'ailleurs, une partie de ses journées à jouer avec son frère.

10 *juin.*—Sans fièvre, l'état général demeurant bien, elle éprouve, en se mouchant, une vive douleur dans l'oreille gauche. Le lendemain, j'examine l'enfant. A gauche, le tympan, bombé dans son quart postéro-supérieur ; par transparence, on voit un fond de caisse rouge foncé, lie de vin ; au premier abord, on pourrait croire qu'il s'est fait sur le tympan une énorme bulle sanguine.   L'oreille droite, qui n'est le siège d'aucune souffrance, montre, en différents points du tympan et surtout tout autour du manche du marteau, un fin piqueté ecchymotique.

13 *juin.*—Tympan rouge et très bombé, avec un point jaunâtre au centre de cette saillie.   La famille s'oppose à la paracentèse.

16 *juin.*—Conduit plein de muco-pus, qui s'échappe par une fistulette de la partie antéro-inférieure du tympan.

25 *juin.*—Guérison.

VI. Voici maintenant une observation curieuse. Au cours d'une grippe légère, une vieille dame est brusquement prise d'une otite moyenne double hémorrhagique, de type apoplectiforme, avec participation de l'oreille externe. Et la femme de chambre qui la soigne, prend, deux jours après, d'abord une grippe légère, puis une otite hémorrhagique brusque de tous points semblable à la première.

obs. vi et vi *bis.*—Mme P..., 72 ans. Diabétique.

Au huitième jour d'une grippe légère, est prise brusquement d'une violente douleur dans l'oreille droite ; à la suite d'une crise douloureuse, plus forte que les autres, écoulement par le conduit, d'abord de sang pur, puis de sérosité sanguinolente sans pus.

6 *février.*—Bulles sanguines rompues à la surface du tympan. Le marteau a une teinte hémorrhagique.

La membrane tympanique est très bombée.   Paracentèse.

8 *février.*—Le Politzer ne fait sortir de l'O.G. que de la sérosité sanguinolente.

Depuis hier, l'O.D. est prise à son tour.   Début par une hémorrhagie du conduit: suivie d'un écoulement séro-sanguin peu abondant qui dure encore. Tympan rouge foncé, très bombé.   Fait une paracentèse qui ne ramène que du sang.

10 *février.*—Réapparition de douleurs depuis hier : les incisions tympaniques sont déjà cicatrisées.   Fait une nouvelle paracentèse bilatérale : à gauche, une goutte de pus : à droite, rien que du sang.

12 *février.*—Détaché du conduit auditif et de la surface du tympan O. G., une épaisse membrane, due à la nécrose des couches superficielles des téguments dans lesquels s'était fait précédemment l'exsudat hémorrhagique.

14 *février.*—Détaché une même membrane du conduit auditif droit.

20 *février.*—Nouvelle phlyctène hémorrhagique dans le conduit.

25 *février.* -Guérison.

La femme de chambre de cette malade, qui est en relations de service constantes avec elle, est prise, le 8 février, d'une légère grippe à forme rhino-bronchique.

10 *février*.—Douleur subite dans l'oreille gauche.

12 *février*.—Je constate que le quart postéro-inférieur du tympan est recouvert d'une bulle séro-hémorrhagique. Le reste de la membrane est plat et gris, le marteau rose.

14 *février*.—La bulle tympanique prend un aspect réellement hémorrhagique. Je perds alors la malade de vue.

Pour ne pas prolonger cette liste, je terminerai par une observation semblable aux précédentes.

Une femme de chambre sans prodromes de grippe ou de rhume est atteinte assez brusquement d'une otite aiguë hémorrhagique, avec bulle sanguine sur le tympan et les parois du conduit. Et quatre jours plus tard son jeune maître, dont elle s'occupe, est soudainement aussi pris d'une otite semblable, de même type et d'évolution analogue.

OBS. VII et VII *bis*.—M. De...., 16 ans.

18 *avril*.—Sans passé autre qu'une pharyngomycose spontanément guérie depuis un an. Ce malade est brusquement pris d'une crise d'otalgie droite, tandis qu'un écoulement séro-sanguin extrêmement abondant se déclare par le conduit auditif droit.

19 *avril*.—Cet écoulement dure encore. Je constate dans l'oreille droite, à la surface du tympan, ainsi que dans le conduit, plusieurs larges bulles sanguines rompues, baignées de sérosité sanguinolente.

21 *avril*.—Aucune douleur, l'écoulement persiste sans changer de nature. Pas de perforation tympanique : mais la membrane est rouge, érodée, très tendue : l'audition à la montre est de : O. G. = 0,80 et O. D. = 0,03.

22 *avril*.—37° 8 sous l'aisselle. Douleur vive dans l'oreille droite. Fait une paracentèse.

24 *avril*.—Un écoulement muco-purulent s'établit abondant. Pansement à la glycérine boratée.

1ᵉʳ *mai*.—Écoulement insignifiant : le tympan est plat et gris, la perforation bien béante.

6 *mai*.—Tout écoulement a cessé.

24 *juin*.—Perforation close par une cicatrice : mais le marteau est immobile au Siègle et l'audition demeure au-dessus de la cervicale. Montre, O. D. = 0,50.

———

La femme de chambre de la maison, qui s'occupe des vêtements et du linge du malade, et a de nombreux contacts de service avec lui, avait été prise trois ou quatre fois avant lui d'accidents analogues et dans les mêmes conditions ; c'est-à-dire que sans grippe, sans coryza antérieur, dans le cours d'une bonne santé, elle avait ressenti des douleurs vives et subites de l'oreille gauche, avec surdité et écoulement séro-sanguinolent. Ces douleurs persistaient pendant une semaine avec intermittence.

Mon assistant, le Dʳ Laurens, qui voulut bien, en mon absence, examiner cette malade, constata, au huitième jour de la maladie, une grosse phlyctène hémorrhagique sur le quart postéro-supérieur du tympan, et deux autres bulles sanguines sur la paroi du conduit.

Cinq à six jours plus tard, la phlyctène a disparu et le tympan se rétracte peu à peu sans suppuration.

On pourrait évidemment interpréter ces observations comme des faits de pure coïncidence. Une telle argumentation est vraiment facile.

Cependant, cette prétendue coïncidence s'est présentée à moi, en deux ans, dans des conditions tellement précises qu'elle ne laisse pas que de susciter quelque méfiance à son égard. La plupart des associations cliniques, les mieux établies aujourd'hui, n'ont-elles pas été, par les premiers observateurs, considérées comme des faits de coïncidence fortuite?

J'ajoute que cette prétendue coïncidence est d'une *fréquence* qui n'est pas sans mériter qu'on la remarque. De 1897 à 1899, période qui comprend les observations rapportées plus haut, j'ai suivi dans ma clientèle environ 20 otites moyennes aiguës graves. Donc, c'est dans le tiers des cas (7 fois sur 20) que s'est produite cette coïncidence, qui m'en aurait imposé pour de la contagion. On avouera que je suis tombé sur une série tout au moins heureuse.

En outre—et la coïncidence devient ici des plus remarquables—les otites que j'ai observées simultanément chez mari et femme, chez frère et sœur, chez maitre et domestique, avaient exactement le *même type*. Or, quand un individu sain, mis en rapport avec un malade, contracte au contact de ce dernier une maladie d'allures identiques, et que cette constatation se renouvelle dans un tiers des cas observés, on est très en droit de soupçonner en cela une contagion, bien plutôt que de se laisser aller à la croyance trop aisée en une coïncidence.

* *

Une objection beaucoup plus sérieuse pourrait encore m'être faite, qui est celle-ci.

On prend pour contagion, devrait-on me dire, une *maladie* et non une *affection* : la maladie étant un processus morbide envisagé dans toute son évolution ; l'affection étant ce processus considéré momentanément dans une de ses manifestations actuelles ou locales. Ainsi on contracte d'une autre personne une maladie telle que la rougeole, la grippe, même une streptococcie, une pneumococcie ; mais on ne peut recevoir directement d'elle une affection telle qu'une otite morbilleuse, une otite grippale. La localisation d'une rougeole dans l'oreille, la complication otique ne peut être individualisée au point de se transmettre par elle-même à un individu sain.

A cela je répondrai par l'exemple de la pneumonie franche aiguë. Théoriquement, on peut prendre par contagion une infection pneumococcique ; mais un malade pneumonique ne devrait pas pouvoir transmettre directement à son voisin une affection, telle que la localisation de la pneumococcie sur le poumon. Les exemples abondent cependant qui démontrent que la pneumonie est contagieuse ; le pneumocoque se transporte de poumon à poumon. Rien n'empêche donc, par analogie, d'admettre que le streptocoque ne puisse se transmettre d'oreille à oreille. Puisque, bien qu'affection du poumon et non pas maladie, la pneumonie est contagieuse en tant que pneumonie, l'otite moyenne aiguë peut bien de même être contagieuse en tant qu'otite.— Gardons-nous des errements de nos ancêtres qui, pendant des siècles, fermèrent leurs yeux à l'observation des faits par respect pour des théories qui, elles au moins, avaient le privilège de l'âge.

On me dira encore : " Mais comment prendre une otite au contact "d'un otitique ? La caisse du tympan n'est pas en rapport direct avec "le monde extérieur. Que d'une angine on prenne une angine, ou d'un "coryza, un coryza, cela est possible : mais comment admettre que deux "organes aussi profondément situés que les oreilles puissent s'entre-"infecter ?..."

Une telle contagion serait difficile à admettre, en effet, si elle se présentait ainsi. Dans certaines de mes observations, il semble, à première vue, que l'otite ait éclaté soudainement au voisinage d'une autre otite. En réalité tous les malades s'infectaient par la voie classique naso-tubaire : ils commençaient nécessairement par avoir un coryza ; mais celui-ci était tellement atténué, que, cliniquement, il passait inaperçu. Dans le même ordre d'idées ne connaissons-nous pas les mastoïdites soi-disant primitives, à l'origine desquelles un observateur attentif dépiste toujours une traînée de rhino-salpingite latente ? Du reste, pour reprendre ma comparaison, on prend une pneumonie d'un pneumonique, sans présenter le plus souvent de symptômes cliniques de laryngite ; et la contagion semble se faire directement de poumon à poumon, quelque profondément situés que soient ces organes.

*
* *

Il n'est donc pas impossible qu'un individu sain, mis au contact d'un otitique, prenne de ce dernier une otite moyenne aiguë. Cependant, cette manière de contracter une inflammation *primitive* de la caisse du tympan doit être excessivement rare ; et j'avoue que mes observations n'en donnent pas la démonstration.

Dans les faits que je rapporte, contagionnants et contagionnés étaient presque tous atteints d'une maladie protopathique, grippe ou rougeole, sur laquelle était venue se greffer l'affection de l'oreille. Ces otites étaient donc *secondaires*, survenant à titre de complications. Et ce que mes observations tendent à prouver est surtout ceci : étant donné un premier malade atteint de grippe compliquée d'otite, tout autre grippé, mis en contact avec lui, aura grande chance de prendre cette complication otique.

Au reste, l'histoire de ces otites peut être calquée sur celle des broncho-pneumonies.

La broncho-pneumonie est presque toujours une affection secondaire, survenant principalement au cours de la rougeole et de la grippe. Elle n'est pas, comme le crurent longtemps les cliniciens, la localisation sur le poumon de la maladie infectieuse protopathique ; ce n'est pas, comme l'avaient pensé les premiers bactériologistes, le microbe spécifique qui provoque les lésions pulmonaires. Elle est, au contraire, une complication contingente, cliniquement superposée à la maladie générale et bactériologiquement due à une infection secondaire, surtout par le streptocoque.

Remplaçons dans cette donnée le mot de broncho-pneumonie par celui d'otite : et nous ne ferons qu'en registrer une constatation acceptée aujourd'hui par tous les auristes. Ce n'est ni l'agent inconnu de la rougeole, ni le microbe de Pfeiffer qui engendre les otites moyennes aiguës chez les morbilleux ou les influenzés, mais presque toujours le streptocoque.

Or, la contagiosité de la broncho-pneumonie secondaire est démontrée : l'influence nocive de l'encombrement est manifeste. La broncho-pneumonie est d'une fréquence extrême dans les salles d'enfants au cours, par exemple, de la rougeole, alors que cette complication est vraiment exceptionnelle dans la clientèle privée (Collet).

Donc — par analogie — l'otite secondaire qui se comporte comme la broncho-pneumonie doit avoir une même contagiosité.

*
* *

J'ai fait pour m'en convaincre, une enquête auprès d'un certain nombre de confrères et surtout de mes collègues des hôpitaux de Paris chargés du service des contagieux. Voici quels en ont été les résultats.

Rougeole. — M. Descroizilles, chargé du service de la rougeole à l'hôpital des Enfants-Malades, note environ 20% d'otites sur tous les enfants de son service pris en bloc. Dans sa clientèle de ville, la proportion des otites morbilleuses ne dépasse pas 1%. La nocivité de l'encombrement s'affirme donc ici d'une manière saisissante.

Chez l'adulte, l'oreille se prend beaucoup moins facilement que chez l'enfant ; pourtant M. Roger, chargé du service de la rougeole adulte à l'hôpital de la Porte d'Aubervilliers, note 34 otites purulentes aiguës sur 1,081 malades — soit une proportion de 3,14%.

En revanche, plusieurs médecins d'enfants très occupés, entre autres, mon ami le Dr. Carron de la Carrière, me déclarent ne voir pour ainsi dire jamais d'otites aiguës dans leur clientèle de rougeoleux, à condition de faire l'antisepsie naso-buccale dès le début de la maladie.

Scarlatine. — M. d'Heilly, chargé du service de la scarlatine à l'hôpital des Enfants-Malades, note 14% d'otites chez ses malades, proportion qui s'élevait à 25% quand il faisait pratiquer systématiquement des irrigations nasales. En ville, il en voit infiniment moins.

M. Variot, chargé du service de la scarlatine à l'hôpital Trousseau, m'écrit que les otites scarlatineuses sont beaucoup moins fréquentes en ville qu'à l'hôpital.

Chez les scarlatineux adultes de l'hôpital de la Porte d'Aubervilliers, M. Roger note sur 997 malades 3% d'otites aiguës purulentes.

En revanche, plusieurs médecins d'enfants me disent que, parmi leur clientèle l'otite aiguë est rarissime dans la scarlatine. Pour ma part, en deux ans, je n'ai été appelé qu'une seule fois en ville auprès d'une otite scarlatineuse.

Cette statistique — que j'abrège à dessein pour ne donner que les chiffres le plus précis — est très instructive ; elle démontre nettement la fréquence des otites aiguës secondaires à l'hôpital et leur rareté en ville.

Or, il y a lieu de faire à ce sujet, deux remarques très importantes :

1° A l'hôpital on laisse les malades atteints d'otite secondaire dans la salle commune, *sans les isoler ;*

2° Et à très peu d'exceptions près, les otites aiguës observées chez les rougeoleux et les scarlatineux nosocomiaux *ont débuté dans la salle*, quelque temps seulement après l'entrée à l'hôpital.

Cette statistique ne plaide-t-elle pas éloquemment en faveur de la contagiosité des otites aiguës secondaires ?

**
**

Un dernier argument en faveur de la contagiosité des otites aiguës secondaires se tire du caractère des diverses épidémies d'influenza qui se sont succédées à Paris depuis 1889.˙ Certains hivers, la grippe a peu touché l'oreille ; d'autres fois, comme dans l'épidémie initiale et comme dans la dernière, les otites aiguës ont été fréquentes et graves. Or, la grippe se prend surtout par contagion d'individu à individu : que signifient donc ces caractères d'épidémicité, sinon que quand les malades ont seulement la grippe, ils ne transmettent que la grippe, tandis que quand ils sont atteints d'otite secondaire, ils transmettent à la fois leur grippe et leur otite par une double contagion simultanée.

**
**

Mes observations personelles ne sont pas assez nombreuses pour préciser les caractères cliniques de la contagiosité des otites aiguës. Cependant je puis dès maintenant faire deux remarques.

C'est d'abord que la durée de l'incubation de l'otite aiguë semble assez courte. Cette période a été respectivement, dans mes divers cas, de deux, trois, cinq, six et sept jours ; une seule fois seulement de deux semaines.

En second lieu, il est remarquable de voir que l'otite aiguë se transmet en conservant son type clinique, catarrhale, purulente ou hémorrhagique ; son intensité varie, non sa forme.

**
**

Une conclusion pratique se dégage de cette étude : *Il faut isoler les malades, surtout les enfants atteints d'otite moyenne aiguë*, même si elle est primitive et à plus forte raison si elle se surajoute comme complication secondaire à une maladie infectieuse.

Nous avons vu que broncho-pneumonie et otite secondaire ont une même pathogénie. A l'hôpital on a considérablement diminué le nombre de broncho-pneumonies et, ce faisant, restreint la gravité de fièvres éruptives, en séparant des rougeoleux simples, des rougeoleux broncho-pneumoniques.

Il faut agir de même vis-à-vis de l'otite.

Or l'otite aiguë n'est pas moins grave que la broncho-pneumonie. Son apparente bénignité la rend peu suspecte, car elle n'amène pas ordinairement la mort en quelques jours, comme le fait la broncho-pneumonie. Mes collègues des hôpitaux en me transmettant si aimablement leur statistique, me faisaient remarquer que presque toujours les otites aiguës avaient été si bénignes qu'elles n'avaient nécessité aucun traitement chirurgical ; qu'on s'était contenté de leur donner de l'eau boriquée et de la glycérine phéniquée : cependant ils ajoutaient que pas mal d'enfants quittaient l'hôpital suppurant encore. Or, l'avenir de ces oreilles est sombre. Il est exceptionnel que l'otite aiguë amène la mort à sa période d'état : il est fréquent qu'elle la cause quand elle s'est chronicisée. Ces enfants, qui quittent l'hôpital avec des oreilles qui suppurent, vont grossir cette foule d'otorrhéiques qui encombrent les services spéciaux, et qui souvent n'auront d'autre moyen d'éviter la terminaison fatale que l'évidement pétromastoïdien : heureux encore s'ils guérissent sans garder une surdité qui les rende impropres à toute carrière.

Prévenir est mieux que guérir. Il est plus simple d'empêcher une otite aiguë d'éclater que de la traiter ensuite. Pour réaliser cette prophylaxie, l'antisepsie nasale et buccale est une excellente pratique dont les résultats sont encourageants. Mais il y a encore mieux à faire.

L'otite aiguë est contagieuse.

Isolons les otitiques.

SUR DEUX CAS DE COMPLICATIONS ENCÉPHALIQUES (ABCÈS-CÉRÉBRAUX) D'ORIGINE OTIQUE.

PROF. E. J. MOURE, Bordeaux.

Depuis que l'Otologie est entrée dans la voie chirurgicale nous avons de temps à autre l'occasion d'observer des complications otitiques évoluant du côté de la cavité crânienne. Comme cette partie de la pathologie a encore besoin d'être mise au point, nous pensons qu'il est du devoir de tous les chirurgiens de rapporter les faits qu'ils ont l'occasion d'observer de manière à rassembler ainsi des matériaux destinés à élever plus tard un édifice sérieux basé sur des séries d'observations. Ainsi arriveront peu à peu à s'élucider les différents caractères cliniques des diverses complications encéphaliques d'origine auriculaire, qui il faut l'avouer, sont encore aujourd'hui difficiles à diagnostiquer.

En effet, sauf les cas où les lésions siègent dans des points du cerveau susceptibles de réagir à l'extérieur, centres moteurs ou autres, les symptômes sont souvent si vagues et si différents, souvent même si légers qu'il est impossible au clinicien de poser le diagnostic précis et surtout de fixer le moment de l'intervention chirurgicale. Dans quelques cas en effet, en particulier pour les abcès extra-duraux, nous voyons s'établir lentement sans doute, de vastes collections de pus autour de l'encéphale, sans que le malade en éprouve autre chose qu'un peu de gêne ou de mal de tête de temps à autre, quelquefois un peu de torpeur consécutive à la compression cérébrale concomitante, mais ces différents signes sont loin d'être suffisants pour permettre au chirurgien d'intervenir s'il n'est poussé par les circonstances telles qu'une otorrhée ancienne, un trajet fistuleux quelconque pendant l'opération duquel il est conduit sur la région extradure-mérienne.

Dans une autre série de cas le malade éprouve un certain nombre de symptômes indiquant que l'encéphale doit être atteint dans une de ses parties, et lorsqu'à l'opération en partant du foyer otitique, on arrive sur la dure-mère, que l'on rencontre à ce niveau une collection purulente, il est d'usage de borner là son intervention, bien convaincu que les altérations constatées peuvent expliquer les troubles ressentis par le malade et observés avant l'opération.

Très souvent alors l'opérateur voit après l'ouverture de cet abcès extra-dural les phénomènes cérébraux continuer ou même s'accentuer ; son intervention a été insuffisante et il ne lui est pas toujours loisible de pouvoir la continuer, surtout lorsqu'on agit dans la clientèle de ville. Cependant, est-il logique, à moins d'avoir des signes de localisation très nets et même dans ces cas, est-il logique, dis-je, si l'on trouve une lésion extradurale considérable en rapport avec la lésion otitique, d'ouvrir de propos délibéré les méninges et de ponctionner le cerveau risquant ainsi d'exposer le malade à une infection qui n'existait pas auparavant.

En effet lorsque après une opération d'urgence les accidents continuent il y a lieu de se demander, à moins qu'on n'ait trouvé du pus à la ponction cérébrale, si les accidents existaient avant, ou n'ont pas été la conséquence d'une infection chirurgicale. Le fait suivant est encore intéressant à ce point de vue ; la première opération n'a soulagé le malade que pendant quelque temps, puis les phénomènes ont continué à s'accentuer, à se délimiter même, montrant qu'il s'agissait d'une façon certaine d'une lésion encéphalique.

OBSERVATION I.

ABCÈS DU CERVEAU CONSECUTIF À UNE VIEILLE OTORRHÉE RÉCHAUFFÉE PAR LA GRIPPE. CURE RADICALE. ABCÈS EXTRA-DURAL. ARRÊT DE L'INTERVENTION. AMÉLIORATION TRÈS MANIFESTE. CINQ JOURS APRÈS, NOUVEAUX SYMPTÔMES CÉRÉBRAUX ENTRAÎNANT LA MORT EN 48 HEURES. LA FAMILLE AVAIT REFUSÉ UNE 2e INTERVENTION.—(Recueillie et rédigée par le Dr. Brindel, aide du clinique otologique à la Faculté de Bordeaux.)

M.M. 50 ans, est porteur d'une ancienne suppuration de l'oreille gauche. Il a contracté la grippe il y a un mois. Depuis 12 à 14 jours il éprouve des douleurs aiguës très vives dans la région mastoïdienne. Il y a 4 jours se sont déclarés des accidents cérébraux : délire, fièvre sans rémission 39 et 40° et céphalalgies très intenses du côté malade. Depuis deux jours le malade est en demi coma et a des sueurs profuses. La pression de l'apophyse au niveau de l'antre est fort douloureuse. Il existe de la paralysie faciale unilatérale du côté malade.

Le malade est vu pour la première fois en consultation par le Dr. Moure le 5 Novembre. Une intervention est immédiatement décidée mais ne peut être exécutée que le 7 Novembre.

OPÉRATION DU 7 NOVEMBRE, 1898.—Incision dans le pli rétro-auriculaire ; suture pétro-squameuse très marquée. M. Moure agrandit le conduit osseux dans sa moitié supérieure au moyen de la gouge et du maillet.

Première couche de tissu paraissant peu dure. Puis dureté considérable de l'apophyse. D'un coup de gouge la surface externe du sinus latéral est mise à nu. Elle n'est distante que d'un centimètre et demi en arrière du conduit.

Dans une cellule de l'apophyse, sur la paroi inférieure de la brèche mastoïdienne créée par la gouge, existe du pus. L'antre est mis à nu. Il est petit, haut placé, rempli ainsi que la caisse et le canal tympano-mastoïdien, de matières caséeuses et de fongosités. LE TOIT DE L'ANTRE ET DE LA CAISSE N'EXISTE PLUS. La paroi osseuse est détruite sur une assez grande étendue. IL EXISTE DU PUS ET DES FONGOSITÉS SUR LES MÉNINGES. Après curettage elles apparaissent résistantes et on borne là l'intervention.

Curettage soigneux de la grande cavité formée par l'antre, l'apophyse, la caisse et le canal tympano-mastoïdien. Section du conduit membraneux sur toute sa longueur et en son milieu. Relèvement du lambeau inférieur par un point de suture au catgut. Ablation du bord du lambeau supérieur.

Fermeture immédiate de la plaie rétro-auriculaire. Pansement à la gaze iodoformée par le méat.

7 Nov. AU SOIR.—L'intelligence commence à revenir. La fièvre n'est plus que de 38°.

DU 7 AU 10 NOVEMBRE.—L'intelligence revient. Il n'y a plus de fièvre.

18 NOVEMBRE.—Le malade s'intéresse à son état. Il ne souffre plus de la tête. La paralysie faciale persiste néanmoins. L'état général semble bon. Le pansement est renouvelé. Pas de pus. Un purgatif est ordonné.

11 NOVEMBRE.—Le malade se sent bien. Il demande s'il en a encore pour longtemps à être complètement guéri. Il se lève et commence à manger avec appétit.

12 NOVEMBRE.—Brusquement, dans la nuit du 11 au 12 le délire apparaît de nouveau, ainsi que le coma. Le malade porte fréquemment sa main gauche à la tête, sur son pansement. Il ne répond à aucune question.

Le soir il est toujours dans le coma, a 31 inspirations à la minute, 100 pulsations et une fièvre de 39° 2.

Le bras droit est nettement et fortement parésié.

Incontinence d'urine.

Le pansement est refait. Plus de pus.

Respiration stertoreuse.

13 Novembre. I heure du soir.—Même état. Bras droit complètement paralysé. Respiration très bruyante. 51 inspirations à la minute. 147 pulsations. Coma. Les pupilles réagissent un peu à la lumière. Le malade souffre manifestement de la tête, car de temps à autre il porte violemment la main gauche sur le pansement qui environne son oreille.

On propose à la famille une nouvelle intervention qui eût consisté dans une crâniectomie au niveau du lobe temporal, et une ou plusieurs ponctions du cerveau car on se croit en présence de tous les signes d'un abcès de la substance cérébrale.

La famille, forte inintelligente, refuse cette nouvelle intervention bien qu'elle eût été prévenue de sa possibilité avant la première opération.

Le malade meurt le 14 Novembre, 1898. Pas d'autopsie.

Je pourrais rapprocher de ce cas celui que j'ai publié autrefois, dans lequel la lésion extra-durale (abcès) une fois vidée, l'amélioration ne suivit pas et je n'eus pas le temps d'intervenir une seconde fois, la malade étant morte 48 heures après des suites d'un énorme abcès du cerveau dont je pus constater l'existence à l'autopsie.

Donc, la conduite du chirurgien en cas de complications intra-crâniennes (phlébites excepté) peut être quelquefois très difficile à déterminer. En effet, lorsqu'une affection de ce genre est soupçonnée et qu'une intervention est pratiquée, il convient de savoir si en l'absence de tout symptôme de localisation cérébrale et quelquefois même dans ces cas, il s'agit de savoir dis-je si l'existence d'une collection extra-durale ou d'une irritation méningée facile à constater, doit arrêter la main du chirurgien ou si au contraire il doit malgré l'existence de ces lésions, extradurales pousser plus loin son intervention. Il semble logique d'admettre que sauf exception c'est à la seconde hypothèse qu'un chirurgien sage doit s'arrêter, quitte à continuer son opération 24 ou 48 heures après, si les symptômes ne s'amendent pas comme ils devraient le faire, si la lésion unique avait été supprimée.

Quelle que soit la clientèle dans laquelle on opère, hôpital ou la ville, il me paraît que la manière d'agir doit être la même dans les deux cas et si en ville les familles font des difficultés pour permettre au chirurgien de faire une seconde opération, il a somme toute dégagé sa responsabilité et sa conscience en agissant comme je viens de le dire.

Par contre si les lésions constatées à l'extérieur de la dure-mère ne sont pas suffisantes pour expliquer les troubles observés, il ne faut pas hésiter dans ce cas à aller d'emblée plus loin jusque dans l'encéphale, pour chercher la cause des symptômes observés. Quelquefois il sera possible de la trouver, d'autrefois au contraire malgré une intervention radicale les symptômes ne continueront pas moins à évoluer et la mort surviendra malgré l'intervention. C'est surtout dans les cas d'abcès du cerveau, dépourvus de parois, que le traitement devient difficile à appliquer et que l'ouverture de la collection purulente ne suffit pas pour guérir le malade. C'est un fait de ce genre que je tiens à rapporter, il est intéressant à plusieurs points de vue, d'abord par les symptômes constatés à l'aide desquels nous avons pu nettement établir le diagnostic d'abcès cérébral. D'un autre côté les incidents opératoires assez insolites en pareil cas, méritent d'appeler notre attention.

OBSERVATION II.

ABCÈS DU CERVEAU CONSÉCUTIF À UNE OTITE MOYENNE AIGUË SUPPURÉE AVEC MASTOÏDITE. OPÉRATION DE STACKE. PONCTION DU CERVEAU. ÉVACUATION SPONTANÉE DE L'ABCÈS DANS LA PLAIE 10 JOURS APRÈS L'INTERVENTION. AMÉLIORATION PASSAGÈRE. MORT LE 22e JOUR PAR HÉMORRHAGIE DANS LE FOYER DE L'ABCÈS AVEC INONDATION VENTRICULAIRE. AUTOPSIE.—(Recueillie et rédigée par le Dr. Brindel, aide du clinique otologique à la Faculté de Bordeaux).

2 JANVIER 1899.—Gilis L... 36 ans, épicier, contracte un refroidissement et un mal de gorge il y a 17 jours. A ce moment se met au lit avec fièvre. Dès le lendemain se plaint de violent mal de tête et de douleurs dans L'OREILLE GAUCHE. 2 jours après : écoulement par l'oreille et soulagement de la douleur auriculaire (Il y a par conséquent 15 jours).

Le 6e ou le 7e jour après le début de la maladie, nouvelles douleurs auriculaires et CEPHALÉE INTENSES qui n'ont plus quitté le malade. Depuis cette époque (22 xbre 1898, insomnie, inappétence.)

Le 31 XBRE 1898 : début des phénomènes intellectuels. A partir de ce jour il commence à perdre ses idées et a avoir quelques vertiges.

ÉTAT ACTUEL : EXAMEN FONCTIONNEL.

P.C.D.   12 000 §   diminution très notable de la perception
P.C.G.   12 000 §   crânienne et disparition de la perception aux points 2, 3, 4, 5 des 2 côtés

M.O.D.   0,01 cm
M.O.G.   Contact
Diap. Vert.   m.à g.
R.O.D.   +   (un peu mieux entendu avec diapason grave)
R.O.G.   =
Sifflet de Galton :   à droite **1 m** | 4e division du sifflet
à gauche, près |
de l'oreille |

EXAMEN OBJECTIF.—Suppuration à gauche. Petite perforation du tympan au centre. Douleur à la pression sur l'apophyse gauche qui est légèrement soulevée en masse. Pas de douleur à la percussion du crâne.

HÉBÉTUDE.—Débilité. Perte d'appétit. Légère constipation. CÉPHALALGIE FRONTALE INTENSE. Quelques vertiges. PAS DE VOMISSEMENTS. POULS : 80 À LA MINUTE. Donc pas de ralentissement.

Pas la moindre convulsion, contracture, ni paralysie motrice. Température normale 37°.

HÉMIANOPSIE HOMONYME DROITE.
Examen de l'oeil | Egalité des pupilles.
| La pupille réagit moins faiblement.
| Papille un peu congestionnée des deux côtés (Congestion veineuse). Dans son ensemble la papille est plus rosée.
| Tracé du champ visuel : très rétréci sur l'hémisphère où il existe.
Réflexes normaux. Sensibilité normale partout.

PHÉNOMÈNES INTELLECTUELS : Cécité verbale. Aphasie de conductibilité. Amnésie verbale. Examen du Prof. Pitres.

DÉNOMINATION ET RECONNAISSANCE DES OBJETS : On montre au malade une boîte d'allumettes, il ne peut prononcer le mot ni dire à quoi cela sert. Il ne peut non plus désigner une clef, un porte-plume, mais dit : c'est pour fermer, c'est pour écrire. Il reconnaît une montre, il reconnaît l'heure. IL NE PEUT LIRE AUCUNE ÉCRITURE.

Il reconnaît les chiffres, O. 8. 5. La lettre S, mais non les T, I, M, Q, F. Il reconnaît G. I. L. lettres entrant dans son nom. Il ne reconnaît point son nom Gilis formé des lettres qu'il a reconnues séparément. Il arrive cependant à lire son nom propre formé avec des lettres identiques.

LA RÉPÉTITION DES MOTS EST PARFAITE : ainsi il répète : chapeau, parapluie, inconstitutionnellement, quelques mots allemands, etc.

ÉCRITURE SOUS DICTÉE.—On lui dit d'écrire BORDEAUX puis PARIS. Après avoir écrit les quatre premières lettres de chacun de ces noms il s'arrête et est dans l'impossibilité de continuer, bien qu'on lui dicte les lettres. Il écrit les chiffres et les nombres 8, 125, 1899.

ÉCRITURE SPONTANÉE. Le malade écrit son nom tout entier sans hésitation, mais par deux fois veut écrire Bordeaux et s'arrête à la 4e lettre.

ÉCRITURE SUR COPIE. On écrit Bordeaux. Il copie Bordeaux.

EXAMEN DES URINES :—

			Par litre.
Densité	...	... 1033	Albumine traces légères
Urée ...	...	... 27,50	Glucose, 28gr. 45
Acide phosphorique			Pigments biliaires. Néant.
Total ...	...	3.15	EXAMEN MICROSCOPIQUE :
			Urate de soude
			Acide urique
Chlorure de Sodium		4,30	Quelques leucocytes

DIAGNOSTIC : du Prof. Pitres, ABCÈS CÉRÉBRAL, siégeant au niveau du pli courbe.

L'apophyse est légèrement soulevée en masse et douloureuse à la pression. Il existe une petite perforation tympanique au centre de la membrane.

Une intervention est pratiquée le 4 Janvier 1899.

OPÉRATION DU 4 JANVIER 1899.—Incision rétro-auriculaire, dénudation de l'apophyse. Elargissement du conduit auditif osseux, dans sa moitié supérieure, à la gouge et au maillet. Chemin faisant on découvre de petites cellules apophysaires. L'os est congestionné en masse peu dure : la mastoïde est celluleuse. L'antre, petit, est mis en communication avec la caisse et le conduit (opération de Stacke). Le toit de l'antre est nécrosé ; un petit séquestre sépare sa cavité de l'encéphale.

En haut et en arrière de l'ouverture antrale et se continuant avec elle on fait, sur le temporal, une brèche qui met à nu une surface méningée de trois centimètres de diamètre environ. Incision cruciale de la dure-mère. Incision de la pie-mère : cette dernière occasionne l'ouverture d'une petite veine qui s'arrête par la compression.

Une pointe de bistouri longue de 3 cm est plongée en arrière un peu en haut et vers la profondeur dans la substance cérébrale, dans la direction du lobe occipital.

Cette ponction est suivie immédiatement d'un jet considérable de sang veineux, comme si un sinus avait été largement ouvert. Le sang est arrêté par la compression au moyen de gaze stérilisée mais coule de nouveau dès que cesse la compression. On est obligé d'arrêter là l'intervention, de ne point faire de nouvelles ponctions soit dans le lobe temporal, soit dans le lobe sphénoïdal, comme on en avait l'intention, et de laisser la plaie cérébrale tamponnée.

Une mèche de gaze iodoformée bourre la cavité attico-mastoïdienne.   Pansement compressif.

9 JANVIER 1899.—Depuis l'opération l'état général est resté bon ; le malade
ne se plaint de rien. Il cause avec plaisir. Toutefois il a maintenant un peu de
PARAPHASIE. Il ne reconnaît plus l'heure.

LA SENSIBILITÉ GÉNÉRALE EST À PEU PRÈS ABOLIE DU CÔTÉ DROIT DU
CORPS, c'est à dire du côté opposé à la lésion.   Le réflexe testiculaire n'existe plus à
droite.   De plus LE BRAS DROIT EST NETTEMENT PARÉSIE.

On enlève le tampon. Pas de sang. Battements du cerveau normaux.   Les
téguments sont suturés. On laisse une petite mèche de gaze iodoformée vers le
cerveau. Pansement légèrement compressif.

10 JANVIER 1899.—Même état sauf que la sensibilité est revenue du côté droit
depuis hier.

13 JANVIER.—Etat général bon. Pas de fièvre. Appétit. Langue saburrale
mais humide.

Analyse des urines le 14 Janvier :—

Volume des 24 heures ... 1 lit. 100	Albumine : traces légères.
Densité à 15° 1,021	Glucose : Néant.
Reaction : acide	Urobiline.
Couleur, Odeur, Aspect Normaux.	Examen microscopique du sédiment :
Uréa : 26gr. par lit.	rien d'important.

Acide phosphorique total : 2gr. 35 par litre.
Chlorure de sodium   6gr. 80 par litre.

15 JANVIER.—Le pansement est INONDÉ DE PUS qui a coulé jusque sur les
épaules du malade, dans la nuit du 14 au 15.   La plaie est en bon état.   Le pus
vient nettement du cerveau à la partie supérieure de l'incision (lobe temporal) ainsi
qu'on s'en rend compte en réouvrant les téguments.   PLUS D'HÉMIANOPIE.   Le
foyer de l'abcès cérébral qui vient de se vider est drainé au moyen d'un drain de
caoutchouc.

Depuis l'intervention la température n'a jamais atteint 37°. Le 11 janvier au
matin elle a été de 35° 2 centigrades.

DU 15 AU 24 JANVIER.—Le malade est manifestement mieux.   Il a toujours de
la paraphasie, mais il parle et s'intéresse à tout. Il connaît son nom. Il compte
jusqu'à 20. Il mange et reprend des forces. Il est pansé tous les deux jours.

24 JANVIER.—Le malade commence à se plaindre que son pansement lui serre
la tête. Il redevient triste et prend de nouveau un faciès terreux.

25 JANVIER.—Pansement refait. Hernie cérébrale d'assez gros volume. Teint
mauvais. Langue embarrassée. Répond cependant aux questions qu'on lui pose,
compte jusqu'à 19. La paraphasie s'accentue.

26 JANVIER.—Même état le matin. Entre dans le coma à sept heures du soir,
meurt à dix heures. Ce jour-là seul la température s'élève à 38°.

AUTOPSIE LE 27 JANVIER.—Il existe, au niveau du pli courbe, un vaste foyer
d'encéphalite nécrosante (abcès diffus) à l'intérieur duquel on trouve un gros caillot
sanguin noirâtre qui s'étend jusqu'à l'intérieur du ventricule. Au-dessus de la
scissure de Sylvius et dans un point correspondant à la cavité de l'abcès, très
superficielle en cet endroit, la pie-mère est nécrosée sur un tout petit espace et
prête à livrer passage au pus. Les lobes temporaux sphénoïdaux faisaient hernie
dans la plaie crânienne et étaient atteints d'encéphalite diffuse.

En somme le malade est MORT D'HÉMORRHAGIE DANS UN FOYER D'ABCÈS CÉRÉBRAL
AVEC INONDATION VENTRICULAIRE.

On a vu en effet dans ce cas que malgré la compression du cerveau par une lanière de gaze iodoformée introduite dans son intérieur, les phénomènes de compression ont été·très peu manifestes, le malade eût certainement guéri une fois son abcès ouvert, si au lieu de nous trouver en présence d'une collection purulente diffuse non limitée, nous avions eu affaire à un véritable abcès enkysté dont la poche seule aurait été ouverte. Comme il est habituellement impossible de savoir au moment de l'ouverture d'un abcès cérébral si l'on a affaire à un abcès enkysté ou à un abcès formé dans la masse cérébrale, sans membrane limitante, il convient d'observer certaines règles que la prudence nous commande. C'est ainsi qu'à mon sens, on ne doit jamais faire d'injections dans l'intérieur de la cavité cérébrale, car dans mon cas en particulier, une injection n'eût pas manqué de produire ce qu'a fait plus tard la collection purulente elle même, c'est à dire de pénétrer dans les ventricules et amener la mort subite du malade.

Peut-être serait-il possible de reconnaître les abcès ayant une paroi en examinant le pus qui s'écoule par l'orifice du drain ou de la canule placée dans le cerveau. Dans mon cas en effet il était absolument évident que le pus était mélangé de matière cérébrale sphacéléen ce qui me fit craindre dès le début une issue fatale, malgré l'ouverture de l'abcès.

D'un autre côté, il est intéressant de noter ces hernies considérables du cerveau qui ne se traduisent somme toute symptomatiquement par aucune sorte de trouble bien net. L'on connaît du reste des cas assez nombreux dans lesquels on a pu réséquer la portion herniée sans que le malade s'en fût ressenti après sa guérison. Le livre de M. Mignon, contient, à ce sujet un exemple assez typique et fort intéressant.

Il est utile aussi d'établir quelle doit être la ligne de conduite du chirurgien en présence de ces hernies cérébrales, souvent volumineuses; faut il essayer de les réduire, ce qui n'est pas facile ; ou faut il au contraire aider à leur élimination, en appliquant à leur base soit une ligature élastique, soit une ligature à la gaze ou quelquefois au contraire la résection pure et simple avec le thermo-cautère. Tels sont autant de problèmes intéressants qu'il conviendra de resoudre car ils intéressent au plus haut degré le chirurgien auriste qui se trouvera de plus en plus souvent aux prises avec des complications crâniennes consécutives à des otites suppurées.

PROF. LUC.—I thoroughly agree with Professor Moure's views about the steps to be adopted in the presence of extra-dural suppuration ; this is, in fact, one of the most delicate points in cranial surgery. Should we content ourselves with disinfecting the dura and wait, before opening this membrane, till we have proof that there are deeper lesions underneath, or is the dura to be opened at once ?

My experience leads me to consider the former method as the more advisable, for the opening of the dura in the neighbourhood of an infective focus considerably aggravates the prognosis, and I have seen the gravest cerebral symptoms caused by a very limited suppuration of the external surface of the dura, and completely relieved by the simple cleansing of this membrane.

I consider the fact of the absence of a limiting membrane round the cerebral abscess in one of Prof. Moure's cases as anything but a rarity. I have been struck, on the contrary, by the facility and rapidity with which suppurations often spread through the cerebral substance, giving the impression of a fire in a stack of hay, and thus rendering the post-operative treatment of opened cerebral abscesses one of the most difficult tasks in surgical practice.

PROF. GRADENIGO.—Io mi associo completamente alle opinioni espresse da Moure e da Luc, che l'apertura della dura madre è un fatto grave che mette a rischio il malato: essa non si dovrebbe praticare che quando esistano sintomi precisi di complicazioni cerebrali o cerebellari.

La mia esperienza mi porta a ritenere che anche sintomi ritenuti comunemente come valevoli ad assicurare la diagnosi di ascesso cerebrale possono esser provocati da lesioni estradurali. In un mio caso una tipica *amnesia verbale* indizio frequente di ascesso cerebrale temporo-sfenoidale sinistro, era provocata unicamente da un vasto ascesso estradurale.

Specialmente nei casi di circoscritta meningite la apertura della dura-madre è pericolosa. Io ho recentemente osservato due casi nei quali l'esistenza di una leptomeningite otitica purulenta fu dimostrata colla puntura lombare mediante il reperto di pus e di stafilococchi virulenti ; in questi due casi si ebbe la guarigione dopo un largo intervento radicale sul temporale, e l'evacuazione della raccolta estradurale; forse le ripetute punture lombari possono aver contribuito alla guarigione. Ma è molto probabile che se in tali casi fosse stato aperta la duramadre o anche semplicemente fossero state praticate delle incisioni si avrebbe facilitata la diffusione della infezione e si sarebbe prodotta una voluminosa ernia cerebrale, facile ad infettarsi.

DR. HEIMAN.—J'ai observé plusieurs cas d'abcès extradural où les symptômes d'un abcès cérébral ont été latents. Lorsque j'ai hésité à évacuer l'abcès, attendant le développement d'autres symptômes, j'ai perdu souvent mes malades ; à l'autopsie j'ai trouvé un abcès. Cela m'amenait à l'idée d'ouvrir chaque fois la dure-mère et ponctionner le cerveau, lorsqu'après l'évacuation de l'abcès extradural, la dure-mère n'a pas eu de poulsation. En pareil cas j'ai trouvé bien souvent un abcès cérébral. Mais même dans les cas où je n'ai pas trouvé d'abcès, l'incision du cerveau était sans conséquence pour le malade. Un transport d'une infection aux parties saines je n'ai pas jusqu'à présent observé.

DR. BRIEGER.—Man wird bei der Eröffnung des extraduralen Abscesses nicht stehen bleiben wenn zuverlässige Erscheinungen eines cerebralen Heerdes vorliegen. Die explorative Eröffnung des Arachnoi-dealraums von den eiternden Mittelohrräumen aus hat indessen, auch wenn man die Dura vorher incidiert und die Punction durch diese hindurch vermeidet, gewisse Bedenken. Man kann dann die in den extraduralen Heerden vorhandenen, durch keine Desinfection sicher auszuschaltenden Erreger direct in den Arachnoidealraum oder das Gehirn einimpfen. Brieger hat einen solchen arteficiell entstandenen Hirnabscess, entlang dem Punctionscanal, gesehen in einem Falle, in welchem bei umschriebener Meningitis in Folge irrtümlicher Annahme eines Abscesses, das Hirn von einer Stelle aus eröffnet war, welche dem meningitischen Heerde fern lag und bei der Operation normal erschienen war.

DR. LERMOYEZ.—Je considère que la ponction systématique du cerveau à travers un abcès extradural chez un malade otitique, pré-sentant des accidents cérébraux, est un procédé éminemment dangéreux. Ponctionner le cerveau avec un instrument stérilisé qui vient de traverser un foyer pyogène équivaut à ponctionner la substance cérébrale avec un instrument sale : or, il n'y a pas de cause plus puissante d'abcès cérébral expérimental.

A ce sujet, deux remarques sont à faire. D'une part, il faut con-sidérer la rareté extrême de suppurations cérébrales dans le cas d'abcès extraduraux. Pour ma part, j'ai observé à l'hôpital St. Antoine un assez grand nombre d'abcès extraduraux, se traduisant parfois par les accidents de coma grave et prolongé. Dans aucun cas le cerveau ne fut ponctionné à travers la dure-mère et presque tous les malades guérirent, je doute qu'il en eut été de même si le cerveau avait été ponctionné dans chaque cas.

D'ailleurs étant donné la difficulté extrême de dire, chez un malade otorrhéique atteint d'accidents cérébraux : 1°. Quelle est le siège et la nature de la lésion. 2ᵉ. Si cette lésion est sous la dépendance de l'otorrhée; le plus sage auriste n'ouvrira l'abcès crànien que jusqu'à la dure-mère, et traversera celle-ci que si au bout de deux ou trois jours aucune amélioration ne se manifeste.

THE OPERATIVE TREATMENT OF MASTOID INFLAMMATION.

DR. EDWARD BRADFORD DENCH, New York.

MR. CHAIRMAN AND GENTLEMEN,—Owing to the rapid strides which aural surgery has made during the past decade, the operative treatment of mastoid inflammation has commanded more and more attention. An examination of the statistics of the larger hospitals, in New York City, devoted to the special treatment of diseases of the ear, shows that ten years ago the mastoid operation was rarely performed. During the last few years, however, this operation has been performed almost daily.

Another fact of importance is that, while in former years, the treatment of intracranial complications of suppurative middle ear inflammation, was relegated entirely to the general surgeon, at the present day, these operations are performed by the otologist.

Regarding the subject chosen for discussion, that is, "The indications for opening the mastoid process in chronic suppurative otitis media," it is my opinion that the indications for the operation, laid down by Schwartze many years ago, are those followed at the present day. The only difference is that, under improved surgical technique, by which perfect asepsis is secured, the surgeon does not hesitate to act on these indications immediately. For this reason, the number of operations is relatively greater than in former years. If I were asked to give the signs which seemed to indicate the necessity of operative treatment in this condition, I should name simply two : 1st, local tenderness over the region of the antrum, and 2nd, a sagging of the upper and posterior wall of the external auditory meatus, close to the membrana tympani.

When these signs exist, I believe that operative interference is always indicated. Experience has shown that the temperature of the patient furnishes but little indication as to the necessity of operative interference. Spontaneous pain may also be absent, although the mastoid may have undergone extensive destruction.

I have spoken of tenderness over the region of the mastoid antrum, and wish to emphasize this physical sign, in contradistinction to tenderness on pressure over the tip of the mastoid process. I am well aware that many surgeons regard "tip tenderness" as an important diagnostic point. In my own experience, it has proven of but little value. In fact, in healthy individuals, it is almost always possible to elicit a certain amount of tenderness by firm pressure over the tip of the mastoid. In hysterical patients this sign can always be elicited, whether or not the osseous structures are inflamed.

Owing to the increased frequency with which the mastoid operation is performed, it may be well to consider any possible dangers which may arise in the operation itself. My own statistics show that, out of 228 operations upon the mastoid process, in no case could death be attributed to the operation.

Where intracranial complications exist, operative treatment offers the only means of relief, and in my own practice, has been followed by very flattering results. In 13 cases, in which thrombosis of the lateral sinus was present, death followed in but two cases ; one patient died of acute nephritis, which was probably caused by ether narcosis. Death in the second case was probably due to acute pulmonary tuberculosis.

Where there was an epidural abscess, my statistics show that, of 14 cases operated on, all recovered.

Regarding the radical operation, for the relief of a chronic purulent otitis media, with involvement of the mastoid, that is, the Stacke-Schwartze operation, 17 cases have, been operated on. Of these, 12 were cured and 5 improved. From these statistics, it can easily be seen that the mastoid operation is not, in itself, a dangerous procedure, if the rules of aseptic surgery are closely followed. No operation of this character, should be performed, without the strictest antiseptic precautions, both as regards the field of operation and the instruments. If proper care is taken, the exposure of the meninges, either in the middle or posterior cranial fossa, or exposure or opening of the lateral sinus, does not increase, in any degree, the mortality of the operation. On the other hand, I have found that the more extensive and radical the operation, the better the result. I believe, therefore, that in treating these cases, the surgeon who operates most frequently, and most radically, is really more conservative than he who waits for very pronounced symptoms.

A few words may not be amiss in regard to the technique of the operation. In the first place, the ear should be thoroughly syringed with a solution of bichloride of mercury, of a strength of 1-3000. The canal should be firmly tamponed to the fundus with a strip of iodoform gauze. The next step is to shave the head for an area of three inches about the external auditory meatus. The parts should then be thoroughly scrubbed, first with soap and water, and afterwards washed with a solution of bichloride of mercury (1-1000), and finally with a mixture of equal parts of alcohol and ether. Where it is possible, it is wise to cover the entire field of operation with a wet bichloride dressing for a few hours previous to the operation. This dressing should not be removed until the patient is thoroughly under the influence of the anaesthetic. The field of operation should then be surrounded by a towel moistened in a 1-1000 bichloride of mercury solution. All instruments should be carefully sterilized by boiling. It is hardly necessary to say that the hands of the surgeon and of the assistants should receive close attention. The primary incision should lie rather close to the line of auricular attachment, and should extend from just below the tip of the mastoid to just above the external auditory meatus, the soft parts being divided down to the bone. In this manner, a very narrow anterior flap is formed. The anterior flap is pushed forward by means of a periosteum elevator, exposing thoroughly the superior and posterior margins of the bony external auditory canal. The bone is uncovered posteriorly, in a similar manner. All bleeding points are secured by means of artery clamps. The next step is to sever the attachment of the sterno-mastoid muscle. This is best done by means of blunt scissors curved on the flat. The tendinous attachment of the muscle should be divided until the finger can be passed beneath the tip of the mastoid into the digastric fossa. In every case, the mastoid antrum should be first entered. This applies not only to those cases in which perforation of the cortex is present near the region of the antrum, but also, where spontaneous perforation has taken place into the digastric fossa through the internal plate of the mastoid. For removing the mastoid cortex, I prefer either the chisel or the gouge. The bone should first be removed as close to the posterior wall of the bony meatus as possible, and not above the level of the *spina supra-meatum*. The opening in the bone should be gradually deepened until a probe can be passed through the mastoid antrum into the middle ear. The wound should then be explored by means of the probe, to ascertain whether the bony walls are intact. After the mastoid antrum has once been entered, the topography of the process is at once evident. The entire mastoid cortex should then be removed by means of the chisel or gouge, and the tip removed by the rongeur forceps. Great care should be taken to thoroughly curette the *aditus ad antrum*, so as to permit of free drainage of the middle ear through the posterior opening. Experience has taught me that the operator is inclined to do a less radical operation than is absolutely necessary; for instance, after the entire cellular structure of the mastoid has been broken down by the sharp spoon, it is positively necessary to investigate the condition of the bone, especially posteriorly. In my later cases, I have found not infrequently that the bone seemed almost normal. Close inspection, however, revealed the fact that it was a little congested and slightly dark in colour. On using the gouge or rongeur forceps, I have often found a number of cells filled with granulation tissue and sometimes with pus, immediately behind this wall of congested bone. This condition, no doubt, explains the long period of convalescence in some of these cases. The operation should never be considered complete until the osseous tissue is perfectly healthy in every direction.

With reference to any possible accidents, which may occur during the operation, these, I think, are of trifling importance, provided the aseptic precautions, already mentioned, are carried out. I never operate upon a case without expecting to expose or open the lateral sinus or to enter the cranial cavity. Whether the sinus is opened by accident or design, is a matter of comparatively little moment. Its exposure, however, in doubtful cases, is imperative, and if its appearance is not perfectly normal, a free incision should be made into the vessel. No harm can possibly result from this procedure, and many a life which would otherwise be lost, may be saved, by what is apparently, a radical and uncalled-for procedure. The same applies to entering the middle cranial fossa. If surgical cleanliness is observed, the dura mater can be exposed without the slightest danger, and, where any doubt exists in the mind of the surgeon, as to the possibility of intracranial infection, the cranial cavity should always be entered. My own cases, which have terminated fatally, have been those in which I have not done a complete and radical operation.

While I feel certain that these remarks will not receive the endorsement of all members present, experience has taught me that the course outlined, offers the greatest safety to the patient.

DR. KNAPP asked Dr. Dench whether he attached the same importance to tenderness on pressure in acute as in chronic cases.

DR. DENCH answered in the negative.

DR. KNAPP declared himself in accordance with him.

PANOTITE AVEC COMPLICATION CÉRÉBRALE. OPÉRATION. MORT. AUTOPSIE.

DR. DELIE, Ypres, Belgium.

Mademoiselle C, âgée de 40 ans, est une personne nerveuse, d'une constitution délicate. Son père était un alcoolique invétéré ; sa mère est atteinte de strabisme. La famille comptait 12 enfants parmi lesquels un s'est suicidé et un autre fut frappé dans son adolescence, d'une hémorrhagie cérébrale qui le laissa hémiplégique. La malade a souffert pendant son enfance de paraplégie (probablement de nature hystérique). Depuis quelques mois s'est développée une surdité droite progressive, accompagnée de violentes douleurs à caractères névralgiques, inter- mittentes, s'irradiant spontanément dans toute la moitié droite de la tête et s'exaspérant pendant la mastication. Un premier médecin institua un traitement antinévralgique qui ne fut couronné d'aucun succès. En quelques jours la surdité devint complète. Des douleurs vives s'étant déclarées dans le conduit auditif externe, la malade eut recours à un spécialiste. Celui-ci croyant avoir affaire à un abcès du conduit, fit une incision et ramena du sang sans traces de pus. Dès le moment de cette légère intervention chirurgicale qui n'apporta aucun changement à l'audition, la douleur choisit pour siège permanent le con- duit auditif externe : de ce centre elle s'irradia par accès dans toute la moitié correspondante de la tête ; s'augmentant par les tractions sur le pavillon, la parole, la mastication, s'exaspérant la nuit au point de créer des insomnies complètes.

C'est à ce moment que j'eus l'honneur de voir la malade : celle-ci est une personne hyperesthésique, pâle, amaigrie et défaite par l'insuffisance de la nutrition et l'absence de repos. Le pouls est à 100, la température ne s'élève pas au delà de 37°. La fille affirme n'avoir jamais antérieure- ment souffert de l'oreille. Elle ne se rappelle pas avoir eu d'otorrhée.

Etat local.—Le conduit auditif externe droit est complètement obstrué par une tumeur arrondie, à muqueuse normale, sessile sur une base de $1\frac{1}{2}$ ctm. partant de la paroi postéro-supérieure du C. A. E. osseux. Elle offre au toucher une consistance renittente : elle est dépressible dans sa coque externe, mais son fond est dur. Un simple attouchement arrache des cris à la malade.

Un stylet mousse, d'un mm. d'épaisseur, peut s'engager en avant et en bas entre la tumeur et le conduit auditif et parcourir entre eux un espace semi-lunaire. Cette dernière exploration est tellement douloureuse qu'elle provoque un état semi-syncopal avec pâleur des téguments, transpiration froide, vertiges, etc. Grâce à la cocaïne il me fut permis de laver avec l'aide d'une petite seringue aspiratrice, la partie du C. A. située au delà de la tumeur. L'eau injectée ne ramena pas une ombre de pus. L'oreille gauche est tout à fait normale, le diapason vertex est perçu dans l'oreille droite. A droite le Rinne est très negatif puisqu'il y a surdité absolue à l'air et perception prolongée sur la mastoïde. Le Corrade est +.

Quand j'établis une petite lumière dans le C. A. E. en comprimant légèrement la tumeur, la malade entend parfaitement la voix. Je ne pus recueillir le moindre renseignement sur l'état de la caisse : le catétherisme de la trompe est impraticable même sous l'action de la cocaïne, à cause de l'éréthisme nerveux de la malade. Le Valsalva ne donne rien. Le nez, le pharynx nasal et le pharynx sont exempts de phénomènes morbides : la région mastoïdienne présente un aspect physiologique.

Fallait-il voir dans la céphalalgie si intense un simple phénomène d'irradiation directe ou réflexe, dû à l'inflammation de la partie externe de l'oreille, analogue à celle que l'on rencontre dans la furonculose? Avions nous à compter sur une névralgie rebelle du trijumeau sans autre manifestation externe que la douleur? La céphalée, dépendait elle d'une manifestation de syphilis héréditaire du cerveau? Les exacerbations nocturnes, les antécédents de famille justifiaient le soupçon de cette hypothèse : mais il manquait pour sa confirmation un des autres symptômes qui l'accompagnent d'habitude : trouble de la vision ou d'un autre sens, paralysies ou anesthésies locales, vomissements, etc. L'examen minutieux de l'urine écartait toute supposition d'intoxication par albuminurie ou diabète. La diathèse rhumatismale ou urique était inconnue à la malade.

Le seul diagnostic rationnel que l'on pouvait établir était celui de : "*Exostose enflammée du conduit auditif externe chez une personne subhystérique.*"

Je prescrivis un calmant général : je fis instiller dans l'oreille alternativement de l'eau oxygenée et de la glycérine pheniquée tiède ; une chaleur sèche fut entretenue sur toute la région auriculaire malade. Des pulverisations de chlorure d'ethyle pallièrent les crises de douleur. Au bout de 3 jours, n'ayant obtenu aucune amélioration, la malade consentit à laisser enlever l'exostose. Je fis autour de la base de la tumeur, 2 incisions sémilunaires comprenant l'épaisseur de la muqueuse, quelques coups de gouge firent sauter la crête osseuse. J'instituai des installations chaudes de glycérine résorcinée. Pour la nuit injection de morphine. Quatre jours s'écoulèrent sans le moindre amendement, la douleur conservait sa tenacité et ses exacerbations nocturnes. Le 5ᵉ jour il n'y avait pas la moindre trace de pus dans le C. A. E. ; au niveau de l'exostose enlevée la lumière du conduit avait la forme d'un petit disque de 2 à 3 mm. de largeur. La malade heureuse d'avoir récupéré l'audition à droite, espérait se voir débarassée ultérieurement de ses douleurs qu'elle attribuait à une névralgie faciale. Elle rentra chez elle. Son médecin habituel lui donna tous les soins que réclamait son état : celui-ci au bout de quelques jours ne tarda pas à reprendre une tournure inquiétante. Je retrouvai la demoiselle couchée dans son lit, se plaignant de douleurs les plus vives, concentrées dans l'oreille droite, et irradiées dans toute la moitié correspondante de la tête, principalement dans la région temporale à 2 travers de doigts au dessus du pavillon. Le pouls était à 90°, la température qui la veille avait atteint 38.5 remontait aujourd'hui à 39. Il n'existe ni vomissements, ni convulsions, ni cris hydrencéphaliques, ni phénomènes convulsifs ; aucun symptôme pathologique n'est perceptible du côté des yeux, de la langue, de la miction, de la sensibilité générale ou du mouvement volontaire ou réflexe des 4 membres. L'intelligence est absolument intacte, la patiente répond sans hésiter, et correctement à toutes les questions que je lui pose, même quand elles ont rapport à des faits antérieurs ; elle se plaint de douleur à la gorge au moment de la déglutition. Les 2 amygdales sont légèrement enflammées et recouvertes de petites plaques disséminées : un ganglion est tangible vers l'angle de la mâchoire inférieure droite. La peau n'est le siège d'aucun éruption. Il n'existe pas d'otorrhée ; la région mastoïdienne ne présente ni rougeur, ni gonflement, ni douleur spontanée : une pression forte exercée à la base de l'apophyse mastoïde, dénote simplement une sensibilité exagérée, mais ne reveille pas d'acuité dans la douleur. La personne se lève et marche seule ; pendant l'examen et le pansement de l'oreille, *elle a plusieurs vomissements spontanés sans vertige.* Ce phénomène était il provoqué par la douleur de l'exploration de l'oreille, ou par l'état de la gorge ? Constituait il la 1ʳᵉ manifestation d'une complication cérébrale ? Nous nous sommes permis de nous retrancher dans une expectation attentive et prudente, préconisant les grandes irrigations tièdes aseptiques fréquentes du conduit auditif ; l'application de la chaleur humide sur la région auriculaire, le badigeonnage à la glycérine résorcinée dans la gorge, l'usage de l'eau citronnée, le régime lacté, etc. Le lendemain le pouls est à 100, la température à 38·3. Il n'y avait eu ni frissons, ni nausées, ni vomissements.

Pour la 1ʳᵉ fois il s'est montré un peu de pus dans le conduit auditif. L'irrigation fait couler l'eau dans la bouche et le nez, et dénote une perforation du tympan : un léger empâtement sans changement de coloration se déclare sur la mastoïde : le sillon auriculo-mastoïdien est effacé. A l'examen du pus on découvre la présence du pneumocoque. 24 heures plus tard, la température monte à 39, l'insomnie a été complète malgré une injection de morphine : l'hémicrânie s'accentue encore et conserve son summum d'acuité dans la tempe droite. Il y a absence de vertige, de nausée, de troubles oculaires, la suppuration de l'oreille est très minime mais l'empâtement et la sensibilité de la mastoïde semblent s'exagérer encore.

Le jour suivant, la température oscille entre 39·4 et 39·6, le soir *un frisson intense* se déclare et la malade tombe bientôt dans une espèce de somnolence dont il est souvent difficile de la tirer. Le lendemain le thermomètre donne 39·4. Il se manifeste *des nausées, des vomituritions continuelles, l'intelligence est engourdie mais nullement éteinte.* A midi la température est de *40°*, et à 5½ du soir de *40°4* ; il s'est déclaré de *nouveaux frissons; la vision a perdu de sa netteté et par moments l'amaurose est complète sur l'oeil gauche ;* l'examen ophthalmoscopique révèle *de la stase, symptôme de névrite optique.* L'état local de l'oreille droite est stationnaire.

Nous nous trouvions sans aucune doute en présence d'une complication cérébrale, sur la nature de laquelle il fallait établir un diagnostic. Les lésions de l'oreille, otorrhée légère et mastoïdite, suffisaient elles pour expliquer les symptômes graves que nous venions de recueillir ? Sans la fièvre et sans les phénomènes cérébraux, les vertiges et les vomissements auraient pu dépendre uniquement d'une irritation de l'oreille interne. Nous nous rappellions que dans les cas aigus un écoulement d'oreille insignifiant peut s'accompagner de l'explosion de phénomènes cérébraux très-graves, tout aussi facilement que d'un simple catarrhe de la caisse avec céphalalgie ordinaire. Le pneumocoque a été trouvé très souvent dans le pus d'otorrhée, accompagnée de complications cérébrales. Grunert a fourni une statistique de 100 cas de mastoïdites aiguës, qui se sont compliquées d'abcès endocrânéen, et dans lesquelles on n'a trouvé que des lésions insignifiantes du côté de l'apophyse (muqueuse des cellules normales ou simplement gonflées ou infiltrées d'une légère couche de pus). S'agissait il des premières manifestations d'une méningite simple ou purulente, générale ou localisée ? Nous avions de la fièvre, des vomissements, des vertiges, du délire, de l'excitation cérébrale : mais il manquait les convulsions, et la céphalalgie bien que violente, me semblait trop ancienne pour caracteriser une inflammation aiguë, ou sub-aiguë des enveloppes du cerveau. Se préparait il une phlébite, une thrombophlébite du sinus latéral, une pyoémie d'origine otique, dont les symptômes cérébraux ou méningitiformes résulteraient d'une réaction de voisinage des centres nerveux ou de leurs enveloppes ? Les frissons répétés plaidaient en faveur de cette éventualité, mais ils sont isolés : nous n'avons pas ces écarts ou oscillations considérables de la température que l'on rencontre dans les pyoémies. En tout cas, nous ne serions qu'au premier stade de l'inflammation du sinus, celui de la phlébite sans thrombose puisque la veine jugulaire n'est ni vide, ni affaisée, ni thrombosée et qu'il n'existe pas de traces de développement d'une circulation veineuse collatérale sur la mastoïde, aux tempes, dans le cuir chevelu, à la face etc.

Une intervention chirurgicale s'imposait. Elle porterait sur l'apophyse mastoïde et la caisse et éventuellement sur la boîte crânienne. Avec l'accord des 2 confrères traitant également la malade, l'opération fut décidée pour le lendemain. Ce jour-là, il n'y avait pas de pus dans l'oreille ; le conduit auditif était complètement obstrué par un boursoufflement œdémateux de la muqueuse ; un gonflement de nature phlegmoneuse avait envahi toute la région mastoïdienne ; celle-ci est douloureuse au toucher, principalement dans le sillon auriculo-mastoïdien et vers la pointe de l'apophyse. La température est à 39·9, le pouls à 120. La patiente répond aux questions posées ; la parole est libre, la vision est meilleure que la veille, les pupilles sont égales et réagissent normalement. La céphalalgie semble moins vive ; la déglutition est bonne : les vomissements spontanés persistent. La surdité est absolue à droite, le vertige est violent, la perte de l'équilibre est complète et la marche est des plus difficiles même quand on soutient la malade.

OPÉRATION.—Incision semi-lunaire de la peau jusqu'à l'os, parallèlement à l'insertion du pavillon à 1 ctm. en arrière et sur toute la hauteur de ce dernier. Détachement du conduit auditif externe en arrière, de manière à dénuder complètement la face antérieure de l'apophyse mastoïde. Remarqué à la partie supérieure une petite saillie osseuse de 2 mm. de base sur 3 de hauteur occupant toute la profondeur du C. auditif, dirigée de dehors en dedans, et portant vers son milieu un point rugueux, vestige de la crête osseuse que j'avais fait sauter à la gouge. Une seconde incision partant du milieu de la première, se dirige en arrière jusqu'au delà de l'apophyse mastoïde. Les lambeaux sont détachés ainsi que le périoste.

Renversement du C. A. E. en dehors et en avant. Ouverture de l'antre mastoïdien au point d'élection (5 mm. en arrière de la spina supra-meatum ou dans l'angle formé par 2 lignes droites, l'une déterminant le plan horizontal qui passe par la paroi supérieure du C. A. E. ; l'autre, celui qui passe verticalement par la limite externe de la paroi postérieure du même conduit). Dès que la gouge a mordu dans l'os, je vois sourdre le long de la partie tranchante une petite nappe de pus. Celle-ci s'est répétée chaque fois que j'entamais la tablette externe de l'apophyse mastoïde : je n'ai rencontré de pus ni dans l'antre ni dans les cellules mastoïdiennes qui ont été largement ouvertes et enlevées jusque contre le sinus transverse. J'ai fait sauter à la gouge le mur de la logette. La chute de cette lame osseuse fait saillir dans la plaie une petite masse charnue, à surface arrondie et lisse. Je l'enlève à l'anse et je reconnais un petit polype un peu applati de 1 ctm. de long, 5 mm. de large, et 2 mm. d'épaisseur. Ce néoplasme venait de l'attique où il avait été emprisonné. J'ai exploré et ràclé minutieusement la base d'insertion de ce polype ainsi que toute la voûte de l'oreille moyenne. Je n'ai pu découvrir nulle part la moindre trace de carie, ou de fistule communiquante avec les fosses cérébrales. Je n'ai rencontré ni tympan ni osselets. Après avoir établi une large communication entre les cellules mastoïdiennes, l'antre, l'oreille moyenne et externe, j'ai tamponné la plaie à la gaze aseptique et appliqué un pansement légèrement compressif.

Cette première opération n'avait donc découvert qu'une infiltration puriforme de la mastoïde spécialement dans sa tablette externe ; un grand polype de l'attique avec dénudation et prolifération charnue de la paroi supérieure de cette partie de l'oreille moyenne.

L'insignifiance des lésions locales, l'absence de trajet fistuleux entre l'oreille et la boîte crânienne, l'impossibilité de poser un diagnostic plausible de la lésion cérébrale, m'ont décidé à surseoir à une intervention endo-crânienne jusqu'au moment de l'apparition de phénomènes cérébraux plus caractéristiques ou de localisation moins douteuse.

Suites de l'opération. Quelques heures après l'opération s'est déclaré un délire gai avec loquacité exubérante et continue. Le lendemain le thermomètre oscille entre 40° et 41°, la malade affirme ne plus éprouver de douleur de tête ; il n'y a ni vomissements ni frissons. Le pouls est à 120, dur et régulier : la respiration a une tendance à perdre son rythme physiologique. L'intelligence s'obnubile d'une manière intercurrénte. L'audition reste totalement abolie à droite, elle est douteuse à gauche. Il n'est plus guère possible de dire s'il faut attribuer ce dernier phénomène à la boiterie de l'intelligence ou à une lésion auriculaire. La malade a dormi un peu, de temps à autre elle jette des cris plaintifs ; elle mange, boit, urine bien, elle a eu une selle normale ; elle marche convenablement et garde la position assise pendant toute la durée du pansement. Il n'existe aucun phénomène de paralysie quelconque, les réflexes des bras et des membres inférieurs sont plutôt exagérés. La sensibilité générale est conservée avec tendance à l'hyperesthésie : c'est ainsi qu'un simple attouchement de la plaie arrache des cris, et s'accompagne de mouvements spasmodiques de la tête et du bras droit. Il n'existait nulle trace de pus dans les pansements et la plaie était idéalement belle. Rien ne pouvait expliquer l'élévation de la température, l'accélération du pouls, le délire intermittent. L'état de la gorge n'avait duré qu'un jour ; il n'existait ni fièvre éruptive ni pneumonie ; l'absence de frissons répétés, de transpirations, de suppurations apparentes, de complications phlegmoneuses articulaires écartaient la septicémie. La névrite optique m'indiquait l'existence réele d'une complication intracérébrale ; mais ce symptôme pouvait être lié à une affection du cerveau tout aussi bien qu'à une maladie quelconque de ses enveloppes. On le trouve en effet, dans des méningites, l'abcès extra-dural ou du cerveau, les néoplasmes, etc. La névrite se rencontre dans les maladies de la convexité comme de la base; même localisée à un oeil, elle ne peut, isolée, fournir une indication certaine sur l'endroit de la partie lésée du cerveau.

Pouvions nous soupçonner l'existence d'un abcès extra-dural? On l'a vu compliquer une simple otite aiguë dont les manifestations locales ont l'air négligeables et passagères. Parmi les symptômes ordinaires de l'abcès extra-dural, nous relevons *le mal de tête*, qui dans le cas présent, a toujours son summum d'intensité vers la fosse temporale droite, audessus de l'oreille correspondante; *l'existence de la mastoïdite* à infiltration purulente; *l'otorrhée*, qui tout en n'ayant qu'une valeur rélative, est insignifiante plutôt que profuse. Les signes de foyer manquent totalement, mais leur absence n'exclut nullement la possibilité de l'abcès extra-dural. Quant à la température elle est ici très-élevée ce qui, par analogie des faits connus, ferait songer à un abcès qui devrait déjà infecter le sinus ou du moins envahir ses contours. Y-avait-il des phénomènes qui plaidaient en faveur d'un abcès du cerveau? Non, car les symptômes de cette complication sont plutôt ceux de l'affaissement général: la température est ordinairement en dessous de la moyenne, ou du moins subit de grandes oscillations; le pouls est le plus souvent ralenti; les fonctions intellectuelles semblent endormies ou supprimées (coma ou alternance de lucidité et de somnolence); la sensibilité et la motilité générales sont déprimées (anesthésie, parésie ou paralysie de groupes musculaires volontaires ou involontaires). Ces phénomènes isolés ou groupés deviennent surtout manifestes quand l'abcès détruit une partie déterminée du cerveau à laquelle est dévolue une fonction spéciale (trouble de la parole, $3^{me.}$ circonvolution frontale gauche etc). Ces phénomènes font absolument tous défaut dans le cas qui nous occupe. Faut-il songer à une affection du cervelet?

L'existence des vertiges, avec ataxie des mouvements volontaires peut seule attirer notre attention du côté de cet organe. Il faut convenir cependant que le vertige se rencontre déjà dans les affections ou les irritations isolées de l'oreille interne et dans presque toutes les maladies du cerveau. La céphalalgie n'est ici pas exclusivement occipitale; il n'y a pas de vrais troubles de la sensibilité générale. L'hémianopsie signalée fréquemment dans les abcès du cervelet ou la compression des circonvolutions occipitales postérieures, n'a pas été accusée par la malade.

Force nous fut donc de rester encore dans l'expectative plutôt que d'aggraver le cas par une intervention inopportune, plus ou moins aveugle. L'état de la malade a peu varié les jours suivants: la fièvre s'est maintenue: il s'est établi graduellement un coma qui a emporté la demoiselle 7 jours après l'opération.

Autopsie. L'ouverture du crâne, l'incision de la dure-mère, la mise à vue du cerveau, ne s'accompagnent de la découverte d'aucune lésion pathologique, en dehors d'une certaine turgescence des vaisseaux des enveloppes cérébrales. J'enlève le cerveau en incisant la protubérance annulaire tout contre le cerveau sur le plan de la tente du cervelet. L'examen minutieux des fosses cérébrales et surtout de la fosse temporale droite est absolument négatif.

Bulbe. Toute la face antérieure de la protubérance et du bulbe depuis la selle turcique jusque dans le canal rachidien est uniformément recouverte d'un demi mm. d'exsudat fibrino-purulent. Cette couche laiteuse avait envahi les faces latérales du bulbe et respecté sa face postérieure. Tous les nerfs crâniens émergeant de ces organes, ont leur origine baignée dans ce pus épais, crêmeux. Il convient de remarquer toutefois qu'il n'existe aucune trace de pus autour des nerfs auditifs et faciaux tant droits que gauches, soit dans leur parcours en dehors du bulbe jusqu'au crâne, soit dans le conduit auditif interne.

Cervelet. Le pus recouvre la face antéro-inférieure de l'hémisphère droit, seulement dans sa moitié interne jusque vers la limite du tiers externe ou postérieur du sinus latéral (sur lequel elle repose). Le reste de la fosse occipitale en dehors d'une forte injection de la pie-mère n'est le siège d'aucune altération morbide. A gauche, toute la face antéro-inférieure de l'hémisphère jusque près de la protubérance occipitale interne est recouverte de pus.

Examen des sinus.—Le sinus occipital est rempli de sang semiliquide. A droite vers l'union du sinus occipital avec le sinus transverse, il existe un petit caillot de sang, un peu allongé, de 2 mm. de diamètre. Les sinus latéraux tant droit que gauche, les sinus pétreux sont vides et ne décèlent pas le moindre indice d'inflammation ou de suppuration.

Dure-mère du rocher droit.—La dure-mère dans les fosses temporales et occipitales droites ne présente ni déhiscence, ni solution de continuité ni trace de pus ou d'irritation. Elle se détache bien et très facilement de tout le rocher, tant à sa face supérieure ou temporale que postérieure ou sinusienne, occipitale. Remarquons en passant que le ganglier de Gasser et ce qu'il l'entoure dans sa fossette présentent un aspect physiologique.

Conduit auditif interne droit.—Celui-ci est normal.

Rocher droit.—L'os semble complètement sain. Je fais sauter à la gouge la partie du rocher qui sert de voûte à l'oreille moyenne et celle qui recouvre les canaux demicirculaires, je remarque dans l'épaisseur de cette lamelle osseuse la présence d'un liquide louche puriforme. Dans la caisse, les canaux demi-circulaires et le vestibule, il n'y a pas de pus. Celui-ci est également absent dans l'antre, et ce qui reste des cellules mastoïdiennes.

Tous les éléments pathologiques tangibles se résument en une infiltration de pus, logée dans l'épaisseur même de l'os de la voûte de l'oreille moyenne et d'une partie de l'oreille interne, analogue à celle qui existait dans la tablette externe de la mastoïde au moment où la gouge mordait dans l'os.

Examen du cerveau.—Dans le 4me ventricule il y a un liquide louche puriforme. (Les coupes ont été d'abord horizontales, analogues à la coupe de Brissaud fronto-occipitale, et ensuite verticales genre Pittres). L'hémisphère droit ne présente rien d'anormal. Tout au plus pourrait on remarquer une coloration rougeâtre du liquide renfermé dans le ventricule latéral. Dans l'hémisphère gauche, toutes les parois du ventricule latéral sont tapissées d'une épaisse couche de pus fibrineux. Celui-ci est inégalement distribué dans les divers recessus ventriculaires : le prolongement sphénoïdal ou corne inférieure est le plus atteint.

Résumé de l'autopsie.—Nous avons donc trouvé du pus dans le ventricule latéral *gauche*, et le 4ième ventricule, des lésions de méningite purulente dans la presque totalité de la fosse occipitale gauche, sur le pédoncule du bulbe, et dans la moitié interne de la fosse occipitale droite ; une ostéite purulente de la partie du rocher droit servant de voûte à l'oreille moyenne et aux canaux demicirculaires avec le vestibule.

Remarques.—Nous voyons dans ce cas une inflammation purulente des couches superficielles de la mastoïde et de la voûte tympanique se compliquer de méningite purulente et entrainer la mort.

Comme dans les cas de Grunert et de Jansen nous trouvons le pneumocoque dans le pus otorrhéique.

Aucune lésion n'établit un passage direct, par continuité, entre l'oreille enflammée et l'exsudat purulent intra-crânéen. La voie d'infection s'est établie à travers une paroi osseuse intacte par le système circulatoire probablement lymphatique.

Les lésions endo-crâniennes étaient principalement localisées autour du cervelet et dans les ventricules du cerveau *du côté opposé à l'oreille malade.*

Phénomènes correspondants aux lésions de l'autopsie.

I. La névrite optique indiquait l'existence d'une complication cérébrale quelconque.

II. L'explosion violente de phénomènes généraux de nature irritative plaidait en faveur d'une altération pathologique des méninges, soit à la pie-mère, soit à la surface externe des enveloppes du cerveau.

Excitation cérébrale (délire ou exaltation des fonctions intellectuelles, céphalalgie ; vomissements, etc). Irritation générale (insomnie,

Phénomènes quasi paradoxaux.

I. Hémicrànie droite temporale quand les lésions du cervelet et du bulbe auraient dû localiser les douleurs, de préférence à l'occiput et dans la nuque.

II. Hypéridéation délirante avec lésions rigoureusement limitées au mésocéphale et au cervelet, quand on la trouve ordinairement dans la méningite de la convexité (méningite aiguë) ou de la face inférieure des lobes du cerveau (méningite tuberculeuse). Le délire et les troubles de l'intelligence n'ont donc pas été causés par une irritation directe des cellules des élévation de température, fréquence du pouls).

III. L'absence de phénomènes circonscrits a été signalée dans la méningite aiguë.

couches corticales hémisphériques mais par une excitation réflexe partie des organes intra ou peri-cérébraux lésés.

III. Les lésions du bulbe surtout de sa partie antérieure qui est spécialement motrice, et gauche, auraient normalement dû provo-quer des contractures soit générales soit principalement des muscles de la face, de la langue, de l'oeil etc. etc. avec prépondérance du côté gauche.

IV. La variation des symptômes chez le sujet plaidait en faveur d'une suppuration intracrânienne (Lucidité alternant avec somnolence, et manifestations graves d'une affection cérébrale), aucun symptôme ne pouvant en préciser la modalité ou le siège.

V. La présence du pus a été souvent constatée dans les méningites d'origine pyoémique.

VI. Un abcès du cerveau proprement dit, aurait pu être latent et ne s'accompagner d'aucun phénomène spécial, tout en étant même étendu, s'il avait respecté les parties du cerveau auxquelles est dévolu une fonction spéciale (langage, etc,); ou bien il aurait provoqué des phénomènes de dépression générale cérébrale et physique (parésie, paralysie, anesthésie, somnolence, coma, abaissement de la température et du pouls). Les statistiques semblent prouver qu'un petit abcès extra-dural crée plus vite des phénomènes de compression intracrânienne énoncés, qu'un abcès intra-cérébral beaucoup plus considérable. L'absence de symptôme de foyer écartait l'idée d'une collection circon-scrite de nature purulente d'abcès.

THE PETRO-SQUAMOSAL SINUS: ITS ANATOMY AND PATHOLOGICAL IMPORTANCE.

MR. ARTHUR H. CHEATLE, London.

As little or nothing is written in even the best works on otology concerning this sinus, which has most important connections with the middle ear, both from anatomical and pathological standpoints, I have thought the subject of sufficient interest to bring before the Congress. The following British authors have written on the subject: J. F. Knott, of Dublin (*Journal of Anatomy*, vol. xvi., p. 27), who quotes C. Krause, Luschka, Otto, and Sir Charles Bell; Henry Morris ("Anatomy," p. 661), Professor Macewen ("Pyogenic Diseases of the Brain and Spinal Cord," pp. 2 and 8), and Quain ("Anatomy").

Comparative Anatomy.—In some lower animals—dog and calf, for instance—this sinus runs across the roof of the middle ear, making its exit by means of a large foramen between the base of the zygoma and the bony meatal wall, and serves almost entirely for the exit of the intracranial blood, taking the place, in fact, of the sigmoid portion of the lateral sinus.

(Mr. Cheatle here demonstrated on the canvas a photo of the outer aspect of a dog's skull, showing the opening in front of the meatus; one showing the canal which leads from the interior of the skull to the external opening laid open; then the outer aspect of a calf's temporal bone, showing the external opening; the inner aspect of a calf's temporal bone, showing internal part of opening; the outer aspect of temporal bone of a Cebus monkey (v. Fig. 1), showing the external opening; and the inner aspect of preceding (v. Fig. 2), showing the groove and opening).

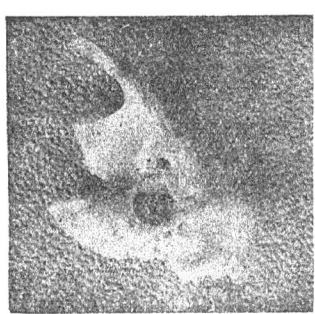
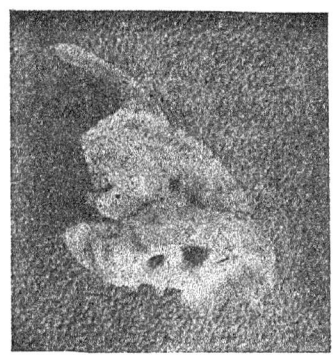
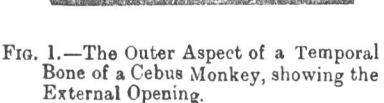

Fig. 1.—The Outer Aspect of a Temporal Bone of a Cebus Monkey, showing the External Opening.

Fig. 2.—The Inner Aspect of Preceding, showing the Groove and Opening.

In the higher forms of monkeys, such as the chimpanzee, gorilla, and orang-outang, the sinus closely resembles the human.

In the Macacus group, the young often have the groove which runs along the petro-squamosal suture, and the anterior external opening, well marked, while in the adult the opening is usually closed or rudimentary, leaving the groove which runs forward to the foramen spinosum. In other varieties, notably in Baboons, Chrysothrix, Cebus, Midas, Hapale, Lemuridæ, and Indri, both the groove and the external opening are well marked, the latter piercing the bone between the large post-glenoid tubercle and the bony meatus. In these the sinus does not take the place of the sigmoid portion of the lateral sinus, as it is also present and well-marked.

Human Anatomy.—In early fœtal life, before the formation of the internal jugular vein, the petro-squamosal sinus carries all the intracranial venous blood, emerging in front to open into the primitive jugular (afterwards the external jugular). It is not to be wondered, then, that this channel, which serves such important duties in early fœtal life, should persist in some form or another in later life. Tho anterior opening usually closes, the sinus or its remains at its anterior extremity forming a connection with the middle meningeal vein. The sinus dwindles to a small size, while the opening into the lateral sinus often persists.

With regard to the persistence of the anterior opening in front of the meatus in adult life, I examined 2,585 skulls in the Royal College of Surgeons' Museum, and among this number I found in twenty-three rudimentary remains, three in the glenoid cavity, three in the zygomatic process itself, six in the base of the zygoma, and eleven just external to the Glaserian fissure, with sometimes a fine groove running outwards, and occasionally bridged over by the junction of the post-glenoid tubercle with the bony meatus. These twenty-three skulls are now, owing to the kindness of the College of Surgeons, in the Congress Museum. I must here say that it is the rule rather than the exception for remains of the sinus to be present in some form or another all through life. In this statement, I am supported by my anatomical friends, Mr. Arthur Keith and Mr. Cadman. Unfortunately, it is impossible in the time allowed for me to describe minutely the different varieties, but in the photographs to be shown directly some idea can be obtained, and some fifty specimens of my own are now in the museum.

In infancy and childhood, the sinus as a rule is well marked, opening into the lateral sinus behind by means of a valve-like opening, and in front joining the middle meningeal vein, while in adult life, although it is often marked, careful search has sometimes to be made. The absence of markings on the bone in the neighbourhood of the suture does not by any means show that the sinus is not present. In infancy and early childhood, in the region of the posterior extremity of the suture, numerous irregularities are often seen ; it is at this spot that a bridge often forms over the posterior end of the sinus, before it opens into the lateral sinus, a common condition in the adult bone.

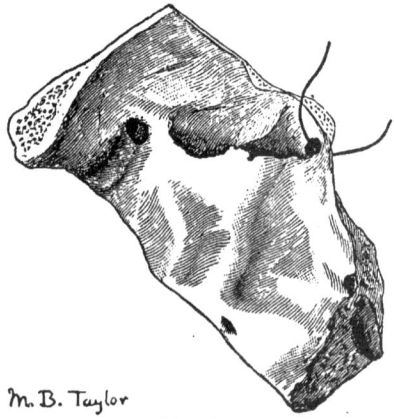

M. B. Taylor

FIG. 3.

Fig 3.—The superior aspect of left temporal bone of a child aged about five years, in whom the anterior opening persisted showing well-marked groove and the inner aspect of the anterior opening.

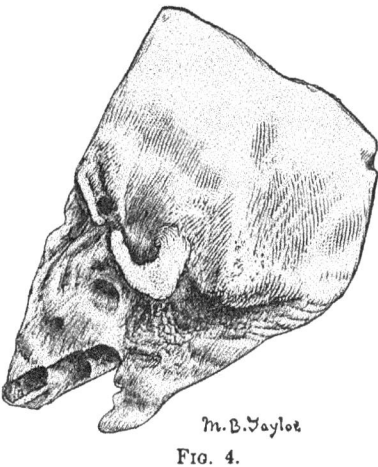

FIG. 4.

Fig. 4.—External aspect of same bone, showing the opening between an unusually large post-glenoid tubercle and the meatus, with a groove running outwards. This is a very rare specimen. Professor Macewen figures a similar one in his book from a ten-days-old infant.

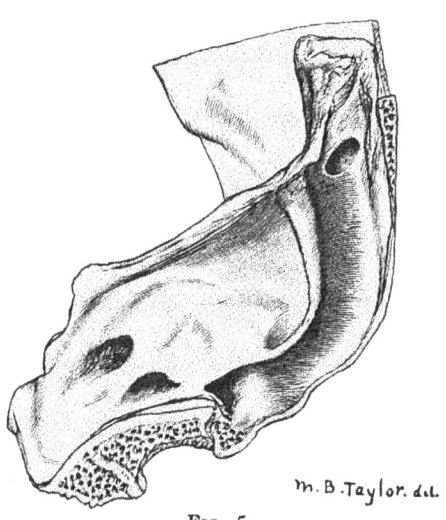

FIG. 5.

Fig. 5.—Right temporal bone of a child, aged five years, showing the valve-like opening in the lateral sinus.

Mr. Cheatle also showed a specimen from a child similar to that in Fig. 5.

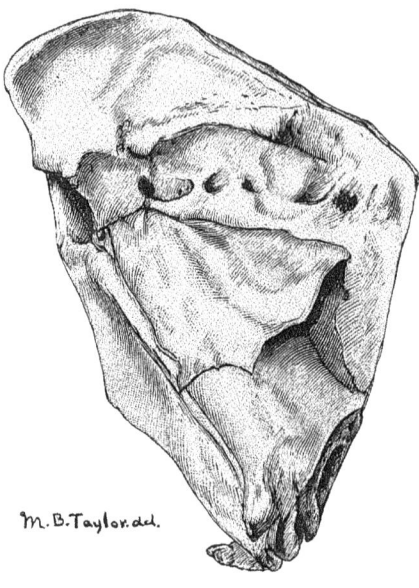

FIG. 6.

Fig. 6.—Superior surface of the left temporal bone of a young adult, the dura mater thrown back to show groove for sinus which lies in the dura mater.

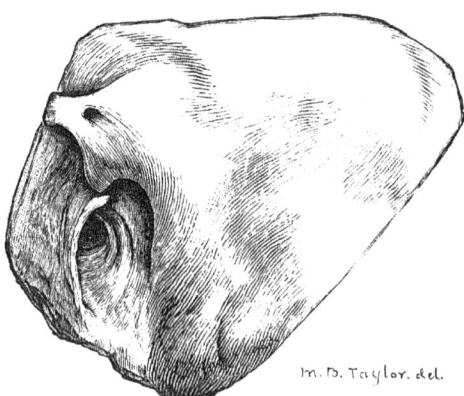

FIG. 7.

Fig. 7.—The outer surface, showing perforation in the zygoma.

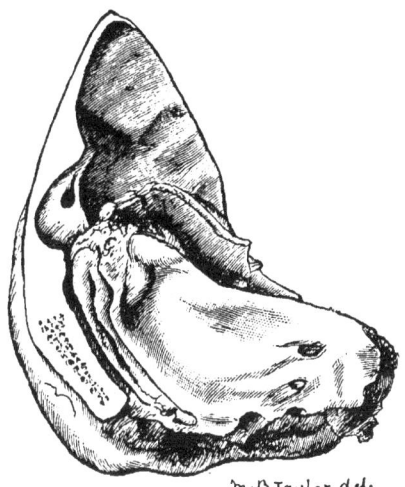

FIG 8.

Fig. 8.—Posterior surface of the same, showing the opening under bridge into the sigmoid groove.

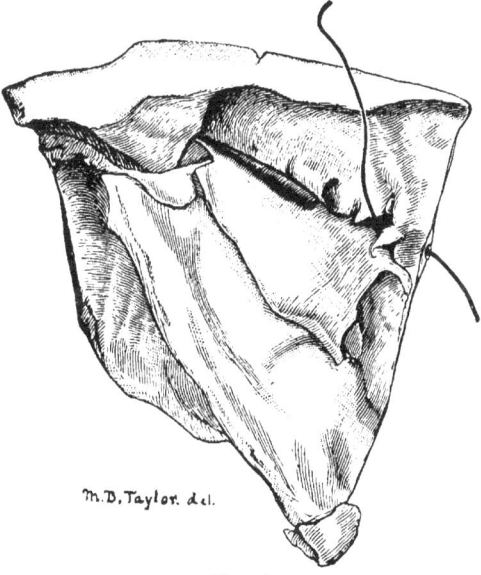

FIG. 9.

Fig. 9.—Superior surface of left adult temporal bone, dura mater thrown back, showing partly-bridged-over groove. The sinus is seen in the turned-back part. There is a wire passed through the anterior opening, which apparently is going to perforate the zygoma.

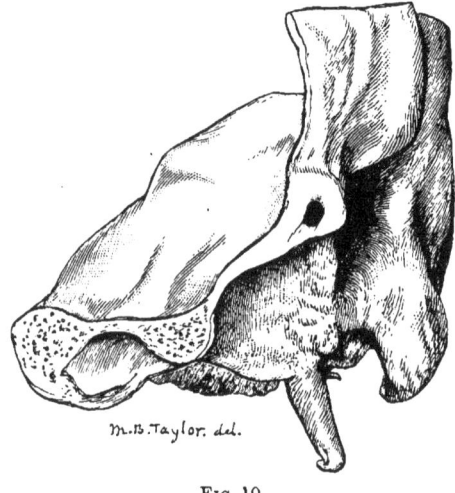

FIG 10.

Fig. 10.—Section through front of preceding specimen, showing canal in the zygoma.

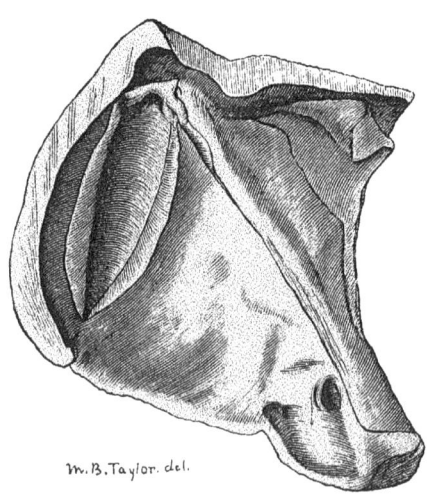

FIG. 11.

Fig. 11.—Posterior aspect of same, showing the opening of the sinus into the lateral sinus.

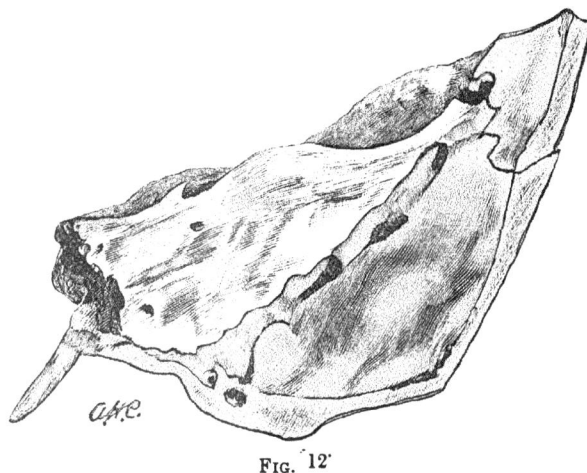

Fig. 12.

Fig. 12.—Adult bone showing deep partly-bridged-over groove opening into sigmoid groove under bridge; no anterior opening.

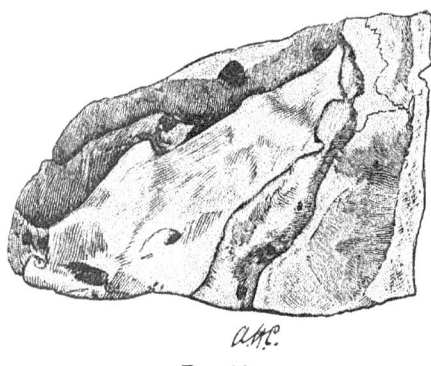

Fig. 13.

Fig. 13.—Adult bone, showing shallow groove partly-bridged-over opening into sigmoid groove; no anterior opening.

A photograph of an adult bone in which the sinus lay under tegmen, and opened into lateral sinus, with no anterior opening, was also demonstrated.

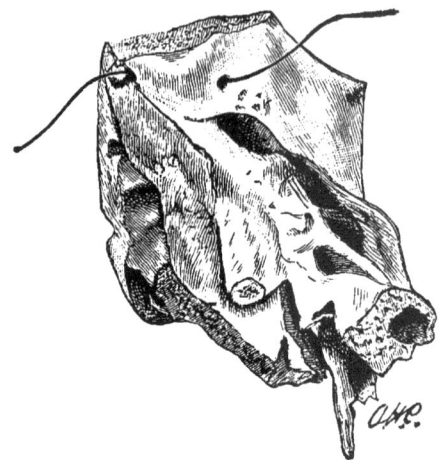

Fig. 14.

Fig. 14.—Adult bone, showing the bridge behind. A common condition ; no anterior opening.

Mr. Cheatle, continuing, said : On looking at the roof of the middle ear in a fresh specimen, after the dura mater has been stripped off, a network of rather large veins can be plainly seen immediately beneath the bone.   From this network several veins emerge through the suture to empty into the sinus.

In children in which the interval between the suture is wide these are sometimes numerous, especially posteriorly.   In the adult a fairly constant one is present, on a vertical level with the membrane ; or more may be present at intervals. These emerging veins receive a fine covering representing the meninges.

(Here two other photographs were shown.   One represented a section through emerging veins, showing extension from the meningeal covering of the sinus, and the other a section through the petro-squamosal sinus with meningeal covering).

Occasionally the openings of fairly large veins can be seen on the cerebral side of the sinus, especially at its anterior part.

Pathological Importance.—It is therefore seen that there is a connection between the veins of the middle ear and those of the meninges, and occasionally, at all events, with those of the temporo-sphenoidal lobe ; and through the meningeal coverings the middle ear is in communication with those of the middle and posterior fossæ. Under these circumstances the importance of this sinus, with its tributaries and connections, from a pathological point of view, is very evident, and explains how infection may spread from the middle ear to the meninges and brain without macroscopical evidence of the connection. Such a state of things is not uncommon, as we all know, in infants and children, in whom, as I have said, the pathway we are considering is well marked, and in whom the membrane may be intact. There is a specimen of mine in the museum, obtained from the post-mortem room from an infant, aged one year, who died of suppurative leptomeningitis without a known cause during an attack of pneumonia. The middle ear was full of pus, containing all sorts of pyogenic cocci, the membrane being intact. I cut sections of the emerging veins, but was unable to find cocci; but this by no means precludes this as having been the pathway. There was no thrombosis. This is by no means the first case of the sort I have seen. Occasionally it is seen in adults, but as a rule a perforation is present in the membrane. It is astonishing, in the face of this close connection of the middle ear with the meninges, that meningitis is not of more frequent occurrence. The explanation may be that the meninges, like the peritoneum, are able to deal with a certain amount of infection, and it is only when the dose is excessive that this resisting power is overcome. This pathway will also explain the presence of a cerebral abscess without macroscopical connection with the diseased middle ear. That the sinus may be the pathway for septic thrombosis of the lateral sinus, I have evidence in two cases.

A. H. Cleveland, of Philadelphia, in the *Archives of Otology*, vol. xxiv., p. 136, 1895, relates the case of a boy, aged six years, who died of pyæmia. At the post-mortem the petro-squamous sinus was found abnormally large and deep, being at one or two points almost entirely bridged over by bony processes. At its anterior extremity necrosis had taken place, and pus had entered the sinus, causing a thrombus, which extended backwards into the lateral sinus. Meningitis was present on the same side.

In St. George's Hospital Museum (No. 33a), and exhibited in the Museum of the Otological Congress (v. Catalogue, No. 696), is a specimen of the dura mater with the lateral and longitudinal sinuses from a man, aged twenty years, who, after suffering with discharge from the right ear for three months, died with symptoms of meningitis, At the post-mortem examination suppurative meningitis was found over the right side, with septic thrombosis of the lateral and longitudinal sinuses. A vein was found which made a direct communication between the tympanum and the lateral sinus, and which would admit the passage of an eye probe.

It may be that we have here one of the pathways which will solve some of the unaccountable intracranial affections met with by the physician, such as the posterior basic meningitis of infants, cerebro-spinal meningitis, and perhaps some cases of tuberculous meningitis, especially when the lining membrane of the middle ear is like the following photograph shown.

It is taken from a section of the lining membrane of the middle ear of an infant who died of tuberculous meningitis and general tuberculosis. Tubercle bacilli can also be seen in another section (to be seen in the museum).

I should like to draw attention to the condition of the middle ears of children who have died of general tuberculosis, including meningeal tuberculosis. There is thin purulent matter in the cavity, often with an intact membrane, and irregular thickening of the lining membrane, which shows on section patches of small-celled infiltration, but no tubercle.

In conclusion, I wish to give my best thanks to the Council of the College of Surgeons, to Professor Charles Stewart, F.R.S., and Mr. Arthur Keith.

DR. KNAPP.—I am sure of speaking the sense of this convention if I express our most hearty thanks to Dr. Cheatle, not only for the instructive demonstration and his important remarks on the petrosquamosal sinus, but also for his untiring efforts in bringing about such an extraordinary, in fact unique, otological museum which we all have admired and studied with keen interest.

My attention has first been drawn to the significance of the petrosquamosal sinus by the case of Dr. Cleveland, of Philadelphia, which Dr. Cheatle quotes, and of which Dr. Cleveland sent me the MS. for publication in the *Archives of Otology* with the remark that in text books of Aural Surgery and also in those of Descriptive Anatomy, nothing, or almost nothing, was to be found. I looked the subject up, and found only a short, but very good description (about 15 lines, small type) in Quain.

I have looked at the six or seven skulls of the Otological Museum in which this sinus is well marked, and the emissary vein with its irregular passage is indicated by bristles. I am sure that now after authoritative attention has been directed to this sinus before this Congress, we shall hear more about it, for I feel sure that by its knowledge we will be enabled to understand many symptoms both *in vivo* and at autopsies which we thus far have found obscure.

CHAIRMAN   -   -   -   PROF. E. J. MOURE.

NOUVEAU TRAITEMENT DES INFLAMMATIONS CHRONIQUES CATARRHALES DU PHARYNX EN RAPPORT AUX MALADIES DE L'OREILLE.

PROF. V. GRAZZI, Florence.

Parmi les maladies du pharynx et particulièrement de cette portion qui a plus de rapport avec l'oreille moyenne, le catarrhe chronique avec ou sans hypertrophie du tissu adénoïde, est sans doute la maladie la plus

importante et la plus rebelle aux traitements proposés ; le nombre de
ceux-ci indique la nullité de leur efficace.

Dans la pharyngite chronique hous avons diverses périodes et à
chacune il faut un traitement particulier ; et celui qui voudrait, pour
une maladie qui dans son parcours produit des effets si variés, proposer
un seul remède se tromperait de beaucoup. Le traitement proposé par
moi, et que j'appelle mécanique ou par écrasement, a un bon succès dans
les premières périodes de la pharyngite catarrhale chronique, c'est-à-dire,
quand il n'y a pas encore des changements étendus dans la structure des
tissus si variés qui composent le pharynx. Ces altérations furent très
bien et diffusément décrites par Faraci dans une communication qu 'on
peut lire à page 214 des Comptes rendus du Troisième Congrès de la
Société Italienne de Laryngologie *(Florence, Tip. Cooperativa, 1899)* ;
et moi je n'en parlerai pas, pour ne pas donner lieu à d'inutiles répétitions.

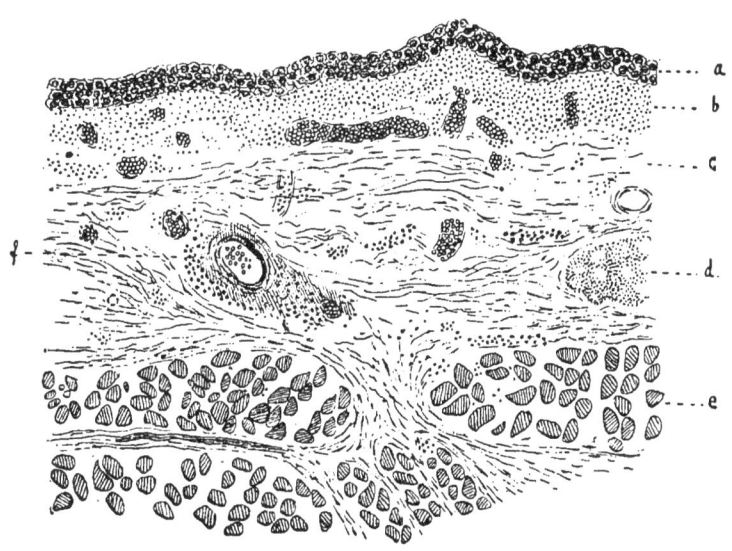

No. 1.—*a*, Epithélium ; *b*, Couche sous-épithéliale ; *c*, Couche sous-muqueuse ;
d, Glande ; *e*, Muscles.

En général la pharyngite chronique produit des altérations remarquables, au commencement dans la partie superficielle et ensuite
s'étend plus profondément. Le tissu qui, plus que tout autre, subit des
changements remarquables dans cette maladie est celui lymphoïde qui
est très abondant dans presque tout le pharynx; en étudiant la structure
normale du pharynx on trouve le tissu lymphoïde dans la partie plus
profonde de la muqueuse *(Poirier, Traité d'anatomie humaine ; Vol.*

IV., pag. 159, L. Bataille et Cie ; Ed. ; *Paris.)* en rapport avec la sous muqueuse et le tissu connectival et l'abondant reseau vasculaire.

Dans les deux dessins ci-joints, le premier représente une section du pharynx prise dans le cadavre d'une jeune fille de treize ou quatorze ans, qui n'avait jamais souffert de maladies à la gorge ; la section est prise en correspondance de la portion moyenne du pharynx ainsi que le démontre l'épithélium pavimenteux. La seconde au contraire fut prise avec la préparation d'un morceau de pharynx que j'ôtai moi-même à une petite fille de Buti près de Pise qui souffrait d'une pharyngite catarrhale chronique avec une énorme prolifération du tissu lymphoïde. Dans ces régions l'épithélium est cylindrique, aussi que le démontre la préparation. (Dessin 2).

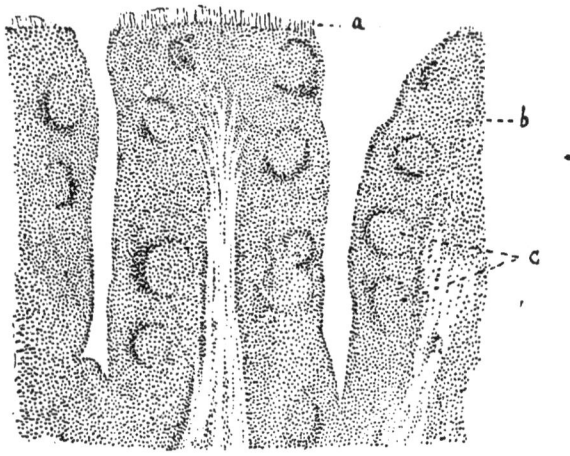

No. 2.—*a*, Epithélium ; *b*, Tissu adénoïde   *c*, Nodule lymphatique.

C'est par la structure normale du pharynx, et en voyant comme dans les premières périodes de la pharyngite catarrhale chronique se produit une étendue prolifération dans le tissu adénoïde, qui amène à des altérations plus graves, c'est-à-dire, à la formation des granulations, aux atrophies, etc., que je pensai à mon nouveau traitement.

Je jugeai qu'il pût être utile d'agir directement sur la muqueuse pharyngienne sans avoir besoin de recourir ni à médicaments qui peuvent en altérer la structure. ni à méthodes caustiques, ni à procès cruents.

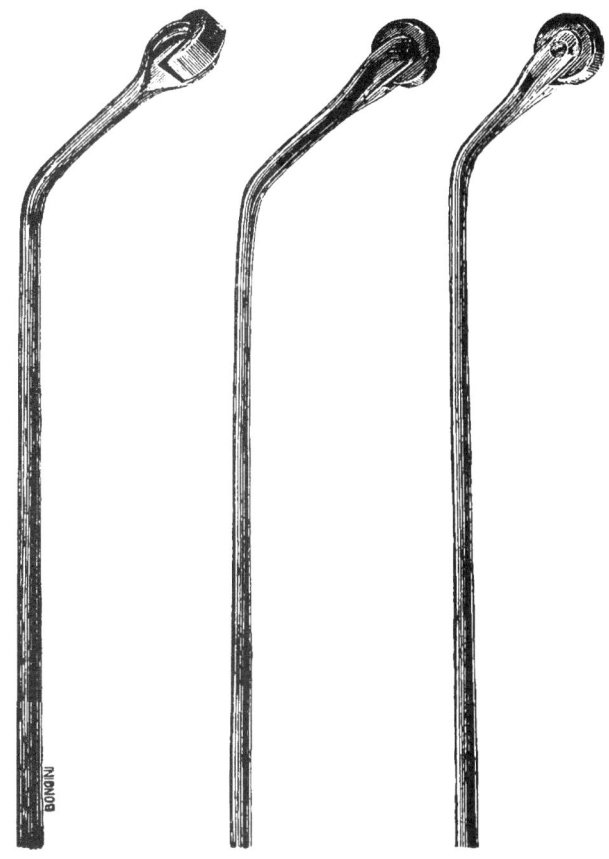

Les substances chimiques (nitrate d'argent, préparations iodiques perchlorure de fer, sulfate et chlorure de zinc) employées en solution trop faible n'ont aucune action sur un tissu vivant. Si on les conseille à doses trop élevées ces médicaments provoquent des inflammations plus ou moins diffuses qui rendent la maladie plus grave et favorisent son développement et sa diffusion à des régions et à des tissus qui encore n'étaient pas attaqués. Avec l'usage de ces substances chimiques on doit encore faire attention à l'ennui qu'on cause au malade en l'obligeant pour des mois, et même pour des années, à avoir toujours dans sa bouche une saveure si dégoutante. Les caustiques d'une espèce quelconque favorisent les procès atrophiques avec toutes les plus graves conséquences en préparant avec plus de célérité le progrès naturel de la pharyngite chronique dont la fin est presque toujours l'atrophie. Ces procédés pour des raisons faciles à comprendre, provoquent la diffusion de la maladie pharyngienne à l'oreille moyenne. Les procès cruents favorisent des adhésions entre les variés tissus pharyngiens, cicatrisations et épaississement connectival. Ces procès sont seulement à recommander dans les cas plus graves de pharyngite chronique avec des volumineuses granulations et étendue et sensible hyperplasie adénoïdienne.   Je crois aussi que dans ces malades le meilleur traitement peut consister dans le ràclement, ou en l'asportation dans les différentes régions du pharynx, ainsi que j'ai pratiqué moi-même, dans cette enfant de Buti, qui put me fournir le matériel pour faire la préparation microscopique qu'on voit dans le Dessin No. 2 du tissu adénoïdien hyperplastique.   Mais ceux-ci ne sont pas certainement les cas les plus fréquents qu'on peut observer dans la pratique journalière.

Dans les adultes cette forme est d'autant plus rare qu'elle est plus fréquente dans les enfants, dans lesquels, pour cette raison et pour bien d'autres, mon traitement ne trouve pas facile application.

Les adultes qui ont eu fréquentes et répétés catarrhes chroniques des fosses nasales avec diffusion de la maladie aux régions, supérieure et moyenne du pharynx : dans ceux qui abusent du tabac, dans les orateurs, en ceux qui ont une profession qui les oblige à rester pendant plusieurs heures au milieu des vapeurs, ou dans un pulviscule atmosphérique irritant, on observe ces cas plus typiques de pharyngite chronique avec hypertrophie des tissus.   Ce sont en effet ces malades qui ont de très grands avantages avec ma méthode thérapeutique.   Ainsi que je l'ai constaté en plusieurs cas où je l'ai employée.

Elle consiste dans la compression ou écrasement méthodique et gradué de la paroi postérieure et de celle latérale du pharynx en toute leur étendue.   Je fais ces manœuvres au moyen de petits soutiens métalliques pliés à angle plus ou moins obtus afin que l'œil de l'opérateur puisse suivre toujours l'extrémité de l'instrument pour pouvoir le faire pénétrer et glisser dans la cavité nasopharyngienne et en bas dans cette portion du pharynx qui a rapport avec le larynx. Ces petits soutiens finissent avec une espèce de fourchette très simple sur laquelle est arrêtée une petite roue.   Les roulettes sont métalliques polies, à angles point aigus de différente grandeur et inclination en rapport à leur soutien pour pouvoir agir, tant soit dans la paroi postérieure, que sur celle latérale.   Les instruments sont facilement désinfectables à la flamme.   Pour appliquer mon traitement dans la pharyngite chronique avec ma méthode on fait asseoir le malade et l'on commence à pratiquer des légères compressions dans la paroi postérieure du pharynx introduisant un de ces instruments que l'on croit, par la grandeur de la roulette et par la courbe de l'angle, plus convenable à la grandeur du pharynx, de la cavité nasopharyngienne, à l'âge du malade, etc.

A cause des dispositions anatomiques des tissus et du système vasculaire sanguin et lymphatique sur lequel a lieu particulièrement la compression, on procède toujours en parcourant avec la roulette de haut en bas.   J'ai vu dans mes expérimentations sur les malades, que nous avons un meilleur effet dans la réduction de l'hypertrophie des tissus et du volume des éléments glandulaires, ne faisant jamais parcourir la roulette en sens contraire, c'est-à-dire, de bas en haut. Quand on veut agir dans le troisième inférieur de la paroi postérieure du pharynx, la roulette se tourne en bas en la faisant parcourir sur les tissus, toujours des parties supérieures à celles inférieures.

Ces manœuvres ne sont pas douloureuses mais pour diminuer ou abolir les mouvements réflexes pharyngiens, dans les premières séances on peut user des anesthétiques locaux. J'ai dit dans les premières séances parceque après plusieurs fois le malade s'habitue à ce traitement et n'accuse aucun malaise à l'exception d'un léger endolorissement à la gorge. Cette sensation aussi est plus forte dans les premières séances que dans les suivantes.

Dans la pharyngite granulaire ma méthode thérapeutique rémplace admirablement les ignoponctions qui pour bien de raisons, inutiles à répéter, ne sont pas exemptes d'inconvénients. En effet, en faisant une légère pression proportionnée au volume de la granulation que l'on veut atrophiser, on voit que peu-à-peu la granulation s'aplatit et que quelquefois en une seule séance on en provoque l'écrasement et la réabsorption.

Quelques uns de ces instruments dont je me sers, sont représentés par le Dessin No. 3 ; on se sert du petit soutien A. pour les parois latérales du pharynx et ceux B. et C. sont l'un plus long et plus gros et l'autre plus court et plus petit, selon le cas où l'on doit opérer. Pour les enfants et pour les individus qui ont l'espace naso-pharyngien restreint j'ai fait construire une autre série de roulettes plus petites et plus courtes dans la partie verticale.

L'action mécanique prolongée et répétée que l'on fait avec ces instruments sur les tissus pharyngiens qui sont le siège d'inflammation chronique et d'hyperplasie diffuse ou folliculaire facilite la réabsorption des exsudats interstitiels et rend plus active et plus accélérée la circulation sanguine et lymphatique. On favorise, de cette manière la chute des vieux épithéliums et rend plus prochaine la formation des nouveaux éléments épithéliales ainsi que se modifient les sécrétions des petites glandes qui en grand nombre existent dans ces régions.

La subtilisation des tissus, la manière de disparaître des granulations et la plus grande activité de la circulation pour les rapports anatomiques qui existent entre la cavité naso-pharyngienne et l'oreille moyenne, font ressentir un avantage remarquable dans le traitement des otites moyennes, catarrhales chroniques. C'est ce que j'ai eu souvent à observer pendant les deux années dans lesquelles j'ai pratiqué ce système thérapeutique, dans cette forme de pharyngite catarrhale chronique que j'ai déjà dit être la plus sensible aux bons effets de ce traitement dans un temps plus ou moins prolongé.

TRAITEMENT CHIRURGICAL DE L'OTITE MOYENNE CHRONIQUE SÈCHE
PAR L'ÉVIDEMENT PETRO-MASTOÏDIEN AVEC ET SANS TUBAGE.

DR. ARISTIDE MALHERBE, Paris.

MESSIEURS,

Je suis heureux d'apporter aujourd'hui au milieu de vous une
nouvelle méthode chirurgicale que j'ai déjà présentée et publiée en
France, mais que je tiens à honneur de vous soumettre.

Je viens donc vous demander la permission de vous exposer cette
intervention que j'ai préconisée sous le nom d'*Evidement petromastoïdien*
et qui a pour but, sinon de guérir radicalement, du moins d'améliorer
dans une très large mesure cette pénible affection, contre laquelle toutes
les ressources de l'art ont été jusqu'à présent employées sans grand
succès : j'ai nommé l'otite moyenne chronique sèche.

Actuellement, Messieurs, les maladies de l'oreille sont entrées dans
le domaine de la chirurgie, grâce aux nouvelles méthodes d'antisepsie et
d'asepsie.

Presque tous les spécialistes sont d'accord qu'il faut aborder l'oreille
moyenne, quand il s'agit de lésions suppurées aiguës ou chroniques,
par la voie mastoïdienne, la seule qui permette d'atteindre ces cavités
dans toutes leurs parties ; il me paraît donc logique, quand il s'agit de
lésions inflammatoires chroniques et scléreuses, de suivre la même voie,
voie essentiellement chirurgicale, et cela pour la même raison.

L'étude de la physiologie, de la structure et du développement des
cellules mastoïdiennes, et surtout de l'une de ces cellules, l'*antre petro-
mastoïdien,*—qui constitue, à proprement parler, une partie régulière et
définie de l'oreille moyenne,—est d'ailleurs de nature à nous expliquer le
bien fondé d'une intervention que viennent légitimer encore l'existence
et la nature des différentes lésions anatomiques caractérisant toute cette
variété d'affections appelées : *otites moyennes sèches.*

Les altérations morbides qui existent dans la caisse, épaississement
de la muqueuse, néoformation de tissu conjonctif, brides membraneuses
reliant les osselets, se continuent dans les cavités mastoïdiennes, où elles
déterminent l'épaississement et la rigidité de la muqueuse et l'hyperos-
tose plus ou moins complète du tissu sous-jacent.

La transmission au labyrinthe des ondes sonores arrivant par la
membrane tympanique, se fait en partie par la chaîne des osselets, en
partie par l'air.

On comprend facilement que des altérations qui ont pour effet de
diminuer plus ou moins la mobilité des organes chargés de transmettre
les ondes sonores et qui atteignent également l'aditus et l'antre, en
réduisant leurs cavités, auront pour résultat de restreindre singulièrement le pouvoir auditif.

En effet, il est permis de considérer l'oreille moyenne comme une
excavation remplie d'air, creusée au centre de la base du rocher.   Par

sa partie antérieure elle se prolonge jusque dans l'arrière-cavité des fosses nasales ; par sa partie postérieure, elle s'étend dans l'épaisseur de la paroi mastoïdienne du temporal. Elle constitue, en somme, un diverticule qui, dans son trajet, se rétrécit et s'élargit tour à tour.

Une première partie de ce diverticule s'étendant de l'arrière-cavité des fosses nasales vers l'angle rentrant du temporal, prend le nom de *trompe d'Eustache*. A ce niveau, le diverticule se dilate brusquement et largement, formant *la caisse du tympan*. Un second rétrécissement très court représente son passage de la portion pétrée dans la portion mastoïdienne ; c'est *l'aditus ad antrum* et se termine presque aussitôt par une dernière dilatation, *l'antre petro-mastoïdien*.

Parmi ces différentes parties, il en est qui présentent une grande importance acoustique, ce sont les *dilatations*. Ce qui caractérise ces dernières, c'est qu'elles renferment de l'air, condition nécessaire à l'audition. L'antre petro-mastoïdien est entièrement formé, ainsi que la caisse, pendant la vie fœtale ; ces .deux cavités peuvent donc être regardées comme la portion la plus importante du diverticule qui constitue l'oreille moyenne.

Les vibrations imprimées à la membrane tympanique arrivent à l'oreille interne aussi par d'autres voies, mais surtout par la fenêtre ovale, au moyen de l'étrier plus ou moins mobile ; celui-ci les reçoit normalement de la chaîne des osselets, de l'air de la caisse et des cellules mastoïdiennes, ou encore, comme cela se passe après l'évidement osseux et surtout après l'évidement avec tubage, de l'air contenu non seulement dans la caisse, mais aussi dans l'antre petro-mastoïdien agrandi, ce qui constitue un appareil de résonnance plus grand pour les sons. Cela est si vrai, que sans vouloir faire ici de l'anatomie comparée, je rappellerai que l'absence de cellules mastoïdiennes est suppléée chez un grand nombre de mammifères par le développement considérable de la caisse du tympan, de telle sorte qu'on trouve, chez ces vertébrés une sorte de balancement entre la cavité tympanique et la cavité mastoïdienne.

Telle est cette partie qui, en raison de son rôle anatomique et physiologique, représente un système particulier qui mérite le nom, que je lui ai donné, de *système tympano-mastoïdien*. Telle est aussi cette partie qui, en raison des différentes lésions qui s'y rencontrent, est susceptible d'être utilement modifiée par l'opération dont je viens vous entretenir, par l'*évidement petro-mastoïdien*.

N'allez pas croire, Messieurs, qu'il entre dans ma pensée de prétendre que tous les cas de surdité chronique soient justiciables de cette intervention chirurgicale. Non, mais il en est un grand nombre, et c'est ce qui m'engage à examiner rapidement devant vous certaines considérations relatives à ce mode de traitement.

Les lésions qui siègent dans l'oreille moyenne, sclérose ou inflammation chronique, prennent surtout de l'importance pour la fonction de

M

l'ouïe suivant leurs relations plus ou moins étroites avec les parties acoustiques principales. C'est ce qui fait les grandes différences de surdité suivant que telle ou telle partie est frappée. En d'autres termes, l'état de la fonction de l'ouïe dépend de la localisation du processus morbide.

Ordinairement, l'aggravation de la surdité, quand la maladie est abandonnée à elle-même, se fait peu à peu, parfois avec rapidité, parfois d'une façon lente et insensible. Le tympan peut être perforé, les osselets plus ou moins mobiles, ce qui est surtout nécessaire à l'audition, c'est l'intégrité des fenêtres et la capacité des cavités moyennes ; et comme, actuellement, il est encore impossible de modifier l'altération de ces fenêtres, tout ce que l'on peut se contenter de faire, quand la lésion n'est pas trop avancée, consiste à favoriser l'intensité et l'amplitude des ondes sonores en augmentant, si possible, la mobilité des osselets et les vibrations de l'air dans toute l'oreille moyenne.

D'une manière générale, on peut dire que dans la grande majorité des affections qu'on englobe sous la dénomination d'otite moyenne chronique sèche, il y a résorption des cavités du système tympano-mastoïdien et par conséquent raréfaction de l'air et *augmentation de la pression* intra-auriculaire, d'où : *diminution des vibrations sonores.*

Le pronostic opératoire, entièrement subordonné à l'état des lésions du système tympano-mastoïdien, ne peut être déduit que de l'étude attentive des différentes parties de l'organe de l'ouïe et de sa fonction auditive. C'est pourquoi j'estime qu'il est indispensable d'examiner les malades d'une façon toute particulière à ce sujet.

La perception atmosphérique de l'acoumètre, du diapason grave et des vibrations musicales amples, comme celles du gong, ne doit pas tomber trop bas si l'on veut avoir un résultat qui soit tout à fait bon. J'en dirai autant de la durée de la conductibilité osseuse du diapason grave qui doit presque égaler la durée de la conductibilité atmosphérique d'une oreille saine.

L'épreuve des pressions centripètes, plus difficilement applicable, donne aussi des résultats dont il faut tenir compte, mais qui ne sont pas sans offrir quelque variabilité dans l'interprétation.

L'abolition de la perception atmosphérique du diapason à note aiguë est un signe extrêmement fâcheux.

Il est absolument nécessaire d'établir le rôle des perceptions des sons aigus et graves, car, dans la surdité d'origine nerveuse, la faculté de perception pour les sons élevés diminue d'abord, tandis que les sons bas sont encore perçus. Il est vrai que dans certaines affections du labyrinthe, la perception des sons bas peut diminuer plus rapidement que celle des sons élevés.

Dans l'otite moyenne chronique sèche au contraire, dans la sclérose, la surdité est généralement plutôt prononcée pour les sons graves, tandis que l'audition est meilleure pour les sons élevés. La diminution des sons aigus paraît être un signe que l'oreille interne commence à participer à la lésion.

Ceci explique pourquoi mon opération donnera des résultats un peu différents, tantôt très bons, tantôt seulement passables, suivant qu'on la pratiquera sur tel ou tel malade, remplissant ou ne remplissant pas les conditions que je viens d'indiquer ; et je puis déclarer que jusqu'à présent, quelque minimes qu'aient pu être certains résultats, ils sont néanmoins incontestables et durables, c'est là déjà une chose suffisamment significative et qu'il convient de retenir. Pour avoir toujours des résultats parfaits, il serait de toute nécessité de ne pas attendre pour opérer que les malades soient trop sourds ; il serait aussi à souhaiter que ceux-ci puissent comprendre qu'ils ont intérêt à ne pas reculer trop loin une intervention qui n'est nullement dangereuse et qui est susceptible de leur donner un très bon résultat, alors que leurs lésions sont encore limitées.

Messieurs, avant de vous exposer la description de mon procédé opératoire, je désire vous dire un mot d'une modification que j'ai introduite depuis quelque temps déjà dans ma technique et qui m'a donné, dans certains cas, des résultats bien supérieurs encore à ceux que j'avais jusque-là obtenus. Pour rétablir l'équilibre de pression intratympanique, qui est souvent rompu, et augmenter les cavités pneumatiques, j'ai eu l'idée de pratiquer, après l'évidement osseux, une communication entre ces cavités tympano-mastoïdiennes et l'air extérieur, constituant un véritable tubage de l'oreille moyenne.

Ce résultat est obtenu à l'aide d'un petit tube en celluloïd pur, incurvé en forme d'U et de la grosseur n° 15 de la filière Charrière ; j'ai l'honneur de vous le présenter.

Ce tube en U, rendu parfaitement aseptique par les vapeurs de formol, est placé par l'une de ses extrémités dans l'antre ; grâce à sa forme, il vient se mettre à cheval, par sa concavité, sur le bord antérieur de l'apophyse mastoïde. L'autre extrémité, taillée en biseau aux dépens du côté convexe, sort dans le conduit auditif externe à travers une ouverture faite dans sa paroi postérieure, réséquée à cet effet, à la jonction même du conduit membraneux avec le conduit osseux.

J'en arrive maintenant à la description des différents temps de cette intervention.

Comme pour toute opération chirurgicale, le malade sera, autant que possible, préparé la veille ; le champ opératoire sera rasé sur une assez grande étendue, puis recouvert d'un pansement antiseptique.

Un aide est chargé d'anesthésier le malade au chloroforme.

Il est bon de faire reposer la tête sur un coussin de sable peu épais, destiné à amortir les chocs.

Un autre aide procède, par un savonnage énergique avec la brosse, à la toilette de l'apophyse mastoïde, du sillon retro-auriculaire, du pavillon sur les deux faces et du conduit auditif externe qui est soigneusement désinfecté à l'aide d'un petit écouvillon.

Le champ opératoire successivement nettoyé avec de l'éther et une solution de sublimé à 1/1000 et garanti par des compresses, je saisis le pavillon de la main gauche, je le rabats en avant en tirant légèrement dessus et avec le bistouri tenu comme une plume à écrire, *j'incise* franchement les téguments et le périoste immédiatement dans le sillon retro-auriculaire, en commençant en haut au niveau de l'insertion du pavillon pour terminer sur le sommet de l'apophyse mastoïde. Cette incision retro-auriculaire a l'avantage de donner une cicatrice absolument invisible.

Je repasse dans la plaie un bistouri court et à pointe rabattue pour achever de sectionner le périoste et *je refoule* celui-ci à la rugine de façon à décoller en avant le pavillon et le conduit, et, en arrière, un lambeau postérieur suffisant pour découvrir toute la surface de l'apophyse. Ce décollement périostique est un temps très important, car il permet de bien voir la région sur laquelle on doit opérer.

Cela fait, je procède à l'*hémostase* ; on rencontre, d'une façon presque constante, une petite artère : l'auriculaire postérieure immédiatement en arrière du pavillon, placée dans le sillon auriculo-mastoïdien et adhérente à la couche sous-cutanée. Il n'est pas rare de couper également une ou deux autres artérioles qui naissent de celle-ci ; l'une est destinée au pavillon de l'oreille, une autre s'anastomose avec la branche postérieure de la temporale, une autre se porte transversalement en arrière pour s'anastomoser avec l'occipitale.

Quelques pinces hémostatiques ou de Kocher arrêtent facilement l'hémorrhagie.

J'introduis alors, par le méat, dans le conduit auditif, une sonde cannelée ou mieux une pince de Kocher dont j'écarte légèrement les mors pour tendre la paroi postérieure et j'incise cette dernière au bistouri dans le sens de la longueur jusqu'à l'entrée du méat. A quelques millimètres de ce point, *je résèque* aux ciseaux deux petits triangles de la paroi jusqu'au conduit osseux, donnant ainsi à la brèche la forme d'un Y dont le sommet répond à l'entrée du méat et dont les deux branches limitent le passage du tube.

Il est important de faire dès le début de l'opération cette ouverture pour le placement du tube ou de la mèche, car elle s'accompagne toujours d'un peu de sang. Un léger tamponnement avec une petite mèche de gaze suffit à arrêter l'hémorrhagie pendant le temps que l'on procède à l'évidement.

Pour pratiquer cet évidement, il est nécessaire de maintenir en avant l'oreille rabattue et d'écarter en arrière le lambeau postérieur. Si l'on confie alors deux écarteurs à un aide, ses mains se trouvent immobilisées pendant toute l'opération et il ne peut plus éponger le sang qui encombre le champ opératoire.

Pour parer à cet inconvénient, j'ai fait construire *mon écarteur automatique*, composé de chaque côté de trois griffes mousses, situées à l'extrémité des deux branches d'une forte pince. Par le rapprochement de ces branches qui fonctionnent à la manière d'une pince hémostatique, on obtient un écartement de plus en plus considérable. Les branches très solides sont légèrement courbes, de façon à se mouler sur la convexité de la tête. J'ajoute que par la compression qu'il détermine, il concourt à l'hémostase des tranches.

J'attaque alors, au lieu d'élection, l'antre à la gouge et au maillet.

Voici, à ce propos, quels sont, suivant moi, les meilleurs points de repère pour sa recherche : *la moitié supérieure du bord postérieur du conduit* qu'il est indispensable de bien voir ou de sentir avec le doigt, et la *linea temporalis*, qui est la continuation de la racine transverse de l'apophyse zygomatique, marquée au niveau du conduit, par une saillie, *spina supra meatum.* L'antre correspond—à la surface de l'os,—à une petite région dont la limite antérieure est une ligne située à un demi-centimètre en arrière de cette moitié supérieure du bord postérieur du conduit et parallèle à ce bord, et dont la limite supérieure est environ deux millimètres plus bas que cette *linea temporalis.* Une autre ligne, située à un centimètre en arrière et parallèle à la première, marquera sa limite postérieure, et une autre ligne horizontale, à un centimètre plus bas, sa limite inférieure.

En ne s'écartant pas de cette région et en avançant lentement, on pénétrera dans l'antre, situé plus ou moins profondément.

Généralement, dans les cas de sclérose vraie, on trouve l'os dur, sec, ne saignant pas ; la cavité de l'antre est, la plupart du temps aussi, petite et ne présentant plus trace de fibro-muqueuse. Presque toujours également, l'aditus est diminué de volume et même est oblitéré.

Après avoir agrandi suffisamment l'antre, je pratique, à l'aide d'un *petit perforateur à main*, muni d'une *mèche*, au niveau même de l'aditus, un canal que je creuse davantage, à l'aide d'une *fraise* montée sur le même perforateur, jusqu'à ce que j'aie pénétré dans la caisse et qu'une communication complète existe entre cette dernière et l'antre petromastoïdien. Cet instrument met à l'abri d'une blessure possible du facial et n'occasionne aucun délabrement. Il suffit seulement de bien connaître la direction exacte de l'aditus, d'avancer lentement et doucement, en garnissant même, pour plus de sûreté, la mèche ou la fraise d'un curseur-protecteur destiné à prévenir toute échappée. L'absence subite de résistance vous avertit que l'on a pénétré dans la caisse.

C'est par ce canal, convenablement agrandi, qu'il sera possible d'introduire les *petits crochets*, les *rugines tranchantes* et les *fines curettes* à courbure spéciale que j'ai fait construire pour cet usage et qui permettent d'explorer la caisse et de détruire les adhérences qui peuvent s'y trouver. Lorsque les osselets sont fortement immobilisés et que les cavités tympano-mastoïdiennes sont peu touchées, j'introduis dans le conduit auditif osseux, en perforant la membrane, un petit crochet qui me sert à fixer le manche du marteau, pendant que j'exerce des tractions du côté de la caisse. Toute cette partie de l'intervention est extrêmement délicate et nécessite la plus grande douceur.

Il peut se faire que parfois, comme cela a lieu dans les otites sèches inflammatoires, l'on soit un peu gêné par le sang ; pour bien éponger, je me sers de petites lanières de gaze stérilisée, très facilement maniables et qui sont susceptibles d'être portées dans les anfractuosités osseuses.

Après avoir, autant que possible, libéré la caisse et donné un peu de jeu à la chaîne des osselets, il faut s'arrêter là.

Je considère comme inutile, et bien plus, nuisible, de vouloir mobiliser la platine de l'étrier ; c'est produire, à coup sûr, en raison de sa situation anatomique, défavorable, la fracture de ses branches et léser souvent la fenêtre ovale, à laquelle il adhère intimement ; d'où la production de vertiges et l'aggravation de la surdité.

Pour terminer, prenant un *tube en U*, j'en introduis une extrémité dans la cavité de l'antre. La concavité du tube vient emboîter exactement le bord antérieur osseux de l'apophyse. Je ramène ensuite le pavillon en place, en faisant pénétrer l'autre extrémité du tube dans l'ouverture ménagée dans le conduit membraneux, en ayant soin que l'extrémité, qui est taillée en forme de biseau, affleure au niveau de la paroi postérieure du conduit, sans toucher à l'autre paroi, ni obstruer la lumière, ce dont il est facile de se rendre compte, en explorant le conduit auditif. Une bonne précaution à prendre consiste à introduire dans l'intérieur du tube, pour empêcher son obstruction, une fine mèche stérilisée ; l'extrémité libre de la mèche ressort au niveau du méat auditif externe. A côté, une autre mèche de gaze stérilisée est placée dans le conduit, pour en maintenir la forme.

Il ne reste plus qu'à terminer l'opération en *réunissant directement* à la lèvre postérieure de l'incision le pavillon à l'aide de six ou sept points au crin de Florence.

Le *pansement* consiste en un *croissant* de gaze stérilisée appliqué immédiatement sur la ligne de suture et en quelques doubles de la même gaze qui viennent recouvrir le pavillon. Ouate stérilisée par dessus et bandes pour maintenir le tout.

Ce pansement est laissé huit jours en place. *Le huitième jour*, j'enlève les points de suture, je retire la fine mèche qui se trouve dans le tube et celle du conduit et je remplace cette dernière par une autre ; nouveau pansement très léger qui reste *deux jours*, au bout desquels la cicatrisation est complète et le malade guéri.

Dans les cas où je ne pratique pas le tubage, je place dans l'aditus et dans l'autre une fine mèche de gaze stérilisée au lieu du tube ; cette mèche passe également par une ouverture faite au conduit auditif et sort au niveau du méat. Elle est enlevée en même temps que les points de suture, au huitième jour.

Quand je laisse le tube permanent ; il persiste pendant un temps assez variable, un léger suintement au pourtour de l'extrémité du tube qui fait saillie dans le conduit ; un simple tampon d'ouate renouvelé tous les jours est le meilleur pansement. Parfois, il est nécessaire de réprimer au nitrate d'argent la présence d'un petit bourgeon charnu. Au bout de 15 à 20 jours au plus, la cicatrisation est absolue par suite de l'épidermisation du trajet du tube.

Chez tous mes opérés, le tube est admirablement toléré ; il ne provoque aucune douleur, ni même aucune gêne. Rien n'est visible extérieurement, même en regardant au niveau du méat auditif. On peut cependant apercevoir, à l'aide d'un spéculum auriculaire, l'extrémité du tube taillée en bec de flûte, qui occupe la place de la paroi postérieure du conduit membraneux.

Messieurs, j'ai opéré actuellement soixante malades par ma méthode, c'est-à-dire l'évidement petro-mastoïdien avec ou sans tubage.

J'ai la ferme conviction, tirée des faits de ma pratique, qu'il faut tenir grand compte pour le choix du procédé, de la diversité des cas de surdité que l'on englobe sous la dénomination générale *d'otite moyenne chronique sèche.*

Dans plusieurs formes d'otites, ce qui domine, c'est la résorption des cavités pneumatiques de l'oreille par un processus sclérosant.

Qu'il s'agisse de *lésions congénitales,* telles que petitesse de la caisse et des niches des fenêtres labyrinthiques, telles qu'étroitesse de la trompe et du pharynx, on trouve dans ces cas, outre l'éburnation des os par l'ostéite condensante, une cavité tympanique presque réduite à sa portion tubaire et dont la partie postérieure forme une masse compacte, scléreuse, privée de vaisseaux, au milieu de laquelle les osselets sont ensevelis.

Qu'il s'agisse, enfin, de *lésions suppurées anciennes,* il existe des adhérences entre la membrane et la paroi labyrinthique. Si les osselets subsistent encore, leur mobilité est diminuée et même abolie, leur revêtement muqueux est devenu entièrement rigide. De plus, les cavités qui entourent l'antre petro-mastoïdien ont subi une transformation complète ; une substance osseuse, dure comme de l'ivoire, s'est substituée à elles, de telle sorte qu'une véritable néoplasie osseuse occupe toute la cavité des cellules, autrefois remplies d'air.

Qu'il s'agisse enfin de *lésions scléreuses,* que celles-ci se développent d'emblée ou bien succèdent à des lésions inflammatoires anciennes, on rencontre un épaississement interstitiel de la muqueuse qui renferme souvent des dépôts calcaires, des ossifications unissant solidement aux régions voisines chacune des parties de l'appareil de transmission ; il existe parfois une néoformation de tissu osseux au niveau de la fenêtre ovale, envahissant plus ou moins la platine de l'étrier, une ankylose des osselets et trop souvent l'ossification de la fenêtre ronde.

Mais là aussi, les lésions scléreuses sont généralisées à tout le système tympano-mastoïdien et contribuent à diminuer sa capacité. La gouge trouve l'apophyse mastoïde dure, éburnée ; l'antre est très réduit de volume, l'aditus est rétréci ou même complètement oblitéré : il n'y a plus trace de muqueuse.

Dans tous ces cas, où il y a manifestement diminution des cavités de l'oreille moyenne, il faut pratiquer *l'évidement petro-mastoïdien avec tubage*. C'est le mode opératoire qui assure de la façon la plus large le fonctionnement de l'annexe pneumatique de l'oreille.

Il n'en est pas de même, au contraire, des *lésions catarrhales* qui n'ont pas encore subi la dégénérescence scléreuse ; dans celles-ci, il n'y a pas diminution, à proprement parler, des cavités de l'oreille moyenne ; ce qui domine surtout, c'est l'inflammation chronique de la muqueuse de la caisse, caractérisée par la néoformation de tissu conjonctif et de vaisseaux ; ce sont des brides membraneuses qui relient les osselets aux parois de la caisse, c'est l'épaississement, en somme, de la muqueuse, qui, lorsqu'elle frappe la fenêtre ovale, est cependant d'un mauvais pronostic. Mais ici, les cavités tympaniques ne sont pas diminuées de volume, l'antre, les cellules mastoïdiennes ont conservé leur dimension, l'os n'est pas dur, il saigne même facilement, en un mot, il n'y a pas de travail d'ostéite condensante.

Souvent, avec le temps, ces lésions deviennent scléreuses ; il est évident qu'alors il faut les traiter comme les lésions scléreuses primitives. Autrement, c'est vers la caisse et son contenu qu'il faut diriger ses efforts ; l'évidement doit surtout tendre à rétablir le fonctionnement des organes de transmission, par la destruction des adhérences et la libération de la caisse. Le tubage ne peut vraiment être utile que s'il existe une obstruction complète de la trompe, ce qui est relativement assez rare.

Ainsi donc une seule et même technique opératoire ne convient pas aussi bien à tous les cas de surdité justiciables de l'intervention. Le choix du procédé à opposer à chaque variété dépend des considérations que je viens d'exposer.

Telle est, Messieurs, cette opération que j'ai tenu à vous présenter avec quelques détails. Lorsqu'elle est pratiquée dans les conditions que j'ai essayé de vous indiquer, elle est susceptible de donner des résultats, dont la constance et la perfection sont loin, je crois, d'être égalées dans toutes les autres méthodes chirurgicales employées jusqu'ici.

Je ne vous parle pas seulement des résultats immédiats, car, ayant suivi presque tous mes opérés, depuis le commencement de l'année 1896, j'ai pu constater, avec entière satisfaction, qu'ils continuent à bénéficier de l'intervention tant au point de vue de l'amélioration obtenue dans l'audition qu'au point de vue de la cessation des bruits subjectifs.

Les résultats éloignés sont donc aussi bons que les résultats immédiats.

Si les divers arguments que je viens de vous exposer ont quelque valeur, je crois pouvoir terminer ma communication en groupant, de la manière suivante, les conclusions principales qui s'en dégagent :

CONCLUSIONS.

1° L'opération que j'ai proposée et décrite sous le nom d'*Evidement petro-mastoïdien* est le traitement chirurgical de choix de l'*otite moyenne chronique sèche*.

Cette intervention, basée sur des considérations de physiologie, de structure et de développement du *système tympano-mastoïdien*, est légitimée par la nature des altérations anatomiques qui caractérisent toute cette variété d'affections.

2° Cette méthode opératoire permet seule d'agir largement sur les organes de la caisse et sur l'annexe pneumatique de l'oreille moyenne.

3° Il y aurait avantage à opérer alors que les lésions n'ont pas encore envahi le labyrinthe, car le résultat opératoire est entièrement subordonné à l'état de ces lésions.

4° Il est indispensable de pratiquer un examen attentif et méthodique des différentes parties de l'organe de l'ouïe et de la fonction auditive.

5° La perception aérienne du diapason grave ne doit pas tomber trop bas, si l'on veut avoir un résultat tout à fait satisfaisant.

6° La durée de la conductibilité osseuse, pratiquée à l'aide du diapason grave, doit être la plus grande possible et tendre à se rapprocher de la durée de la conductibilité atmosphérique d'une oreille saine.

7° La diminution et surtout l'abolition de la perception aérienne du diapason à note aiguë sont des signes extrêmement fâcheux.

8° Il ne faut pratiquer l'opération que sur une oreille à la fois. C'est toujours, à moins de contre-indications, l'oreille qui entend le plus dur ou qui est atteinte de bourdonnements les plus violents que le chirurgien doit opérer de préférence.

9° Les différents temps de l'opération sont :

a) L'incision rétro-auriculaire, le décollement du pavillon et du conduit et le refoulement du périoste.

b) L'hémostase et la résection de la paroi postérieure du conduit.

c) L'évidement osseux à la gouge et au maillet.

d) L'agrandissement de l'aditus et la communication large avec la caisse.

e) La mobilisation des osselets et la libération de la caisse.

f) Le placement du tube en U et des mèches.

g) La réunion immédiate de la plaie par la suture du pavillon.

h) Le pansement.

10° Le huitième jour, les fils sont enlevés et, le dixième jour, tout est terminé.

11° Les sons à tonalité élevée bénéficient, dans une plus grande proportion, de l'amélioration acquise.

12° Les bruits subjectifs résultant d'une lésion de l'appareil de transmission et d'une augmentation de la pression intra-tympanique, disparaissent ou diminuent progressivement à la suite de l'intervention.

13° Grâce au tubage qui réalise une communication permanente entre les cavités tympano-mastoïdiennes et l'air extérieur, la pression intra-auriculaire est réglée et par là même les vibrations sonores sont augmentées.

14° L'évidement petro-mastoïdien avec tubage est indiqué dans tous les cas où il y a diminution et résorption des cavités de l'oreille moyenne, comme cela a lieu dans les otites à lésions sclérosantes et à ostéite condensante. Il assure d'une façon plus complète le fonctionnement de l'annexe pneumatique de l'oreille.

15° L'évidement petro-mastoïdien simple doit être préféré dans les formes hyperplasiques de l'otite, sans lésions chroniques du tissu osseux.

16° Dans les cas d'évidement avec tubage, le tube en celluloïd parfaitement aseptique n'occasionne aucun trouble ; il est invisible et ne provoque aucune douleur ni même aucune gêne.

17° L'amélioration obtenue par l'intervention reste acquise dans la suite.

PROF. FARACI. Mi sorprende come il Dr. Malherbe ottenga dei risultati acustici col trattamento chirurgico dallo stesso eseguito nelle otiti sclerosanti.

Io ho costantemente trovato che quando dopo l'operazione segue una reazione infiammatoria di una certa entita, il risultato acustico conseguito poco alla volta si perde, perchè si vengono a ristabilire le condizioni anatomo-patalogiche rimosse con l'operazione. Ora, è possibile non avere una reazione infiammatoria di lunga durata in un operazione come quella pràticata dal Dr. Malherbe ? Aggiungo che io non ho trovato nelle molte operazioni che me eseguite alcuna difficoltà nello scoprire la staffa dal condotto specialmente con la resezione del segmento postero-superiore del annulo timpanico. L'operazione per il condotto ha inoltre il vantaggio di non deturpare la disposizione anatomica dell' orecchio medio, il quale rimane quasi normale, e di assicurare meglio un risultato acustico permanente.

Dr. SUAREZ DE MENDOZA.—Je voudrais demander à M. Malherbe quel était l'état de la trompe dans les cas où il a obtenu les meilleurs résultats. Car voulant me faire une opinion sur son opération, j'ai opéré depuis deux ans 11 malades. Dans ce nombre huit avaient les trompes absolument perméables et chez eux le résultat, je dois le dire **a** été absolument nul.   Chez les trois autres il y a eu un mieux sensible, mais ce mieux n'a pas déposé celui obtenu auparavant par des paracenthèses répétés ou par des myringodectomies. Ma religion pour le moment est que le résultat obtenu n'est pas suffisant pour m'autoriser à faire courir aux malades le risque de semblable intervention.

DR. MALHERBE.—Les résultats obtenus par mon opération restent constants ; c'est du moins ce qui résulte de mon observation personnelle, car j'ai des malades que j'ai opérés en 1896 et dont l'audition n'a pas baissé.   Contrairement à ce qui se passe après les perforations tympaniques qui se referment avec persistance, ou les opérations par le conduit qui déterminent presque toujours la formation d'adhérences qui sont loin d'améliorer l'ouïe.

Dans mon procédé j'ai pour but d'augmenter l'annexe pneumatique de l'oreille qui est fortement atteinte dans la sclérose, et de libérer la caisse dans les cas d'origine inflammatoire.   L'état de la trompe n'a donc un intérêt clinique que dans ces derniers cas.   Le nombre de mes opérés (60) est déjà suffisant pour permettre de juger de la valeur de cette intervention.   Beaucoup de mes malades, satisfaits d'un premier résultat sur une oreille, n'ont pas hésité à se faire opérer l'autre.

Je ne sais si M. Suarez (de Mendoza) qui dit avoir opéré onze malades (dont trois, de son propre aveu ont eu un résultat) a suivi ma technique.   Je ne le crois pas, car elle est assez délicate et nécessite au moins qu'on l'ai vue, les descriptions étant forcément incomplètes.

ASCESSI DELLA FACCIA.

PROF. AVOLEDO, Milan.

La nostra specialità si è ormai affermata togliendo alla chirurgia generale molta parte dell ricco materiale che già essa possede. E questo risultato lo si deve alla accurata osservazione di tutti i fatti clinici che si presentavano, cosi la chirurgia cranica per gli ascessi cerebrali si è fatta strada per merito degli otologi che ne osservavono le origini. Fino dallo scorso anno mi fu presentata una paziente che portava una fistola cronica della faccia e propriamente in corrispondenza del margine anteriore del massetere e del decorso del facciale e mi si demandò se essa non avesse rapporti coll'orecchio medio, che da tempo suppurava.   Non ho potuto a tutta forma dare una risposta, ma osservando attentamente l'orecchio medio potei capire che si trattavo di una raccolta di fungosità e che pertanto consigliava il paziente di curarsi.   Durante la cura ebbi anche occasione di levare un piccolo sequestro osseo, e fu dopo l'ablazione di quest'ultimo che osservai come il liquido con cui veniva lavato l'orecchio usciva costantemente ed in gran copia dalla fistola la quale in capo a pochissimi giorni guariva.   Mi pareva questo un fatto isolato e non me ne occupai gran fatto, senonchè dopo cinque o sei mesi non si presentò anme un bambino con un vero ascesso grande come una noce nella stessa regione ; il paziente era convalescente di un morbillo ed aveva suppurazione acuta da entrambi gli orecchi medii.

Dapprima credetti che l'ascesso rappresentasse pure una localizza-zione secondaria del morbillo e quindi senza attribuirvi alcun valore patogenico, ne praticava l'incisione lo raschiamento e la disinfezione. Ebbi occazione di osservare lo stesso fatto accenato nel primo caso, che cosi il liquido che lavava l'ascesso usciva dall'orecchio, mi persuasi dunque che non děbbono essere poi cosi rari questi ascessi e che cosunque bisognava ben tenerne conto, specialmente per il pronostico.   Qui bisogna ricordare anatomicamente che l'aponeurosi che ricopre i muscoli è quella che può guidari negli atti operativi, e se questi ascessi sotto aponeurotici, conviéne aprire da parte della bocca, se sono sopraaponeurotici conviene aprire da parte della cute e gli ascessi osservati da me sono appunto sopraaponeurotici. Ora quello stratogrambo cellulare che copre l'aponeurosi si continua fin verso la parete inferiore del condotto e fa capo a tutto il tessuto che circonda la articolazione Io credo che sia de questa parte che il pus può portarsi in basso ed in avanti e costituirvi un vero canale fino a formare un ascesso, forse nella regione dove ha maggior difficolta a progredere e facilmente segue il decorso del facciale fuori del foro stilomastoides.* Per se stessa è questa un osservazione (per quanto ho potuto cercare) di poco momento ma posso assicurare che la litteratura non ha mai registrato fatti identici e che è del massimo interesse per il paziente poter guarir si di una fistola del viso a cui generalemente nessun medico attribuisse l'origine ad un orecchio o che suppura o che forse non suppura più ma che ha in se le ragioni per la diffusione del pus.

ABCÈS ANTÉRIEURS DE LA MASTOÏDE ET FURONCULOSE DU CONDUIT AUDITIF EXTERNE.   (Etude de diagnostic.)

DR. LOUIS BAR, Nice.

Les abcès des cellules limitrophes antérieures de la mastoïde con-stituent une variété d'abcès qui peut être confondue avec un abcès furonculeux ou sudoripare† et dont Lubet-Barbon et Broca‡ ont essayé de fixer les éléments de diagnostic.   Ce n'est donc point un rareté que d'apporter quelques observations personnelles, mais c'est une occasion favorable pour reprendre l'analyse minutieuse des symptômes en vue d'un diagnostic difiérentiel souvent aussi important qu'extrêmement difficile à poser.

---

* Faccio anche osservare che nè l'uno ne l'altro dei pazienti ebbero mai sintomi morbosi di parte della parotida.

† Simon Duplay.   Maladies de l'appareil auditif en Traité de Chirurgie. 1891, p. 618.

‡ Broca et Lubet-Barbon.   Les suppurations de l'apophyse mastoïde et leur traitement, p. 62.

Voici quatre cas :—le 1ᵉʳ et le 2ᵉ sont des exemples de ces abcès en pleine évolution et d'un diagnostic longtemps difficile ; le 3ᵐᵉ est un exemple de la terminaison de ces abcès ; le 4ᵐᵉ indique comment ils débutent.

Mme R...., que notre distingué confrère et ami Dr. Vivan (de Monte Carlo) nous a prié d'observer avec lui, est une jeune femme bien portante, légèrement anémique, qui très rapidement a été prise de douleur violente dans le conduit auditif externe gauche avec irradiation à la face, inflammation du méat, suppuration légère, état fébrile à peine notable quoique précédé de frissonnement. Adénite praetragienne : Traction douloureuse du conduit. Au moment où nous voyons la 1ᵉʳᵉ fois la malade (4ᵉ jour) le conduit auditif externe très fortement tuméfié par un gonflement non accuminé, douloureux au toucher, sans rougeur vive, plus marqué à la paroi postérieure, laisse sourdre à travers la tuméfaction une petite quantité de pus provenant de la caisse par une petite perforation. La malade a beaucoup souffert avec exacerbations vespérales. Le pouls et la température sont en accord parfait, à peine légèrement au dessus de la normale. Au 10ₑ jour de la maladie la tuméfaction s'étant journellement accrue au point d'obstruer complètement le conduit nous pratiquons une large incision sur la tuméfaction postéro-supérieure. Il ne sort que du sang mêlé au pus ordinaire qui s'écoule. La douche d'air ne provoque rien. Soulagement des douleurs. Traitement par alcool boriqué à saturation, comme pour la furonculose, et pour remplacer les lavages boriqués qui ne font rien. Vers le 15ᵉ jour de la maladie la mastoïde devient douloureuse, empâlée vers son sommet ; le pli rétro-auriculaire persiste un peu effacé. Agitation nerveuse. Lavage au lysol 1%. Gouttes calmantes morphinées. Calomel tous les jours 0.10 grammes.

Après 5 semaines la guérison s'annonce par disparition de la tuméfaction du méat, après laquelle on voit enfin le tympan encore perforé et la paroi postéro-supérieure siège de l'abcès. Celui-ci ne s'est pas ouvert dans le conduit mais derrière le tympan. La question de trépanation de la mastoïde a été subordonnée à la marche symptomatique et par suite évitée.

Pendant toute la durée de la maladie nous avons constaté la surdité à la montre, le signe de Weber, des bourdonnements, bruits divers, battements.

Remarques : Tuméfaction des parois du conduit auditif externe, région osseuse, avec maximum au segment postéro-supérieur. Douleur intense avec irradiation faciale. Engorgement ganglionnaire praetragien ; oedème péri-mastoïdien ; mastoïde douloureuse. Etat fébricitant du début, puis état normal du pouls et de la température. Agitation nerveuse. Durée de l'affection.

Observation II.—Mme. D . . . d'un tempérament sanguin est prise après une rougeole d'un écoulement d'oreille qu'un erysipèle de la face, survenu tout à coup, semble un instant modifier en bien. Elle nous est adressée par notre distingué confrère et ami Dr. de Langenhagen de Menton et nous constatons à notre premier examen (3ᵉ semaine de maladie) : Tuméfaction rouge du conduit auditif externe, portion osseuse, tympan invisible, pus abondant, rougeâtre. Douleur à la pression mastoïdienne. Rougeur congestive du rhino-pharynx. Pouls normal, température normale. La douche d'air n'augmente pas l'écoulement de pus qui sort du méat. Incision à travers la tuméfaction. Il sort du sang et du pus. La douche d'air en provoque une plus grande sortie. Lavage au lysol 1%, au sublimé 1/4,000. Alcool boriqué à saturation. La mastoïde reste douloureuse, l'écoulement persiste ; empâlement ; battements, bruits entotiques ; surdité. Weber positif ; pas d'état fébrile ; oedème périmastoïdien. Sept semaines après le début de la maladie, la tuméfaction disparait et laisse voir la localisation primitive aux cellules limitrophes sans perforation dans le conduit. La suppuration disparait et l'audition revient. Douche d'air, etc.

Remarques : Tuméfaction indolore du conduit, surtout paroi supéro-postérieure. Ecoulement abondant. Aucun état général manifeste. Oedème péri-mastoïdien. Guérison sans intervention autre que l'incision de la tuméfaction.

Observation III.—M. T . . . 29 ans, vient consulter pour surdité et écoulement rare, mais fétide de l'oreille droite ; dure depuis plusieurs mois ; scrofulose ; le malade ne se souvient d'aucun fait ou épisode grave de l'oreille. L'écoulement et la surdité ont paru insidieusement s'établir. Un examen minutieux nous fait remarquer en nappe et au segment postéro-supérieur du conduit un polype sessile qui cache l'entrée d'une fistule osseuse où le stylet pénétre à 3^{mm} de profondeur. Il parait s'enfoncer vers l'aditus, à 2^{mm} en avant du tympan, 3^{mm} à 4^{mm} au dessus du canal de Fallope. Ablation du polype. Curettage ; cauterisation au Chlorure de Zinc 1/50. Lavages au lysol 1%. Observation est faite au malade qu'un traitement général, analeptique : Quinquina, Arsenic, Glycerophosphate aidera puissamment à la guérison ou amélioration notable. Deux mois après en effet, la guérison s'affirme. La suppuration n'a plus reparu depuis les premiers jours ; l'ouïe est allé de 1,5cm., du début à 35cm ; disparition de tout bruit. La fistule parait se rétrécir de plus en plus, comblée par du tissu de cicatrice.

Remarque : Etablissement d'une fistule suite d'abcès antérieur de la mastoïde, lequel a evolué insidieusement.

Observation IV.—Mlle: W . . . . 18 ans environ, d'un tempérament nerveux et arthritique, ayant déjà eu de l'angine glanduleuse avec poussée congestive du côté des trompes d'Eustache, est prise à la suite d'un coup de froid d'otalgie violente avec irradiation à la nuque et à la face. Diminution de l'ouïe ; Weber positif ; battements pulsatils, exascerbations vespérales et après chaque examen. Le début de la maladie remonte quatre jours environ lorsque nous la voyons. Traction douloureuse du pavillon ; engorgement léger mais sensible des ganglions parotidiens. Sur la paroi antéro-inférieure du conduit cartilagineux tuméfaction, qui parait être le reliquat d'un furoncle. La paroi postéro-supérieure du conduit auditif osseux est rouge, douloureuse à la pression du stylet. Congestion du hyle de Gellé. Tympan de couleur naturelle, mais retracté. Gêne de la mastication ; sensibilité et fourmillement de la face du côté de l'oreille malade. Léger état fébrile ; douleur vive intra-auriculaire paroxystique jour et nuit. Malgré les bains d'oreille boriqués, les gouttes morphinés à 0,10/10, des sangsues appliquées derrière le pavillon ; purgations au calomel, pédiluve, l'état continue à empirer ; en plus, douleur à la pression de la mastoïde dont la face externe ainsi que le pavillon sont le siège de rougeur et d'un léger empâtement. Enfin pendant un jour douleur pharyngienne et rougeur vineuse côté droit, c'est à dire du côté de l'oreille malade. Vers le 12e jour le tympan devient couleur feuille morte, moins concave et nous proposons l'intervention. A ce moment la famille est obligée de partir pour Paris ; nous avons appris par son médecin, que l'état s'était prolongé, et qu'il y avait un commencement de nécrose au point malade.

Remarques : Rougeur postéro-supérieure du conduit. Empâtement mastoïdien et engorgement parotidien ; douleur spontanée et provoquée. Irradiation faciale. Congestion pharyngienne, passive, douloureuse.

Des cas de ce genre où le symptomatologie est si peu précise, sont moins rares dans la pratique médicale que Mignon* parait le supposer. Tous les Otologistes en citent des exemples, ou réservent dans leur traité

---

* Mignon. Des principales complications septiques des Otites moyennes suppurées, p. 306.

général d'otologie quelques considérations spéciales et il y a non seulement à établir le diagnostic entre ces abcès et la furonculose, mais aussi
à savoir si un furoncle a été le point initial apparent de cette variété
d'abcès, si un abcès de ce genre a provoqué l'éclosion d'une furonculose,
si enfin il s'agit purement et simplement de l'une ou de l'autre de ces
affections.

Des conséquences thérapeutiques en découlent. Quelques soins
bien ordonnés guérissent une furonculose ; il faut au contraire lutter
énergiquement contre l'inflammation des cellules mastoïdiennes, quelquefois même par une intervention chirurgicale importante parer à une
nécrose ménaçante ou à des complications encéphaliques redoutables.

Il faut rapporter à l'anatomie et à la physiologie de l'oreille, la
plupart des considérations sérieuses qui sont relatives à la connaissance
du diagnostic de ces abcès. Nous savons en effet que le conduit auditif
externe est tapissé sur toute son étendue par un revêtement cutané
absolument semblable à la peau dans la portion cartilagineuse ; solidement fixé au périoste, délicat et de plus en plus simple dans la région
osseuse, au point que les anatomistes ont cru longtemps que les éléments
glandulaires faisaient complètement défaut dans cet endroit. Les
recherches de Buchanan et v. Tröltsch ont montré qu'il y a aussi de
glandes dans la portion osseuse et d'après v. Tröltsch la couche glandulaire s'étend de la paroi postéro-supérieure de la portion cartilagineuse
dans le conduit osseux sous la forme d'un coin triangulaire de plus d'un
millimètre de long dont la pointe est dirigée vers la membrane du
tympan. Comme dans toute région à glandes pilosebacées, les microbes
du furoncle ainsi que Loewenberg* l'a montré, peuvent établir leur
quartier dans cette couche glandulaire et parmi les Staphylococcus
albus, aureus et citreus observés, on trouvera principalement le
Streptococcus pyogenes albus qui d'après Kirchner† serait le véritable
microbe de la furonculose de l'oreille. Mais cette même région ou
segment postéro-supérieur du conduit osseux est celle des cellules limitrophes de la mastoïde. D'après von Tröltsch‡ et Politzer§ les cavités
cellulaires situées entre les lamelles de la paroi supérieure du conduit
auditif se présentent en nombre et en grandeur variable ; en relation,
en partie avec la caisse du tympan, en partie avec les cellules
mastoïdiennes. On y trouve parfois des modifications qui proviennent
de la propagation du processus inflammatoire de l'oreille moyenne ; un
abcès intra-cellulaire se forme, désorganise la lamelle osseuse, tuméfie le
revêtement du conduit à l'instar d'un furoncle ou d'une hydrosadénite
et comme ceux-ci s'ouvre dans le conduit. En pareille occurrence la
furonculose et l'abcès antérieur peuvent avoir des signes semblables.

Comme l'écoulement purulent est généralement peu important dans

---

* Loewenberg. Monatsschrift für Ohrenheilkunde, 1887.
† Kirchner. Deutsche Med. Wochenschift. 1888. No. 67.
‡ v. Tröltsch. Lehrbuch der Ohrenheilkunde (Cinquième édition 1873).
§ Politzer. Dissection anatomique et histologique de l'organe auditif (1898) (Traduction Schiffers).

la furonculose et au contraire très abondant et longtemps continu dans la mastoïdite, on a pensé qu'il y avait là un excellent signe différentiel. D'après nos observations personnelles, nous ne pensons pas qu'il en soit toujours ainsi ; nous croirions plutôt aux éléments différentiels que peut fournir l'étude microscopique du pus et du bourbillon furonculeux lequel contient les microbes plus haut signalés tandis qu'avec diverses mastoïdites appartient le pus des Otites moyennes avec ses streptocoques, pneumocoques, staphylocoques pyogènes, et le bacille encapsulé de Friedlander, ainsi que l'ont indiqué les recherches bactériologiques de Neller* et Zaufalt.   En pareille circonstance aussi il faut penser que la forme et la couleur de la tuméfaction inflammatoire prêtent également à confusion car s'il est vrai que le furoncle se présente acuminé et non point arrondi comme l'abcès, avec un point blanc à son sommet—sans coloration spéciale ; dans le conduit cependant sa forme particulière change par manque d 'espace et la peau qui le recouvre acquiert un aspect plus ou moins congestif et inflammatoire qui laisse des doutes ; doutes d'autant plus sérieuses qu'à ce moment le méat est comblé par le gonflement inflammatoire et l'examen de la tuméfaction de même que celui du tympan, devient impossible par suite de cette obstruction.   Il arrive même que l'inflammation peut retentir sur les parties voisines, gagner le tissu cellulaire et le périoste, occasionner un gonflement oedémateux de la région parotidienne, de la peau de la mastoïde, et déterminer enfin une tuméfaction qui écarte le pavillon.   "S'il y a," dit Schwartze,‡ "gonflement inflammatoire avec douleur compressive et tumeur fluctuante sur l'apophyse mastoïde, on ne peut attribuer ces signes à une périostite.   Les inflammations furonculeuses du méat donnent lieu à un gonflement oedémateux de la région mastoïdienne qui disparait rapidement après l'incision du furoncle et n'aboutit jamais à la formation d'un abcès."   Il arrive aussi que les ganglions périauriculaires sont seuls atteints par l'engorgement inflammatoire.   Si cet engorgement a lieu au début même de la maladie, on a toute raison d'en rapporter la cause à la présence d'un furoncle, si cet engorgement n'arrive qu'en pleine période d'état de la maladie, on ne pensera qu'à une ostéopériostite du conduit secondaire à un furoncle ou à un abcès antérieur de la mastoïde, car ces adénites ne peuvent avoir d'autre origine que les lymphangites du conduit et du pavillon qui se jetent tous dans les ganglions praetragiens, parotidiens, rétro-auriculaires ou mastoïdiens.   Les lymphatiques de la caisse se perdent dans les lacunes lymphatiques du voisinage.   Enfin d'après Leuterd,§ lorsqu'il s'agit d'un abcès ouvert de l'apophyse mastoïde par perforation de la paroi postérieure du conduit, il faudra se souvenir que

---

* Neller. Recherches bactériologiques sur les otites moyennes aiguës.   Annales des maladies de l'oreille etc., 1883.

† Prager Medezin. Wochenschrift 1887, 1888 1889.

‡ Schwartze. L'oreille, maladies chirurgicales, trad. Ratel, P. 154.

§ Leuterd. " Ueber periauriculäre Abscess." Archiv für Ohrenheilkunde. No. 40 à 43.

les phénomènes inflammatoires sont surtout prononcés au niveau du sillon qui sépare le pavillon de l'oreille de l'apophyse mastoïde, tandis que dans les abcès ayant pour point de départ cette dernière la rougeur et la tuméfaction envahiront toute la région mastoïdienne. Cet avis est d'ailleurs celui de Simon Duplay* qui écrit : " Dans la périostite simple, le gonflement est diffus, le sillon qui existe entre la conque et l'apophyse mastoïde a disparu ; dans l'inflammation des cellules mastoïdiennes, le gonflement est plus circonscrit, le sillon qui existe entre la conque et l'apophyse persiste."

On peut tirer quelques indices encore des connaissances exactes de la circulation artérielle et veineuse. L'oreille externe et l'oreille moyenne reçoivent en effet le sang artériel de branches diverses issues de la carotide externe. C'est pourquoi, dans la mastoïdite aussi bien que dans la furonculose ou les diverses otites, les malades éprouvent des bourdonnements d'oreille, des battements violents, etc., qui sont le résultat de la propagation inflammatoire au voisinage du tympan dont les vaisseaux sont gorgés de sang. ' La déplétion veineuse se fait par des veines qui se jettent dans les jugulaires mais celles de l'oreille moyenne se jettent en outre dans le plexus pharyngien, sinus pétreux etc., d'où la céphalée gravative ainsi parfois qu'une stase veineuse pharyngienne qui est le propre de la mastoïdite, chose qui ne saurait avoir lieu dans la furonculose du conduit auditif externe.

L'analyse exacte de la douleur spontanée ou provoquée fournit des renseignements les plus précieux pour le diagnostic d'abcès antérieur mastoïdien et de furonculose. Par sa précocité, par sa violence, par son siège, par sa continuité, elle fournit des renseignements de première valeur. Le moindre attouchement avec la pointe du stylet, la traction du pavillon, arrache des cris au malade s'il s'agit d'un furoncle. Le gonflement des cellules limitrophes forme une tumeur à peu près indolente à la pression. C'est que l'innervation du conduit auditif externe est exquise, son revêtement cutané si adhérent au conduit, innervé par les fibres du trijumeau, du pneumogastrique et du plexus cervical traduit un gonflement aussi rapide que celui du furoncle par des douleurs d'une acuité étonnante spontanée, ou provoquée, accompagnée quelquefois d'un malaise général, lypothymie, anxiété cardiaque. Les cellules mastoïdiennes au contraire et principalement les antérieures innervées faiblement par le facial, par le trijumeau mais d'une manière remarquable par le nerf de Jacobson (branche du glossopharyngien) traduit son inflammation et le développement lent de son abcès par une sensibilité plus obtuse et aussi par une sensibilité spéciale due à la IXe paire, savoir une constriction gutturale une exagération de la sensibilité gustative, toute chose que le furoncle n'occasionne jamais.

Pour terminer, nous remarquerons encore que si parfois dans la furonculose, il y a un mouvement fébrile, c'est tout à fait exceptionnel.

* S. Duplay. Traité de Chirurgie. T. 4, P. 725. Paris, 1891.

Dans toute mastoïdite un état général plus ou moins grave est la règle. Le frisson initial ne manque pour ainsi dire jamais, et si quelquefois, plus fréquemment même qu'on ne saurait le croire, la température est normale ou du moins au dessous de 38° une observation attentive biquotidienne fait constater alors et d'une manière à peu près constante, une discordance remarquable entre les degrès thermométriques et le nombre des pulsations artérielles.

Disons enfin que le traitement local peut à son tour aider à l'affirmation du diagnostic. Nous avons dit déjà que l'incision du furoncle est très rapidement suivie de la disparition du gonflement inflammatoire de même que l'alcool boriqué à saturation aide puissamment à une guérison prompte, mais ne guérissent pas la mastoïdite antérieure. Pour la cure de celle-ci il est non seulement utile d'inciser le pseudo-furoncle, mais aussi de faire une véritable trépanation de l'apophyse.

En resumé :—

Les Otologistes s'accordent pour trouver le diagnostic entre un abcès des cellules limitrophes de la mastoïde et le furoncle du conduit auditif osseux très difficile et parfois imprécis.

En pareille occurence un diagnostic semblable ne peut être dégagé que de la connaissance parfaite anatomo-physiologique de la région et de l'observation clinique.

Or l'une et l'autre nous apprennent :—

1.   Que la nature microbienne du pus est différente dans les 2 cas.

2.   Que la lymphangite et l'adénite préauriculaire précoce est la règle dans toute affection furonculeuse du conduit—qu'elle est tardive et exceptionnelle dans l'inflammation abcédale des cellules limitrophes, ceci par suite d'un double système lymphatique différent pour l'oreille moyenne.

3.   Que le gonflement oedémateux périmastoïdien efface le sillon rétro-auriculaire dans la furonculose et conserve ce sillon rétro-auriculaire dans la mastoïdite et y demeure circonscrit.

4.   Que le sinus pharyngien est souvent l'occasion d'une stase veineuse et pénible du pharynx dans la cellulite.

5.   Que par un système d'innervation différent dans les deux cas, la douleur spontanée et provoquée est plus violente dans la furonculose, obtuse en général dans l'abcès antérieur de la mastoïde, mais que dans la cellulite antérieure il y a souvent une parésie faciale et une exagération de la sensibilité gustative due à son innervation particulière, signe qui lui appartient en propre.

6.   Qu'enfin dans les cas rares mais possible où l'état général sans fièvre demeure sans réaction, la discordance fréquente et continue entre le pouls et la température est un signe très favorable au diagnostic de pseudo-furonculose, ou abcès antérieur de la mastoïde.

Résultat des Exercices acoustiques chez les Sourds-Muets.

Dr. A. Costiniu, Bucharest.

Permettez-moi, Messieurs, de vous rapporter ici les résultats, que j'ai obtenus, en traitant par des exercices acoustiques 10 sourds-muets, dont 6 garçons, 3 filles et une dame âgée de 23 ans, du nombre de 26 que j'eus à soigner. Je ne vous parlerai pas de ces 16, parce-qu'il faut avouer que je n'ai rien obtenu. Les uns d'entre eux étaient déjà personnes bien âgées, et les autres après quelque temps ne voulu-rent plus continuer le traitement.

Je traite en ce moment par la même méthode encore 13 enfants, les résultats seront publiés plus tard. Comme méthode je me suis servi à peu près de celle décrite d'Urbantschitsch.

J'ai employé la voix parlée en lui donnant différentes intensités; souvent j'ai fait des mains un sort de cornet, par laquelle la voix arrive à l'oreille. Très rarement, je me suis servi du tube acoustique parce que j'ai observé qu'il modifie le timbre de la voix. En outre, je fais faire jouer par une personne placée à distances de plus en plus éloignées (jusqu'à 20 à 30 mètres) de différents instruments (Trompette, Violon-celle, Tambour, etc.) Les résultats ont été assez satisfaisants. Dans 5 cas je suis arrivé à faire entendre les sons de la trompette placée à 30 mètres, les autres instruments jusqu'à 18 mètres.

Comme j'ai eu seulement des malades à traiter en ville, les exercices ont été faits par différents membres de la famille, même par des petits enfants âgés de 10 ans. La variation des voix c'est une chose capitale.

Autant que possible je parle à mes malades de côté, pour les habituer à entendre sans regarder la personne. Quand il y a des malades qui sont habitués à lire sur les lèvres de celui qui parle, alors je tâche de perfectionner cette langage. Dans ces cas il faut leur parler à voix mi-haute, et la prononciation d'une fréquence moyenne. Je commence par faire entendre à mes malades des voyelles, une ou deux par séance, celle-ci est répétée 2 à 3 fois par jour et dure chaque fois 20 minutes; quand une voyelle détermine une sensation auditive précise et quand les malades la prononcent bien, je passe à d'autres voyelles, puis aux con-sonnes, ou monosyllabes, enfin aux mots et aux phrases. J'avoue qu'il faut une persévérance extraordinaire, tant de la part du médecin, que du malade et de sa famille. Il arrive souvent un certain degré de con-fusion, lorsque les malades connaissent déjà plusieurs voyelles et con-sonnes. Il faut alors revenir toujours sur ses pas, répéter sans cesse et insister sur les sons mal prononcés. La plus grande confusion se fait entre les voyelles e et i, entre o et u; entre les consonnes b, p, m, entre d et b. Pour les mots, c'est naturelle d'employer ceux qui peuvent intéresser plus le malade. Il m'est arrivé à trois reprises de voir des malades qui jusque-là entendaient et prononçaient bien différentes lettres et même de mots, brusquement dans l'espace de 24 heures, ne plus entendre et prononcer difficilement. C'est là un côté désagréable, tant pour le malade qui perd la confiance, que pour le médecin. Il faut alors recommencer le travail et après 2-3 semaines, on arrive au niveau où on l'avait commencé. Pourquoi ce changement ? Je ne peux pas encore l'expliquer.

Les femmes mettent plus d'intérêt à ces exercices que les hommes ; chez une d'entre elles j'ai observé des phénomènes nerveux ; céphalalgie, insomnie ; une autre âgée de 24 ans, qui est devenue sourde à l'âge de 11 ans, et chez laquelle les exercices donnaient des résultats peu appréciables, perd toute patience après 2 mois ; 7 jours de reflexion plus tard, elle se décide de recommencer.

Tous ces 10 malades, pouvaient prononcer au commencement quelques voyelles, même des mots.

Chez 3 d'entre eux, j'ai trouvé de végétations adénoïdes ; après leur ablation et plus tard douches de Politzer l'audition devint meilleure et les exercices avancèrent à merveille. J'ai observé au commencement chez ceux qui pouvaient écrire et lire, que si on leur criait à l'oreille, ils comprenaient assez bien quelques mots et pouvaient même les reproduire soit par la voix, soit par écrit.

La controle par l'écrit, je l'ai toujours employé pour me convaincre qu'ils comprennent ce qu'ils entendent.

Deux filles qui ne savaient pas écrire ont appris en même temps la prononciation et l'alphabet. Dans aucun cas la surdité n'était pas totale. Ordinairement l'oreille qui entendait le mieux dès le commencement reste toujours la meilleure ; cependant l'inverse a eu lieu 2 fois.

Chez tous mes malades je leur ai fait ou des douches de Politzer ou le cathéterisme pendant longtemps, avec des interruptions. Tous ces 10 malades sont devenus sourds après la naissance (entre 2 et 11 ans).

Voilà en quelques mots leurs observations :—

E. B. fille âgée de 16 ans, devint sourde à l'âge de 6 ans, à la suite d'une scarlatine. A l'oreille droite, trace d'audition de la voix parlée, à une distance de 15 c.m., à gauche moins encore. Les membranes du tympan ; opaque à gauche, presque normale à droite. La fille parait assez intelligente. Elle ne sait pas écrire. Peut prononcer des voyelles, et plusieurs mots. Elle est déjà habituée à lire sur les lèvres, mais ne parvient que difficilement à répéter.

On commence les exercices le 24 Mai 1898, le progrès assez rapide pour l'oreille droite, moins pour la gauche. Après 3 mois l'audition devient tout à coup plus mauvaise, la malade devient triste et irritable ; avec beaucoup de peine, je la persuade de continuer le traitement. Ce mauvais état dure 3 semaines, puis l'amélioration s'accentue de nouveau et au mois de Février 1899 (10 mois) elle peut prononcer des phrases, entend la voix parlée à 1,20 de côté, et la trompette à 15 mètres. Elle parle mieux de face que de côté ; l'oreille droite est la meilleure. Elle a appris en même temps l'alphabet et à l'écrire.

J. L. 12 ans. sourd-muet depuis l'âge de 2 ans à la suite de rougeole. Sait écrire et lire mais ne peut prononcer que les voyelles, a, o ; très intelligent. Trace d'audition aux deux-oreilles. Entend même la tonnerre. A la distance de 5 c.m., après une répétition de 6 fois, il entend la voyelle a, qu'il reproduit par écrit.

Les exercices ont duré depuis le mois de Juin 1897 jusqu'au mois de Novembre 1898 époque à laquelle il parle bien et entend de même ; les instruments de musique, il les entend jusqu'à 12-20 mètres. Il est employé dans un atelier de menuiserie.

H. L. la soeur du précédent âgée de 10 ans, sourde depuis l'âge de 3 ans, à la suite d'un accident de voiture. L'audition très diminuée pour l'oreille gauche est nulle du côté droit. Peut prononcer des voyelles. Les exercices commencés en même temps avec son frère sont continués jusqu'au mois de Novembre 1898. Elle entend assez bien à gauche, moins à droite ; peut prononcer des mots et quelques phrases. Au commencement cette malade était très nerveuse, avait de la céphalalgie et de l'insomnie. Quand elle peut prononcer le mot, *mama*, elle a commencé à pleurer de joie.

Mme. G. âgée de 24 ans, sourde depuis l'âge de 11 ans à la suite d'une fièvre typhoïde. Cette malade parle assez bien et peut soutenir une conversation à voix mi-haute, quand on lui parle en face. *Vestige d'audition.* Après 2 mois d'exercices elle perd la patience et le traitement est interrompu pendant 7 jours ; mais on recommence, et au bout de 9 mois, elle peut soutenir conversation de côté même à une distance de 1 mètre. Les différents instruments sont entendus jusqu'à la distance de 25 mètres.

V. C. 15 ans, sourd depuis l'âge de 4 ans à la suite d'une rougeole. Rinne positif à droite, négatif à gauche. Une montre est entendue à la distance de 5 c.m. à droite. Végétations adénoïdes surtout du côté gauche. Par une seule douche de Politzer, l'audition est rendue meilleure. Ablation des végétations. Il peut prononcer alors presque tout ce qu'il entend. Après 10 mois de traitement, il entend et parle bien. Les instruments, il les entend à plus de 30 m. de distance.

A. V. 14 ans, devenu sourd à l'âge de 6 ans à la suite d'une scarlatine. Peut prononcer toutes les voyelles et même des mots. L'oreille gauche est meilleure que la droite ; végétations adénoïdes très prononcées. Opération, quelques douches de Politzer, l'audition s'améliore du côté droit. Exercices pendant 17 mois.

Aujourd'hui le malade entend bien à la distance de 2 mètres. Les instruments, il les entend et les distingue à 30 mètres.

F. C. 13 ans, sourde depuis l'âge de 4 ans, à la suite d'un accident de voiture ? C'est un type d'adénoïdienne. Peut prononcer quelques mots peu difficiles. L'oreille gauche est meilleure que la droite. Au commencement du traitement elle est irritable—après 19 mois d'exercices, l'audition et la parole sont bonnes ; je lui ai appris, en outre, à écrire l'alphabet. Opérée et douchée au Politzer.

F. J. N. 14 ans, sourde depuis l'âge de 3 ans. L'oreille droite entend mieux que la gauche. Peut prononcer les voyelles a, e, o, et quelques mots. Exercices pendant 12 mois. Résultat bon. Parle même des phrases et entend bien à 2 mètres. Le 2e mois du traitement le malade n'entendait plus, mais dix jours plus tard l'audition était revenue.

F. M. C. 13 ans, sourd depuis l'âge de 5 ans à la suite d'une fièvre typhoïde ; oreille droite meilleure que la gauche au commencement, plus tard c'est l'inverse. Peut prononcer quelques voyelles a, e, o. Après 19 mois d'exercices, il entend et peut parler des phrases entiers à 1 mètre, entend les instruments à 20 mètres.

F. N. 14 ans, sourd depuis l'âge de 3 ans à la suite d'une scarlatine. Peut prononcer *mama*, *apa* (eau) et les voyelles *a*, *o*. Audition meilleure pour l'oreille droite ; à gauche, il y a perforation du tympan. Exercices pendant 18 mois. Résultat excellent surtout pour le côté droit, peut parler des mots et phrases courtes.

On voit, d'après ces observations, qu'avec de la patience on peut obtenir par cette méthode quelquefois des résultats satisfaisants.

Mais seulement, il faut observer qu'il faut mettre beaucoup de temps et surtout beaucoup de persévérance.

Je crois que cette méthode ne donne pas des résultats chez les personnes déjà âgées, et chez ceux qui n'ont pas de la patience. Comment faut il interpréter ces résultats ? Je ne peux pas encore donner une explication, mais je crois que cette gymnastique fréquente des oreilles y contribue en bonne partie.

Une autre question que le temps va résoudre c'est, si ces bons résultats seront maintenus pour toujours.

DR. DIDSBURY demande à M. Costiniu pourquoi dans ses exercices acoustiques il ne s'est pas servi de l'appareil micro-téléphonique de Dussaud, plus facile à employer que tout autre procédé : voix, harmonium, trompettes, etc. Ce procédé étant beaucoup moins fatigant pour le médecin et permettant de faire entendre des sons bien déterminés et fixés à l'avance sur les rouleaux de l'appareil enregistreur.

DR. HEIMAN. La question d'exercices de sourds-muets pour les apprendre à parler a été discuté au Congrès international de Moscou, et la plupart de médecins ont exprimé une opinion défavorable pour ces exercices. Quant à moi, j'en ai fait plusieurs avec des enfants de 8-12 ans pendant 6 mois. J'ai réussi que les enfants parlaient quelques mots, mais en 2-3 semaines ils ont tout oublié.

PROF. GRAZZI.—In Italia e stato molto studiata la questione degli esercizi acustici nella cura del sordo mutismo ed il Vice Direttore dell'Istituto dei sordomuti di Siena, andò a Vienna ed a Monaco di Baviera per studiare sul posto la questione, ma tornò in patria molto scoraggiato.

DR. GARNAULT.—J'ai fait des exercices phonatoires que j'ai poursuivis pendant quelque temps sur des malades préalablement améliorés par la mobilisation de l'étrier. Les résultats ont été quelquefois positifs mais peu marqués et peu durables.

SIXTH MEETING.

FRIDAY, AUGUST 11TH, AT 10 A.M.

CHAIRMAN · - - - PROF. LUCAE.

THERAPY OF THE TYMPANIC MUCOUS MEMBRANE.

DR. M. A. GOLDSTEIN, St. Louis, U.S.A.

In the consideration of tympanic therapy, a comparison of the mucous membrane of the nasal tract with that of the ear as to anatomical and physiological characteristics reveals many points of similarity; and pathologically the condition of the naso-pharynx is of greatest moment in its relation to aural affections. Too much stress, therefore, cannot be laid on the direct association of the naso-pharynx with the tympanic cavity.

Otologists frequently overlook the importance of active therapeutic measures directed to the nose and naso-pharynx, and the intimate relations of these areas to the ear should ever be kept in mind.

This subject is considered from two points of view:—1st, Catarrhal, non-suppurative otitis media, where an intact membrana tympani exists; 2nd, Suppurative otitis media, associated with perforation of the drum membrane.

The author advocates the use of rectified petroleum oils, properly medicated, and injected through the Eustachian catheter directly into the tympanic cavity. In chronic catarrhal otitis media, where no sclerosis has been definitely established, this injection is followed by massage of the drum by Siegle's otoscope attached to some massage device, and operated either by hand, compressed air, or electric motor. The time for massage which is considered most favourable is immediately following injection into the tympanum. Continued inflation of the middle ear is also employed to insure penetration of the injected oily fluid.

A plea is offered against the too liberal and too frequent use of the syringe. As a dressing in suppurative otitis, nosophen is substituted for boracic acid and iodoform.

Operative interference should not be attempted until milder measures have been given a thorough trial.

As the nose is the natural gateway to the upper respiratory tract and to the ear, so too may we regard the mucous membrane lining the tympanic cavity and contiguous with that of the naso-pharynx as *the* factor of greatest value in the consideration of middle ear diseases.

The proper moisture, filtration, and temperature of the air we breathe depends on the normal anatomical and physiological functions of the nose, and especially its lining mucous membrane; so, too, the well-being of the middle ear cavity is preserved when the adjacent mucous membrane of the Eustachian tubes and naso-pharynx is in a healthy condition.

The etiology of more than 70 per cent. of all affections of the tympanic cavity may be found in some disturbance of the delicate mucosa lining the nasal and post-nasal passages. Wherever a pathogenic micro-organism is the factor in rhino-pathology, experience has taught us to carefully guard against the easy and natural invasion of the middle ear cavity by such a host.

In the application of our therapeutic resources for the relief of nasal, post-nasal, and pharyngeal affections, too much stress cannot be laid on the direct associations which these structures bear to the tympanic cavity.

On the other hand I would offer the criticism, that Otologists frequently overlook the importance of active therapeutic measures directed to these accessory areas which must be undertaken in the successful treatment of the middle ear cavity. I have often heard prominent confrères assert that they employ no spray, no douche, no cleansing of the naso-pharyngeal tract whatever in the treatment of catarrhal and suppurative conditions of the middle ear cavity. The plea has often been advanced that otology should be distinctly disassociated from rhinology and laryngology. There are often those who look with disfavour on the Otologist of to-day who includes the treatment of diseases of the nose, naso-pharynx and larynx in his professional field.

It is one of the purposes of this paper to emphasize the importance of the intimate relations of this trio of specialities in medicine in order that the best therapeutic results may be obtained. Where we are dealing with catarrhal and suppurative middle ear processes, the causes in by far the majority of cases may be attributed to some lesion in the nose or naso-pharynx, or some pathological change of the mucous membrane lining these areas.

While my subject is confined to the consideration of the therapy of the tympanic cavity, this area is so dependent on the well-being of the adjacent structures and its therapy is so often made difficult by the pathological influences of this tract, that a brief consideration of these factors is essential.

One factor which is frequently responsible for our inability to successfully treat the tympanic cavity is its inaccessibility. The calibre of the Eustachian tube leading to the tympanic cavity is mechanically a very small one; the distance from the naso-pharynx is comparatively great; the naso-pharyngeal orifice of the tube is reached by instruments and medications with some difficulty, and the obstacles which pathological changes in the nasal passages produce are numerous.

I would arbitrarily divide my subject into two sections, first, the therapy of the tympanic cavity where the membrana tympani is intact, and where our efforts are directed mainly through the natural channels; second, where perforations of the membrana tympani are present, admitting of direct medication of the tympanum from the external auditory canal.

This classification carries with it a subdivision of the pathology affecting the ear. Thus, in a general way, we may consider the catarrhal and non-suppurative affections of the middle ear cavity together with an intact membrana tympani; suppurative otitis media together with the usual perforation of the membrane.

In no class of cases has the variation in therapy been so pronounced in recent years as in the treatment of catarrhal affections of the middle ear. Of the most prominent of these therapeutic measures inflation, either with the air bag as first suggested by Politzer, or by the intervention of the Eustachian catheter has been most generally employed; injections of fluid medications either in an aqueous or an oily menstruum have been applied to the middle ear cavity; puncture of the drum membrane by a modified hypodermic syringe needle, and injection into the tympanic cavity of pepsin solution, as suggested by Cohen Kysper, has had its day; the vapors of ammonium chloride, chloroform, ether and numerous volatile oils have been used, the Eustachian bougie has been advocated where changes in the mucous membrane of the tube diminishing its calibre have ensued; the pressure probe of Lucae still affords successful results in some cases; massage of the drum membrane by apparatus ranging from the hand masseur of Delstanche to the electric masseur engine of Chevalier Jackson are the latest aspirants for recognition in tympanic therapy. Many of these treatments have proven of service in selected cases, but to many of us the treatment of this class of chronic diseases of the ear still yields but moderate results, when taken as a whole.

Rational therapeutics find no better field for practice than in dealing with the chronic inflammations of the middle ear cavity, whether catarrhal or suppurative in character. Hypertrophic catarrh of the middle ear is almost invariably associated with similar pathological changes in the nose and naso-pharynx. Chronic naso-pharyngeal catarrh, septal and turbinal obstructions, adenoid growths, hypertrophy of the faucial tonsil and the several acute inflammations of the pharynx accompanying the exanthemata are the main etiological factors of this form of aural catarrh. The mucous membrane lining the Eustachian tube assumes the same hypertrophic condition as that found in chronic nasal and post-nasal catarrh; the tube is narrowed in calibre and is often completely stenosed; the air supplied to the tympanic cavity is cut off, and the drum collapsed, in many cases to such an extent that its inner mucous surface is in direct contact with the inner wall of the tympanum; exudations of serum and mucus are poured into this largely diminished area of the tympanic cavity. With the continuation of this hypertrophy and its many accompaniments, the drum-head becomes thickened and opaque and adhesions by fibrous bands and tissues, of the membrana tympani to the inner wall of the tympanum, and subsequent ankylosis of the ossicles, become imminent.

As atrophic rhinitis may be considered the sequel of hypertrophic rhinitis, so sclerotic or adhesive otitis, may be regarded as the sequel of hyperplastic or hypertrophic otitis.

Anatomically and pathologically we deal here with aural conditions analogous to those of the nose. It is logical and rational to conclude, therefore, that the form of treatment which yields most favourable results in these pathological affections of the nose should be applicable to similar affections of the ear.

For some time I have used purified petroleums as a base for my medications in the treatment of non-suppurative middle-ear catarrh of the hypertrophic form, and have even found this therapy of occasional advantage in mild sclerotic otitis media.

The applications to the tympanic cavity are made as follows :—A short hard rubber Eustachian catheter is introduced in the usual manner and snugly fitted into the nàso-pharyngeal orifice of the Eustachian tube. To the cone-shaped end of the catheter, the tip of a glass-barrel syringe, two inches in length and one inch in diameter is tightly fitted. The syringe is loaded with the desired medication, and with the catheter and syringe properly adjusted, the patient's head is tilted well backwards, inclined toward the ear to be medicated and the piston gradually pressed home. In the majority of cases, after six or eight drops have been delivered, the patient will state that he feels an unusual fulness in the ear. The syringe is then detached and the cone-shaped tip of the compressed air apparatus adjusted; a few short taps and then a steady air pressure continued for eight or ten seconds is given. This insures the penetration of the tympanic cavity by the fluid. I have convinced myself on numerous occasions of the penetrability of this fluid by applying it not only in chronic catarrhal conditions of the middle-ear where the membrana tympani is intact, but also in the treatment of middle-ear cavities, suppurative or non-suppurative, where perforations of the drum membrane existed; where such perforations are present this dark coloured oily fluid may be found on examination exuding from the auditory canal.

I have employed the drugs which have given the best results in their application to hypertrophy of the nasal mucous membrane ; iodine, menthol, carbolic acid, eucalyptus, pinus canadensis, etc.

It is understood, of course, that the auscultation tube is employed in these inflations, in the first place to determine the patulency of the Eustachian tube, in the second to detect the bubbling sound which is made by the injected fluid as it enters the tympanic cavity. The many difficulties of properly reaching the tubal orifice as the result of various nasal obstructions produced by enlarged turbinals, septal deflections and thickenings, spurs and growths, are overcome by operative intervention.

Where the examination of the patient has determined the fact that the Eustachian tube offers obstruction to the free passage of air or fluids, or where irregularities in the nasal passages occur to prevent satisfactory catheterization I have used continued vapour-inflations with good results.

For this purpose I employ a globe hand nebulizer, to which is attached a short flexible shaft armed with a glass nasal tip. I avail myself of the most excellent suggestion of Dundas Grant ; namely, that of directing the patient to blow through a narrow-calibred tube. When the Eustachian tube is patent, I usually succeed in obtaining a continuous and considerable vaporization of the tympanic cavity by this means. It is understood that a continuous air current is used in connection with the vaporizer instead of the usual rubber inflation ball.

Following the injection or vaporization of the tympanic cavity by such medicated petroleum products, I apply the aural masseur, either operated by hand or by compressed air. I assume that as the contents of the tympanic cavity are brought into contact with these oily vapours or solutions, that it has a tendency to soften the fibrous bands and adhesions, and that this is an opportune time to apply massage to the drum-membrane.

The results of this plan of treatment have proven superior to so many of the older therapeutic suggestions, as to the rapidity with which improvement has been noticed, and also from the fact that this course of treatment has frequently proven successful when the usual methods have failed.

It is in that large class of cases of chronic suppurative otitis media where the constant presence of purulent secretions threatens the destruction of the soft tissues of the tympanum, where ossicular necrosis is imminent, and where an extension of the inflammatory products to the accessory spaces of this cavity is possible, that conservative otology should be practised. Here the radical operator, with his often too active interference, frequently promotes unfavourable results.

A question which has often been of considerable bacteriological interest is the fact that micro-organisms can be retained within the area of the middle ear cavity for so long a time without giving rise to a further extension of the inflammatory process. We come in contact almost daily with suppurations of the middle ear which have existed for months and years without indication of tissue destruction, and without causing the patient any inconvenience beyond that of discharge. This fact should appeal to us as one of much clinical value. Here is a cavity lined with mucous membrane which, microscopically is very similar in structure with that of the Eustachian tube and its naso-pharyngeal orifice. This continuity of tissue extends from the naso-pharynx to the tympanic cavity, as well asto the attic, antrum, and mastoid cells. Bacteriologically, we know that micro-organisms find an especially favourable habitat on mucous membrane, and that this suitable culture medium, supplemented by a moist serous surface, and a fairly uniform temperature, such as is found in the tympanum, offers the best possible opportunity for the rapid spread from an infected focus.

We know furthermore that over 70 per cent. of the suppurative affections of the tympanic cavity are due to an extension and infection from the naso-pharynx via Eustachian tube. Through this section of the mucous tract an extension of infection to the tympanic cavity is rapid ; conversely, in the chronic forms of suppurative infection of the middle ear an extension to the more vital areas of the attic, antrum, and mastoid, is slow. It would be interesting to determine the reason for this decided difference in the tendency of micro-organisms to spread ; on the one hand the rapid spread from the naso-pharynx via Eustachian tube to the tympanic cavity ; on the other the slow progress from the tympanic cavity via attic and antrum to the mastoid cells.

I do not assume that even the most radical enthusiast would undertake operative procedures for the relief of chronic suppurative otitis media until he had given a fair trial to milder measures. It is to the application of these therapeutic measures that I desire to direct your attention.

In a brief paper recently published I attempted to compare the two systems of treatment which have in recent years been given every practical test ; one, the so-called "dry treatment ; " the other, the irrigation and syringing with various antiseptic solutions. In summing up the advantages and disadvantages which either of these methods might afford, I have considered the pathological status of the affected area, the character of the discharge and the size of the perforation, as factors.

From a close comparison of these two methods I believe that the constant use of the syringe and irrigation of the auditory canal are distinctly contra-indicated in active suppurative cases where large perforations of the membrana tympani exist, and where a free entrance of the fluid into the tympanic cavity is so easily effected. In the first place the mucous membrane of the tympanic cavity, bathed in purulent secretions, affords an excellent supply of infectious material which the force of the current from the syringe or douche may wash into the remote and healthy areas of this cavity and thus mechanically produce an infection of the attic or antrum where none had previously existed. I think I can substantiate the assumption that many of the cases requiring mastoid interference or ossiculectomy have been unconsciously produced by the too liberal use of the syringe as a cleansing agent in suppurative otitis media.

Otological literature contains frequent references and admonitions as to the indiscriminate use of the nasal douche, especially when handled by the patient himself, and points to a subsequent infection of the tympanic cavity as the result of this procedure. If this is so frequently possible by the carrying of the fluid through the entire tract of the Eustachian tube, how much more readily can a similar result ensue when the syringe is brought directly into contact with the tympanic cavity through a large perforation of the membrane.

The second factor contra-indicating the use of aqueous fluids in these conditions is the pathological status of the tympanic cavity itself. The tympanic cavity during a suppurative otitis is constantly bathed by purulent secretions, resulting in a sodden, boggy surface, and this is accentuated by the addition of aqueous fluids. It is this very stimulation and irritation of the mucous membrane by the fluids with which it is brought into contact, that causes granulation and polypus formation. It should be our object to *extract* fluid from this area and not to add to the already existing serous or purulent infiltration.

Where the discharge is viscid, tenacious and copious the application of the syringe with a gentle current of a mild warm antiseptic fluid may be advocated to clear the auditory canal *to the surface of the membrana tympani.* Beyond this point, however, it is my opinion that the syringe should not be used in suppurative conditions of the tympanic cavity.

Clearing the auditory canal of these copious discharges may be just as readily accomplished by the cotton mop and by the use of solutions of peroxide of hydrogen. This obviates the necessity of the syringe and the considerable pressure of the current of fluid which is often necessary to dislodge these ropy, purulent shreds.

The "dry dressing" in surgery has found general favor of late. Its advocates and enthusiasts claim for it a more rapid healing, a more natural covering, less irritation of the injured surface, and less danger from infection of the surrounding areas. The use of the syringe usually produces an infiltrated surface and unintentionally aggravates that condition of "bogginess" of the mucous membrane which it is our purpose to subdue.

For clearing the auditory canal of pus or muco-purulent discharges, I have found a small tuft of sterilized cotton wound about the end of a probe or cotton-carrier, frequently renewed and gently applied as a mop, a more effective cleansing agent than a large current of antiseptic fluid.

If but a small perforation exists and the cotton tuft cannot find its way through this perforation into the tympanic cavity, there is always a possibility of retention of the purulent matter and a tendency to prolonged suppuration. In suppurative otitis media of a chronic character where no pain or discomfort exists I employ the Eustachian catheter in connection with a nebulizing or vaporizing apparatus, thus accomplishing the three-fold result of inflating the middle ear cavity, of clearing the tympanum of pus and forcing it by a medicated compressed-air current through the perforation, and of medicating the middle ear cavity more effectually and with less unfavourable possibilities than by the use of an aqueous fluid. My nebulized fluid consists of iodine, 3 grains, carbolic acid, 5 grains, and benzoinol or albolene, 1 ounce. This I use in conjunction with a Globe hand-nebulizer, the supply tube of which is fitted with a special tip which in turn is snugly adjusted to the proximal end of the Eustachian catheter. In this way my medicated vapour is insured a thorough penetration of the tympanic cavity and the inflation may be continued *ad libitum*. The most simple index for determining the volume of vapour which reaches the middle ear cavity in this manner is to watch the vapour as it passes out of the auditory canal. I have frequently succeeded by this steady inflation, continued for five minutes at a time, in forcing the residue of the purulent matter through small perforations of the membrana tympani in a single sitting, and long-standing cases of suppurative otitis media have yielded to this treatment where all other methods have failed.

An antiseptic powder, lightly insufflated, completes this treatment. Boracic acid, which has for so many years been the sheet anchor of otologists in the treatment of suppurative conditions of the middle ear, is hardly of sufficient antiseptic strength to meet all the demands of modern therapy ; iodoform is objectionable, first because its germicidal action is often questionable, second, because of its disagreeable odour; and third, as it possesses a tendency to stimulate granulations ; my preference has been for nosophen, as it meets the majority of the requirements of an ideal powder dressing in the ear, being more potent than boracic acid in its antiseptic qualities, odourless and less irritating than iodoform, and with no tendency to clog (cake).

Where the discharge is profuse I add to this treatment a gauze packing, selecting narrow strips of plain sterilized gauze in preference to that of iodoform as previously advocated.

I would also take this occasion to state that in the evolution of medications employed in the treatment of the mucous membrane of the upper respiratory tract and of the ear, it is my opinion that oil sprays and vapours, in their various combinations, will soon gain the upper hand.

In the consideration of this paper I have simply recorded several experiences from practical work, which, by comparison with the various therapeutic measures with which I have become familiar, have offered better possibilities, and in conclusion, I desire to emphasize my plea against the indiscriminate use of the syringe; against the indifference frequently observed in medication of the nasal passages and naso-pharynx when treating the ear; against too hasty operative steps when milder measures, if given a fair trial, would succeed; and in favour of petroleum preparations in preference to aqueous solutions as a basis for sprays and vapours; of the "dry dressing" in suppurative otitis, and especially of massage, prolonged inflation, and medicated petroleum injections into the tympanum, all effected at the same sitting.

DR. LEDERMANN—I rise to endorse the remarks of the reader of this interesting paper, and wish to emphasize the importance of treating pathological lesions in the nose and naso-pharynx in cases of chronic middle ear catarrh. It has been my custom for the last few years to treat the mucous membrane of the Eustachian tube and middle ear in a manner similar to that practised upon the nose and naso-pharynx.

The intimate association of these cavities is readily seen in cases of acute otitis following a catarrhal condition of the nose and post-nasal spaces.

Suitable aeration of the tube and middle ear is the most important factor in the treatment of these cases. For this reason we must first attack any obstruction of the nose or naso-pharynx. After these passages are free, we may then with impunity apply our oily applications in suitable strength.

It is always advisable to begin with weak solutions. Iodine, in combination with menthol—about five grains of the former to ten of the latter to the ounce of any oily menstruum, preferably benzoinol—has acted satisfactorily in my hands. These proportions can be increased as the chronicity of the case warrants.

The solution may be applied through the catheter by means of the air bag, or compressed air-apparatus. If the latter is employed, we must not at first apply too much pressure. About ten to fifteen pounds should be the initiative force. After a number of treatments this may be increased. It is advisable to apply some form of massage to the drum and ossicular chain before employing the Eustachian medication, so as to loosen the ankylosis if feasible.

In suppurative conditions cleanliness plays a very important part. Too much moisture, however, stimulates the degenerative process, and constantly the speaker employs a saturated solution of boracic acid in alcohol. The dehydrating properties of the alcohol, together with the deposit of the acid after the alcohol has evaporated, accomplishes the purpose of dry treatment, without damming back any of the discharge, as would be apt to occur if the canal were tightly packed with the acid.

Trichloracetic acid has proven an active medicament in the speaker's hands in treating hypertrophic lesions of the tympanic mucous membrane.   The use of cocain must always precede its application, as the latter is very painful otherwise.

DR. WM. L. BALLINGER.—The paper presented by Dr. Goldstein is most admirable, and in most points meets with my approval.   I wish to protest, however, against the inference that existing hypertrophy of the mucosa of the middle ear or nose can be materially reduced by the topical application of vapours or oily emulsions, as described in the paper. When hypertrophy is present there is permanent thickening of the tissues, and it can only be removed by caustic or surgical measures. The value of topical measures in true hypertrophy is limited to their influence upon the vascular and lymphatic circulation.   In this way the local nutritive processes may be so modified as to reduce the vascular engorgement, and to accelerate the lymphatic flow, thereby establishing a better nutritive process in the mucosa.   The local engorgement being reduced, and the hypertrophic process checked, the conduction apparatus of the middle ear is in a measure restored to its normal activity.

DE L'INFLAMMATION PRIMITIVE DE L'APOPHYSE MASTOÏDE.

DR. THEODORE HEIMAN, Warsaw.

Parmi la quantité si variée d'affections de l'appareil acoustique, que j'ai traitées et observées jusqu'à présent, j'ai très rarement rencontré la périostite primitive de l'apophyse mastoïde ; et je n'ai jamais constaté un seul cas d'inflammation idiopathique ni de suppuration limitée aux cellules de l'apophyse.

Les cas très rares de périostite primitive de l'apophyse mastoïde, que j'ai constatés, et qui ont donné naissance à un abcès sous-périostal, étaient toujours consecutifs à des traumatismes ; une fois seulement l'erysipèle détermina une suppuration primitive ; quant aux cas qui n'aboutirent pas à la suppuration, mais sont disparu complètement ou produisirent l'épaississement et l'hyperplasie du périoste, ils provenaient, soit du traumatisme, ou étaient la conséquence d'un refroidissement, de la syphilis ou de l'artritisme.   Un certain nombre de cas confondus de prime abord avec une inflammation primitive, après un examen plus minutieux, se montra être la suite d'affections purulentes ou exsudations récentes ou peu accentuées de la caisse, d'inflammations dans le conduit acoustique externe, les parties molles recouvrant l'apophyse mastoïde ou les parties voisines.

Les cas isolés d'inflammation et de suppuration primitive des cellules mastoïdiennes se montrèrent être toujours la suite d'affections de la caisse et du périoste de l'apophyse mastoïde soit disparu, soit encore existant.

Pas plus dans la littérature otiaţrique ancienne que dans nombre d'ouvrages récents, il n'y a pas la moindre mention de l'inflammation primitive du périoste et de l'os de l'apophyse mastoïde (Toynbee, Wilde, Itard, Bonnafont, Triquet, Kramer, v Tröltsch, Hartmann, Bing, etc.) Quant à ceux qui décrivent ces formes morbides (Politzer, Schwartze, Bürkner, Gruber) ils considèrent également la première forme comme rare, et la seconde comme exceptionelle. Les cas isolés d'inflammation du périoste et de l'os de l'apophyse mastoïde, ont été cités dans différentes publications par Jacoby, Roosa, Ely, Voltolini, Knapp, Kirchner, Hatz, Blau, Schwartze, Christinek, Williams, Ménière, Kretschman, Bezold, Politzer, et d'autres. A l'examen critique de ces cas, on constate que plus d'une fois le diagnostic a été erroné et que ce n'étaient en réalité que des inflammations secondaires. Comme exemple, je citerai quelques uns de ces cas. Politzer rapporte un cas de périostite primitive purulente de l'apophyse mastoïde ayant pour origine une inflammation de la lèvre supérieure du malade, qui gagna le pavillon, les parties molles de l'apophyse mastoïde et s'étendit à l'apophyse. A mon avis ce n'est que la plus simple inflammation secondaire de l'apophyse mastoïde, et cette inflammation aurait été primitive, si elle avait débuté par le périoste de l'apophyse. Kretschmann dans son travail indique clairement que le malade avant l'apparition de la périostite, souffrait d'une inflammation parasitaire de l'oreille externe ; nous devons par conséquent admettre que dans ce cas, la cause de la périostite de l'apophyse mastoïde était une affection primitive de l'oreille externe ; du reste l'auteur lui-même admet cette hypothèse. Schwartze donne un cas d'inflammation de l'os même de l'apophyse chez un enfant de 9 mois, aggravée de syphilis héréditaire ; mais l'auteur dit aussi qu'il y avait une suppuration dans l'oreille et perforation de la membrane du tympan. Schwartze mentionne également dans son Anatomie Pathologique de l'Oreille (page 110) un cas d'inflammation primitive purulente des cellules de l'apophyse mastoïde, qui lui a été communiqué verbalement par Zaufal et qui se termina mortellement à la suite de l'inflammation des sinus cérébraux. Toutefois Zaufal, autant que l'on en peut juger considère ce cas comme la suite d'une inflammation de l'oreille, provoquée par des pneumocoques.

D'après Zaufal l'abcès mastoïdien peut provenir dans des cas un certain temps après la cessation de troubles de ce genre de la caisse, et le retour de l'ouïe à état normal. Aussi strictement parlant, le cas de Zaufal cité par Schwartze ainsi que ceux qui lui sont analogues, ne peuvent être considérés comme des inflammations primitives de l'apophyse mastoïde, attendu que le point saillant de l'affection de l'apophyse mastoïde, est comme nous le voyons, toujours, une affection antérieure de la caisse. Bezold prétend, que nous avons assez souvent l'occasion d'observer des accumulations de pus dans l'apophyse mastoïde, où la matière se déverse sous le périoste ou sous les parties molles de l'apophyse et ces accumulations se développent à la suite de suppurations récentes ou anciennes de la caisse ; en outre il n'est pas nécessaire qu'il y ait eu perforation préalable de la membrane du tympan. Roosa est presque du même avis. Bezold explique l'origine de ces suppurations tardives de l'apophyse mastoïde par le fait que dans l'affection de l'oreille, presque simultanément est atteinte l'apophyse mastoïde ; toutefois le développement de l'état morbide dans cette dernière, ou plutôt sa réaction n'apparaît qu'au bout d'un certain temps, probablement par suite de l'influence de facteurs propices favorisant le développement des produits morbides renfermés dans l'apophyse.

J'ai recueilli dans ma propre pratique quelques cas qui à première vue peuvent être considérés comme des affections inflammatoires primitives de l'apophyse mastoïde, et que pourtant, je suis obligé de considérer comme secondaires, consécutives.

Pendant l'épidémie d'influenza qui régna chez nous en 1889, je fus appelé auprès d'une jeune femme, qui à la suite de l'influenza fut atteinte d'une otite gauche externe et moyenne (affection caractéristique dans les cas de cette maladie : otite externe bulleuse, hémorragique et otite moyenne) avec violentes douleurs dans l'oreille ; l'apophyse était sensible à la palpation. Après l'application des remèdes appropriés, en 3 jours les douleurs cessèrent, les vésicules du conduit auditif externe et de la membrane du tympan s'ouvrirent ou se résorbèrent ; au bout de quinze jours la malade se sentait tout-à-fait bien ; la membrane était pâle, on apercevait encore à sa surface quelques vaisseaux sanguins hyperhémiés.

L'ouïe auparavant considérablement affaiblie (la malade au 3e jour de la maladie ne percevait le tictac de la montre ni par la voie osseuse ni par la voie aérienne, quant à la conversation à haute voix elle la percevait au maximum à 1 mètre) s'améliora au point qu'elle entendait bien la montre par la voie crânienne ; par la voie aérienne à 8cm. de l'oreille, la parole à 5 mètres. Cet état dura 10 jours, la malade entra en convalescence, et continua à vaquer aux soins du ménage. Ayant par hasard regardé par la fenêtre, elle ressentit presque immédiatement de violentes douleurs mastoïdiennes à droite, de légers picottements dans l'oreille, puis des frissons et une forte fièvre. En examinant l'oreille de la malade le soir même, je trouvai la membrane droite du tympan un peu trouble, à la suite de l'inflammation ; on apercevait le manche du marteau et sa courte apophyse. L'audition était presque normale. L'apophyse mastoïde ainsi que les parties molles qui le recouvraient ne présentaient pas le moindre changement objectif, la pression exercée sur l'apophyse en augmentait la sensibilité. Des douleurs violentes au fond de l'apophyse mastoïde, une forte fièvre (40-39°), avec rémission légère le matin (39°-38,7°), tel fut l'état presque ininterrompu pendant 5 semaines. Tous les moyens thérapeutiques tels que le froid, la chaleur sous diverses formes, les sangsues, la teinture d'iode, la paracentèse de la membrane du tympan à 2 reprises ainsi que la médication interne (bromure, salol, codeine, morphine) demeurèrent sans effet, ou n'apportèrent qu'un soulagement momentané. Je m'étais décidé à ponctionner la membrane du tympan, supposant l'existence d'une sécrétion de la caisse, que je ne pouvais constater, vu l'opacité de la membrane ; la douche d'air ne fournissait aucun indice. Chaque fois, je n'obtenais qu'une goutte de sang provenant de la membrane du tympan. Pendant tout le temps, l'audition demeura presque normale à gauche. Au bout de cinq semaines survint une infiltration inflammatoire de l'extrémité inférieure de l'apophyse et des parties molles avoisinantes du cou, et en même temps l'oreille laissa couler une grande quantité de pus, qui, comme le démontra l'examen, avait perforé la membrane du tympan dans le haut de la partie postéro-supérieure Malgré la suppuration, les douleurs mastoïdiennes persistaient, quoique moins violentes, et la fièvre céda pour la première fois. Devant la persistance de la douleur et de l'oedème des parties molles, je pratiquai l'ouverture de l'apophyse mastoïde ; au fond je ne trouvai que deux gouttes de pus ; une partie de ses cellules étaient détruites et remplies de granulations, le reste de l'os était rouge. Dès ce moment l'état de la malade commença à s'améliorer ; six semaines plus tard la plaie était cicatrisée.

Un lieutenant colonel, âgé de 46 ans, au cours de l'été de 1893, fut atteint d'un rhume de cerveau et remarqua qu'il entendait de moins en moins par l'oreille droite A l'examen je constatai des symptômes de catarrhe aigu de la trompe d'Eustache et de la caisse droite, avec exsudat séreux insignifiant. Il n'entendait le bruit de la montre que par l'application contre le pavillon, le diapason à 4cm. de l'oreille, la voix à 1.50 m. La perception crânienne était amplifiée, Rinne négatif. J'appliquai la douche d'air au moyen de la sonde, le malade se remit complètement après 2 semaines, et partit guéri. Quatre mois après il revint, se plaignant des bruits dans l'oreille droite, de la surdité et des douleurs au voisinage de l'apophyse mastoïde droite et dans la région occipitale du même côté. Ces symptômes s'étaient déclarés la semaine précédente, à la suite de grandes fatigues aux manoeuvres. La membrane du tympan était normale sauf un léger refoulement. La douche d'air excluait l'existence d'un gonflement de la trompe ou d'exsudats dans la caisse. La douche d'air appliquée pendant 2 semaines fut abandonnée car elle n'eut aucun effet sur la surdité et les bruits Cependant la douleur dans l'apophyse mastoïde augmentait graduellement et dura sans interruption pendant 6 semaines ; elle privait le malade de sommeil, et le plus souvent était intolérable. La pression du doigt sur l'apophyse mastoïde n'en augmentait guère la sensibilité. Tous les moyens thérapeutiques échouèrent ou ne procurèrent qu'une amélioration passagère. Une quadruple ponction de la membrane du tympan n'amena pas dans la caisse la moindre trace de sécrétion. On n'observa pas le moindre changement objectif sur les parties molles de l'apophyse mastoïde, pas plus que dans son voisinage. Six semaines après, apparaissaient les frissons, le malade eut la fièvre, sa figure prit une teinte jaune terreuse. Au bout de quelques jours on reconnut l'existence d'une infiltration dure envahissant la région mastoïdo-occipitale ainsi que presque toute la partie postéro-latérale du cou, et presque simultanément le conduit auditif externe livra passage à une grande quantité de pus.

Malgré tout, les douleurs persistaient dans l'apophyse. Trépanation de l'apophyse mastoïde, la couche externe était sensiblement hypertrophiée, un certain nombre des cellules mastoïdiennes étaient remplis de pus et de granulations ; et ne formaient qu'une cavité. Je fis donc une incision large et profonde le long du bord postérieur du muscle sterno-cléido-mastoïdien ; sous l'aponévrose moyenne du cou il y avait une forte infiltration purulente. Alors seulement cessèrent les douleurs et les autres symptômes graves. La plaie guérit en 3 mois, l'audition revint à normal.

Un homme de 57 ans fut, sans raison apparente atteint de bruits dans l'oreille gauche, compliqués de légers picottements et de violents maux de tête à l'occiput, maux qui gagnèrent par la suite l'apophyse mastoïde gauche. L'examen des oreilles indiqua une légère hyperémie du tympan gauche, l'épreuve de l'ouïe révéla une légère diminution de l'audition à gauche. Les douleurs de la région occipitale gauche durèrent presque sans interruption pendant 4 mois.

La ponction à deux reprises de la membrane du tympan ainsi que d'autres traitements locaux ou généraux, ne servirent pas à grand'chose. Quelques jours après la seconde ponction de la membrane du tympan, je vis une quantité minime de pus sortir de la caisse sans que cela exerçat la moindre influence sur les maux de tête et sur l'apophyse mastoïde. Aucun changement sur les parties molles de l'apophyse mastoïde. Au bout de 4 mois et demi, les douleurs étant devenues intolérables le malade consentit à l'ouverture de l'apophyse mastoïde. Les cellules étaient remplies de granulations, avec très peu de pus. J'ouvris l'apophyse jusqu'à l'antre. Après l'opération les douleurs cessèrent, la plaie se cicatrisa, deux mois et demi après, l'ouïe était revenue à l'état normal.

J'eus l'occasion de constater d'autres cas similaires, mais je me contente de citer ces trois observations. Comme nous le voyons, l'affection de la caisse était insignifiante, non invetérée, et il était facile de méconnaitre ses rapports avec les altérations de l'apophyse mastoïde.

Il est vrai, que j'ai traité il y a quelques mois un malade que l'on pourrait considérer comme atteint d'une inflammation primitive de l'apophyse mastoïde, chez lequel l'inflammation se développa comme une ostéite condensante, ce cas lui-même n'est pas typique.

Je fus appelé auprès d'un malade atteint depuis un mois d'une otite moyenne gauche aiguë ave: sensibilité de l'apophyse mastoïde à la pression, dans la région correspondant à l'antre mastoïde ; le tout accompagné de fièvre violente à caractère pyæmique, et d'un affaiblissement général. Je pratiquai l'ouverture de l'apophyse mastoïde sur une grande étendue ; je trouvai un abcès sous-dural, et mis à nu la dure-mère dans la région du sinus transversal. Pendant l'opération je remarquai la surface irrégulière presque stalactiforme de l'apophyse, ainsi que sa dureté et son volume qui atteignait 2 centimètres avant que je n'eusse découvert le foyer purulent dans l'apophyse. J'avais en un mot devant moi le tableau de l'apophyse mastoïde sclérotique que nous rencontrons souvent dans les affections purulentes chroniques de la caisse. Le malade qui était intelligent, affirmait qu'il n'avait jamais souffert de l'oreille, fait confirmé par la marche de la maladie après l'opération, ainsi que le retour rapide de l'ouïe à l'état normal, et la cicatrisation de la membrane du tympan. Toutefois, une quinzaine d'années auparavant le malade avait reçu un coup de sabot sur l'oreille et l'apophyse mastoïde gauche, dont il avait souffert pendant plusieurs mois avec complication de légères douleurs dans la région du traumatisme. L'oreille resta indemne. Nous avions par conséquent affaire ici à une inflammation ancienne de l'apophyse mastoïde d'origine traumatique que je considère non comme primitive, mais comme la suite de l'inflammation périostique de cette région.

Probablement, plus d'un cas analogue à ceux que j'ai cités a été considéré comme une inflammation primitive de l'apophyse mastoïde. D'après ce que nous avons dit, on est convaincu que les cas d'inflammation primitive de l'apophyse mastoïde, même par ceux qui les ont décrits, ne peuvent pas être renfermés dans cette catégorie, vu qu'un certain nombre d'entre eux constituaient des états morbides secondaires ; par contre il existe un certain nombre de praticiens sérieux qui mettent en doute l'existence de l'inflammation primitive de l'apophyse mastoïde en général. Bezold prétendait à l'origine que tout en n'excluant pas la possibilité de l'affection de l'apophyse mastoïde du côté de la trompe, ou par la circulation du sang, surtout au cours des maladies générales, même à l'autopsie, on ne pouvait se prononcer en faveur de la primordialité des altérations de l'apophyse mastoïde, aussi doit on être très circonspect dans le diagnostic sur le vivant.

Avec le temps Bezold finit par se convaincre que les cas d'inflammation purulente idiopathique de l'apophyse mastoïde sans participation de la caisse, sont généralement douteux.

Roosa dit que certains cas décrits sous le nom de périostites primitives de l'apophyse mastoïde, après examen attentif, se sont montrés douteux, vu que c'étaient des formes morbides dans lesquelles le périoste de l'apophyse mastoïde était plus sérieusement atteint que la muqueuse des autres parties de l'oreille moyenne, et où l'affection dans la caisse était presque à son déclin, alors que dans le périoste la maladie avait atteint son plein développement.

J'observai les mêmes faits chez mes malades porteurs d'inflammation des cellules de l'apophyse mastoïde. Weil cite de nombreux exemples d'erreurs de diagnostic. Enfin Buck doute que nous ayons même le droit de parler de périostite primitive de l'apophyse mastoïde, et dit qu'il n'a jamais rencontré un cas que l'on puisse en toute conscience rapporter à cette catégorie. Les cas d'inflammation apparents chez les enfants s'expliquent par le fait, que chez eux le pus se fraye plus facilement le chemin de la caisse par l'apophyse mastoïde que par la membrane du tympan.

Théoriquement, l'inflammation mastoïdienne primitive est possible par la voie des vaisseaux sanguins et lymphatiques, au moyen desquels les éléments morbides c.à.d. les microcoques passent d'un foyer déterminé dans l'apophyse mastoïde et c'est par là que pourrait survenir l'inflammation primitive dans la syphilis, la tuberculose, la scrofule, la diphthérie, la scarlatine, le typhus. L'inflammation primitive de l'apophyse mastoïde offre une certaine analogie avec l'ostéomyélite aiguë. Comme Kocher l'a démontré le premier, l'étiologie de cette maladie est la suivante, les microcoques pathogènes doivent d'un point quelconque de la peau, des poumons, des organes digestifs pénétrer dans le sang et par son entremise, pour des raisons anatomiques, se fixer dans les vaisseaux de la moelle des os, s'y développer et provoquer les inflammations purulentes, resp. septiques avec participation de l'os et du périoste. D'après les expériences de Colzi, les microcoques arrivent le plus souvent de la peau dans le sang, plus rarement par d'autres voies.

Le traumatisme facilite le développement de l'ostéomyélite. Peut-elle provenir d'un refroidissement, cela n'a pas été prouvé jusqu'à présent, mais on peut supposer que l'inflammation peut avoir cette origine. Elle se développe également à la suite d'exanthèmes aigus et de suppurations de différents organes.

Donc, tout foyer purulent peut déterminer une myélite aiguë par le contact avec les bacilles pyogéniques. Et par suite pour que l'ostéite primitive de l'apophyse mastoïde survienne, il doit exister avant tout un foyer purulent sur ou dans l'organisme, d'où les germes pyogéniquespar la voie sanguine gagneraient l'apophyse mastoïde. Et cependant, personne rapporte d'observations de cette nature, non plus que de celles où l'inflammation primitive de l'apophyse mastoïde, se développerait sous l'influence d'exanthèmes aigus. Politzer, qui dans son manuel présente le tableau clinique détaillé de la périostite et de l'ostéite primitive de l'apophyse mastoïde comme cause originelle de l'inflammation de l'os lui-même, ne parle que du traumatisme, du refroidissement et de la syphilis ; sans signaler d'autres maladies contagieuses. A mon avis les affections de ce genre débutent toujours par une inflammation modérée du périoste ou bien de la caisse qui attaque l'os ultérieurement.

Toutefois B. Fränkel a rencontré dans l'inflammation de la cavité pharyngienne et presque toujours dans le pharynx à l'état normal le staphylocoque pyogène doré et blanc ; si c'était là un des facteurs provoquant l'inflammation primitive de l'apophyse mastoïde, et si ce microcoque sortant du pharynx s'introduisait par le sang dans les cellules de l'apophyse mastoïde, il serait difficile de s'expliquer la rareté de cette inflammation. Il est peu probable que les microbes après avoir abandonné la cavité naso-pharyngienne laissent indemnes la trompe d'Eustache et la caisse, et y perdent leur vitalité, pour la retrouver dans les conditions favorables, dans l'apophyse mastoïde.

On reconnaît l'existence de la périostite primitive de l'apophyse mastoïde, lorsque l'on observe un gonflement douloureux, dur, strictement limité, dont le revêtement cutané n'est que peu ou non attaqué par l'inflammation, lorsqu'il y a manque de symptômes d'inflammation du côté du conduit auditif externe, de la membrane du tympan, de la caisse, et des autres portions du temporal et des parties molles avoisinantes, et enfin lorsqu'on peut exclure absolument toute lésion récente de l'oreille ou des parties molles de l'apophyse. Quant à savoir si le gonflement disparaît ou s'il donne naissance à la suppuration, c'est une question secondaire. Malgré l'affirmation de Roosa et de Buck je suis d'avis que l'existence de ce genre ne saurait être mise en doute ; ils sont rares il est vrai, mais tout médecin auriste les constate de temps en temps dans la pratique. Pour plus d'exactitude, je ferai remarquer que je ne range pas dans cette catégorie d'inflammation, les cas où l'on constate simultanément l'existence d'un état purulent des parties molles recouvrant l'apophyse (phlegmon).

Je crois inutile d'ajouter que l'inflammation, l'infiltration et la suppuration des glandes lymphatiques sur l'apophyse mastoïde, ainsi que le gonflement douloureux du périoste et des parties molles, rencontrées çà et là dans les inflammations circonscrites du conduit auditif externe, n'ont rien de commun avec la question qui nous occupe.

Le diagnostic de l'inflammation primitive des cellules de l'apophyse mastoïde, repose sur l'existence de violentes douleurs persistantes au fond de l'os, sur l'absence de toute altération du côté du périoste et des parties molles de l'apophyse mastoïde ainsi que du côté de l'oreille externe, de la caisse et de la membrane du tympan. Lorsqu'au moment du premier examen, il existe un gonflement ou une suppuration de l'apophyse mastoïde, ou bien lorsqu'il y a des altérations de la caisse, le diagnostic devient impossible ; n'oublions pas non plus que l'inflammation de l'apophyse mastoïde est en général difficile à reconnaître. Politzer est d'avis que si après l'incision de la peau jusqu'à l'os la douleur ne cède pas, l'existence d'une suppuration profonde dans l'os devient vraisemblable. Toutefois cela ne préjuge pas selon moi, la primordialité de la lésion osseuse. D'autre part comme le prétend Politzer à bon droit, les douleurs répétées et persistantes dans l'apophyse mastoïde, sans modifications apparentes de la surface externe, et sans que rien ne réveille la présence de pus dans la caisse, ces symptômes dis-je ne prouvent pas encore que l'on soit en présence d'une inflammation purulente de l'apophyse, attendu que ces symptômes s'observent au cours de scléroses dans les névralgies mastoïdiennes. L'absence de sensibilité de l'apophyse dans les cas d'affection de l'oreille externe ou de la caisse n'exclut pas son état inflammatoire. Mais, même l'existence de tous les symptômes caractérisant l'inflammation purulente de l'apophyse mastoïde, ne révèle pas toujours l'existence de cette altération et ne permet nullement de diagnostiquer une inflammation primitive. Comme exemple je citerai en quelques mots le cas suivant.

Il y a quelques années je soignai à l'hôpital un militaire, qui sans raison apparente, avait depuis quelques jours des frissons, une forte fièvre et de vives douleurs dans l'apophyse mastoïde droite. La membrane du tympan était normale. Quatre jours après, l'état du malade n'ayant pas changé, et que les douleurs mastoïdiennes devenaient intolérables, devant l'échec de moyens ordinaires, je perforai la membrane du tympan, sans cependant obtenir la moindre sécrétion. Après avoir attendu quelques jours je pratiquai l'ouverture de l'apophyse mastoïde, vu la persistance de la douleur et de la fièvre. L'apophyse mastoïde était complètement saine, ses cellules vides, et sa muqueuse brillante et d'un aspect gris-jaune. L'opération n'influa pas sur les accidents, le malade succomba quelques jours plus tard et à l'autopsie on reconnut une infection typhoïdale.

Schwartze dit à bon droit que le seul véritable signe d'une inflammation purulente des cellules de l'apophyse mastoïde est la présence du pus dans l'os que l'on vient d'ouvrir.

En résumant ce que nous avons dit concernant la périostite et l'ostéïte primitives de l'apophyse mastoïde, nous arrivons aux conclusions suivantes :—   .

La périostite primitive de l'apophyse mastoïde, est sans aucun doute une maladie rare apparaissant sous une forme clinique distincte. L'ostéite primitive de l'apophyse mastoïde, existe théoriquement, mais tous ceux qui en font mention la considèrent comme une affection excessivement rare, attendu que les cas décrits jusqu'ici reposent sur des erreurs de diagnostic, et que les auristes très compétents, doutent de l'existence de cette affection.   Quant à moi personnellement, sur une quantité de malades malgré l'examen le plus attentif, je n'ai constaté aucun cas absolument net, que l'on put, sans hésitation prendre pour une ostéite primitive de l'apophyse mastoïde, attendu que l'anamnèse qui permettrai d'exclure les lésions récentes de la caisse ou des parties voisines de l'apophyse mastoïde, surtout chez les sujets d'intelligence bornée, est le plus souvent inexacte et trompeuse, attendu que l'examen de l'inflammation de l'apophyse mastoïde est généralement malaisé et qu'enfin, même au point de vue théorique nous possédons de données insuffisantes pour expliquer l'origine de cette forme morbide, que nous nous bornons à reconnaître par analogie, pour toutes ces raisons, l'ostéite primitive de l'apophyse mastoïde, doit être considérée comme un produit artificiel qui en réalité n'existe pas.

BIBLIOGRAPHIE.

Bürckner.   Lehrbuch der Ohrenheilkunde 1892, page 270, avec indication des sources des cas isolés.

Ménière.   Revue mensuelle de laryngologie 1887, No. 17.

Roosa.   Lehrbuch der praktischen Ohrenheilkunde, 1889, page 282, et suivantes ; édition allemande.

Gruber.   Lehrbuch der Ohrenheilkunde, 1888, page 483.

Jacoby.   Zur Casuistik der primären und secundären Periostitis und Osititis des Proces. mastoïd.   A. f. O. T. 16.   Page 286.

Williams.   Ein Fall primärer Periostitis des Warzenfortsatzes. Z. f. O. T. xvii.

Voltolini.   M. f. O. T. 11.

Politzer.   Lehrbuch der Ohrenheilkunde.   Ed. 3, 1893.   Page 414, et suivantes.

Weil.   Zur operativen Behandlung der Eiterung im Mittelohr und Warzenfortsatz.   Würtembergisches   med.   Correspond. 1891, No. 6.

Schwartze.   A. f. O. T. 19, page 231.

du même.   Pathologische Anatomie des Ohres, 1878, pages 110-111.

Zaufal. Fälle von genuiner acuter Mittelohrentzündung veranlasst durch den Diplococcus pneumoniæ und complicirt mit Abscess des Proc. mast. Prager med. Wochenschrift 1889, No. 36.

Kretschmann. A. f. O. T, 23, page 234.

Bezold. Ueberschau über den gegenwärtigen Stand der Ohrenheilkunde, 1895.

Buck. Diseases of the Ear, page 355.

Bezold. Primäre Erkrankung des Warzentheiles, etc., dans le Manuel de l'Otiatrie de Schwartze, T. 2, page 326.

Schwartze. Die chirurgischen Krankheiten des Ohres, 1885, page 308, et suivantes.

COMPLICATIONS OTIQUES DE L'OZÈNE.

DR. P. LACROIX. Paris.

Pendant de nombreuses années, le rôle étiologique de l'ozène, dans la genèse des maladies de l'oreille, a été considéré comme accessoire, et l'on pensait alors que le coryza atrophique retentissait rarement sur l'organe de l'ouie.

Ces idées anciennes, bien que déjà battues sérieusement en brèche par des travaux récents, ceux de Wyss, de Genève, par exemple, ne sont pas encore actuellement, peut-être, tout à fait abandonnées, tant est puissante la force de l'habitude et de la tradition.

Aujourd'hui, nous désirons montrer à notre tour que, bien au contraire, l'ozène se complique très fréquemment de lésions otiques, méritant véritablement, dans certains cas, le nom d'Ozène de l'Oreille.

Il nous semble difficile, en effet, de ne pas donner cette désignation à l'observation clinique dont nous allons parler maintenant, laquelle d'ailleurs sert de point de départ à notre étude.

C'est un cas certainement type d'ozène de l'oreille. Il éclaire la pathogénie des autres symptômes auriculaires observés au cours de l'atrophie des cornets.

Voici cette observation :

Une jeune fille de 14 ans, ozèneuse depuis plusieurs années, a été atteinte à différentes reprises de troubles otiques transitoires caractérisés par des douleurs, des bourdonnements et de la surdité.

Un jour ces phénomènes se reproduisent à nouveau, mais plus intenses cette fois ; finalement ils aboutissent à une sorte d'otite moyenne aiguë droite.

L'examen de l'oreille montre un tympan légèrement congestionné, dépoli, catarrhal et refoulé au dehors par du liquide accumulé dans la caisse. Nous pratiquons à ce moment, une perforation artificielle de la membrane tympanique avec l'aiguille à paracentèse, et, lorsque le malade exécute ensuite la manœuvre de Valsalva, il s'écoule par la perforation quelques gouttelettes d'un liquide muco-purulent mêlé de stries sanguinolentes venues des lèvres de la plaie tympanique.

Avec un tampon d'ouate monté sur tige, la sécrétion est épongée et nous constatons avec surprise que le liquide ainsi extrait de l'oreille moyenne répand une odeur nette et absolument caractéristique, semblable à la punaisie nasale : l'odeur si spéciale de l'ozène !

En observant cette sécrétion de plus près, nous constatons la présence de petites lamelles cornées odorantes pouvant être comparées dans une certaine mesure aux croûtes nasales.

L'examen des fosses nasales, et du pharynx dénonce les lésions classiques de l'ozène.

Ces phénomènes otiques, d'ailleurs, disparurent assez rapidement, sous l'influence d'un traitement approprié et tout rentra bientôt dans l'ordre, après évacuation du liquide de l'oreille moyenne.

Le coccus de Löwenberg n'a pas pu être recherché.

* *
*

Partant de cette observation qui semble bien être une ozène véritable de l'oreille, nous nous sommes demandé quelle pouvait être la fréquence et l'importance des complications otiques de l'ozène en général, et nous avons alors fixé spécialement notre attention sur tous les ozéneux qu'il nous a été donné de rencontrer.

Si l'on interroge superficiellement les malades, ou si on leur laisse l'initiative d'attirer eux-mêmes l'attention du médecin sur leur oreille, il est fréquent de méconnaître les troubles et les lésions de l'organe de l'ouïe.

Assez souvent, en effet, la surdité et les bourdonnements sont ou unilatéraux ou peu développés encore, et les malades, tout entiers aux inconvénients de l'odeur nasale, n'y attachent que peu d'importance jusqu'au jour où elles déterminent une diminution trop sérieuse de l'acuité auditive.

Il est donc nécessaire d'insister auprès du malade, de l'interroger soigneusement sur la présence possible de surdité et de bourdonnements permanents ou transitoires, uni ou bilatéraux, et même de pratiquer l'examen de l'audition.

Il est indispensable enfin de jeter un coup d'œil sur l'organe lui-même au travers du spéculum.

Dans ces conditions et ainsi recherchées, les complications otiques de l'ozène apparaissent comme extrêmement fréquentes. Souvent même tel sujet qui pendant longtemps avait eu l'oreille indemne, voit à un moment donné les bourdonnements ou la surdité apparaître.

Histologiquement nous nous trouvons en présence d'une même muqueuse ; la muqueuse de l'oreille moyenne prolonge la pituitaire et elle présente dans sa structure les mêmes cellules cylindriques vibratiles.

En clinique, sur 42 ozéneux que nous avons ainsi examinés systématiquement, sans tenir compte des réponses parfois un peu hâtives des intéressés, nous en avons trouvé 30 d'entre eux porteurs de complications otiques diverses, légères ou sérieuses—souvent légères, il est vrai—mais indéniables.

Ce chiffre représente les trois quarts des cas.

Au point de vue de la nature elle-même des complications otiques de l'ozène, nous avons rencontré :

Une fois la sclérose grave de l'oreille ; elle a dû être, nous le pensons, simplement aggravée par l'ozène, mais en aucune façon causée par elle.

Les autres cas se sont traduits par une otite moyenne chronique à forme catarrhale, généralement bilatérale. Le tympan y apparaissait dépoli, grisâtre, plus ou moins rétracté.

Les troubles fonctionnels étaient constitués par une surdité, sérieuse dans deux cas, moyenne dans quatre, moins importante chez huit autres malades. Les quatorze derniers se plaignaient seulement de bourdonnements et de surdité transitoires.

Tel est donc la bilan des complications otiques de l'ozène : légères ou sérieuses, elles sont indiscutablement très fréquentes.

En raison de leur aspect clinique et tenant compte de l'observation rapportée ci-dessus, nous pensons que les lésions de la rhinite atrophique se propagent à l'oreille moyenne, pour constituer une véritable otite chronique ozéneuse, avec les sécrétions et l'odeur spéciale de la punaise et que cette affection mérite le nom *d'ozène de l'oreille.*

Exostose du Conduit Auditif Droit.

Dr. Rutten, Namur, Belgium.

Messieurs,—Ne voulant pas abuser de votre temps trop précieux, je ne ferai que résumer les particularités qui distinguent l'exostose de l'oreille que j'ai l'honneur de vous présenter.

Cette anomalie osseuse est d'abord remarquable par son gros volume. En effet, elle mesure 15 mm. en longueur et jusqu'à 12 mm. en épaisseur. Elle remplissait complètement le conduit auditif externe à tel point qu'il fut impossible d'introduire le plus petit stylet entre la paroi et la tumeur. Ce qui plus est : par la compression l'excroissance avait détruit les téguments et avait occasionné de l'ostéo-périostite du canal. Cette suppuration secondaire, compliquée de la rétention du pus dans l'oreille moyenne avec commencement de symptômes cérébraux, a forcé le patient de se laisser opérer.

L'exostose se distingue en dehors de ses dimensions extraordinaires, par la durée très longue qu'elle a séjournée dans l'oreille sans occasionner aucun ennui. Son développement a passé inaperçu. Le porteur de l'excroissance, âgé de 38 ans au moment de l'opération, tonnelier de profession, a servi dans l'armée et n'a jamais souffert d'écoulement de l'oreille. Sept ans avant l'opération il est venu me consulter pour la surdité de ce côté. A ce moment, l'exostose obstrua déjà complètement le conduit, et le malade fut fort étonné quand je lui fis toucher au petit doigt le corps dur qui ne fut éloigné de l'ouverture du conduit que de quelques millimètres. Il ne se douta pas même de sa présence.

A cette époque, l'opération que je proposais, ne fût pas acceptée, bien que j'eusse indiqué le danger d'une suppuration, complication éventuelle possible qui s'est présentée sept ans après. On peut donc dire avec quelque certitude que la tumeur a mis pour se développer une durée de quinze à vingt ans.

L'exostose, de consistance de l'ivoire, est comme vous le constaterez, pédiculée. Recouverte d'une mince peau transparente, elle avait son point d'implantation à la paroi postérieure occupant toute la partie du conduit.

L'ablation a été faite dans la narcose, sans décoller le pavillon, au moyen de la gouge. Les suites de l'opération ont été heureuses en ce sens que j'ai obtenu une amélioration immédiate de l'ouïe et la guérison de l'écoulement après quelques jours de traitement.

En terminant, je me permets de poser une question aux confrères ici présents ou du moins à ceux qui ont examiné la belle collection de crânes porteurs d'exostoses que le Dr. Cheatle a exposés : comment on explique la fréquence extraordinaire des exostoses du conduit auditif, sur un nombre relativement minime de pièces ?

Comme on le sait, ces crânes intéressants, très bien conformés et ne présentant aucune autre déformation osseuse que l'exostose, le plus souvent dans les deux conduits à la fois, ont été trouvés réunis dans un même endroit au Pérou. De plus, toutes ces excroissances dont la plupart sont de belles exostoses pédiculées, d'autres des hyperostoses, ont leur point d'implantation sur le bord de la paroi inférieure, s'étendant exceptionnellement jusqu'à la paroi postérieure, à la partie correspondant aux cellules mastoïdiennes qui est le siège de prédilection des exostoses du conduit, comme l'a démontré le Prof. Politzer sur des pièces anatomiques, à la Société Autrichienne d'Otologie (séance du 20 Mai 1895). Le savant professeur a prouvé en plus qu'il y a participation de l'apophyse mastoïde, qui se transforme parfois au point d'être totalement éburnée. Il serait intéressant de rechercher à l'autopsie des crânes du Prof. Cheatle jusqu'à quel point l'apophyse mastoïde participe à cette transformation. Cet examen pourrait nous éclairer en grande partie sur la cause réelle de ces excroissances osseuses.

Malgré que la partie osseuse du conduit soit logée assez profondément, je ne suis pas loin de croire, me basant d'abord sur le nombre extraordinairement élevé de crânes qui présentent cette déformation osseuse des deux côtés et qu'on ne trouve que dans une même région et ensuite sur le siège du point d'implantation, qui est surtout la paroi inférieure au moins pour les exostoses pédiculées ; qu'il faut chercher la cause dans une irritation artificielle de l'os.

Doit on expliquer cette mutilation très douloureuse par la coquetterie ? Ou ces sauvages avaient ils les mêmes notions de médecine que les " sauvages " de notre temps qui percent les oreilles des enfants et les font suppurer le plus longtemps possible, dans le seul but de prévenir les affections oculaires et de dériver ainsi les mauvaises humeurs de la tête ?

Il est difficile de se prononcer.

On Extraction of the Stapes.

Prof. Politzer. Vienna.

Gentlemen,—I had intended to read a paper on extraction of the stapes, giving a critical review of the value of this operation when performed in the different pathological conditions of the middle ear, but the time is so limited and the number of papers to be read so large, that I am sure you will agree with me that it will be better only to give a short resumé of the subject.

1. Simple mobilization of the stapes only leads to a temporary improvement in hearing. When the improvement is more lasting it is due to a tearing of the adhesions.

2. Better results are obtained by dividing the adhesions formed between the branches of the stapes and the walls of the niche of the fenestra ovalis.

3. The operation of extraction of the stapes is founded on the results of experiments made on animals. Flourens, Kessel, Ricardo, Bobey, Grinaert, and Garnault have found that in birds and rabbits after the extraction of the columella and the stapes respectively, a new membrane is formed which closes the fenestra ovalis. My own experiments on rabbits have confirmed this fact, and in addition I have found by microscopical examination that no pathological changes are produced in the labyrinth.

4. Extraction of the stapes in cases of so-called sclerosis of the middle ear, is, according to my experience and that of Prof. Blake, a perfectly useless operation, because, as shown by my investigations, there is in these cases a proliferation of the bony tissue of the labyrinth capsule which, even after the stapes has been removed, effectually closes up the fenestra ovalis.

5. The results of extraction of the stapes in cases of non-suppurative middle ear catarrh with the formation of adhesions, are still too few to enable us to form a definite opinion as to its value.

6. In cases of chronic middle ear suppuration, we have at hand a good number of observations, where the stapes has been removed either intentionally or accidentally during the performance of the radical operation. Even when the immediate effects in a certain number of these cases have been favourable, but little is known about the ultimate results. Panse is of opinion that extraction of the stapes may be performed without danger to the hearing during the course of a chronic suppurative otitis media. But against those cases in which the hearing was improved must be placed a series of cases in which it was destroyed.

The latter result is well-shown in the following case which came under my observation two years ago. During a radical operation performed by one of my assistants the stapes was accidentally removed. The patient, who was a pale, emaciated and delicate child two years of age, died of tuberculosis several months after the operation. Examination of the microscopical sections showed the following:—In sections which pass through the niche of the fenestra ovalis and vestibulum, the inner wall of the tympanic cavity is seen to be covered by a granular mucous membrane composed of round cells. The granulation mass fills the niche of the fenestra ovalis, and passing forward from here through the fenestra into the vestibulum, fills out the whole cisterna perilymphatica, it is also firmly fused with the utriculus and surrounds it on all sides. The wall of the utriculus itself shows inflammatory thickening. In the superior and posterior semi-circular canals the condition is normal, but in the horizontal semi-circular canal the connective tissue network is in a state of inflammatory infiltration, invaded by round cells and intersected by dilated vessels. More conspicuous changes are found in the *cochlea*, here the inflammatory proliferations have entered both scalæ of the cochlea, —reaching as far as the tip—principally however, the scala tympani. The infiltration starts mostly from the inner side of the cochlear canal, and from the lamina spiralis, and shows the same structure as the connective tissue proliferation in the vestibulum.

This case, the first in which the labyrinth has been examined histologically after extraction of the stapes, is of great importance in helping us to determine the indications for the removal of the bone in suppurative otitis media. It shows the possibility of the inflammation spreading into the labyrinth, and may possibly give us the explanation of the impairment of hearing which often follows extraction of the stapes. I, therefore, for one, am against the performance of this operation during the course of a chronic suppuration of the middle ear.

On the other hand, in cases in which the suppuration has passed off and has left adhesions between the branches of the stapes and the niche of the fenestra ovalis, there is, I think, a distinct future for the operative extraction of the stapes with a view to improving the hearing.

This opinion is based upon observations made by others, and also upon a case which I have had under observation since 1897. In this case the stapes was accidentally extracted during the removal of crusts from this region. Vertigo accompanied by severe vomiting suddenly ensued, but disappeared after 24 hours. A cicatricial membrane formed over the fenestra ovalis, after which the hearing was materially improved. This improvement is still maintained, and is considerably increased by the introduction of a pledget of cotton-wool moistened with vaseline.

PROF. LUCAE. Politzer's case reminds me of a very serious case observed in the Berlin University Ear Clinic. When I was away from Berlin a radical operation was performed in a case of old purulent discharge, without any dangerous symptoms, and unintentionally a luxation of the stapes was produced. The purulent inflammation extended to the internal ear and brain, and was followed by fatal purulent meningitis.

UEBER DIE HEILERFOLGE DER VIBRATIONSMASSAGE.

PROF. OSTMANN, Marburg.

Nach länger dauerndem Verschluss der Tube, sowie nach entzündlichen Erkrankungen des Mittelohres bleiben nicht selten Schallleitungsstörungen zurück, deren Beseitigung mit den vorhandenen Mitteln keineswegs immer gelingt.

Die Störungen können an sehr verschiedenen Punkten des leitenden Apparats ihren Sitz haben und sehr verschiedener Art sein : Ausgedehnte oder totale Verkalkungen, Verlust, Atrophie, hochgradige Wölbungsanomalien oder Verwachsungen des Trommelfells; sclerosirende Entzündung und narbige Schrumpfung der Paukenschleimhaut wie Kalk und Knochenablagerungen in derselben ; Ankylose der Gelenke, abnorme Fixationen und Adhäsionen der Gehörknöchelchen, sowie insbesondere die mannigfachen Veränderungen an den Labyrinthfenstern. Wir sind nicht immer im Stande, anzugeben, welche dieser pathologischen Veränderungen im Einzelfall der Schwerhörigkeit zu Grunde liegt, noch haben wir ein einheitliches Mittel zu ihrer Beseitigung. Aber einzelne dieser Veränderungen, die bleibende und bisher unheilbare Schwerhörigkeit bedingten, scheinen durch eine in neuerer Zeit mehr in den Vordergrund getretene Behandlungsmethode günstig beeinflusst werden zu können, nämlich durch die *Vibrationsmassage des Schallleitungsapparates*, zumal wenn man dieselbe mit einer zweiten vielumstrittenen Behandlungsmethode, *den methodischen Hörübungen* combinirt.

Ich habe in dem letzten Jahre dieser combinirten Behandlungsmethode meine besondere Aufmerksamkeit zugewandt, und habe sie bisher an einigen Personen erprobt, die zuvor von mir und Anderen für unheilbar schwerhörig erklärt worden waren.

Ich will in Form einer vorläufigen Mittheilung in Kürze über meine bisherigen Erfahrungen, über die Indikationen, Art der Anwendung und Aussichten der Behandlung berichten.

Verminderte Leitungsfähigkeit der Knöchelchenkette verbindet sich sehr häufig mit Verlagerung des Hammers und Einziehung des Trommelfells.

Die ersten Versuche von Politzer, Lucae und Anderen, aus denen sich im Laufe der Jahrzehnte die Vibrationsmassage des Schallleitungsapparates entwickelt hat, suchten durch Luftverdünnung im äusseren Gehörgang das eingezogene Trommelfell nach aussen zu ziehen, um so wieder normale Schallleitungsbedingungen herbeizuführen. Diese Versuche haben das angestrebte Ziel nicht erreicht und konnten es nicht erreichen.

In der Folgezeit entstanden dann eine Reihe von Apparaten, welche in schneller Aufeinanderfolge Luftverdünnung im äusseren Gehörgang herbeizuführen vermochten. Von diesen ist der bekannteste der Delstanche'sche Raréfacteur. Die Wirkung dieser Apparate kann eine so kräftige werden, dass von mehreren Seiten die Nothwendigkeit von Schutzvorrichtungen in Gestalt von Nebenöffnungen oder Manometern im zuführenden Schlauch hervorgehoben wurde.

Man hat über den Wert des Raréfacteurs und der ihm ähnlichen Instrumente sehr verschieden geurteilt; ich glaube das Resultat seiner nunmehr jahrelangen Anwendung ist das, dass die mit ihm erzielten thatsächlichen Erfolge hinter den gehegten Erwartungen im Allgemeinen weit zurückgeblieben sind.

Der Weg zur Vibrationsmassage war gefunden, so bald man der Luftverdünnung im äusseren Gehörgang eine Luftverdichtung folgen liess! Die zu diesem Zwecke construirten Apparate hat man Tympanovibrator, Vibrationsmasseur, Vibrometer genannt und den Vorgang als solchen auch Pneumo oder Oscillationsmassage. Die bisher construirten Massageapparate sind zahlreich und mit der Zeit immer mehr für machinellen Betrieb eingerichtet, sei es dass die Hand, der Fuss, Wasser oder Elektricität die treibende Kraft bildet.

Im Laufe der letzten Jahre hat man die Vibrationsmassage bald als unfehlbares Heilmittel gegen alle möglichen Formen von Schwerhörigkeit gepriesen, bald aus mehr oder weniger zutreffenden Gründen ihr jede Wirkung auf den Schallleitungsapparat und damit auch jede Heilwirkung abgesprochen.

An einer ernste wissenschaftliche Prüfung der mechanischen Leistung der Massageapparate überhaupt wie ihrer Wirkung zunächst auf den normalen Schallleitungsapparat hatte jedoch keiner gedacht, und doch waren derartige Untersuchungen unbedingt erforderlich, um die Grundsteine zu einer tieferen wissenschaftlichen Erkenntniss der Wirkung dieser vielumstrittenen Heilmethode zu legen, ihre Indikationen und Contraindicationen aufzustellen und das Mass wie die Art ihrer zweckmässigsten Anwendung zu bestimmen.

Ich habe durch meine experimentellen Arbeiten die hierfür erforderliche Grundlage gegeben, und habe gezeigt, dass die Ansicht derer unzutreffend ist, die der Heilmethode desshalb jede Wirkung absprechen, weil eine Bewegung des Schallleitungsapparates überhaupt oder nur in sehr beschränktem Umfange zu Stande komme. Gerade das Gegentheil ist beim normalen Ohr der Fall, der gesammte Apparat bis zur Platte des Steigbügels gerät in die ausgiebigsten Schwingungen, so dass bei Anwendung allzu starker Luftdruckschwankungen sogar Trommelfell wie Bänder des Apparates in offenbar unzweckmässiger Weise gedehnt und in der Paukenschleimhaut Blutextravasate erzeugt werden.

Die weitere Fortführung dieser Untersuchungen hätte logischer Weise darin bestehen müssen, die Wirkung der Massageapparate an Gehörorganen zu prüfen, die Personen entstammten, die durch Schallleitungsstörungen schwerhörig waren. Solche ganz frischen Präparate haben mir jedoch bisher nicht zur Verfügung gestanden; ich habe deshalb die Untersuchungen nach dieser Richtung noch nicht weiter fortführen können.

Die pathologisch-anatomischen Veränderungen, welche nicht wenigen und zwar gerade den schwersten Fällen von Schwerhörigkeit zu Grunde liegen, wie z. B. die Ankylose des Steigbügels, lassen es jedoch von vornherein als ausgeschlossen erscheinen, dass die Vibrationsmassage in solchen Fällen noch einen Heileffect haben sollte; denn man wird nicht erwarten können, einen durch Knochenneubildung etc. fixirten Stapes wieder schwingbar zu machen.

Diejenigen, welche gleich im Anfang auf diesen Punkt hinwiesen und deshalb der Vibrationsmassage jede Wirkung absprachen, bleiben mit Bezug auf derartige Fälle gewiss allezeit im Recht, aber hoffentlich im Unrecht, wenn sie meinten, die Wirkungslosigkeit der Massage für alle bisher unheilbaren Fälle von Schwerhörigkeit durch Schallleitungsstörung annehmen zu müssen.

Wir sind nun wohl in der Lage, mit hinreichender Sicherheit eine Ankylose des Steigbügels intra vitam zu diagnosticiren, aber wir vermögen nicht, die Ursache der Ankylose zu erkennen. Bei der Voraussage aber, welche Wirkung die Vibrationsmassage in einem Fall von diagnosticirter Ankylose haben wird, kommt es nicht so auf die Diagnose als solche als auf die der Veränderungen an, welche der Feststellung des Steigbügels zu Grunde liegen. Wir können daher nicht im Voraus sagen, wie die Massage im Einzelfall

wirken wird, sondern können nach meinen Erfahrungen eine
Auskunft darüber erst nach einer wenigstens 8-14 tägigen Probe geben.
Dies ist ein Uebelstand, der sich aber vor wesentlicher Verfeinerung der
diagnostischen Methoden kaum beheben lassen dürfte. Sehr viel klarer
liegen von vornherein die Verhältnisse, wenn das Trommelfell sichtbare
Veränderungen zeigt. Ein hochgradig atrophisches Trommelfell oder ein
solches mit ausgedehnten Narben oder flächenförmigen Verwachsungen
mit der Labyrinthwand wird in den ersteren Fällen die Vibrationsmassage contraindiciren, in den letzteren die Behandlung von Anfang
an ziemlich aussichtslos machen, denn ein atrophisches Trommelfell
wird durch die Massage nur gedehnt und gezerrt, und somit für die
Schallaufnahme noch ungeeigneter gemacht; flächenförmige Verwachsungen aber werden nicht gelöst werden. Es bleiben somit für die
Anwendung der Vibrationsmassage diejenigen Fälle übrig, in denen das
Trommelfell von normaler Dichte oder verdickt ist und der Unter-
suchungsbefund auf eine der Schwerhörigkeit zu Grunde liegende reine
Schallleitungsstörung hinweist.

Es dürfte kaum zweifelhaft sein, dass eine kräftige Vibrationsmassage auch auf den Hörnerv einzuwirken vermag, doch möchte ich
bis zum Beweis nicht annehmen, dass die Perceptionsfähigkeit der
erkrankten Nervenfaser gesteigert werden kann. Im Gegentheil habe
ich bei versuchsweiser Anwendung der Massage bei reinen Erkrankungen des schallempfindenden und voller Gesunkenheit des schallleitenden Apparats bisher nur eine Verschlechterung der Hörfähigkeit
unmittelbar nach der Massage eintreten sehen.

Nach meinen experimentellen und klinischen Erfahrungen kommen
bei der Heilwirkung der Massage zwei Faktoren in Betracht; die
mechanische Erschütterung der Knöchelchenkette und die vermehrte
Blutzufuhr zur Paukenschleimhaut.

Bezüglich des letzteren Punktes habe ich an lebenden Hunden und
Katzen nachgewiesen, dass es bei übermässig starken Luftdruckschwankungen zur hochgradigen Injection und Ruptur der Schleimhautgefässe
kommt. Eine erhöhte Blutzufuhr zur Schleimhaut tritt nun schon
auf, wenn man mit 2 mm. Kolbenverschiebung schnell massirt,
denn darauf deuten die Angaben der Massirten hin, dass sie nach
dem Aufhören der Massage ein lebhaftes, einige Zeit fortdauerndes
Wärmegefühl im Ohr empfinden. Diese Wirkung lässt sich vielleicht
vortheilhaft verwerthen gegen den Beginn von Ernährungstörungen
der Schleimhaut. Sind dagegen schon weitgreifende pathologische
Veränderungen derselben eingetreten, so wird allein die mechanische
Wirkung der Massage noch in Frage kommen können, um den durch
die verdichtete Schleimhaut festgewordenen Schallleitungsapparat
beweglich zu machen.

Ich werde zeigen, dass selbst bei jahrelang bestandener, von mir
und Anderen nach vielfachen therapeutischen Versuchen für ganz

unheilbar erklärter Schwerhörigkeit, es durch allerdings länger fortgesetzte Massage gelingen kann, nicht unerhebliche Besserungen zu erzielen ; aber die Erfahrungen, die ich an den bisher massirten Fällen gesammelt habe, weisen mich doch darauf hin, dass der volle Wert der Vibrationsmassage erst bei der Behandlung frischerer Fälle zu Tage treten dürfte, wo die zur Feststellung der Kette führenden Veränderungen noch nicht völlig consolidirt sind, eine Beseitigung derselben auf andere Weise aber nicht hat erzielt werden können. Nehmen wir einen Fall von akuter Mittelohrentzündung, der nach völliger Abheilung eine Hörschärfe von 4-5 m. für Flüstersprache aufweist, ohne dass es gelingt, die Hörfähigkeit durch Lufteinblasungen oder andere therapeutische Massnahmen zu heben. Die Untersuchung ergäbe eine völlige Integrität der Nerven. In solchen Fällen versuche man die Vibrationsmassage, von der ich in dem ersten von mir massirten Fall eine ganz überraschende Wirkung gesehen habe.

Eine Dame war von mir im Jahre 1897 an doppelseitiger, subakuter Mittelohrentzündung behandelt worden, ohne dass es mir gelang, durch irgend ein Mittel die Hörschärfe über circa 3 m. für Flüstersprache zu heben. Desgleichen waren Ohrgeräusche bestehen geblieben, die im Frühjahr 1898 sich zu unerträglicher Höhe steigerten. Die Patientin suchte mich von Neuem auf, und nachdem ich nochmals mich vergeblich bemüht hatte, durch Lufteintreibung etc., eine nennenswerthe Besserung herbeizuführen, machte ich ihr den Vorschlag, versuchsweise die Vibrationsmassage anzuwenden. Ich massirte im Hinblick auf meine experimentelle Prüfung der Wirkung meines Massageapparates mit 2 mm. Kolbenverschiebung täglich 5 Minuten bei 1000-1200 Stossen in der Minute, und nach vierwöchiger Anwendung war das Hörvermögen beiderseits normal, und die Ohrgeräusche traten nur noch zeitweise des Morgens nach dem Erwachen in sehr geringer Stärke auf. Die Heilung hat bis jetzt, also 1¼ Jahr Stand gehalten.

. Ein so werthvolles Heilmittel schien mir der ernsten praktischwissenschaftlichen Prüfung werth, und so wurde der Fall der Ausgangspunkt einiger Untersuchungen, über deren Ergebniss ich Ihnen heute berichten möchte.

Um die Grenzen der Leistungsfähigkeit der Vibrationsmassage zu erkennen, habe ich sie bei diesen Untersuchungen bisher der schwersten Aufgabe gegenüber gestellt, indem ich nur solche Fälle massirt habe, welche Jahre lang hochgradig schwerhörig und von mir und Anderen specialistisch durchgebildeten Aerzten für unheilbar erklärt waren.

Um den durch die Massage unbedingten Fortschritt zu erkennen, kam es vor Allem darauf an, eine durchaus sichere Grundlage der Beurtheilung der jeweiligen Hörfunktion zu gewinnen.

Durch die genaue Prüfung derselben mittelst der continuirlichen Tonreihe von Bezold-Edelmann, wurde diese Grundlage gewonnen, nachdem ich durch eigene Uebung und Schulung der Kranken gelernt hatte, die Fehlerquellen zu vermeiden, die auch bei dieser Untersuchung das Resultat wesentlich beeinträchtigen können. Dem gemäss wurde in jedem Falle nach Feststellung des Befundes an Ohr, Nase und Rachen bestimmt :—

1. Die obere und untere Grenze der Hörempfindung.

2. Die Hördauer für C, c, c^I, c^{II}, c^{III}, c^{IV}, c^V, im Vergleich zu derjenigen des normalen Ohres.*

3. Die Hörfähigkeit durch Knochenleitung (Weber'scher und Schwabach'scher Versuch.†

4. Das Verhältniss der Hörfähigkeit durch Luft-und Knochen-leitung (Rinne'scher Versuch).

5. Die Hörfähigkeit für Flüsterzahlen und Flüsterworte von hohem, mittlerem und tiefem Tonklang.

Nachdem so vor Beginn der Massage eine sichere Unterlage für die Beurtheilung ev. Veränderungen der Hörfunktion geschaffen war, wurde unter Ausschluss jeder anderweitigen Behandlung methodisch massirt.

Die Methode der Anwendung : Mit dem elektrisch betriebenen Massageapparat wurde bei 2 mm. Kolbenverschiebung täglich wenigstens 10 Minuten, im Fall 1 einige Zeit selbst bis 25 Minuten so schnell massirt, dass 1000-1200 Stösse in der Minute erfolgten. Die höchste Zahl der an einem Tage auf das Trommelfell geworfenen Massagewellen dürfte somit zwischen 25 und 30 Tausend liegen. Einige Zeit wurde vor der schnellen Massage mit 2 mm. Hubhöhe auch ganz langsam mit 4 mm. Kolbenverschiebung massirt.

Selbst bei dieser sehr ausgedehnten und intensiven Massage wurden *objectiv* ausser einer geringen Füllung der Hammergriffgefässe *keinerlei Reizerscheinungen* wahrgenommen ; *subjective Beschwerden wurden von den Kranken niemals geäussert: nur ein Gefühl der Wärme,* welches längstens ¼ Stunde anhielt, wurde in der Tiefe des Ohres gefühlt.

Die bei allen Kranken bestehenden, sehr intensiven subj. Ohrge-räusche erfuhren niemals eine Steigerung, wohl aber mit der Zeit eine wesentliche Verminderung, doch sind sie bei keinem der Massirten bisher gänzlich geschwunden ; wie früher machten sich auch nach zwei und drei monatlicher Massage Schwankungen in der Intensität der Ohrgeräusche bemerkbar, doch wurde auch auf den Höhepunkten die frühere Intensität gewöhnlich nicht erreicht.

Sämmtliche Kranke empfanden eine mehr oder weniger erhebliche Besserung, welche für sie besonders dadurch deutlich hervortrat, dass sie Töne und Geräusche, welche sie lange Jahre nicht mehr gehört

---

* Man lernt relativ schnell, die Stimmgabeln in annähernd gleich starke Schwingungen durch An-schlagen mit dem Klöppel zu versetzen; man könnte somit ein für alle Mal einen mittleren Wert für die Hördauer des normalen Ohres festsetzen, wodurch diese äusserst zeitraubenden Untersuchungen in sehr erwünschter Weise abgekürzt würden. Ich habe es jedoch bei diesen rein wissenschaftlichen Untersuch-ungen vorgezogen, in jedem Fall die Stimmgabeln vor meinem normalhörenden Ohr ausklingen zu lassen, um so die Fehlerquellen des mittleren Wertes zu vermeiden.

† Für die Prüfung der Knochenleitung wie für den Rinne' schen Versuch wurde eine kleine belastete c-Gabel mit Fuss, ev. c^{I}verwandt.

hatten, wieder zu hören vermochten; auch ihre nächste Umgebung bemerkte diese Verbesserung und objectiv konnte Art und Umfang mit grösstmöglicher Genauigkeit durch die in Intervallen von einen Monat wiederholten genauesten Hörprüfungen mittelst der continuirlichen Tonreihe etc. nachgewiesen werden.

Die einzelnen Fälle will ich nur ganz kurz charakterisiren, da diese Mittheilung nur eine vorläufige sein soll; die genaue Darlegung behalte ich mir für den III. Theil meiner experimentellen Untersuchungen zur Massage des Ohres vor.

Fall 1. Frau Dr. X. hat angeblich seit 1895 zunehmende Schwerhörigkeit beiderseits bemerkt. Von dieser Zeit an bestand beständiges, zuweilen ungemein starkes Ohrensausen. Sie wurde bis Anfang 1896, wo sie in meine Behandlung trat, in Dortmund, Marburg, und Heidelberg behandelt, ohne dass die erhebliche Schwerhörigkeit und die Ohrgeräusche eine Besserung erfuhren.

1896 bestand beim Eintritt in meine Behandlung ein sehr starker chronischer Katarrh der Nase, und des Rachens. Die rechte wie die linke Nase waren für Luft schwer durchgängig, rechts in Folge starker diffuser Schwellung der Schleimhaut und insbesondere erheblicher hinterer Hypertrophie der unteren Muschel, links in Folge ausgedehnter Verwachsung der unteren Muschel mit der Nasenscheidewand.

Beide äusseren Gehörgänge normal; rechtes Trommelfell normal gewölbt, links leicht eingezogen, Gewebe beider derb, fleckig getrübt, glanzlos, Trommelfelle in allen ihren Theilen beweglich, doch erscheint die Beweglichkeit etwas verringert, insbesondere folgt der rechte Hammergriff nur sehr träge. Entzündliche Erscheinungen fehlen.

Beide Tuben öffnen sich bei mittlerem Drucke, Luftstrom voll, Blasegeräusch laut, etwas scharf, von einzelnen grossblasigen Rasselgeräuschen in der Tubenmündung begleitet.

Die *Hörprüfung* ergiebt beiderseits eine bedeutend stärkere Herabsetzung der tiefen wie hohen Töne, Knochenleitung um 6 Sec. verlängert, Weber vorwiegend nach links, Rinne beiderseits − .

Von Flüsterzahlen nur die hohen Klangcharakters in der Nähe gehört. Bei Verschluss der äusseren Gehörgänge angeblich keine Verstärkung des Tones bei Zuleitung desselben durch Knochenleitung.

Beständige, zuweilen sehr starke Ohrgeräusche, Brausen.

1896 bestand die Behandlung wesentlich darin, dass die Dauerentzündung der Schleimhaut in Nase und Rachen beseitigt, die hintere Hypertrophie rechts, die Verwachsung links entfernt wurden. Kurze Zeit nachdem wurde der Catheter ohne Erfolg angewandt.

Herbst 1897 Versuch mit der Drucksonden Behandlung, welche jedoch wegen zu erheblicher Schmerzhaftigkeit nach kurzer Zeit aufgegeben werden musste. Hörschärfe hatte seit 1896 keine wesentliche Veränderungen erfahren. Laute Conversationssprache wird von der Kranken, auch wenn sie nicht vom Munde abliest, verstanden. Ohrgeräusche wie vor. Tuben relativ weit und frei; Luftstrom voll und laut, Blasegeräusch scharf.

Diagnose: Chronischer Mittleohrcatarrh beiderseits; abgelaufen mit Fixation der Knöchelchenkette; schallempfindender Theil, so weit nachweisbar, frei.

Herbst 1898 erneute Untersuchung; wesentlich der gleiche Befund an Ohr Nase und Rachen wie nach der Behandlung im Jahre, 1896.

Die Hörprüfung mit der continuirlichen Tonreihe ergiebt einen Hörumfang *rechts* von E der grossen Octave bis O, 1 der Galtonpfeife ;
links von Gis der Contra-Octave bis O, 1 der Galtonpfeife ;
bei stärkstem Anschlag der Stimmgabeln.

Die Hördauer rechts für e, c^i, c^{ii}, c^{iii}, c^{iv}, links für C, c, c^i, c^{ii}, c^{iii}, c^{iv}, gegenüber der normalen, diese gleich 100 Secunden gesetzt, zeigt Tafel I in den Feldern 1.

Stimmgabel c von der Höhe des Scheitels vorwiegend nach links ; Schwabach + 5 Sec ; Rinne rechts wie links negativ.

Fl. r. "8" in 15 cm. ; links in 25 cm. Es wurde nunmehr unter Ausschluss jeder anderweitigen Behandlung fast täglich durchschnittlich 10-15 Minuten mit 2 mm. Kolbenverschiebung sehr schnell massirt, und in Abständen von ungefähr je einem Monat die Hörfunktion von Neuem in der oben angegebenen Weise festgestellt. Die Resultate der Prüfungen bezüglich der Hördauer für C, c, c^i - c^{iv} sind in der Tafel I. dargestellt, so dass die nach $3\frac{1}{2}$ Monaten erreichte Hörverbesserung sofort übersehen werden kann, wenn man die Höhe der ersten Felder mit der der letzten vergleicht.

Die Weite des Hörumfangs war gleichfalls auf beiden Ohren beträchtlich gewachsen ; rechts von E der grossen Octave bis C der Contra-Octave ; links von Gis der Contra-Octave bis C der Contra-Octave.

Diese Hörverbesserung erleichterte der Kranken das Sprachverständniss erheblich ; sie war am Schluss der Behandlung fähig, und ist es bis jetzt geblieben, eine hinter ihrem Rücken kaum mittellaut geführte Unterhaltung sicher zu verstehen. Die subjectiven Ohrgeräusche hatten eine wesentliche Besserung erfahren und waren zuletzt so schwach, dass sie in keiner Weise mehr belästigten. 4 Monate nach Beendigung der Behandlung klagte die Kranke, dass die Geräusche nach einer länger währenden Erkältung zeitweise wieder etwas zugenommen hätten ohne indess die frühere Höhe zu erreichen. Auf vielfache interessante Einzelheiten versage ich es mir, an dieser Stelle einzugehen.

Fall 2. Frau K., seit 10 Jahren nach sehr starker Erkältung langsam zunehmende Schwerhörigkeit, welche durch mehrfache Behandlungen (Catheter, Politzer'sche Luftdouche) nicht gebessert worden ist. Während des letzten halben Jahres weitere Verschlechterung bemerkt. Links beständiges Ohrgeräusch von mässiger Stärke, welches mit Wasserrauschen verglichen wird.

Befund 9.10.98. In Nase und Rachen keine bemerkenswerthen krankhaften Veränderungen. Linkes Trommelfell mit Ausnahme kleinerer Abschnitte in der Hammergegend verkalkt, leicht eingezogen, mit dem Hammer, wenn auch schwer, beweglich.

Entzündliche Erscheinungen fehlen. Das rechte Trommelfell weniger ausgedehnt verkalkt, normal gewölbt, gleichfalls mit dem Hammergriff in allen Theilen beweglich, ohne entzündliche Erscheinungen Beide Ostia Tubae pharyng. im postrhinoskopischen Bild weit, die vorderen Tubenlippen blass ; Tuben öffnen sich bei geringstem Druck. Luftstrom sehr voll, Geräusch laut, etwas scharf, ohne Nebengeräusche. Knochenleitung um "7" verlängert ; beim Weber'schen Versuch wird der Stimmgabelton (c) im linken Ohr vornehmlich gehört.

Rinne mit c ausgeführt l.-18 Sec., r.-16 Sec.

Flüsterzahlen r. (Residualluft) "3" in 50 cm., l. "3" in 5 cm. Catheter bringt geringe, schnell vorübergehende Besserung ; auf die Ohrgeräusche hat die Luftdouche keinen Einfluss.

Prüfung mit der continuirlichen Tonreihe ergiebt bei stärkstem Anschlag einen

Hörumfang auf dem rechten Ohr von A der Subcontra-Octave bis O, 1 des Galton-pfeifchens; auf dem linken Ohr von D der grossen Octave bis O, l des Galtonpfeifchens.

Die Hördauer für C. c, c^i—c^iv auf beiden Ohren im Verhältniss zur normalen, diese gleich 100 Secunden gesetzt, zeigen die Felder 1 der Tafel II.

Es wurde nunmehr unter Ausschluss jeder anderweitigen Behandlung 1½ Monate fast täglich circa 10 Minuten mit 2 mm. Kolbenverschiebung sehr schnell, zeitweise auch nachher noch 2-3 Minuten mit 3 u. 4 mm. Kolbenverschiebung langsam (circa 150 Stösse in der Minute) massirt. Das Resultat der Massage, so weit die Hördauer für die Töne C—c^iv in Frage kommt, ist aus der Höhe der Felder 2 in Tafel II. ersichtlich. An Hörumfang hatte die Kranke vom 9-10-98 bis zum 29-11-98 gewonnen: rechts von A der Subcontra-Octave bis zum C dieser Octave, links vom D der grossen Octave bis zum E der Contra-Octave.

Das Ohrensausen war am Tage verschwunden, Nachts wurde es noch empfunden, aber nicht sehr störend.

Nach dem Protokoll, welches die Kranken selbst über ihre Wahrnehmungen während der Massage führten, schilderte die Patientin die Verbesserung ihrer Hörschärfe mit den Worten: "Jetzt verstehe ich im Nebenzimmer, wenn die Kinder Abends in den Betten um Wasser bitten oder sonstige Wünsche haben, während ich früher in das Schlafzimmer gehen musste zu fragen. Zu meiner grossen Freude höre ich jetzt auch das Anklopfen an die Thür stets, wenn Jemand kommt, was früher selten der Fall war." Diese Worte sind am 18-11-98 ohne jede Beeinflüssung niedergeschrieben.

Die Hörprüfung für Flüsterzahlen "3" ergab gegenüber dem Anfang keine Veränderung.

Fall 3. Fräulein H. 20 Jahr; mittelkräftig, blass. Im 6ten Jahre Scharlach; im 13^ren Diphtherie mit nachfolgender Gaumensegel u. Accommodationslähmung. Seit der Diphtherie hat grosse Neigung zu Catarrhen der oberen Luftwege, Nase und Rachen, bestanden. Im 15ten Lebensjahr zuerst Schwerhörigkeit rechts bemerkt; das linke Ohr wurde stets für normal gehalten, obgleich auf diesem zeitweise Wochenlang Ohrgeräusche bestanden haben. Eiterung ist nie beobachtet worden. Patientin wurde in den letzten 5 Jahren wiederholt specialistisch behandelt, ohne dass eine Besserung des Ohrleidens erzielt wurde. Am 19-10-96 wurden Flüsterzahlen "2, 20, 6" rechts dicht am Ohr; links "6, 8" in 5 m. gehört; am 27 Juli, 1898, wurde rechts "6" in 30 cm; links "7" in 1½ m. verstanden; nach Catheter trat eine schnell vorübergehende, geringe Hörverbesserung auf. 1896 wie 1898 wurde Patientin ausser an dem Ohrenleiden gleichzeitig an chronischem Rachenkatarrh behandelt, ohne dass Besserung des ersteren Leidens erzielt wurde.

Am 20, October 1898 ergab die Untersuchung folgenden Befund.

Ohr. Beide Gehörgänge weit, gerade gestreckt, R. Trommelfell glanzlos, mässig eingezogen, Gewebe dick, im hinteren Abschnitt starke, halbmondförmige Trübung, im Lichtkegelgebiet zwei kleinere Verkalkungen, Trommelfell in allen Theilen beweglich.

L. Trommelfell glanzlos, stärker eingezogen als rechts, Gewebe grauweiss, dick, im hinteren Abschnitt die gleiche sehnige Trübung wie rechts, alle Theile beweglich, continuirliches, zeitweise sehr starkes Sausen links seit Juli 1898.

Die Prüfung der Hörfunktion mittelst der continuirlichen Tonreihe etc., ergiebt einen Hörumfang:

Rechts vom G. der grossen Octave bis O, 1, der Galtonpfeife.

Links vom A der Contra-Octave bis O, 8 der Galtonpfeife.

Die Hördauer rechts für c-c^iv, links für C, c-c^iv, im Verhältniss zur normalen, diese gleich 100 Secunden gesetzt, ist aus den Feldern 1 Tafel III. ersichtlich Beim Weber'schen Versuch wird der Stimmgabelton c (kleine belastete Gabel mit Fuss) vorwiegend rechts, aber auch links gehört. Schwabach + 14 Sec., Rinne $\frac{\text{r. ci}-\text{11 Sec.}}{\text{l. c.}-\text{23 Sec.}}$; Flüstersprache rechts " 3 " in 15 cm, " 8 " in unmittelbarer Nähe des Ohres, links " 3 " in $\frac{1}{2}$ m. .

Tuben : *L. Tube* öffnet sich nur bei starkem Druck, Luftstrom dünn, Blasegeräusch leise, continuirlich, ohne Nebengeräusche; nach Catheter keine Verbesserung. *R. Tube* öffnet sich bei sehr viel geringerem Druck, Luftstrom voll, lautes, continuirliches, etwas scharfes Blasen ohne Nebengeräusche.

Nase : Nasenathmung nicht wesentlich erschwert : Schleimhaut beider Nasenhöhlen befindet sich im Zustande der Dauerentzündung ; mit der Sonde vermag man dieselbe über beiden unteren Muscheln tief einzudrücken ; Sekretion dick, schleimig, mässig stark.

Rachen : Schleimhaut der pars oralis wie nasalis im Zustande mässiger Dauerentzündung ; Rachenmandel schwach entwickelt, überragt den oberen Choanenrand nicht ; Einlagerung adenoiden Gewebes sehr gering. Beide Ostia Tubae pharyng. eng ; vordere Tubenlippen blass-roth.

Diagnose: Chronischer Mittelohrkatarrh beiderseits.

Patientin wurde nun bis zum 3 Mai 1899 mit kurzen Uu erbrechungen täglich mit 2 mm. Hubhöhe 10 Minuten massirt. Der Erfolg bezüglich der Hördauer für C-civ ist aus den Feldern 2, 3, und 4 der Tafel III. ersichtlich ; der Hörumfang war *rechts* vom G bis zum D der grossen Octave, links von A der Contra-Octave bis zum G. der Subcontra-Octave gewachsen. Das Sausen bestand auch nach Beendigung der Massage noch fort, wenn es auch im Ganzen so stark vermindert war, dass es Patientin häufig nur hörte, wenn sie ihre Aufmerksamkeit auf dasselbe richtete.

Hierdurch mag es wohl bedingt sein, dass die Patientin ihres Erachtens eine nicht unwesentliche Besserung des Ohrenleidens erfahren hatte, wenngleich auf Grund der Stimmgabeluntersuchungen von einer solchen kaum gesprochen werden kann. Eine objectiv nachweisbare wesentliche Erweiterung hatte nur der Hörumfang am unteren Ende der Tonscala erfahren.

Fall 4. Fräulein B., 32 Jahre alt, ist seit ungefähr 10 Jahren immer schwerhöriger geworden, trotzdem sie an verschiedenen Orten in der verschiedensten Weise specialärztlich behandelt worden ist. Sausen hat nicht immer und in wechselnder Stärke bestanden.

Im Jahre 1897 wurde Patientin von mir zum ersten Male untersucht und für unheilbar erklärt ; deshalb auch s. z. keiner Behandlung unterzogen.

Ende December 1898 kam sie wieder ihres Ohrenleidens wegen zu mir, weil sich dasselbe dauernd verschlechtert hatte. Patientin hörte jetzt so schwer, dass man sich mit ihr nur mittelst eines Hörrohres unterhalten konnte, wobei die Worte noch deutlich und langsam gesprochen werden mussten.

Anfang Januar 1899 wurde folgender Befund erhoben :

Ohr. Beide äussere Gehörgänge normal ; R. Trommelfell normal gewölbt, zeigt erhöhten Glanz, in der Umgebung des Umbo scheint die hyperämische mediane Paukenwand rosa hindurch ; Beweglichkeit aller Theile des Trommelfells erhalten. Das linke Trommelfell zeigt wesentlich denselben Befund; insbesondere ist auch hier die starke Hyperämie der medianen Paukenwand sichtbar. Zeitweise sehr starkes Sausen.

Tuben öffnen sich beiderseits bei sehr geringem Drucke, Luftstrom sehr voll ;

Blasegeräusch laut, scharf, ohne Nebengeräusche. Nase und Rachen ohne Abweich-ungen ; beide Ostia tubae pharyng. weit ; vordere Tubenlippen blass.

Die Prüfung der Hörfunktion ergab einen Hörumfang : *rechts* vom G. der Contra-Octave bis 3, 6 der Galtonpfeife.

Links vom A der Contra-Octave bis 2, 2 der Galtonpfeife.

Die Hördauer für die Octaven C-c^{iv}, beiderseits im Vergleich zu normalen Hördauer, diese gleich 100 Secunden gesetzt, zeigen die Felder 1 der Tafel IV.

Weber unbestimmt ; Rinne $\frac{\text{r. für } c_i - 23 \text{ Sec.}}{\text{l. für } c - 12 \text{ Sec.}}$; Schwabach + 5 Sec.

Bei Verschluss der äusseren Gehörgänge keine Tonverstärkung.

Flüstersprache wird nicht gehört ; nur mittellaut gesprochene Zahlen in unmittelbarer Nähe des Ohres.

Diagnose : *Sclerose beiderseits.*

Vom. 2. 1.99 ab, wurde Patientin mit geringen Unterbrechungen täglich 15 Minuten mit 2 mm. Hubhöhe des Kolbens sehr schnell zeitweise ausserdem mit 4 mm Hubhöhe 4 Minuten langsam massirt.

Den Erfolg der Massage ergiebt das Untersuchungsresultat vom 3 Febr. 1899, welches auf Tafel IV. dargestellt ist.

Bei einem noch im Fortschreiten begriffenen Fall von Sclerose ist immerhin ein gewisser Erfolg zu verzeichnen. Sehr bemerkenswert war, dass auf beiden Ohren die starke Hyperaemie der medianen Paukenwand schwand, somit auch objectiv eni Zeichen der Besserung festgestellt werden konnte. Die Ohrgeräusche haben an Intensität verloren, sind jedoch nicht völlig geschwunden, dagegen sind die früher bestandenen zeitweisen Schwindelanfälle in der Folgezeit ganz ausgeblieben.

Der Hörumfang war rechts nicht gewachsen ; links von A bis F der Contra Octave und im oberen Tonumfang von 2, 2 bis 1, 8 der Galtonpfeife.

Die Hörschärfe hatte sich soweit gehoben, dass man sich mit der Patientin un-terhalten konnte, wenn man in der Nähe des linken Ohres mit etwas erhobener Stimme sprach. Die Behandlung wurde fortgesetzt und mit methodischen Hörü-bungen combinirt.

Dies sind die Erfolge, welche bisher bei unheilbaren Fällen von chronischer Schwerhörigkeit in Folge chronischen Mittelohrkatarrhs und Sclerose des Mittelohres von mir erzielt worden sind. Es sind so wenige Fälle, dass man auf Grund derselben ein abschliessendes Urtheil in keiner Weise wird fällen können ; aber bei ihrer Behandlung sind doch im Allgemeinen Erfahrungen gesammelt worden, welche schärfer wie bisher die Indikationen wie Contraindicationen und einige andere wesentliche Punkte erkennen lassen.

Ich will versuchen, dieselben in Kürze aufzuführen. wobei ich jedoch nicht unterlassen möchte, zu bemerken, dass weitere Prüfungen den einen oder anderen Punkt wohl ändern könnten.

Die Vibrationsmassage ist indicirt : Bei chronischer Schwerhörigkeit in Folge Schallleitungsstörung nach erfolglosem Versuch der sonstigen Heilmittel.

Ausgenommen sind die Fälle von Schwerhörigkeit, in denen Atrophie, ausgedehnte Verwachsungen, hochgradige Einziehungen des Trommelfelles bestehen.

Die Vibrationsmassage ist contraindicirt : Bei Schwerhörigkeit in

Folge von Erkrankung des schallempfindenden Apparates, sowie bei allen akuten Entzündungen des schallleitenden Theils.

Die *Voraussage*, welchen Heilerfolg ihre Anwendung haben wird, ist stets *unsicher*; erst die *versuchsweise* tägliche Anwendung während wenigstens 2 Wochen giebt darüber Aufschluss; nach 4 wöchiger Massage scheint zuweilen der durch sie überhaupt erreichbare Erfolg erzielt zu sein.

Dieser Erfolg scheint um so grösser zu sein, je weniger die auf andere Weise nicht zu beseitigenden Schallleitungshindernisse consolidirt sind. Die besten, ja vollkommene Erfolge dürften demnach dann erzielt werden, wenn man bei relativ frischen Leiden, bei denen die Hörschärfe auf andere Weise sich nicht in erwünschter Weise hat heben lassen, als ultima ratio die Massage anwendet, wobei es allerdings für den Bestand der erzielten Heilerfolge vor Allem darauf ankommen dürfte, dass Nase, Rachen wie Tubae gesund bzw. zuvor geheilt sind.

Die Anwendung hat, wenn möglich, täglich in der Weise zu geschehen, dass mit 2 mm. Hubhöhe des Kolbens sehr schnell 5-15 Minuten massirt wird.

Die Massage ist völlig schmerzlos und bei richtiger Anwendung niemals von Reactionserscheinungen gefolgt.

Die durch die Massage erzielte verbesserte Schallleitung wird für den Kranken am nutzbarsten, wenn man ihn gleichzeitig täglich 5-10 Minuten lang methodischen Hörübungen unterzieht. Die Kranken erwerben so von Neuem eine Summe von Hörbildern, welche ihnen während der langen Dauer ihrer Schwerhörigkeit ganz oder theilweise verloren gegangen waren, und gewöhnen sich wieder daran, zu hören, statt vom Munde abzulesen. Durch zweckmässige Combination dieser beiden Methoden scheint man bezüglich des Sprachverständnisses Erfolge erzielen zu können wie sie insbesondere bei fortschreitender Sclerose bisher nicht erzielt worden sind.

Im Archiv für Ohrenheilkunde werde ich später des Näheren darauf zurückkommen.

DR. F. ROHRER wished to mention, that the first to use methodical pneumatic massage in the treatment of diseases of the Ear was Prof. Delstanche of Brussels.

PROF. POLITZER, kann die optimistischen Anschauungen Prof. Ostmann's nicht theilen. Die Heilung von Fällen im Beginne leichter Catarrhe ist nicht beweisend für die Anschauung Ostmann's. Wenn aber Ostmann behauptet dass man auch in chronischen Adhaesivprocessen und Sclerosen, mit vorgeschrittener Schwerhörigkeit *Heilung* durch die Vibrationsmassage erzielen kann, so muss dem widersprochen werden. Dass *Besserungen* durch die verschiedensten Methoden der Massage (Delstanche, Lucae's Drucksonde, electromot. Massage) bei Sclerose und bei Adhaesivprocessen nach abgelaufenen Mittelohreiter-

ungen erzielt werden, ist bekannt, und verweist Politzer auf die ausführrliche Publication seines vor zwei Jahren in Moskau gehaltenen Vortrages über diesen Gegenstand, auf welche Prof. Ostmann eben so wenig reflectirt hat, wie darauf, dass wir die Einführung der Massage Prof. Delstanche verdanken. Aber die Besserungen die wir bei Adhaesivprocessen im Mittelohre erzielen, sind in den meisten Fällen vorübergehend. Dies schränkt aber keineswegs den hohen Werth der Massage ein, da eine auch durch Wochen oder Monaten andauernde Besserung ein grosser Gewinn für den Kranken ist. In diesem Sinne muss die optimistische Auffassung Ostmann's über die ja längst bekannten Vortheile der Massage, eingeschränkt werden.

DR. FELIX COHN :—In a meeting of this kind, it is most necessary that on a subject of such importance as the cure of deafness by a certain method, everyone should give their experience. While I have been delighted to hear of the favourable results obtained by Prof. Ostmann, I regret that I am not in a position to speak so favourably of the electrical vibratory massage. I have not been using the apparatus for one year only, as Prof. Ostmann has, but for three years, ever since it was first made by the firm of Reiniger, Gebbert, and Schall.

When I first received the apparatus, I was enthusiastic in the hope of being able to cure a number of my deaf patients. After having used the apparatus, my hopes of curing deafness waned, but I still hoped to be able to cure cases of tinnitus. I am sorry to say that my hopes, even in this direction, were not verified. Although using the apparatus for three years, I cannot find that even cases of tinnitus are benefited by electric vibratory massage. Shortly after the massage, a patient claims that the noises appear to be diminished or gone, but in a few minutes they appear to return in the same strength as before.

It is true that I have not used the apparatus for so long a time at one sitting as Prof. Ostmann, not for twenty-five minutes, but only for five minutes at a time. It is possible that his method of using the apparatus may account for his more favourable results. I regret, therefore, that I cannot speak favourably of the results obtained in deafness, and even in tinnitus, by the use of electric vibratory massage, but on the contrary, I have found that my results have been more favourable by the use of the Delstanche apparatus, and the explanation is obviously that the excursions of the membrane and ossicles are wider, and the force obtained more powerful, even if the vibrations are slower than with the electrical apparatus.

DR. DUNDAS GRANT referred to the mechanical vibration applied to the spine which he had already described. He endeavoured to produce vibration without acoustic stimulation. The treatment was apparently indicated in cases of better hearing in a noise, but the probable result could only be ascertained by empirical trial. In a certain number of cases which were not improved by other means, this form of treatment produced improvement in hearing and relief from tinnitus.

PROF. LUCAE : Ich kann nur die Bedenken theilen, die Politzer gegen die Ostmann'sche Behandlungsmethode ausgesprochen hat. Die pneumatische Vibrationsmassage ist zunächst bereits längere Zeit vor Ostmann von mir angewendet worden und zwar auch mit electromotischer Kraft. Meine zweijährigen Erfahrungen stehen denen von Ostmann direct entgegen, insofern ich bei nicht wenigen, namentlich nervösen Personen eine, nicht selten andauernde Zunahme des Ohrensausens erlebt habe. Selbst Ohnmachten und Erbrechen kamen vor, was jedenfalls durch den *Lärm des Apparates* bedingt war. Weit bessere Resultate sah ich mit dem einfachen *Delstanche*'schen Apparate namentlich in Verbindung mit der von mir angegebenen Druck-Sonde (Pressure-Probe), welche allerdings wenn sie schmerzlos sein soll, weit *grössere* Uebung von Seiten des Arztes erfordert, als die pneumatische Behandlung.

DR. M. A. GOLDSTEIN : I desire to express myself in favour of aural massage in selected cases, whether this be effected by the original hand-masseur of Delstanche or by some modification of the machine-masseur.

I take issue with the essayist in the matter of the prolongation of this massage; no matter how mild the massage, the air-tight pressure of the Siegle speculum, and the continued vibratory action, is sure to produce hyperaemia and undue congestion of the parts.

In my paper I briefly outlined an additional feature to aid massage, consisting of first injecting the tympanic cavity with medicated liquid petroleums, via Eustachian tube, and then applying the masseur while the fluid is still in contact with the tissues of the tympanum, the thus softened tissues yielding more readily than when the massage alone is applied to a dry tympanic cavity.

DR. J. M. E. SCATLIFF : As an advocate of *passive motion* (frequently spoken of as massage) as a remedy for sclerotic and other conditions of the middle ear with consequent ankylosis, or crippled movement of the ossicular joints, I think it is of great importance to bear in mind that *compression* ought to be alternated with *rarefaction* of the air in the external auditory meatus in order to get the full benefit of this line of treatment and a more perfect movement of the joints in this chain. By this method of procedure the base of the stapes is tilted and the fenestra ovalis pressed upon in its anterior and posterior parts (segments) respectively, and the internal ear affected in both its important divisions : the head of the malleus is rotated upon the incus and a very perfect form of passive motion is the result.

PROF. OSTMANN betont, dass man in der für den Vortrag gegebenen Zeit nicht auch noch geschichtliche Daten bringen könne, deshalb habe er, um nicht gegen einzelne ungerecht zu werden, von solchen ganz abgesehen.

Was die Bemerkung des Herrn Professor Politzer betrifft, Ostmann hätte von Heilungen gesprochen, so muss er einen derartigen Eindruck dahin richtig stellen, dass mit Rücksicht auf seine eigenen Untersuchungsergebnisse er nicht éinmal in allen seinen Fällen von Besserung sprechen könne, vielmehr seien einzelne Fälle in dieser oder jener Tonlage überhaupt nicht gebessert. Von einer Heilung habe Ostmann somit keineswegs gesprochen, sondern er habe bei seinen Versuchen wesentlich die Absicht gehabt, auf wissenschaftlicher Basis nach dem Körnchen Gold zu suchen, was in dieser Behandlungsmethode enthalten zu sein scheint.

Wenn Prof. Lucae Ohnmacht, Erbrechen, und andere schwere Erscheinungen bei Anwendung der Vibrationsmassage gesehen habe, so wird man nach Ostmann's Ansicht derartige unangenehme Zufälle nur bei nicht richtiger Indikationsstellung auftreten sehen und zwar dadurch, dass die Vibrationen zu stark durch den Schallleitungsapparat hindurch gehen und somit eine unzweckmässige Wirkung auf den schallempfindenden Apparat stattfindet.

Bezüglich weiterer Bemerkungen bemerkt Ostmann, dass bei 2 mm. Kolbenverschiebung und selbst ausgiebigster Massage niemals eine andere Reaction als eine ganz leichte Hyperaemie der Schrapnell'schen Membran gefunden wird. Die Patienten selbst empfinden eine ganz leichte Wärme, welche gewöhnlich noch eine kurze Zeit nach Aufhören der Massage andauert. Selbstbehandlung hält auch Ostmann für durchaus verwerflich.

Die Drucksonde wirkt nach Ostmann's experimentellen Untersuchungen (cfr. Archiv für Ohrenheilkunde) selbst bei normalem Schallleitungsapparat auf diesen ganz ausserordentlich schwach, weil sie ihren Angriffspunkt an einem für Erzeugung von Schwingungen des Schallleitungsapparats sehr ungünstigen Punkte findet.

CHAIRMAN - - - - DR. KNAPP.

RESOLUTION—

The following resolution was proposed by the President, Prof. Urban Pritchard, seconded by Dr. Arthur Hartmann (Berlin), and after being submitted to the Meeting in English, French, and German, was carried by a very large majority, viz.:—

"That the Members of the Sixth International Otological Congress are of opinion that at all General Medical Congresses, Otology and Laryngology should be represented by separate and full Sections."

Des Bourdonnements Provoqués par l'Insuffisance Aortique.

Prof. Eeman, Ghent.

L'on a souvent reproché à la spécialisation en médecine, de fixer tellement l'attention du médecin sur tel ou tel organe, qu'il est exposé à perdre de vue les rapports unissant cet organe à d'autres parties, à l'ensemble de l'organisme.

C'est un danger qu'il était certes utile de signaler, mais je suis sûr que tous les spécialistes savent l'éviter à l'heure actuelle. Nous avons tous cette conviction profonde que nos connaissances spéciales en otologie doivent être greffées sur des connaissances suffisantes en médecine générale.

Il me parait cependant, qu'il s'attache un grand intérêt à tout ce qui établit l'existence de rapports étroits entre notre spécialité et la médecine interne ; c'est ce qui me détermine à vous dire quelques mots des bourdonnements provoqués par l'insuffisance aortique.

Que les maladies du coeur (organiques ou fonctionnelles) puissent déterminer des manifestations symptomatiques du côté de l'appareil auditif (des bourdonnements surtout), c'est un fait clinique bien connu. Mais il m'a semblé que le rôle de l'insuffisance aortique, n'a point été jusqu'ici estimé à sa juste valeur. Je ne crois plus aujourd'hui comme je l'ai fait longtemps, et comme beaucoup d'entre vous le font peut-être encore, à l'extrême rareté des cas de bourdonnements provoqués uniquement par l'insuffisance aortique.

Voici ce qui me parait correspondre à ce sujet à la réalité des faits cliniques. A côté des cas où il existe, avec les bourdonnements, une insuffisance aortique classique, facile à diagnostiquer, il y a des cas d'insuffisance aortique fruste, latente, qui échappent souvent au diagnostic.

Ces cas, sur lesquels je désire particulièrement attirer votre attention, ne s'accompagnent point des signes classiques de l'insuffisance aortique ; vous chercherez en vain l'hypertrophie considérable du ventricule gauche, vous ne constaterez point le souffle diastolique caractéristique au niveau du 2e espace interchondral droit. Le pouls radial ne ressemblera point au pouls de Corrigan, et par voie de conséquence le tracé sphygmographique ne sera point celui que l'on recueille dans l'insuffisance aortique typique. Il semble que dans ces conditions, on ne puisse songer à une insuffisance aortique, et cependant elle existe, se trahissant par un signe objectif, d'une extrême valeur au point de vue du diagnostic : ce signe précieux c'est le pouls capillaire à la région de l'ongle.

Et encore, Messieurs, faut il se placer dans des conditions un peu spéciales pour découvrir ce phénomène ; l'inspection directe de la région de l'ongle, suffisante dans les cas classiques, ne donne pas nécessairement un résultat positif; il faut dans bien des cas recourir au petit artifice que voici. L'observateur exerce à l'aide du doigt une pression modérée sur l'extrémité libre de l'ongle à examiner.

Il provoque ainsi une anémie de la partie moyenne de la région sous-ungéale; cette zône anémiée se distingue aisément des parties sus- et sousjacentes dont la coloration est restée normale.

C'est aux limites supérieures et inférieures de cette zône d'anémie artificielle, qu'il faut rechercher et étudier le pouls capillaire. On constate très bien dans ces conditions, une diminution d'étendue de la zône anémiée, à chaque systole ventriculaire, et l'accroissement de cette zône au moment précis où s'opère, en raison de l'insuffisance aortique, le retour, le reflux diastolique du sang dans le ventricule gauche.

Le bourdonnement lié à cette forme d'insuffisance aortique, est habituellement de caractère pulsatile; il peut être absolument intermittent, perçu à chaque systole ventriculaire; d'autrefois il sera continu, mais avec renforcement périodique plus ou moins net, renforcement synchrone avec la systole ventriculaire. Dans les cas de ce genre, il n'y a point de diminution appréciable de l'acuité auditive, si l'on examine le malade à un moment où le bourdonnement est atténué ou nul. L'intensité du phénomène est en effet très variable d'un moment à l'autre, et il en est de même nécessairement du pouls capillaire. Je dois même faire remarquer que le phénomène du pouls capillaire, tout comme le bourdonnement, peut disparaître pendant des périodes de temps plus ou moins longues; nous en déduirons cette conclusion qu'il ne faut se prononcer sur l'existence ou l'absence du pouls capillaire qu'après des examens répétés.

Il convient aussi de rechercher ce phénomène au niveau de chaque doigt des deux mains, pour la raison qu'il est inégalement accusé aux différents doigts.

L'absence des signes classiques habituels de l'insuffisance aortique, surtout l'absence du grand signe stéthoscopique, porte à admettre qu'il s'agit d'une insuffisance aortique fonctionnelle du genre de celles que nous voyons survenir dans des conditions cliniques bien différentes, p.ex. dans les maladies infectieuses aiguës, le typhus abdominal.

J'ai tenu à vous signaler ces faits pour la raison que je vous indiquais tantôt, parce qu'ils démontrent une fois de plus, que dans bien des circonstances de sa pratique, l'auriste doit faire un examen absolument méticuleux et complet de tous les appareils et organes de l'économie. Mais je vous les ai signalés aussi en raison des conséquences thérapeutiques qu'on en peut déduire.

Vous savez tous, Messieurs, combien sont embarrassants les cas de bourdonnements constituant une manifestation isolée, chez des sujets dont l'oreille ne présente aucune espèce d'altération appréciable.

Les recherches qui conduisent au diagnostic étiologique sont longues et délicates, parceque des causes très multiples, très diverses peuvent être la source de ces phénomènes. Nous devons même avouer, que dans un certain nombre de cas, l'enquête étiologique la plus habile, la plus patiente, la mieux conduite, ne donne pas au problème une solution satisfaisante, ou même une solution quelconque. Dans un certain nombre de ces cas, cette difficulté clinique sera écartée, parceque, recherchant et découvrant le phénomène du pouls capillaire, on aura dépisté une insuffisance aortique latente. On sera, tout naturellement amené dans ces conditions à substituer à une thérapeutique empirique, ou purement symptomatique, un traitement rationnel visant directement la cause du bourdonnement.

DR. DUNDAS GRANT considered many forms of sclerosis as really arthritis of the stapedio-vestibular articulation of osteo-arthritic, rheumatic, or sometimes syphilitic nature. Osteo-arthritis was sometimes infective as from suppuration in other organs, sometimes toxic as from intestinal sepsis. Suppuration in other organs required appropriate treatment and good results were often obtained from the use of aloetic purgatives or long-continued small doses of calomel. The otologist must in this disease study the general condition and not confine his exertions to local treatment.

SULLA POSSIBILITÀ DI RIAPRIRE LA FINESTRA OVALE NEI CASI DI ANCHILOSI OSSEA DELL'ARTICOLAZIONE STAPEDIO-VESTIBOLARE.

TYRIDANOIXI-OVALIS.

PROF. GIUSEPPE FARACI, Palermo.

Sin dal 1895 studiando clinicamente e sperimentalmente l'utilità della stapedectomia, tutte le volte che questo ossicino è affetto da impotenza funzionale, volsi l'attenzione alla possibilità di riaprire, con opportuni strumenti, la finestra ovale anche in quei casi in cui l'immobilità della staffa si dovesse ad anchilosi ossea dell'articolazione stapedio-vestibolare. Questo nuovo studio mirava a dare una maggiore applicazione pratica alla stapedectomia, collo estendere i benefici effetti di tale operazione a tutti gli infermi che si trovano ad avere ancora normale l'apparecchio di percezione del suono, qualunque siano le condizioni anatomo-patologiche della staffa o dell'articolazione stapedo-vestibolare.

E poichè molti e gravi erano i pericoli da temersi per tale operazione secondo Schwartze,* Politzer † e qualche altro i quali ritengono,

---

* Handbuch der Ohrenheilk (Bd. 11, 5,777, 1893).

† Trattato di Otologia. Ediz. 3a F. Enke, Stuttgart, 1893. Rivista critica pel Dott Eugenio Morpurgo (Bollettino delle malattie dell' orecchio, della gola e del naso, ginguo 1893).

ignoro se tuttora, che la caduta di piccoli frammenti ossei nel vestibolo, determini una laberintite purulenta e la consecutiva possibilità di una meningite, e poichè d'altro canto l'importanza fisiologica che Goltz e Breuer attribuivano al vestibolo doveva per lo meno farmi ritenere come assurda temerità quella di penetrare con gli strumenti chirurgici fin dentro il vestibolo, volli tuttavia dare una larga base sperimentale a questo nuovo studio, onde potere con molta esattezza controllare quanto di vero vi fosse nelle affermazioni dei suddetti autori.

Il numero delle esperienze, a tale scopo da me praticate, ascese a quattordici ed eseguite sopra otto conigli, due gatti, e quattro cani.

Non potendo naturalmente operare sopra animali la cui articolazione stapedo-vestibolare fosse sede di quelle alterazioni anatomo-patologiche per la quali l'operazione dovrebbe essere indicata, ho pensato di avvicinarmi al trauma-chirurgico da praticarsi nell'uomo, operando in maniera da spezzare non solo la base della staffa. ma di resecare anche una piccola parte dell'orlo della finestra ovale.

Non parlo qui della tecnica operativa eseguita sui diversi animali, nè voglio esporre in tutti i dettagli le singole operazioni avendole già minutamente descritti nel mio libro*, mi limito semplicemente a riassumere le conclusioni alle quali sono venuto.

1° L'apertura della finestra ovale con lo spezzamento della base della staffa *(thyridanoixi ovalis)*† non è un'operazione pericolosa, e se nessuna infezione accompagna l'atto operativo, non si ha mai una laberintite purulenta come hanno supposto Politzer, Schwartze e qualche altro, nè si provoca alcun disordine funzionale come era da temersi in seguito alle ipotesi di Goltz e Breuer.

2° I frammenti caduti nel vestibolo dànno luogo a fenomeni reattivi di nessuna entità che hanno per effetto la formazione di connettivo attorno a questi frammenti quali rimangono incapsulati da questi processi neo-formativi, senza che ciò comprometta la tessitura e la funzione delle parti molli del vestibolo. Basta infatti osservare il preparato istologico qui annesso per convincersi del fatto suesposto.

Esso rappresenta una sezione della cavità vestibolare dell'orecchio interno di un coniglio da me operato di *thyridanoixi ovalis.*

Al posto della staffa mancante osservasi un tessuto di neo formazione connettivale, formatosi a spese del periostio del vestibolo e del promontorio. Le membrane vestibulari, ripiegate da una parte per effetto della preparazione conservano la tessitura normale.

Notasi solo di patologico la presenza di due frammenti della staffa distrutta incapsulati da fibre connettivali e situati, uno in vicinanza dei bordi della finestra e l'altro dal lato opposto aderente alla parete interna del vestibolo. Questi due frammenti sono uniti altresì da fibre connetti-

---

* Chirurgia dell'orecchio medio ed esame critico della conseguenze dei varii atti operativi relativamente alla facoltà uditiva (Società Editrice Dante Alighieri, Roma, 1895).

† Credo di'potere bene definire con questa parola il nuovo genere di operazione.

Q

vali -che formano una specie di diaframma nell'interno della cavità.

È interessante che io faccia rilevare come l'animale, da cui fu tolto il preparato, non presentasse mai durante sei mesi di osservazione, disturbi nell'equilibrio e nell'attitudine del càpo, e che la funzione acustica del medesimo rimanesse discretamente conservata.

3° Nonostante la gravità maggiore del trauma chirurgico, rispetto a quello della stapedectomia, è possibile osservare, come in questa ultima, che i processi neo-formativi che devono sostituire la staffa mancante, rimangono circoscritti al periostio del vestibolo e delle pareti della nicchia della fossetta ovale, e si ottiene al posto della staffa la formazione di una membrana sottile, che gode un ottimo potere di trasmissione per l'onda acustica.

4° La forza uditiva rimasta, sia quantitativamente che qualitativamente, non differisce da quella riscontrata negli animali operati di rimozione *in toto* della staffa e quindi anche dal punto di vista acustico questo nuovo genere di operazione è consigliabile.

5° Queste esperienze lasciano soltanto un punto oscuro a delucidare, cioè l'influenza che i prodotti di neoformazione connettivale (per quanto limitati nel vestibolo) possano spiegare nella produzione dei rumori endotici, e quindi conchiudevo colla scorta dei risultati delle mie esperienze, col ritenere non azzardata una tale operazione nell'uomo, e che a questa si potrebbe ricorrere in quei casi che ad una grave sordità con apparato di percezione normale, si accoppiasse la presenza di gravissime paracusie, ben inteso mettendo in pratica rigorosamente tutte quelle cautele antisettiche che tale operazione richiede.

Venuto quindi fin da allora a tali conclusioni acquistai il convincimento di poter tentare questa operazione nell'uomo, non appena si fosse presentata l'opportunità di farla.

Fu solo quest'anno che potei attuare la mia idea e non voglio privare i colleghi della conoscenza dei risultati ottenuti, potendo col loro contributo scientifico stabilire fin d'ora l'utilità o meno della *thyridanoixi ovalis* nell'uomo.

L'operata è stata una ragazza di nome Leonarda Barbera di anni 15 ricoverata nell'orfanotrofio dei poveri a Palermo. *Storia.* Sin dall'infanzia ha sofferto di suppurazione cronica intermittente nell'orecchio sinistro, di continue paracusie ed accessi intercorrenti di vertigine. In questi ultimi due anni tanto i rumori che le vertigini acquistarono una intensità tale da obbligare l'inferma a stare spesse volte al letto. Nulla di ereditario nella famiglia, l'ammalata non ha sofferto processi febbrili acuti, non è stata contagiata da sifilide.

L'esame funzionale dell'orecchio ammalato è stato il seguente : Orologio a contatto ; Ut 0 ; Ut¹ ¹⁰/₅₀ * ; Voce afona e parlata0 ; sente solo il linguaggio forte in vicinanza dell'orechio ; Galton 4.7 ; Rinne negativo ; Weber a sinistra. L'orecchio destro è in condizioni normali.

---

* Esprimo con una frazione la durata della sensazione rispetto ad un udito normale.

Esame elettrico.—Si ottiene reazione dell'acustico con 8 M. A. tanto alla chiusura del catode che alla chiusura dell'anode—Nessuna reazione all'apertura del catode ed all'apertura dell'Anode. La reazione ottenuta dura pochi secondi e provoca nell'ammalata la sensazione di un sibilo.

Esame obbiettivo.—Distrutta completamente la membrana timpanica, vedesi solo il martello retratto in dentro e fissato al promontorio. La mucosa della cassa trasformata in tessuto cicatriziale. Mancante la branca verticale dell'incudine e le branche della staffa. La fossetta ovale é letteralmente coperta da un tessuto fibroso di neo-formazione in maniera da non potersi stabilire se la base della staffa trovasi o no a posto. Rimpicciolita la nicchia della fossetta rotonda per la presenza di uno spesso tessuto connettivale. In corrispondenza dell' *aditus ad antrum* mastoideo notasi la presenza di scarso essudato purulento.

Diagnosi clinica.—Esito di otite media purulenta cronica, carie delle paret dell'antro mastoideo, impotenza funzionale dell'apparecchio di trasmissione del suono.

Operazione.—Il 24 Novembre 1898 procedetti all'operazione con la quale mi proponevo di raggiungere un duplice scopo. 1° distruggere il processo di carie che si trovava nelle pareti dell'antro mastoideo. 2°. Aprire una via al passaggio dell'onda acustica nel laberinto.

Dopo aver distaccato il martello dal promontorio ed eseguita la tenotomia del tensore del timpano, estrassi quest ossicino assieme al corpo dell'incudine la cui articolazione si trovava solidamente anchilosata su quella del martello.

Resecai allora con la mia pinza osteotoma, tutta la parete esterna dell'attico timpanico, dell'antro mastoideo e dopo avere per bene vuotata quest'ultima cavità dalle granulazioni ivi esistenti ne cauterizzai le pareti con una soluzione al 10 per 100 di acido idroclorico.

Ciò fatto cerco di soddisfare la seconda indicazione. Dopo avere vuotato la fossetta ovale dal tessuto fibroso che la riempiva, constato che la base della staffa trovasi a posto, mi adopero in tutti i modi per mobilizzarla, però inutilmente, essendo solidamente anchilosata. Stabilisco allora di riaprire la finestra rompendo la base della staffa, la quale cosa viene da me praticata con molta circospezione, limitandomi a praticare un forellino più piccolo dell'ordinaria apertura della finestra ovale.

L'ammalata tollerò benissimo l'operazione, non vi furono inconvenienti nè complicazioni di sorta, tranne un pò di vertigine che dopo mezz' ora circa era del tutto cessata. Ripetei l'esame funzionale dell'orecchio operato e medicai come di regola.

Risultato. Il risultato acustico immediato è stato il seguente : Or. $^{30}/_{200}$; voce afona 0.40 ; voce parlata m. 3 ; Galton 4, 2 ; Ut $^{20}/_{50}$.

12 Dicembre.—Continua la suppurazione. Or. 0.03 ; Ut $^{10}/_{50}$ Ut¹ $^{15}/_{50}$. Weber a sinistra ; Galton 4.0 ; Voce afona 0.05 ; voce parlata m. 1 ; diminuiti i rumori e la vertigine.

15 gennaio 1899.—Voce afona m. 3 ; Or. $^{40}/_{200}$; Ut¹· $^{10}/_{50}$ Ut. $^{20}/_{50}$; Galton 4.0 ; guarita completamente la suppurazione.

1 Giugno.—Continua il miglioramento acustico come nell' ultimo esame, cessati definitivamente i rumori e la vertigine.

Come vedesi il risultato non poteva essere più soddisfacente tanto dal punto di vista acustico che funzionale, e posso anzi affermare che tale esito ha superato la mia aspettativa di fronte alla gravità delle condizioni anatomo-patologiche dell' orecchio operato.

Nè credo che valga a menomare l'importanza di tale operazione il fatto che trattasi di un'operazione isolata, perchè io trovo in questo la conferma più completa di quanto ebbi a dimostrare sin dal 1895 nelle numerose mie osservazioni esperimentali, specialmente per quanto riguarda la funzione acustica intorno a questo soggetto.

Ho ottenuto infatti, subito dopo l'operazione, un miglioramento considerevole dell'udito a cui tenne dietro una grave diminuzione del medesimo e fu solo dopo circa un mese che la funzione acustica potè ripristinarsi e rimanere stazionaria.

Questi cambiamenti sono in rapporto con le modificazioni istologiche che si svolgono nella finestra ovale in seguito all'operazione.

Nel 1° tempo rimane un'apertura completamente libera al passaggio dell'onda acustica e ciò spiéga la facoltà di potere udire subito dopo l'operazione. Debbo però fare rilevare che finora non ho trovato in seguito all'operazione, tanto nelle mie osservazioni sperimentali che cliniche quella profonda anestesia acustica post-operatoria della durata di 8 giorni di cui parla Straaten,* e nemmeno quel vero periodo di iperestesia di cui parla Botey †.

Non escludo tuttavia la possibilità che questi fenomeni possano avverarsi però nulla hanno da vedere con la natura dell'operazione in sè stessa ed io suppongo che ciò dipenda pinttorto dalla maniera di operare e dalla pressione in cui vengono a trovarsi gli elementi nervosi del laberinto in seguito all'operazione, analogamente a quello che succede negli elementi specifici della retina dopo l'estrazione della cateratta. Se la fuoruscita della perilinfa in seguito all' operazione, è scarsa e la pressione endolaberintica si mantiene entro certi limiti fisiologici, la funzione degli elementi nervosi rimane inalterata e non è difficile che un tale leggiero squilibrio nella pressione agisca eccitando la funzione del nervo per cui si avvera quella speciale iperestesia di cui parla Botey ; se invece la fuoruscita della perilinfa é stata maggiore e la pressione endolaberintica scende al disotto di dati limiti gli elementi nervosi cessano dal funzionare perchè non si trovano più in quelle condizioni di pressione indispensabile al loro funzionamento e non è difficile che avvenga l'anestesia acustica riscontrata da Straaten.

In un secondo tempo in cui per l'attività neo-formativa del periostio della cavità vestibolare e della capsula laberintica la finestra ovale viene ripiena da un tessuto di neo-formazione giovane costituito in gran parte da cellule linfatiche, la funzione acustica deve necessariamente ridursi essendo questo nuovo tessuto poco adatto alla trasmissione dell'onda sonora.

Solo in una fase tardiva, quando cioè il tessuto embrionale si é trasformato in connettivo definito con la formazione di una membrana

---

* Ueber die Mobilisation und Extraktion des in der Fenestra ovalis fixirten Steigbügels und die Folgen für das Gehör, 1894 pag 7.

† Annales des maladies de l'oreille, du nez et du larynx 1890 pag 38.

che gode di un sufficiente potere trasmissivo, l'udito ritorna in maniera stabile, e, come ho dimostrato in un altro lavoro, il ritorno della funzione acustica può essere maggiore o minore di quella avuta in seguito all'operazione, a seconda che la nuova, membrana è formata soltanto dal periostio del vestibolo o invece vi concorre l'attività neo-formatrice della capsula laberintica, dappoichè nel primo caso questa è sottile, trasparente ed elastica, nel secondo invece é spessa e poco vibratile.

Dal punto di vista funzionale questo caso ci fornisce dati interessanti : Anzitutto ci dimostra, nonostante il lieve traumatismo a cui vanno esposte le parti molli del vestibolo, nonostante l'attività dei processi istologici che vi si svolgono, che l'operazione non dà luogo a disturbi nell'equilibrio e non produce stimolazione abnorme negli elementi specifici del nervo acustico, che anzi tanto la vertigine quanto i rumori possono venire mitigati ed anche scomparire come è avvenuto nel caso da me operato.

Questa operazione dimostra ancora l'interessante fatto della innocuità, anche quando nell'orecchio medio si trovino focolai di carie e di processi purulenti cronici.

Credo quindi abbastanza giustificata l'affermazione che la *thyridanoixi ovalis* é un'operazione non solo praticabile nell'uomo ma anche consigliabile tutte le volte che rimanga ancora normale l'apparecchio di percezione del suono e che per le gravi condizioni anatomo-patologiche dell'articolazione stapedo-vestibolare, non sia possibile la stape dectomia.

DR. GARNAULT : Je regrette que M. Faraci ne nous dise pas comment il a procédé pour faire son opération, parceque je n'ai pu réussir, probablement en raison de ma manière défectueuse de procéder, à obtenir un bon résultat. J'ai perforé la platine de l'étrier avec un excavateur des dentistes et les résultats ont été défectueux.

PROF. POLITZER remarked that in his experiments on rabbits, he found that in the most of them a part of the bony border of the footplate of the stapes remained in the oval window. The method recommended by Faraci to break the footplate of the stapes, and his opinion, that the introduction of sterilized instruments into the vestibulum, or of bony particles penetrating into the vestibulum were not dangerous to the hearing, could not be approved, as they might cause inflammation and suppuration. Politzer saw a case in which during an operation of dividing the connective tissue in the niche of the oval window, the needle penetrated into the vestibulum ; the patient was seized with sudden vertigo and deafness from which he has never since recovered.

DR. NUVOLI trova estremamente sorprendente che le vibrazioni aeree prodotte dal tic-tac d'un orologio da tasca possano comunicarsi al liquido labirintico senza l'intermediario della membrana e della catena. Perquanto sieno in ottime condizioni il nervo acustico e la conduzione delle ossa, sarà sempre estremamente difficile, se non impossibile, che vibrazioni aeree prodotte da un suono sì debole, possano mettere in vibrazione un solido o un liquido.

DR. HERMAN KNAPP : In America the removal of the stapes has had a fair trial (Jack, Blake, etc.). The results have been that the operation is not very difficult, nor followed, as a rule, by grave symptoms ; the improvement as to acuteness of hearing and tinnitus has been very insignificant.

PROF. FARACI: Rispondo al Dr. Garnault che la prima parte delle sue osservazioni é fuori proposito perchè nei miei esperimenti non ho parlato di estrazione della staffa nei conigli ma di frattura della staffa ed apertura della finestra.

Se poi l'estrazione della staffa è, o no, possibile nei conigli è una questione che non è il momento di discutere.

Riguardo ai risultati contrari ch'egli ha avuto ciò non infirma il risultato da me ottenuto.   In queste operazioni bisogna tenere gran conto delle condizioni del nervo acustico ed io in un altro mio lavoro sono venuto a queste conclusioni, cioè in seguito alla mobilizzazione o ablazione della staffa, si possono avere uno dei seguenti risultati o nessuno risultato, o un peggioramento, o un miglioramento a seconda se il nervo acustico è più o meno affetto.   Bisogna quindi vedere come si opera ed in che condizione si opera. Infine sulla possibilità che un' onda acustica possa trasmettersi attraverso una membrana connettivale molto spessa, è un fatto innegabile. Io ho parlato solo di debole potere uditivo constatato nell' animale.

Rispondo al Dr. Nuvoli con poche parole : Il fatto esiste, vuol dire che le nostre conoscenze fisiopatologiche sulla conduzione del suono lasciano molto a desiderare.

UEBER DIE BEHANDLUNG DER KATARRHALISCHEN ADHAESIVPROCESSE IM MITTELOHRE, MITTELST INTRATYMPANALER PILOCARPININJECTIONEN.

DR. FR. FISCHENICH, Wiesbaden.

Die Fortschritte der modernen Ohrenheilkunde sind hauptsächlich auf dem operativen Gebiete zu suchen ; das Hauptinteresse konzentrirt sich seit einer Reihe von Jahren auf die Vervollkommung der operativen Technik der infolge von akuten oder chronischen Mittelohreiterungen auftretenden vielfachen Komplikationen.   Die hier erzielten Erfolge rechtfertigen dieses Interesse vollkommen, machen aber auch eine gewisse Einseitigkeit in den Darbietungen unserer Fachpresse und Special-versammlungen erklärlich.   Mit weit weniger Glück hat die Chirurgie versucht sich auf dem Gebiete der chronischen katarrhalischen Mittelohr-erkrankungen hervorzuthun ; ich will nicht die verschiedenen operativen Eingriffe der Reihe nach aufzählen, welche zur Verbesserung des Gehörs und zur Beseitigung störender Nebengeräusche bei den erwähnten Erkrankungen empfohlen worden sind, ich möchte nur erwähnen, dass nach meiner Ueberzeugung und Erfahrung, operative Eingriffe vorläufig wenigstens keine hervorragend nennenswerthen Chancen bieten. Die sonst üblichen Behandlungsmethoden, wie Lufteinblasungen, Luftverdünnung, Massage jeder Art u.s.w. haben nur eine Zeitlang Erfolg und versagen bei den vorgeschritteneren Fällen mehr oder weniger. Die Einleitung von Dämpfen ins Mittelohr wird anscheinend wenig mehr geübt und nur die Injektion medikamentöser Flüssigkeiten findet noch Anwendung; die Anzahl der hier empfohlenen Mittel ist Legion, vom einfachen Natr. bicarbonicum bis zum Vaselin und Paraffin der Neuzeit. Meine Erfahrungen mit den verschiedenen Mitteln sind nicht derartige gewesen, dass sie zur Fortsetzung dieser Therapie hätten ermuthigen können. Erst als ich anfing das Pilocarpinum muriaticum konsequenter Weise bei den adhaesiven Mittelohrprocessen zu verwenden, hatte ich Erfolge zu verzeichnen, welche nicht nur weit über dem Niveau des bis dahin Erreichbaren standen, sondern auch dauernder Natur waren. Bevor ich Ihnen meine Erfahrungen über die intra-tubale Pilocarpinbehandlung, welche sich auf die Dauer eines Zeitraumes von 4 Jahren erstreckt, mittheile, muss ich zunächst einige historische Daten geben. Politzer empfahl zuerst das Pilocarpin muriat. auf dem Kongresse in Mailand 1880 und zwar bei frischer Labyrinthsyphilis in der Form von subkutanen Injektionen; 1885 veröffentlichte er seine Resultate und betonte die Unwirksamkeit des Mittels bei den mit Affection des Labyrinthes verbundenen trockenen Mittelohrkatarrhen; er sistirte die Behandlung, wenn nach 8-10 Injektionen kein Erfolg zu bemerken war. Im 16ten Bande der Zeitschrift für Ohrenheilkunde berichtet Kosegarten zum ersten Male über äusserst günstige Resultate, welche er bei der Behandlung der chronischen Processe im Mittelohr erzielte, die Politzer als mit Affektion des Mittelohres komplicirten Mittelohrkatarrhe nennt, auch er injicirte das Pilocarp. muriat. subkutan und machte mit vollem Rechte Politzer gegenüber auf die Nothwendigkeit einer weit längeren Behandlungsdauer aufmerksam. Ob Kosegarten das Mittel auch bei den reinen Sklerosen ohne Labyrinthaffektion anwandte, geht aus seiner Arbeit nicht hervor. Im Jahre 1893 erschienenen Lehrbuche gibt Politzer an, dass er befriedigende Resultate durch die Injection von Pilocarpin. muriat. ins Mittelohr bei chronischen Processen erhielt, in welchen noch leichte Schwellung der Tubentrommelhöhlenschleimhaut bestand; die subkutanen Injektionen erwiesen sich als werthlos. Skirmunsky berichtet im Jahre 1894 auf der Versammlung russischer Aerzte in St. Petersburg über das Mittel in der Ohrenheilkunde und bespricht auch seine Anwendung bei trockenen Katarrhen, seine Resultate waren nicht günstig, doch war sein Material nicht bedeutend und die Behandlungsdauer nicht ausreichend. Aus dem Mitgetheilten erhellt, dass die Ansichten über den Werth des Pilocarpin. muriat. bei der Behandlung des chronischen Mittelohrkatarrhes auseinander gehen;

ich gestatte mir daher meine eigenen Erfahrungen über das Pilocarpin welches ich als ein hervorragendes Mittel bei der Behandlung der chronischen Adhaesivprocesse im Mittelohre—sei es mit, sei es ohne Labyrinthbetheiligung—schätzen gelernt habe, in Folgendem zusammenzufassen. Zunächst muss ich erwähnen, dass ich im Anfange nur Fälle von möglichst reiner Mittelohrsklerose behandelte, später auch solche mit Betheiligung des Labyrinthes; ebenso muss ich erwähnen, dass die ausgewählten Fälle theils solche waren, welche schon lange von mir ohne wesentlichen Erfolg behandelt worden waren, theils solche an denen von anderer fachmännischer Seite alle üblichen Behandlungsmethoden versucht worden waren.

Die Schwerhörigkeit war meist eine hochgradige; in vielen Fällen wurde nur noch die Flüstersprache, in anderen die laute Sprache am Ohre vernommen. Die erzielten Besserungen schwankten zwischen dem Zwei bis Zehnfachen der vorhandenen Hörschärfe; die Zahl der Injektionen variirte je nach der Schwere der Erkrankung zwischen dreissig und fünfzig; benutzt wurde eine 2% wässrige Lösung von Pilocarp. muriat. Die Anfangsdosis betrug 6-8 Tropfen für jedes Ohr und wurde im Laufe der Behandlung auf 10-12-16 Tropfen gesteigert; in der gesteigerten Dosis glaube ich zum nicht geringsten Theil die Erklärung für meine günstigen Resultate zu finden. Die Resorptionsfähigkeit der Paukenhöhlenschleimhaut ist eine ausserordentliche hohe, am Morgen nach der Injektion ist meist keinerlei Flüssigkeit mehr nachweisbar; wenn dagegen noch Flüssigkeit in höherem Grade vorhanden, sistire ich die Injektion und beschränke mich auf die Lufteinblasung. Die Technik der Injektion ist einfach und die allgemein übliche: ein elasticher Paukenhöhlenkatheter mit centraler möglichst weiter Oeffnung wird durch den massiven Ohrkatheter soweit im Tubenkanal vorgeschoben, bis man sich durch die Probe überzeugen kann, dass die Luft frei in die Paukenhöhle hineindringt; dann wird injicirt und mit einem kleineren Ballon, dessen Ansatz möglichst der Oeffnung des elastischen Catheters angepasst ist, unter mässigem Drucke die Flüssigkeit in die Paukenhöhle gepresst. Bei grösseren Flüssigkeitsdosen muss das Hineinpressen in mehreren Absätzen geschehen. Ich pflege sowohl vor als nach der Injektion zu katheterisiren. Die unmittelbare Folge der Injektion ist meist etwas Schwindel und im Anfange hier und da ein leichter Schmerz; es empfiehlt sich daher den Patienten nicht sofort zu entlassen und ihm eventuell horizontale Lage bis zum Nachlassen der Erscheinungen zu verordnen. Nur im Beginne meiner Erfahrungen mit dieser Methode erlebte ich dreimal eine heftigere Reaction bestehend in einer starken Hyperämie des Trommelfelles—in dem einen Fall sogar einen Bluterguss in dasselbe—mit stärkeren Schmerzen, die aber nach einigen Stunden nachliessen; irgend eine üble Nachwirkung erfolgte nicht. Eine leichtere Hyperämie am Hammergriffe, am Trommelfell selbst und in

der Umgebung desselben ist fast nach jeder Injektion nachweisbar ;
ebenso tritt nach einiger Zeit Speichelfluss und gelinde Schweiss-
absonderung auf. Die störenden Ohrgeräusche verschwinden nur in
einer kleineren Anzahl der Fälle vollständig ; dagegen wird allgemein
angegeben, dass das Benommensein und das schwere Gefühl im Kopfe,
über welches eine Anzahl von Patienten klagt, eine ganz erhebliche
Besserung erfährt. Ich möchte nicht verfehlen auf die guten Dienste
aufmerksam zu machen, welche mir die Methode bei der Sklerose hochgradig chlorotischer Individuen geleistet hat. Die bis zur Unerträg-
lichkeit gesteigerten Geräusche verbunden mit starken Kopfschmerzen
verschwanden schon nach mehreren Injektionen vollständig. Solange
die Injektionen vorgenommen werden, klagen die Patienten manchmal
über Verschlechterung des Gehörs ; es ist rathsam die Hörprüfung
nicht sofort nach dem Sistiren der Injektionen zu machen, sondern
erst noch etwa 8 Tage lang Lufteinblasungen vorzunehmen, bis jeder
Rest von Flüssigkeit geschwunden ist. Ohne auf Krankengeschichten
einzugehen will ich ganz kurz den Verlauf eines charakteristischen
Falles von progressiver Sklerose skizziren, um daran anknüpfend
einige Thatsachen hervorzuheben, welche wichtig sind. Es handelt sich
um eine Patientin, bei der ich die verschiedenen Behandlungsmethoden,
auch die Massage sowie die Injektion medikamentöser Flüssigkeiten ins
Mittelohr mit Anfangs vorübergehenden, später konsequent negativem
Erfolge versucht hatte. Ich sistirte daher jede Therapie, und sah sie
erst 3 Jahre nach der letzten Behandlung wieder ; die Schwerhörigkeit
hatte weitere rapide Fortschritte gemacht, die laute Sprache wurde
beiderseits nur am Ohre vernommen, Rinne negativ, Kopfknochenleitung
eher verlängert ; die Ohrgeräusche hatten einen ausserordentlich
quälenden Charakter angenommen. Nach 35 Injektionen ergab sich
beiderseitige Hörweite von 5 Metern ; die Geräusche waren viel
erträglicher, der Kopf freier geworden ; die nach einem halben Jahre
vorgenommene Untersuchung zeigt, dass die Besserung Stand gehalten
hat. Dreissig Injektionen im folgenden Jahre steigerten die Hörschärfe auf 7 Meter ; die Untersuchung ergab ein halbes Jahr später
dass die Hörschärfe auf 10 Meter angelangt war ; die Ohrgeräusche
waren minimal. Das Gehör liess im Laufe des Jahres infolge einer
Influenzaattake etwas nach, wurde aber durch eine nochmalige
Behandlung wieder auf die alte Höhe gehoben und hat bis jetzt Stand
gehalten. Die Beurtheilung dieses Falles, der gewissermassen als
Schema für den Verlauf der meisten anderen Fälle betrachtet werden
kann, führt zu folgenden Ergebnissen : —1. Es wird bei einer
einmaligen Pilocarpinkur ein gewisses Maximum von Hörschärfe
gewonnen. 2. Dieses Maximum kann bei einer wiederholten Behandlung später überschritten werden. 3. Das nach dem Ende der
Behandlung zu verzeichnende Hörresultat ist meist nicht das definitive;
die Wirksamkeit des Mittels muss ich insofern als eine kumulative

bezeichnen, als auch nach Beendigung der lokalen Behandlung eine weitere Besserung der Hörkraft stattfindet. Versuche, welche ich zur Kontrolle anstellte, überzeugten mich ferner, dass die einfache subkutane Injektion bei Weitem nicht die Wirkung der Injektion ins Mittelohr erreicht. Ueble Vorkommnisse ausser den schon erwähnten, habe ich niemals beobachtet, mit der fortschreitenden Technik liessen sich kleine Uebelstände immer mehr vermeiden ; in der grossen Anzahl behandelter Fälle habe ich nur zweimal ein vollständiges Ausbleiben jeglichen Erfolges beobachtet, es waren dies Kranke, bei denen schwere Labyrinthveränderungen nachweisbar waren. Eine eigentliche Kontraindikation existirt, meiner Meinung nach, nicht, doch ist es gut bei Herzleidenden eine gewisse Vorsicht in der Dosirung zu beobachten. Nebenbei möchte ich auf die ausserordentlich günstige Wirkung der intratubalen Pilocarpininjektionen bei allen Tubenkatarrhen mit Schwellung der Schleimhaut, die schon einige Zeit besteht, aufmerksam machen ; es genügt mehrere Male einige Tropfen der Lösung langsam durch die Tuben zu giessen, um den Weg gänzlich frei zu machen. Im Allgemeinen wird man sich mit Kosegarten die Wirkung des Pilocarpins auf das Mittelohr so erklären müssen, dass es durch die immer wiederkehrende Hyperaemie zur Lockerung des starren Gewebes kommt, sowie zur Erweichung und Durchfeuchtung der Adhäsionen, wodurch der Leitungsapparat wieder schwingungsfähiger wird und vorhandene Exsudate zur Resorption gebracht werden. Ich bin aber geneigt nach meinen Erfahrungen mit dem Pilocarpin an eine beinahe specifische Wirkung des Mittels in der Paukenhöhle zu glauben, die es vor anderen medikamentösen Flüssigkeiten voraus hat. Jedenfalls betrachte ich die Sklerose nicht mehr als das noli me tangere, für welches sie vielfach bei den Ohrenärzten gilt. Leider gelingt es in vielen Fällen nicht, dem Patienten, der schon durch so vieler Aerzte Hände gegangen ist, und wie diese, auch selbst den Glauben an eine dauernde Besserung verloren hat, das nöthige Vertrauen zu einer neuen Behandlung und wie ich immer wieder betonen muss, auch die nöthige Ausdauer aufzuzwingen. Den Herren Kollegen glaube ich aber die Pilocarpintherapie, mit den von mir angegebenen Modifikationen auf Grund eines Materiales empfehlen zu können, welches sich auf 120 Fälle beläuft.

PROF. GRADENIGO: Sono dolente di non poter esser d'accordo col collega Fischenich sopra l'efficacia della pilocarpina. Poichè si continua a raccomandare le injezioni ipodermiche nella cura della sclerosi e dell' otite interna, devo dichiarare che io non ho mai avuto risultati da questo trattamento, e che tutto quanto si può ottenere colla artificiale sudazione, si ottiene molto più semplicemente e senza dover sottomettere l'organismo a una vera intossicazione, coi bagni a vapore.

Rispetto al trattamento intratimpanico devo dire che non solo nei pochi casi, nei quali io l'ho praticato, ma anche nei malati nei quali la

cura fu fatta da altri colleghi, e io ho avuto occasione di esaminare i
malati prima e dopo del trattamento, non ho potuto constatare
miglioramenti. Credo che poi l'uso di questo alcaloide non sia del tutto
indifferente per le condizioni generali.

PNEUMOMASSAGE UNTER HOEHEREM DRUCKE.

DR. P. J. MINK, Zwolle, Holland.

Die Kette der Gehörknöchelchen ist, wie die Physiologie uns lehrt,
als ein federndes Hebelsystem zu betrachten, das zwischen Trommelfell
und Membrana ovalis eingeschaltet ist.

Die Leichtigkeit mit der die Trommelfellbewegungen, mittelst dieses
Apparates zum Labyrinthe fortgeleitet werden, ist von bestimmendem
Einfluss auf das Hören.

Die Beweglichkeit des federnden Systems in seiner Gesamtheit ist
daher ein Faktor von der höchsten Bedeutung. Von physischem Standpunkte würde sie durch einen bestimmten Wert, den Elasticitätscoëffi-
cienten, vorzustellen sein. Etwaïge Rigidität der Gehörkette findet
dann in einer Vergrösserung dieses Wertes seinen Ausdruck.

Unser therapeutisches Streben muss in diesem Falle darauf
gerichtet sein, diesen Wert zur normalen Grösse zurückzuführen, d.h.
zu verkleinern.

Man hat versucht durch Luftdruckschwankungen im abgeschlossenen Gehörgange, dieses Ziel zu erreichen. Meistens sind es
kleinere Kräfte, die bei dieser Pneumomassage angewandt werden.
Achtet man nur auf den Einfluss den diese kleinen Erschütterungen auf
die vitalen Verhältnisse der Teile ausüben mögen, so ist gegen diese Art
des Verfahrens nichts einzuwenden. Betrachtet man die Sache aber
von rein mechanischem Standpunkte, so ist von diesen kleineren
Kräften meistens nicht viel zu erwarten. Die Zahl kann nicht ersetzen,
was man der Grösse nicht zumuten darf. Millionen von kleinen
Schwingungen die innerhalb der Grenze der federnden Kraft einer
Feder liegen, werden nichts von der Elasticität dieser Feder rauben ;
eine einzelne Schwingung aber, die diese Grenze überschreitet, ist im
Stande den Wert des Elasticitätscoefficienten zu verkleinern.

Zwar ist die Gehörkette einer Feder aus einem Stücke nicht gleich
zu setzen. Wenn aber die angewandten Kräfte die Kette als Ganzes
nicht in Schwingung versetzen, so werden die Verbindungen zuerst
betroffen werden, welche die beweglichsten, somit die normalsten sind,
während die rigideren unbeeinflusst bleiben können. So kann man sich
z.B. vorstellen, dass Bewegungen, die dem Trommelfell mitgetheilt
werden, in einem leichtbeweglichen Amboss-Stapesgelenke ihr Ende
finden, indem ein kräftiger befestigtes Stapesköpfchen als fixer Punkt
fungiert. Die gewöhnliche Pneumomassage würde in diesem Falle

einen Zustand der Lockerung und sogar der Abschleifung in dem
betreffenden Gelenke provocieren können. Ich bemerke hierbei dass
Rudolf Panse solch einen Befund bei den von ihm näher studierten
Fällen von Stapesankylose mehrere Male hat constatieren können.
Solch eine partielle Lockerung in der Gehörkette kommt aber der
Hörfunktion nicht zu gute, ja kann dieser unter Umständen selbst
schaden. Nur eine grössere Beweglichkeit der Gehörkette als Ganzes
wird für das Hören nützlich sein.

Will man daher den Wert des Elasticitätscoefficienten einer rigiden
Gehörkette auf rein mechanischem Wege vom Trommelfell aus
verkleinern, so hat man auf folgendes zu achten :—1° muss die
angewandte Kraft die Gehörkette solcherweise angreifen, dass diese
sich, ihr gegenüber als Einheit verhält, 2° muss diese Kraft so weit
gesteigert werden, dass die Elasticitätsgrenze der Gehörkette, sei es
auch um ein Minimum, überschritten wird.

Zweckmässig ist es daher, eine konstante Kraft auf das Trommelfell
einwirken zu lassen, die so gross ist, dass diese Elasticitätsgrenze nahezu
erreicht ist. Jetzt kann man durch hinzugefügte kleinere Druckerhöhungen jedesmal die Grenze um ein weniges überschreiten, und auf
wirksame Weise den pathologisch erhöhten Widerstand beeinflüssen.

In Bezug auf die Art der Kraft womit man die Kette in Spannung
bringen will, ist es am rationellsten den Weg zu folgen, der uns von der
Natur vorgezeigt ist, nl. Luftdruck im äusseren Gehörgange. Auf
der am meisten schonende Weise, wird hierdurch der Hammergriff
einwärts bewegt, das Sperrzahngelenk in Wirkung gesetzt, und die
Kette im ganzen so gespannt, wie es ihrem Zwecke das Ueberbringen
von Trommelfellschwingungen zum Labyrinthe, am besten entspricht.

Es fragt sich nur wie gross die durch Luftdruck auf das Trommelfell anzuwenden de konstante Kraft im Einzelfalle sein muss.

Ich habe bei einer Reihe von Personen auf das Trommelfell einen
langsam ansteigenden Luftdruck einwirken lassen. Es zeigte sich dass
bei normalem Gehörorgan sehr bald, meistens schon bevor $\frac{1}{4}$ Atmosphär
Druck erreicht war, Schmerz in der Tiefe des Ohres auftrat. *Wo eine
Rigidität der Gehörkette angenommen werden konnte, wurde aber im
Allgemeinen ein viel höherer Druck ertragen.* Bei den Fällen wo eine
erhöhte Schleimsekretion in Tuba, und Paukenhöhle vorlag, traf dieses
nicht immer zu. Bei den Fällen von ausgesprochener Sklerose, die ich
bis jetzt zu untersuchen Gelegenheit hatte, habe ich diesen Satz dagegen
immer bestätigt gefunden. Selbst eine gewisse Gesetzmässigkeit war
unverkennbar, indem bei den weiter fortgeschrittenen Fällen auch ein
höherer Druck ertragen wurde, bevor das Schmerzgefühl auftrat. Bei
inveterirter Sklerose, wo es nahe lag, eine Stapesankylose anzunehmen.
habe ich selbst mehr als 1Atm. Druck anwenden können, ohne dass
dieser Tiefenschmerz verspürt wurde.

Ich neige deshalb sehr dazu anzunehmen, dass, wenigstens bei

Sklerose, etwa durch Luftdruck auftretender Schmerz, an der Fenestra ovalis empfunden wird. Immerhin wünsche ich mir noch eine durch grösseren Zahlen belegte, auch von anderen beigebrachte Bestätigung, bevor dieser Causalnexus, zwischen auftretender Schmerz und Rigidität der Gehörkette, bei Sklerose, als allgemein giltig, vorzustellen ist.

Noch andere Fragen, über die ich mich hier nicht verbreiten kann, harren ihrer Lösung, bevor die Sache in ihrer ganzen Ausdehnung klar zu Tage liegt. Vorläufig aber betrachte ich das durch Luftdruck auftretende Schmerzgefühl in der Tiefe des Ohres als ein Zeichen, dass die Elasticitätsgrenze der Gehörkette nahezu erreicht ist.

Ich erachtete mich daher zu Heilungsversuche auf folgender Weise berechtigt : Eine Luftreservoir wurde mittelst eines dickwandigen, elastischen Schlauchs, mit dem Gehörgange in luftdichte Verbindung gebracht. Durch eine Schraubevorichtung wurde dann der Druck langsam erhöht bis Patient angab, beginnende Schmerzhaftigkeit zu spüren. Ein kreuzformiges metallenes Rohr war im Schlauche eingeschaltet und brachte den abgeschlossenen Luftraum einerseits mit einem Manometer, anderseits mit einem kleinen dickwandigen Gummiballon in Verbindung. Dieser Ballon lieferte bei Zusammenpressung die kleinere Druckerhöhungen, die nötig waren um die schon erreichte supponirte Elasticitätsgrenze der Kette zu überschreiten. Immer vom Schmerzgefühl geleitet, konnte man diese Druckerhöhungen grösser oder kleiner gestalten. Irgendwelche stärkere Schmerzempfindungen wurden strengstens vermieden.

Anfänglich wurden einmal wöchentlich auf diese Weise 50-100 Massagebewegungen unter höherem Drucke ausgeführt, und später dasselbe mit grösseren Zwischenräumen längere Zeit hindurch.

Mehrere Male betrug der konstante Druck mehr als eine halbe Atmosphär. Nachteile habe ich von dieser Art des Verfahrens nicht gesehen. Die schrecklichen Folgen bei Drucksteigerung und Druckabnahme auf das Gehörorgan, wovon neuerdings Alt, Heller und Mayer in Wien berichteten, beziehen sich jedenfalls auf andere Umstände.

Das so gefürchtete Einreissen des Trommelfells ist mir niemals vorgekommen, auch nicht bei dem 1 Atmosphäre übersteigenden Drucke, wovon die Rede war. Leichte Schwindelerscheinungen ohne weitere Bedeutung, habe ich beim vorsichtigen Vorgehen nur ausnahmsweise gesehen. Konstant war nur eine stärkere Injection der Trommelfellgefässe unmittelbar nach der Behandlung, die sich bald verlor ohne Folgen zu hinterlassen. Manchmal folgte auf den Eingriff ein kurzes Stadium von Gehörverschlechterung, dass durch Application des Katheters aufzuheben war oder einer Verbesserung Platz machte.

Die Zahl der so behandelten Fälle ist noch gering. Ich verfüge aber schon jetzt über einige höchst erfreulichen Resultate, sowohl in Bezug auf der Hörfunktion, als auf die subjektiven Geräusche. Ich betone dass diese Erfolge erzielt wurden, nachdem die gewöhnlichen Behandlungsmethoden fehlgeschlagen hatten.   Zu seiner Zeit hoffe ich hierüber näher zu berichten.   Nichtsdestoweniger möchte ich den Herren Collegen, die sich meines Verfahrens bedienen wollen, vorläufig ein sehr vorsichtiges, tâtonnierendes Vorgehen ans Herz legen.   Es bedürfen einige Momenten eines genaueren Studiums in Bezug auf die richtige Auswahl der Fälle, die dieser Behandlung zugänglich sind.   Es liegt daher die Gefahr vor sich ein unrichtiges Urteil über den Wert dieses Vorgehens zu bilden.

Vorläufig möchte ich seine praktische Anwendung reserviert wissen für nicht zu weit fortgeschrittene Sklerose ohne Complicationen.

Inzwischen kann ruhig weiter gearbeitet werden, um die Grenzen zu bestimmen, die bei dieser Methode innegehalten werden müssen.

Auf dieser Weise vorgehend, wird es sich am besten herausstellen, welcher Platz der Pneumomassage unter höherem Drucke in unserem Heilverfahren zukommt.

Ich bezwecke mit dieser vorläufigen Mitteilung, Mitarbeiter zu gewinnen um dieses Ziel im Interesse der zahllosen Ohrenleidenden, sobald wie möglich zu erreichen.

DR. CHEVALIER JACKSON.—While unable to fully understand all that Dr. Mink has said, I should like to state the results of my experience.

In my earlier trials of pneumo-massage all my cases were made worse by it.   This I attributed to too great pressure, and to the forcing inward of the stapes.   After further trials and observations, I came to the conclusion that to get satisfactory results it is essential to be gentle and to avoid compression.   To thump and pound at the membrana tympani, and treat it as an orthopaedic surgeon would an ankylosed knee joint, I feel convinced is to produce flabbiness and relaxation of the membrana tympani.   The higher the pressure, the greater the harm in my opinion.   Compression, if the pressure be high, is likely to do harm, immediate or remote, by forcing the stapes inward.   Massage in any form has, in my hands, always done harm in cases in which there has been labyrinthine involvement.

ON PNEUMATIC TREATMENT OF THE DISEASES OF THE EAR.

DR. G. NUVOLI, Rome.

In order to get as clear an idea as possible of the pneumatic treatment as practised by means of the ear-pump, worked by an electric motor, I have made an anatomical study of the effects of this treatment on the auditory organ in the dead body.

As we know, by means of this pump, the air in the external auditory canal is condensed and rarified with rapid alternations, and the tympanic membrane is consequently propelled either inwards or outwards in such a way as to assume a very rapid, regular movement, which may be repeated two or three hundred times a minute generally without any disturbance or injury.

The whole of the endotympanic movement may be observed through apertures made in the roof or sides of the tympanic cavity.

The tympanic membrane is then seen to be in rapid oscillatory motion, the culminating point of which corresponds to the *umbo*, which may have an excursion of a millimetre and a half. Whilst the handle of the hammer is propelled outwards, the head is propelled inwards, and vice versa, the whole of the small bone turning on a horizontal axis, placed exactly above the short process. When the head of the hammer, revolving on the above-mentioned axis is propelled inwards, the horizontal portion of the articular surface of the anvil is struck vertically, from above downwards, by the corresponding articular surface of the head of the hammer; the anvil, however, sliding, transforms this vertical movement into a horizontal one.

The movement of the long process of the anvil differs according to whether it is united to the stirrup or not. In the latter case, this process, remaining constantly parallel with the handle of the hammer, follows the movements of the hammer, but with more limited oscillations, its lower extremity receding from, or approaching the oval window. When, however, the long process of the anvil is united to the stirrup, their point of union remains perfectly motionless, at least to the naked eye, because the stirrup opposes a vigorous resistance to the shock of the movement, and then the anvil works backwards and forwards, turning on an axis, which passes through the extremities of the long and short processes and connects them. The whole movement above described becomes greater, if the tendon of the *tensor tympani* be cut ; whereas, if this muscle be laid bare and stretched, the curvature of the membrane is increased and the movements produced by the pump become most limited.

To discern the movement of the stirrup caused by the pump, observations must be made from the vestibulum, the latter being first cut in half and emptied of its liquid and membranous contents.

With the aid of the frontal mirror, let the eye be fixed on some luminous point in the outline of the stirrup, then, provided the anatomical piece be normal, the point will be seen to acquire minimal vibrations during the application of the pump, which vibrations can only be measured with the aid of the most accurate mathematical instruments If a hole be pricked between the *margin* of the stirrup and that of the oval window, and a bristle be introduced into this hole, it will be observed that the bristle acquires a vibratory movement, or if, with a file, a very tiny hole be made corresponding to each of the three semi-circular canals and the eye be fixed on a luminous point in this hole, produced by the endolabyrinthine liquid reflecting the light from the mirror, then also a vibratory movement may be discerned in the luminous point. Without one of these two methods it is impossible to detect the slightest movement of the vestibular surface of the stirrup and of the endolabyrinthine fluid.

By making a suitable opening in the posterior wall of the tympanic cavity, so as to disclose the round window, the vibration communicated to the membrane of this window by the said liquid may be seen.

In this way the pneumatic treatment, applied in the manner above described, gives a regular vibrating movement to all the parts forming the middle and inner ear.

With respect to the clinical results, I may say that our diagnostic means do not allow us to judge, in an absolute manner, *a priori*, in which cases this treatment may be advisable.

Experience will show that it is very useful in many cases, whilst having little or no effect in others.

From the above described anatomical observations we may draw the conclusion that the pneumatic treatment will be useful in chronic non-suppurative diseases of the middle ear, where adhesions are forming, which are an obstacle to the free movement of the membrane and of the little bones, provided that these connections be limited, recent, and easily stretched, especially when they are situated in or around the articulation of the anvil with the hammer, or between this articulation and the *attic*.

Having seen that even in the normal ear the movements of the stirrup caused by the pneumatic pump are extremely limited, we can easily draw the conclusion that this treatment will be inefficacious in cases of *anchylosis* of the stirrup.

With respect to the consequences of putting the labyrinthine fluid into vibration, the only thing we can be sure of is, that it does not harm. Probably it may turn out useful in recent, slight and limited alteration of this liquid, if we recollect the usefulness of *massage* and especially vibratory massage in the diseases of other nerves.

Finally we must not forget the prudence, which here as always, has to guide the surgeon.   This treatment especially in the beginning must be only continued for a few minutes, and the compression and rare-faction of the air must not be exaggerated, because it may happen that instead of a moderate and gradual extension of the connections we find ourselves confronted with a rupture of the same or a bursting of the membrane.   In this case the patient would have intense and immediate pain, giddiness, endo-tympanic hæmorrhage, and acute suppurative otitis.

20TH CENTURY PROGNOSIS IN CHRONIC CATARRHAL DEAFNESS.

DR. SARGENT SNOW, Syracuse, N.Y.

GENTLEMEN,—The unfavourable, but time-honoured prognosis given in chronic catarrhal deafness has made it a subject rather shunned by modern writers, but the importance and frequency of the problem impels me to place before the Sixth International Otological Congress a few more hopeful conclusions born of my personal experience.

For many years this affection has baffled the skill of foremost Otologists, each apparent success being overcome by the progressive nature of the disease, until gradually it has taken a place in the list of non-preventable and incurable maladies ; even now it does not seem safe to assume that those almost totally deaf can be improved, but we must admit, that recent advances have changed our prognosis in other conditions ; why not in that great body of chronic catarrhal cases where for instance words in a forced whisper can still be heard ten inches or more.

A study of the anatomy of the parts shows us the intimate relation of the nasal and aural membranes both by continuity and sympathy ; what benefits the nose is in the right line to benefit the ear in some degree. It matters not whether we have to deal with an hypertrophy or a sclerosis, our first duty is to relieve the nasal passages of all abnormal conditions.

During the past ten years, I have been consulted by many people whose deafness, by tests, duration, and degree was surely the result of a chronic catarrhal state, and whose intelligence enabled them to appreciate the whys and wherefores of the persistent line of treatment necessary in such deep-seated cases. A large number have been under observation five, three, and two years, giving a good opportunity for impartial judgment on the methods in vogue at the present day, and I feel certain that the general principles of treatment as employed by advanced authorities, that all pathological conditions within the nose and naso-pharynx must first be removed, etc., are correct and reliable.

The idea is rational, and it is my experience, and a thought that led me to select this subject, that the reason we still have so many failures is that either we have overlooked some point of obstruction or contact in the upper portion of the nose that is acting as an irritant or we should go further and advise our patients to submit from year to year if necessary, to hygienic care and a tonic treatment with stimulating vapours to the tube and middle ear.

Of late we have been led to expect too much from purely nasal operative work, when with eighty per cent. of such cases recurring catarrhal inflammations yet remain as an important causative factor. In early adult subjects, where the deafness is of only one or two years' standing, it is true that the removal of turbinate pressures, ethmoidal

R

disease or adenoids may be followed by good results without special attention being paid to the middle ear. But, with those cases giving a history of five, ten or twenty years' impairment of hearing, we are sure to find that the inflammatory action within the ear and Eustachian tubes will continue if we do not also institute a thorough and persistent course of after treatment.

Chronic catarrhal deafness is a preventable disease. In every one of these patients we will find, besides their nasal trouble some functional disorder or an habitual and gross transgression of nature's laws :—Unseasonable clothing, improper diet, poor portal circulation, warm baths, exposure to draughts night or day, and too little arm exercise are among those most prominent, and it is against these our great fight has to be made. I say "great fight" for here our judgment and skill are most taxed ; these errors must be corrected, the surface reaction improved by cold baths and each habit scrutinized, for, when membranes have once been in a state of chronic congestion, dietary and other excesses or the taking of a slight cold will produce a profound impression on the already weakened blood vessels.

A few patients afflicted with chronic otitis media give no history of nasal trouble ; but we will invariably find the post-nasal or Eustachian membranes in some stage of inflammation or atrophy, frequently pale and relaxed, but very sensitive. This class need little operative work, but the parts require stimulation. Their life must be looked into and so regulated that they are better able to resist colds and throw off congestions. Even those showing sclerotic states are capable of some improvement.

Assuming that our patients are sensible and intelligent people, it is just and expedient that we go quite into detail in explaining nature's method of repair and the different steps of treatment. No further encouragement or promise is necessary, if we make the points clear. An ignorant, unreasonable patient is not a favourable one, for he fails to appreciate the obstacles to be overcome, and the great need of regular and careful attention. I believe that our best policy is to be honest. Surrounded as these people are by bad climatic influences, and tempted by the good things of life to an unhealthful indulgence, we do wrong to encourage them in thinking that they will have no relapses, but we can assure them that these relapses will be much more tractable and easily subdued if their membranes have once been relieved of abnormal conditions.

To get favourable results in chronic catarrhal deafness, it is absolutely necessary that we first, do most thorough nasal work ; second, study habits and environment, correcting all that tend to induce recurring congestions of the membrane ; and third, give persistent treatment to the middle ear and watch the general health.

When all removable causes have been taken care of, and the parts healed, a vapour of camphor and iodine by interrupted jets, applied through the Eustachian catheter, serves well the treble purpose of strengthening relaxed or atrophied membranes, increasing ossicular mobility, and absorbing inflammatory products. These treatments should be gauged according to the individual case in hand. Some every day, some twice a week, but each with the most particular care, using the auscultation tube to make sure that the vapour reaches the tympanic cavity until the relaxed blood vessels are toned up, and we cease to get more improvement in the hearing.

A rest from active treatment can then be permitted, but the patient should be instructed to report again at the office as soon as an increase in deafness is noted. These periods of rest may become longer and longer until three to six months are allowed.

An interesting feature is that many times after these periods of rest, we can press the improvement further than at our previous attempts seemed possible, and to a point where the disease is surely under control or good hearing established. Protracted effort with the stimulating vapour is a great aid in this last portion of the treatment and we find that Nature's power to regenerate membrane and function is truly wonderful if tonic applications are steadily made.

Chronic catarrhal deafness in itself is not so formidable a disease, but the fact that the patient is adding to it so many days in each year is why we are baffled.

We must not expect too much improvement in hearing during or soon after the nasal operative stage, for there may still remain very sensitive nasal and tubal membranes, dependent often on some disorder of the general system that requires careful attention before we can get our vapours well into the middle ear, but if we keep courage and follow the above plan we will find that eighty per cent. of those that have been given an unfavourable prognosis, because they failed to improve from a six or eight weeks' course of sprays and inflation, can be taken up and very satisfactory results obtained.

I would plead for a more sanguine, a more regular, and a more persistent treatment and observation of these patients. It is true that we may temporarily have to assume the attitude of a medical adviser and perhaps exhaust some energy in teaching them personal hygiene, but I doubt if we as Aurists, discharge our full obligation if we look only at the surgical aspect of the case. They are in desperate straits, looking to us for help, and we must have a broad conception of our duties. Instead of sending them away in a state of resigned discouragement to become the prey of some quack, let us show them that Otological progress in this the last of the 19th century allows a more favourable prognosis in the dawn of the 20th.

In an article by the Author before the American Rhinological, Laryngological and Otological Society, May, 1898, under the title

"Modern Possibilities in Chronic Catarrhal Deafness," detailed reports of the time required and methods used in some obstinate cases, representing three distinct ages and periods in life, were made. Quoting from the same I would again say :—

"The question does not seem to be so much whether we have an atrophic or hypertrophic condition, but did the deafness primarily occur as a catarrhal inflammation, or is there so much fixation of the ossicles as to preclude a possibility of relief except through operative work on the auditory structures.

"If examination shows that the trouble be a catarrhal process, each year's added experience has given us more courage to make a favourable prognosis.

"Many practitioners are opposed to the treatment of deafness in particular, and catarrhal affection in general. This influence is felt in families, and in those cases where prompt, energetic measures are imperative, may become pernicious. Their opposition is honest, and comes from the unfavourable prognosis given by authorities for whom they and the Author have great respect. We maintain that the conclusions of these authorities were based on experiences obtained under auspices much less favourable than the present ; their every effort on the ear was hampered by recurring catarrhal inflammations, which to-day we can in a great measure control."

DR. LEWIS TAYLOR expressed his appreciation of the paper just read, believing it to be one of the most important we had heard. The important point to be considered was the length of time necessary for treatment. These patients came to us with a disease existing for many years. They wanted to be cured at once. When asked the length of time needed for treatment in cases of catarrhal deafness, we should say promptly that it was a question of a lifetime. The conditions causing these troubles continued, therefore every year, or often every year, a certain amount of treatment should be followed.

Many cases were due to climatic conditions, these conditions also continued. So we could say to our patients " so long as you live in a climate causing such trouble you must expect that trouble to continue." As to treatment, one word expressed much, cleanliness.

Cleanliness of the nasal passages by antiseptic sprays, cleanliness of life and habits, and care of the general health. He believed the treatment of catarrhal conditions in children was entirely too much neglected. We should begin early, and continue carefully so long as needed.

DR. C. R. HOLMES : The subject which Dr. Snow has so carefully presented is well worthy of our most careful attention, because the affection is so universal, especially in the United States. The symptoms being as a rule slight, and seldom associated with much if any severe pain, the patient is more likely to neglect himself till the pathological changes are well advanced. As well stated by Dr. Taylor, the patients must be informed that a cure cannot be accomplished in a few weeks or months, but must be a matter of a lifetime, and that his mode of living will, in a great measure, determine whether or not the disease shall be controlled.

Sur la Mobilisation et l'extraction de l'étrier.

Dr. Garnault, Paris.

Monsieur le Président, Messieurs : Je veux, au sujet de cette opération que j'ai faite actuellement 107 fois depuis cinq ans, par la voie que j'ai définitivement adoptée : décollement du conduit membraneux, ablation du mur de l'attique et évidement de la paroi postérieure du conduit osseux, suture immédiate de la plaie après l'opération, tamponnement par le conduit, vous parler plus spécialement de deux cas qui me paraissent d'un grand intérêt, en raison des résultats obtenus, de la nature de l'affection traitée, et des circonstances qui s'y rapportent.

Le premier cas est celui d'un malade actuellement âgé de 72 ans, M. Rondeau, opéré par moi au mois de Novembre 1896. Au dire du malade, la dureté de l'ouïe pour le côté opéré, remontait en arrière à une trentaine d'années, et sa surdité était devenue très forte depuis 15 ans. Une grosse montre, qui est entendue par une personne normale à 8 ou 9ᵐ n'était plus entendue par la voie de l'air, au voisinage immédiat de l'oreille ; par contre elle était très bien entendue par la voie crânienne, ainsi que des montres notablement plus faibles. De l'autre côté, cette même montre était entendue à 30 ct. La voix chuchotée n'est pas même entendue dans le voisinage immédiat de l'oreille. Pour la voix ordinaire, le malade ne la comprend que si on lui parle très fort et très près de l'oreille.

L'épreuve de Rinne, avec le diapason, est très nettement négative. Le tympan ne présente aucune trace de suppuration ancienne ou récente.

J'ai enlevé le pansement intérieur au bout de 8 jours, les suites opératoires furent excellentes, puisque le malade pouvait se promener dès le 3ᵉ jour ce qui est la règle pour les malades qui ne sont pas trop éprouvés par le chloroforme.

Je trouvai un étrier assez mobile, son muscle tenseur, normal, ne fut pas sectionné. Je mobilisai encore l'étrier, en lui faisant subir des mouvements d'oscillation, au moyen d'une petite palette. Dès que le pansement interne fut enlevé l'audition fut portée à 25 cent. L'audition pour la voix chuchotée fut portée à 3 mètres. Par la suite, l'audition pour la montre à pu monter à 35 cent. et l'audition pour la voix a été également augmentée. En somme, l'amélioration pour la voix a été proportionnellement plus considérable que pour la montre. C'est plus souvent le contraire qui se produit, surtout dans les cas où l'étrier est assez mobile. Depuis cette époque, l'audition de l'autre oreille a continué à s'abaisser progressivement, aujourd'hui elle ne sert plus à rien, et le malade, qui est très mélomane, peut entendre la musique au théâtre et même le dialogue, s'il est convenablement placé, uniquement avec son oreille opérée. M. Rondeau avait subi un traitement par la douche d'air près d'un spécialiste de Paris, M. le Dr. Ménière* sans aucun résultat. M. Rondeau fut nettement détourné de tout traitement ultérieur, de toute intervention, par les médecins qui l'ont soigné.

Le second malade dont je veux vous parler, est Mlle. Lem..., âgée de 40 ans, qui se trouve actuellement près de nous, dans le " Examination Hall," et que je désire instamment soumettre à votre examen direct. Elle a subi en Juillet 1897 la mobilisation de l'étrier du côté droit et en Juillet 1898 l'extraction de ce même osselet du côté gauche. C'est un cas d'otite sèche, à forme progressive, sans que jamais se soit produit aucune suppuration ; il semble même n'avoir jamais existé de catarrhe. L'épreuve de Rinne est fortement négative des deux côtés, la perception crânienne pour les montres, même petites, est bonne. MM. les Drs. Natier et Lubet-Barbon, qui furent consultés, détournèrent la malade de tout traitement, de toute intervention et ne lui laissèrent aucun espoir. Au moment où j'opérai le côté droit, la grosse montre était entendue à 20 centm. Je trouvai l'étrier fortement ankylosé, les tentatives de mobilisation n'aboutirent qu'à la rupture des branches. Je fis la circoncision de la platine de l'étrier avec une palette tranchante, sans grand espoir d'avoir produit un résultat effectif, car il s'agissait évidemment ici d'une ankylose osseuse. M. Gellé et moi avons signalé presque simultanément, il y a plusieurs années, à la Société de Biologie qu'un degré très élevé d'audition était compatible avec l'ankylose osseuse de l'étrier. J'ai en effet trouvé dans mes opérations bien des cas d'étrier ankylosé, où l'audition après l'opération était beaucoup meilleure que dans des cas à étrier mobile. L'épreuve de Rinne et la perception crânienne du son de la montre étant égales d'ailleurs. C'est pour ces raisons que je n'attache, plus, pour déterminer s'il y a lieu d'opérer, une grande importance aux épreuves, d'ailleurs incertaines, qui ont pour but de déterminer le degré de mobilité de l'étrier.

Chez ma malade, l'audition pour la montre passa, dès l'extraction du tampon intérieur, de 20 ct. à 1 m. 50 ct. et s'est très régulièrement maintenue aux environs de ce chiffre avec de faibles alternatives. Les bourdonnements, qui étaient assez gênants, ont complètement disparu depuis l'opération. Encouragée par ce premier résultat, la malade fit opérer l'oreille gauche, qui cependant entendait la montre à 1 mètre, le 7 Juillet 1898. L'étrier que je m'attendais à trouver très ankylosé. comme celui de l'autre côté, céda au premier contact énergique, et son extraction fut suivie de l'écoulement du liquide labyrinthique. Aussitôt après l'opération, se manifesta du vertige, mais assez léger, et qui disparut complètement au bout de trois semaines. A l'ablation du pansement intérieur, l'audition était nulle ; elle reparut, excellente, un seul jour, le 30 août, disparut et reparut à nouveau le 24 Sept., à ce moment elle dépassait 3 mètres. L'amélioration pour la voix était très considérable. Au bout de 5 jours chute de l'audition, puis à partir du commencement d'Octobre, se manifestèrent des alternatives d'audition très médiocres et d'audition excellente. Lorsque je revis le 14 Mai 99 cette malade, après une longue absence, elle présentait une audition de 5 mètres, 5½, et même 6 mètres, pour ma montre dans les meilleurs moments, 40 cent. seulement dans les pires. Ces alternatives, qui ont été déjà observées et signalées par Kessel, dans des conditions semblables, sont brusques, rien ne les fait prévoir, elles ne semblent obéir à aucune loi et on ne voit pas la relation qu'elles pourraient avoir avec les causes ordinaires de la congestion de l'oreille. La malade a marqué très soigneusement sur

---

* Si pour ce malade, ainsi que pour le suivant. je cite expressement les médecins qu'ils ont consultés, c'est pour que l'on puisse vérifier dans les notes médicales, qui ont été certainement conservées l'exactitude de mes observations, au sujet du degré de la surdité.

des calendriers que je fais passer sous vos yeux, les bons jours, par des traits noirs. M. Gellé que j'appelai en consultation, en mai dernier, fut comme moi d'avis qu'il s'agissait de phenomènes vasomoteurs se développant sous l'influence de la moindre cause dans un organe irrité et mal guéri, qu'il fallait appliquer des toniques nerveux et assurer d'une façon définitive l'assèchement de l'oreille. En effet, si jamais les deux oreilles n'avaient présenté d'écoulement depuis l'époque de l'opératio n, cependant à l'occasion d'un voyage que fit la malade pour venir d'Algérie en France, l'oreille gauche présenta un écoulement séreux plutôt que purulent, et dépourvu de fétidité. J'instituai un traitement électrique, je fis du massage externe et des applications d'alcool fort à l'intérieur. La malade eut d'abord une période de 15 jours excellente et sans interruption. Mais bientôt se produisit une inflammation profonde du conduit membraneux qui débuta en avant et se propagea en arrière entrai ant un suintement assez abondant du fond de l'oreille et un abaissement notable de l'audition ; et à partir de ce moment les bons jours se firent rares ainsi qu'en témoigne le calendrier. J'espère qu'ils reviendront lorsque l'irritation de l'oreille sera calmée, mais d'ores et déjà je tiendrais infiniment Messieurs à recueillir vos avis sur les causes des phénomènes et sur les moyens d'y remédier.

J'ai chosi ces cas typiques pour vous en parler avec détails ; mais chez beaucoup d'autres malades, dont l'histoire est à mon avis plus banale, j'ai obtenu des résultats aussi bons et même meilleurs dont quel-ques uns se maintiennent depuis 4 et même 5 ans. Plusieurs de ces cas favorables sont connus du Dr. Luc qui se trouve ici, notamment celui de M. Chap. d'Auray, opéré en novembre dernier et chez lequel l'étrier a été enlevé sans que cette opération ait été suivie ni de surdité immédiate ni de vertiges ; de Mdlle. P. de Tours, malade du Dr. Luc qu'il m'a chargé d'opérer et dont l'audition est passée de 15 à 75 centimètres. Et Messieurs, je veux ici rendre d'une façon très spéciale mon hommage de gratitude et d'affection (il me permettra ce mot) à notre éminent con-frère Luc. Sachant combien j'ai à cœur de mettre au jour tous les résultats que peut donner cette méthode d'opération, il m'a fait, chose rare, opérer ses propres malades, sa sympathie m'a soutenu et si, dans ces tentatives, il faut le dire aussi hautement, nous n'avons pas toujours rencontré la victoire, nous n'avons pas renoncé à l'espoir de pouvoir un jour mieux préciser dans quel cas il faut combattre, dans quel cas s'abstenir.*

Bien que l'ankylose osseuse de l'étrier ne soit pas un obstacle absolu à l'audition, il est certain que dans ces cas où la plaque qui forme le plancher de la fenêtre ovale est très épaissie, au point même de remplir presque la fenêtre ovale dans certains cas, il y a lieu de penser, qu'en perforant cet obstacle on améliora l'audition, lorsque la perception crânienne est bien conservée. M. Panse n'est guère satisfait des résultats obtenus. M. Faraci l'est beaucoup plus. Quant à moi, les deux tenta-tives que j'ai faites ont donné les résultats les plus médiocres, bien que

---

* Au moment ou je corrige ces épreuves (20 mars 1900) je revois Mlle P., malgré plusieurs poussées récentes d'influenza, elle entend à 1m. 25 ma montre ; c'est là je pense une reponse triomphale aux adversaires de l'operation.

j'aie cependant obtenu une amélioration passagère.   Peut-être mon insuccès, que je crois pouvoir attribuer en partie au développement d'un bouchon fibreux très épais dans le trou opératoire est il dû en partie également à une manière défectueuse d'opérer, au moyen d'un excavateur de dentiste.

Voici quels sont les principaux desiderata et les principales conclusions qui se présentent à mon esprit.   1° on peut, dans certains cas favorables d'otite sèche, à évolution lente, même invétérés, même héréditaires, et chez lesquels la diminution de l'acuité auditive, peut être très considérable, obtenir des résultats extrêmement favorables pour l'audition, par la mobilisation ou l'extraction de l'étrier.   Mon expérience prouve déjà qu'ils peuvent se maintenir au moins cinq années. 2°. J'estime que la meilleure façon d'opérer est celle que j'emploie depuis cinq ans, qui consiste à décoller le conduit membraneux, à faire sauter à la gouge le mur de l'attique, à évider la paroi postérieur du conduit osseux, puis aussitôt après l'opération suturer complètement les lèvres de la plaie.   Chez une personne saine sans trace de scrofulose, de tuberculose, et de syphilis, cette opération, en somme simple et sans gravité, guérit très rapidement.   Cependant, je le reconnais facilement, il peut se produire un suintement séreux et même purulent, des granulations et des brides cicatricielles.   Je ne dirai pas avec Stacke que l'évolution de l'opération est sous la seule dépendance des soins antiseptiques employés pendant l'opération, et de la perfection avec laquelle ont été pratiqués les pansements.   Mais ces conditions ont assurément une très grande importance.   Il y a des opérés qui suppureront malgré tous les soins que l'on peut prendre, d'autres qui guériront avec une extrême facilité. Stacke dit expressement que si on réussit à faire utilement pour la surdité des interventions opératoires dans l'oreille moyenne, c'est son procédé que l'on devra employer ; en effet les opérations de plus en plus précises, fines et délicates que nous faisons sur les fenêtres, ne peuvent, à mon avis se faire justement, avec la précision et la sûreté nécessaires, que si l'on opère par cette voie, au grand jour, dans un champ opératoire largement ouvert.   Dans bien des cas, l'étrier est caché derrière le bord de la paroi postérieure du conduit complètement ou en partie, et on est toujours gêné par l'exiguité du champ, la difficulté d'y opérer en s'éclairant et l'obstacle que crée le moindre épanchement sanguin. Assurément le mode opératoire que je préconise, produit une réaction plus vive et plus durable des organes profonds, mais ces phénomènes le plus souvent passent assez vite et il est bien douteux que chez ces malades, où l'opération n'améliore pas l'audition, toute autre méthode opératoire eut pu arriver à ce but.   Enfin, dans certains cas d'otite sèche, où les organes nerveux sont intacts et ne réagissent pas, je crois que l'irritation déterminée par cette méthode opératoire, lutte, au moins pour un certain temps, contre l'évolution du processus de sclérose.

3° Quels sont les cas qu'il faut opérer ?   C'est là la grosse question, le grand desideratum, et j'avoue qu'après avoir cherché avec le plus grand soin à résoudre cette question pendant plus de deux ans, j'ai été ensuite pris de découragement. Des, cas qui me parraissaient devoir donner des résultats excellents en ont donné de bien médiocres; d'autres, au contraire, sur lesquels je fondais peu d'espoir, en ont donné d'excellents. Il est nécessaire pour opérer que l'épreuve de Rinne soit très fortement négative, et que la perception crânienne pour la montre soit très bien conservée. Nous disons, au moins pratiquement, que ces signes indiquent l'intégrité des nerfs acoustiques. Il y a beaucoup à dire à ce sujet, mais ce ne sont pas ces moyens qui nous indiqueront comment réagira le malade. La vérité est que quelques cas (un petit nombre à la vérité) de ce genre, ont donné un résultat médiocre. Cependant il y a un très grand intérêt à préciser cette question qui dépend encore trop du flair clinique de l'opérateur. Je n'ai pas encore une expérience suffisante pour dire quand on doit enlever ou seulement mobiliser l'étrier.

4° Résultats. Je n'ai pas les éléments suffisants pour établir à l'heure actuelle une statistique scientifique de mes opérations, mais il est définitivement acquis que l'on peut obtenir des résultats très favorables pour l'audition et les bourdonnements : les résultats peuvent aussi être médiocres. M. Luc en connait de ce genre parmi les malades qu'il a bien voulu me faire opérer; en tout cas, la probité du médecin est strictement engagée à mettre le malade au courant de la question.

Je crois que cette conclusion éclectique mettra beaucoup de gens d'accord; il s'est en effet formé deux camps, dans les uns se rangent ceux qui contestent toute valeur à cette opération, dans l'autre, ceux qui prétendent qu'elle réussit toujours, que l'on peut actuellement préciser d'une façon certaine les conditions dans lesquelles elle doit réussir; la vérité est dans le troisième camp, qui, je l'espère, sera bientôt le plus nombreux.

OTITE MOYENNE SUPPURÉE AVEC THROMBOSE DU SINUS LATÉRAL, ET ABCÈS DU CERVELET. ÉVIDEMENT DU ROCHER. MISE À NU DU SINUS. LIGATURE DE LA JUGULAIRE SUIVIE DE L'OUVERTURE DU SINUS. PONCTIONS DU CERVEAU ET DU CERVELET À LA RECHERCHE D'UN ABCÈS. MORT DE LA MALADE : À L'AUTOPSIE, ABCÈS CÉRÉBELLEUX.

DR. GEORGES LAURENS, Paris.

Le cas que j'ai observé m'a paru digne d'être relaté au triple point de vue de la symtomatologie; du traitement chirurgical que j'ai appliqué, traitement qui a été logique, rationnel, mais insuffisant; de l'examen anatomo-pathologique qui l'a suivi et qui déroutant complètement la clinique a confirmé la succession des actes opératoires.

Nous savons tous les difficultés de diagnostic des complications crànio-cérébrales des otites et nous poserions volontiers le schème suivant, autant qu'il est possible toutefois de faire rentrer la chirurgie dans une formule. Nous distinguons 3 cas : 1. Le diagnostic de la lésion est ferme, presque mathématique. 2. Il est incertain et douteux. 3. Il est impossible.

A cette triple formule clinique peut correspondre le corollaire chirurgical suivant : dans le premier cas, l'otologiste va droit au but, dans le second, il se laisse surtout guider par les lésions, dans le troisième enfin il doit être explorateur et rien de ce qui est mastoïdien ne doit rester étranger à sa gouge et à son maillet.

C'est dans cette dernière variété clinique et thérapeutique que rentre l'histoire de ma malade et dont voici le résumé :—

Femme àgée de 48 ans, entrée à l'hôpital Saint-Antoine dans un service de médecine le 9 avril 1899 pour un abattement général et une céphalalgie diffuse.

Le lendemain, 10 avril, elle est examinée pour la première fois par M. Lermoyez. Sa température est de 39°. Elle repose dans le décubitus dorsal, dans une demi-prostration dont on la tire cependant assez facilement, mais elle répond aux questions qu'on lui pose pour retomber ensuite dans sa somnolence. On apprend qu'elle a une otorrhée ancienne du côté gauche, tarie depuis quinze jours, et c'est de l'arrêt de cet écoulement que date la céphalalgie.

Localement on trouve l'oreille droite normale, l'oreille gauche est remplie de pus fétide ; la caisse est bourrée de fongosités. L'apophyse n'est ni douloureuse à la pression ni tuméfiée. Les mouvements de la tête s'exécutent normalement. Mais la pression du doigt éveille une douleur vive en deux points : l'un à la partie supérieure du triangle pharyngo-maxillaire, l'autre dans la région rétro-mastoïdienne : en ces deux points, un peu d'empâtement profond, mais pas de fluctuation. L'exploration du cou ne dénote rien de particulier sur le trajet de la veine jugulaire gauche.

Dans le cours de cet examen, la malade accuse une douleur de tête violente localisée surtout à la région occipitale et au vertex, et elle est prise de baillements continuels. Pas de troubles de la sensibilité ni de la motilité des membres, mais exagération des réflexes rotuliens et légère trépidation épileptoïde. Pas de diplopie ni de troubles oculo-moteurs, les pupilles réagissent à la lumière ; l'examen ophthalmoscop-ique n'a pas été pratiqué. L'examen des viscères montre leur intégrité parfaite : il n'y a eu ni vomissements ni constipation.

Il est donc permis, en présence de ce tableau symptomatique, de rattacher à l'oreille les accidents cérébraux, mais à quel ordre appar-tiennent-ils ? On hésite entre méningite et complication sinusale. A vrai dire, je ne cherche pas à approfondir les finesses d'un diagnostic bien difficile dans le cas particulier, le temps presse, l'état cérébral est grave, il y a de toute évidence une complication endo-crânienne à rechercher d'une manière urgente et j'insiste vivement pour ouvrir l'apophyse de la malade. Celle-ci refuse d'abord, accepte ensuite, mais des considérations d'ordre particulier surgissent, qui font différer l'intervention.

Aussi le lendemain, la situation s'aggravait, la température était de 40° le soir, 38° le matin, la prostration était complète, la malade ne pouvait répondre et c'est à peine si elle pouvait ouvrir les yeux quand elle entendait parler. On constatait une parésie du facial inférieur gauche. Le pouls était un peu petit, mais régulier et à 100. Ce jour-là encore, il est impossible d'opérer.

Le lendemain seulement, 12 avril, trois jours après l'entrée de la malade à l'hôpital, l'autorisation est donnée d'intervenir. Mais alors, les accidents se sont précipités et le dénouement ne paraît plus qu'une question d'heures. Le coma est absolu, il y a incontinence des réservoirs, le pouls est filiforme, à 120. La température est de 40°. Même douleur à la pression, au niveau des points précités et qui provoque de légers mouvements de défense.

Malgré cet état général alarmant, que tous pensent à une méningite d'origine auriculaire, je fais la part possible d'une erreur de diagnostic et me décide à l'opération. Avant de prendre le bistouri, je me trace la conduite suivante : ouvrir l'apophyse et la caisse, aller ensuite droit au sinus, si le vaisseau est reconnu sain, défoncer les parois supérieure et postérieure de l'antre et explorer le cerveau et le cervelet.

Dans un premier temps opératoire, je trépane la mastoïde au lieu d'élection : l'os est dur, éburné et la gouge me mène sur le sinus qui est logé dans toute l'apophyse, et se met en contact intime avec la paroi postérieure du conduit : le vaisseau est très volumineux. En présence de cette apophyse scléreuse, je prends un fin burin et sculpte l'antre qui est extrêmement petit, profond et du volume d'un pois. A la curette j'enlève le pus, les fongosités et les amas caséeux et fétides qui le remplissent, puis faisant sauter la paroi externe de l'aditus je pénètre dans la caisse, en extrais les osselets cariés, les polypes et débris putrides qu'elle renferme et termine par la toilette de cette portion évidée du rocher. En aucun point du squelette je n'avais trouvé de déhiscence, de fistule ou de région cariée qui communiquât avec la cavité crânienne.

Donc, ou bien le sinus seul était en cause, ou il existait une complication endo-crânienne, à distance, indépendante du foyer mastoïdien : peut-être que les deux ordres de lésions coexistaient.

Je résolus donc : 1, d'explorer le sinus, 2, de mettre à nu la dure-mère au niveau du cerveau et du cervelet, de l'inciser si je ne trouvais pas d'abcès extra-dural et de ponctionner les deux organes encéphaliques.

Revenant donc au sinus latéral, je trouvais sa paroi bleu violacée, de coloration normale. Pas d'abcès péri-sinusal. Le vaisseau ne présentait aucune pulsation, il était assez dépressible. Plusieurs ponctions avec la seringue de Pravaz ne ramènent pas de sang ; quand l'aiguille est retirée, le liquide s'écoule en bavant du point ponctionné et non pas avec un jet abondant et sous pression comme on l'observe quand le sinus est sain. Devant cette thrombose oblitérante, je me prépare à ligaturer la jugulaire.

Je liais donc la veine, facilement : elle n'était pas thrombosée, je fis un pansement cervical au collodion et revins au sinus que j'incisais suivant sa longueur et sur une étendue de deux centimètres. J'enlevais des caillots et tamponnais.

J'avais donc constaté une thrombose partielle du sinus, mais insuffisante pour expliquer les troubles cérébraux observés. Il était donc de toute nécessité de pénétrer dans la cavité crânienne et d'explorer cerveau et cervelet. La route était toute indiquée : entrer dans le cerveau par la paroi supérieure de l'antre, dans le cervelet par sa paroi postérieure. Malheureusement cette voie simple, commode, sus-attico-antrale, et que j'ai l'habitude de suivre m'était fermée par le tamponnement du sinus qui avait saigné abondamment et dont l'hémorrhagie avait nécessité l'emploi d'une mèche qui absorbait tout le puits mastoïdien.

Aussi, pour aborder le cerveau, partant du sinus avec la pince-gouge, je morcelais un large fossé crânien me conduisant à un demi-centimètre au-dessus de l'antre. Dans ce trajet, la dure-mère était saine. Ayant ainsi réalisé une sorte de trépanation sus-attico-antrale, j'incisais la méninge en croix et ponctionnais avec le bistouri le cerveau dans trois directions, en avant, en arrière, en dedans. Aucune goutte de liquide ne sortit par l'orifice ponctionné.

Me dirigeant en bas, sous le sinus, toujours avec la pince-gouge, je mis à nu la dure-mère cérébelleuse, saine comme la précédente. J'enfonçai le bistouri dans la profondeur du cervelet, en dedans, en avant en arrière : la ponction fut blanche.

Ayant épuisé la série des interventions, ne trouvant ni phlébite du sinus, ni abcès extra-dural, ni collection suppurée intra-encéphalique, je pensais que le diagnostic qu'on avait posé de méningite était exact et croyant à la méningite suppurée de la base, je fis un lavage du cerveau, et du cervelet, voulant tenter dans la cavité encéphalique et avec la grande séreuse intra-crânienne ce qu'en chirurgie abdominale on pratique dans les péritonites.

Par les deux incisions dure-mériennes je fis pénétrer le bec d'une canule adaptée à un bock à irrigation et je lavai l'hémisphère cérébral et cérébelleux avec un litre d'eau tiède bouillie. Cette irrigation ne ramena ni sérosité, ni pus, mais fut bien tolérée par la malade : il n'y eut aucune modification du rythme respiratoire, le pouls monta il est vrai à 160, mais il me fut difficile de rapporter cette ascension au lavage ou à l'injection de sérum que j'avais fait pratiquer.

En terminant, en effet, le récit de cette observation, j'ajouterai que l'opération qui dura une heure et demie ne put être pratiquée qu'avec une anesthésie modérée. Pendant toute sa durée, on faisait une injection continue de sérum artificiel, des injections sous-cutanées d'éther et de caféine ; grâce à tous ces moyens, à la faible dose de chloroforme employé seulement au début et au moment de la ligature de la jugulaire, le choc opératoire fut réduit à sa plus simple expression. Mais la malade ne sortit pas du coma et mourut quatre heures après l'intervention.

L'autopsie devait révéler une surprise : aucune trace de méningite, mais un abcès de l'hémisphère du cervelet correspondant à la lésion otique, abcès volumineux, antéro-inférieur, bien enkysté avec membrane pyogénique. La face postérieure du rocher était normale, pas de plaque de méningite, pas de carie osseuse.

La moralité que je tirais personellement de ce cas fut d'abord une satisfaction d'être intervenu par une série d'actes opératoires qui devaient me mener au but, et d'autre part l'ennui de l'avoir manqué. La seule excuse que je pourrais invoquer est la voie suivie pour aborder le cervelet.

Habituellement, pour aborder cet organe, ainsi que le cerveau, je suis la voie sus et rétro-antrale : en faisant sauter le plafond de l'antre et sa paroi postérieure il est facile de rencontrer les deux organes encéphaliques. Dans le cas actuel je dus me frayer un passage sus et sous-sinusal et cette pratique que je ne suis jamais me valut une fausse route.

CLOSING MEETING.

FRIDAY, AUGUST 11TH, AT 3 P.M.

CHAIRMAN   -   PROF. URBAN PRITCHARD.

The PRESIDENT, Prof. Urban Pritchard, opened the Meeting by saying that he was glad to be able to communicate a pleasant fact to all present, viz.:—That an invitation had been received from France to. hold the next Congress there, and that the City of Bordeaux had been recommended. It was also proposed that the President-Elect should be Dr. Moure, of Bordeaux. This proposition was carried by acclamation.

The President then called upon the Hon. Sec. Gen., MR. CRESSWELL BABER, to read the list of names which it was suggested should form the Organization Committee for the next Congress. They were as follows:—

AMERICA.

Dench,	New York.	Randall,	Philadelphia.
St. John Roosa,	,,	Holmes,	Cincinnati.
H. Knapp,	,,	Pierce,	Chicago.
Clarence Blake,	Boston.	Daly,	Pittsburg.
Orne Greene,	,,	Barkan,	San Francisco.
Goldstein,	St. Louis.	Roaldes,	New Orleans.
Bryan,	Washington.		

AUSTRIA-HUNGARY.

Politzer,	Vienna.	Böke,	Buda-Pesth.
Pollak,	,,	Szenes,	,,
Morpurgo,	Trieste.	Zaufal,	Prague.
Habermann,	Graz.		

BELGIUM.

C. Delstanche,	Brussels.	Coosemans,	Brussels.
Capart,	,,	Delie,	Ypres.
Huguet,		Schiffers,	Liege.
Goris,		Eeman,	Ghent.

British Empire.

Arthur Cheatle,	London.	Cresswell Baber,	Brighton.
A. E. Cumberbatch,	,,	W. Milligan,	Manchester.
Sir W. Dalby,		A. Bronner,	Bradford.
G. P. Field,		D. R. Paterson,	Cardiff.
Dundas Grant,		George Stone,	Liverpool.
W. Hill,		P. McBride,	Edinburgh.
Jobson Horne,		Thomas Barr,	Glasgow.
Macnaughton Jones,	,,	A. W. Sandford,	Cork.
E. Law,		C. E. FitzGerald,	Dublin.
Urban Pritchard,	,,	J. W. Barrett,	Melbourne, Aus.
St. Clair Thomson,	,,	Birkett,	Montreal, Canada.

Denmark.

Schmiegelow,	Copenhagen.	Holger Mygind,	Copenhagen.

France.

Chatellier,	Paris.	Lermoyez,	Paris.
De la Charrière,	,,	Lubet-Barbon,	,,
Gellé,		Loewenberg,	,,
Ménière,		Gougenheim,	,,
Baratoux,		Moure,	Bordeaux.
Luc,	,,	Lannois,	Lyons.
Castex,	,,	Noquet,	Lille.

(With power to add to their number).

Germany.

Lucae,	Berlin.	Körner,	Rostock.
Jansen,	,,	Röpke,	Solingen.
Hartmann,	,,	Kirchner,	Wurzburg.
Bezold,	Munich.	Brieger,	Breslau.
Stacke,	Erfurt.	Kümmel,	..
Passow,	Heidelberg.		

Holland.

Guye,	Amsterdam.	Moll,	Arnheim.
Zwaardemaker,	..	Van Anrooij,	Rotterdam.
Meyjes,			

Italy.

Grazzi,	Florence.	Chiucini,	Rome.
Avoledo,	Milan.	De Rossi,	,,
Bobone,	San Remo.	Ferreri,	,,
Brunetti,	Venice.	Cozzolino,	Naples.
Putelli,	,,	Gradenigo,	Turin.
Secchi,	Bologna.	Masini,	Genoa.
Faraci,	Palermo.	Poli,	..

RUSSIA AND POLAND.

Benni,	Wàrsaw.	Stepanoff,	Moscow.
Heiman,	,,	Von Stein,	..
Orloff,	Kieff.	Scott,	
Pietkowski,	Lublin.		

SPAIN.

Sune-y-Molist,	Barcelona.	Sota-y-Lastra,	Seville.
Botey,	,,	Moresco,	Cadiz.
Verdós,	,,	Casanova,	Valencia.
Gonzalez Alvarez,	Madrid.		
Uruñela,	,,		

NORWAY AND SWEDEN.

Uchermann,	Christiania.	Ceterblad,	Stockholm.
Hörbye,	,,	Lagerlöf,	..

SWITZERLAND.

Secretan,	Lausanne.	Schwendt,	Basle.
Rohrer,	Zürich.	Siebenmann,	..

The Committee was appointed.

PROF. POLITZER, President of the Lenval Prize Jury, was next asked to give his report, which he did in the following words —:

"I have the honour in the name of the Jury for the Lenval Prize, elected at the Congress in Florence, to give you our decision on the award of this prize.

The Lenval Prize (Capital 3,000 francs) was founded by Baron de Lenval, at the suggestion of our honoured colleague, Dr. Benni, of Warsaw, in the year 1880, the four years' interest of this sum to be awarded to the author of the most marked progress in the practical treatment of affections of hearing, accomplished since the last Congress, or to the inventor of a new apparatus, easily portable and considerably improving the hearing-power of deaf persons.

The Jury of the Lenval Prize has decided to propose to the Congress that this year the prize shall be awarded to a distinguished Otologist for his instrumental treatment of the affections of the middle ear, by which he has materially improved our methods of treatment in this direction.

It is with the greatest pleasure that I have the honour in the name of the Jury to proclaim the name of our nominee for the Lenval Prize,

DR. CHARLES DELSTANCHE, of Brussels."

On the proposition of the Chairman, this recommendation was carried by acclamation.

PROF. GRAZZI proposed that the President should be requested to send a telegram to Dr. Charles Delstanche announcing the award.

On the proposition of DR. EEMAN, seconded by DR. HARTMANN, it was resolved that the Jury for the Lenval Prize to be awarded at the next Congress consist of the present Jury, with the addition of Dr. Moure, of Bordeaux. The list is as follows :—

Prof. Politzer (Vienna), President.
Dr. Benni (Warsaw).
Dr. Gellé (Paris).
Prof. Pritchard (London).
Prof. St. John Roosa (New York).
Prof. Kirchner (Wurzburg).
Prof. Grazzi (Florence).
Dr. Moure (Bordeaux).

PROF. URBAN PRITCHARD : "This brings us to the end of our business, the thought of which bears with it feelings both of pain and pleasure; pain, because we are parting from many friends ; and pleasure, because of the happy memories which this week will leave behind ; to say nothing of the personal gratification to those of us who are now relieved of the strain of arranging the proceedings. The greatest pleasure of all is that of feeling that everything has gone off so well.

I think, as a rule, the President of a Congress has too large a share of its credit. The President is, after all, but the top stone of a pyramid, no larger, no better than any of the others. To carry forward this simile, we may say that the layer on which this stone rests, fitly represents the other officers of the Congress. First, there is that one to whom we are indebted in a very special way, for does he not hold the purse strings ? I allude, of course, to Mr. Cumberbatch, our good Treasurer. Then comes our great Organizer, Mr. Cresswell Baber, the Secretary General. Again, we have Mr. Field, our Vice-Chairman of the Reception Committee, one who, not content with what he has already done, is yet going to do more for us to-morrow, and his Secretary, Mr. Lake. Then there is the Vice-Chairman of the Dinner Committee, Mr. Mark Hovell, and his Secretary, Mr. Lawrence, who have been working so energetically behind the scenes, and the fruit of whose labours in one department we are to enjoy this evening ; and there are also Dr. Dundas Grant and Mr. Yearsley, to whom we are indebted for the excellent arrangements made for the excursions.

And last, but assuredly not least, there is the Museum Committee. When the idea of the Museum was first mooted, I was delighted, but I was still more delighted when Mr. Ballance undertook the Vice-Chairmanship of the Committee which was appointed to carry it out The thing grew and grew, and finally assumed proportions that entailed a great deal of hard work, the heaviest part of which fell on Mr. Arthur Cheatle and Dr. Jobson Horne. The result has proved well worth the labour however; nor will the good end with the Congress; for the Catalogue remains, a most valuablé work of reference to all Otologists.

This goodly layer of stones is yet resting on a larger base; namely, the Members of the Congress. For unless friends had rallied around us from near and from far, the gathering could not have been a real success in the true sense of the word.

In conclusion, we desire to bespeak your indulgence for all the sins of omission and commission which we know, alas, only too well, have occurred in spite of all our care. Our troubles have arisen chiefly owing to the number of communications received, and I should like to suggest to the Organization Committee of the next Congress, that all communications be printed and circulated before the Meeting, when they might be read only in abstract, thus allowing more time for discussion. I much regret that it was impossible to have any of those papers read that were sent in after time, and even more, that some few had to be omitted which arrived before the closing date.

Before closing the business of our Congress, one or two friends would like to make a few remarks."

PROF. GRAZZI: "When Dr. Delstanche in addressing the closing speech to me at the last Congress, alluded to Dr. Pritchard, he said: 'I hope that the President who will reunite us in London in four years' time, will also meet with unanimous approbation.' I feel sure that the wishes expressed by Delstanche have been fully realized. No one can understand better than I, the feelings of our beloved President. I am sure that his heart beats tumultuously, and that all the cells of his brain are in movement. I am very pleased that the London Congress has greatly surpassed that of Florence, and for this success the honour must be principally accorded to Prof. Urban Pritchard, who has been able to gather round him such a large number of Otologists, great not only in number but also in merit.

"Under the direction of Prof. Pritchard, it has been possible to get together such a collection of preparations, specimens and instruments, as we have never yet seen, and it is a source of sorrow to everybody that this collection must now be dispersed. In a didactic sense especially, it would have been of great importance to have left it intact, and the Museum would have been a most splendid and useful memento of our Congress. Allow me to add that it would also have proved a monument worthy of our President, and one to which I would have given the name of 'The Pritchard Museum.'

"There are other colleagues to speak after me, so I will not occupy much of your time. Only very few words are necessary in which to say that our President, for his knowledge and sympathetic manner merits all our gratitude, having conducted our Meetings so splendidly that we may imitate but cannot surpass him. He must be very pleased that his anxious work has attained such success, and I am quite sure, at this solemn moment, that I am interpreting the grateful expressions of us all, in giving our best thanks to Prof. Pritchard."

DR. BENNI : "Gentlemen—Allow me in the name of the foreign members of your Congress to express all our gratitude and admiration for the detailed, thorough, and in one word, most excellent way in which all the technical difficulties of the Congress, all the manifold necessities of its members have been foreseen, solved, and attended to. Our admiration is sincere, and our gratitude great, to the Organizer and the Organization Committee."

PROF. POLITZER : "Mr. President and Gentlemen—In every Congress there is always one outstanding feature which remains in our memory for ever ; it will, I think, be allowed by every one here present that the outstanding feature of this Congress has been the Museum. I have attended every Otological Congress up to the present, and also seen every important museum in the world, and I do not hesitate to say that I have never before seen such a magnificent and well-organized museum, and I doubt if it will be possible to see such a one again. This result is due to the exertions of Mr. Cheatle, ably assisted by Dr. Jobson Horne. Those of us who have had to arrange specimens in the Museum will join with me in giving unlimited praise to these two gentlemen for their never failing urbanity, their suavity of temper, and their amiable behaviour in the midst of very trying circumstances. I take upon myself to express to these gentlemen the thanks of the Congress for their incessant and indefatigable labours which have so materially helped to render this Congress such a great success."

MR. CRESSWELL BABER, replying for the Organization Committee, thanked Dr. Benni for his kind remarks, and expressed a hope that the results of the Congress would be an encouragement for the future study of Otology.

The President then called upon Mr. Cheatle to make a few remarks.

MR. ARTHUR CHEATLE : "I thank you on behalf of the Museum Sub-Committee for all the many kind expressions towards us. If we have given pleasure we are amply rewarded, and will undertake to do it again if you will only give us a little rest."

THE PRESIDENT : "I thank Prof. Grazzi for his kind words. I hope the Congress has stimulated, and will stimulate us the older ones, and still more the younger ones, to work the harder, both for the science of the subject, and also for that which is its aim, viz., the relief of human suffering, and the saving of human life.

I pronounce the Congress closed."

COMMUNICATIONS NOT READ.

EXPERIMENTELLE UNTERSUCHUNGEN UEBER DAS CORTICALE HOERCENTRUM.

DR. FERDINAND ALT, Vienna.

Nach einer Zusammenstellung der bisher vorliegenden Thierversuche und anatomischen Studien, sowie der klinischen Beobachtungen und der pathologischen Befunde, welche für die Verlegung des corticalen Hörcentrums in den hinteren Bezirk der ersten, beziehungsweise in die hinteren zwei Drittel der ersten und zweiten Schläfenwindung sprechen, berichtet der Vortragende über seine gemeinsam mit dem Privat-docenten Dr. Arthur Biedl ausgeführten experimentellen Untersuch-ungen über das corticale Hörcentrum.

Wir haben unsere Arbeit damit eingeleitet, dass wir bei jungen Hunden einseitige und doppelseitige Zerstörung der Schnecke ausführten und das Verhalten dieser Thiere bei Hörprüfungen neben normal hörenden Hunden genau beobachteten. Später zogen wir zum Vergleiche jene Thiere heran, bei welchen wir die Exstirpation der Rinde eines Schläfenlappens, beider Schläfenlappen oder eines Schläfen-lappens und die Zerstörung der gleichseitigen Schnecke vorgenommen hatten. Als Instrumente zur Hörprüfung wurden herangezogen: Pfeife, Trompete, Harmonika, Galton Pfeife, Ratsche, Glasglocke, Radfahrglocke, und improvisirte Geräusche, so z.B. Hämmern auf einem Blechschirm, Aufwerfen von Metallstücken auf Tische, Detonationsgeräusche durch Zerschlagen unbrauchbar gewordener Glühlampen. Diese mannigfaltigen Hörprüfungsmethoden erwiesen sich als nothwendig und hinreichend. Denn wir konnten uns bald überzeugen, dass normal hörende Hunde sich sehr rasch an einen erzeugten Schallreiz gewöhnten, dass sie mitunter nur das erste oder zweite Mal auf einen gellenden Pfiff stutzten und sich umwandten, das dritte Mal auch nicht die geringste Bewegung des Kopfes oder der Ohren ausführten. Wir konnten uns ferner überzeugen, dass normal hörende Thiere, wenn ihre Aufmerksamkeit durch irgend etwas abgelenkt war, mitunter auch ohne jeden nachweisbaren Grund eine Stunde lang für jeden Schallreiz theilnahmslos blieben, so dass unerfahrene Beobachter leicht gut hörende Thiere für taub gehalten hätten.

Aus allen diesen Umständen können so viele Fehlerquellen erwachsen, dass die geradezu unglaubliche Incongruenz in den Berichten der einzelnen Experimentatoren auf diesem Gebiete einigermassen begreiflich wird. Wir waren bestrebt, durch eine möglichst grosse Reihe von Versuchen und durch 1½ Jahre hindurch fortgesetzte Beobachtungen alle Fehlerquellen zu eliminiren.

Wir haben im ganzen 41 Versuche ausgeführt. Exitus (durch Meningitis und durch Nachblutung) kam im ganzen sechsmal vor. Die Operation wurde unter der peinlichsten Asepsis ausgeführt. An jedem einzelnen Thiere wurden zwei Operationen vorgenommen, entweder Exstirpation der Rinde eines Schläfenlappens und dann des anderen oder einseitige Exstirpation des Schläfenlappens und nachträgliche Zerstörung der gleichseitigen Schnecke. Der Zeitraum zwischen beiden Operationen betrug gewöhnlich vier Wochen. Der Operationsmodus war folgender : —

Durch die Mitte des Musculus temporalis wird ein 6cm. langer Schnitt geführt, der den Muskel in seiner Mitte quer durchtrennt, die beiden Theile des Muskels werden nach aufwärts und abwärts zurückgeschoben und durch Haken fixirt. In dem Schädeldach über dem Schläfenlappen wird mit Hammer und Meissel eine kleine Lücke geschaffen und sodann der ganze Knochen über dem Temporallappen mittelst Kneipzange entfernt. Die Dura wird hierauf sorgfältig über dem ganzen Schläfenlappen abgetragen und die Rinde des ganzen Schläfenlappens in einer Dicke von 2—3 Mm. möglichst parallel zur Oberfläche exstirpirt. Wir gingen nach vorne bis an die Fossa Sylvii, nach rückwärts bis an den Occipitallappen (von dem in vielen Fällen unabsichtlich ein Theil mitentfernt wurde), nach abwärts bis an den Gyrus Hippocampi.

Bei unseren Untersuchungen kam es uns nicht darauf an, durch Exstirpation einzelner Rindenpartien eine genaue Localisation des corticalen Hörcentrums beim Hunde festzustellen, wir gingen vielmehr von der feststehenden Thatsache aus, dass die Rinde des Schläfenlappens als centrale Endausbreitung des Nervus 8 gilt, und suchten durch Exstirpation der ganzen Rinde des Schläfenlappens an einer grossen Zahl von Thieren, die wir durch lange Zeit beobachteten, Erfahrungen zu sammeln, welche der geradezu unglaublichen Incongruenz in den bisher in der Litteratur vorliegenden einschlägigen Beobachtungen ein Ende machen sollten.

Die Zerstörung der Schnecke wurde folgendermassen ausgeführt : Freilegung der Bulla ossea, Entfernung der äusseren Wand derselben mit Hammer und Meissel sowie mittelst Knochenzange, Abbrechen der unteren Schneckenwand durch Zerstörung der Promontorialwand um das runde Fenster herum, Zerstörung der Schnecke durch eingeführte nadelförmige Instrumente. Alle ausgeführten Eingriffe wurden durch die nachträgliche Autopsie der Thiere controllirt beziehungsweise verificirt.

Unsere Versuche waren zunächst darauf gerichtet, die Ausfallser-scheinungen zu studiren, welche bei einseitiger Exstirpation der oben bezeichneten Partien des Schläfenlappens auftreten. Bei Besprechung der beobachteten Ausfallserscheinungen halten wir die Aufzählung der einzelnen Versuche für unzweckmässig und sehen davon ab, erstens, um immerwährende Wiederholungen zu vermeiden, zweitens, um jene Fehler zu eliminiren, die bei der Beobachtung *eines* Thieres unvermeidlich sind. Wir schildern demnach im Folgenden das Ergebnis unserer Beobachtungen, wie es in jedem typischen Falle ausgeprägt war.

Der Hund ist gleich am Tage nach der Operation ganz munter, er läuft umher, frisst und trinkt (nur in einigen wenigen Fällen, in denen wir gelegentlich der Operation auch Theile des Hinterhauptslappens mitnahmen, trat contralaterale Hemiopie ein, das Thier stiess beim Gehen an, ein Symptom, das bald vorüberging).

Der Hund reagirt in den ersten 2 Tagen nach dem Eingriffe auf Schallreize von geringer Intensität, leisen Zuruf, Schnalzen, Pfeifen mit den Lippen gar nicht. Bei Geräuschen von grösserer Intensität, wie durch Pfeife, Harmonika, Ratsche, Galton Pfeife etc., wendete er den Kopf zuerst nach der operirten Seite, selbst wenn sehr intensive Schallreize auf der contralateralen Seite erzeugt wurden. Befand sich die Schallquelle auf der contralateralen Seite, so versuchte das Thier, den Kopf über seinen Rücken hinweg nach der contralateralen Seite zu drehen, wobei Kopf und Hals in eine unnatürliche Stellung gerathen. Wenn man ihm das Ohr der operirten Seite mit Gazestreifen und Watte verschliesst reagirt er auf schwache Schallreize gar nicht, auf starke, sehr schlecht.

Am dritten und vierten Tage wendet der Hund auf Schallreize von der operirten Seite her den Kopf ziemlich prompt nach der Schallrichtung. Dagegen blickt er bei Schallreizen von der contra-lateralen Seite noch immer nach der operirten Seite, stutzt dann, als ob er über die Schallrichtung nicht orientirt wäre, und versucht dann wieder in der oben beschriebenen Weise über seinen Rücken hinweg den Kopf nach der Schallrichtung zu drehen. Wenn wir das Thier an einen Tisch banden und nun von der contralateralen Seite her ein wahres Höllenconcert auf mehreren Instrumenten aufführten, dauerte es oft $\frac{1}{2}$-1 Minute, bis der Hund über die Schallrichtung orientirt war und nach derselben blickte.

Am 5ten und 6ten Tage ist die Reaction auf Schalleinwirkungen von der operirten Seite eine sehr prompte. Bei Schallreizen von der contralateralen Seite verhält sich der Hund noch so, dass er den Kopf nach der operirten Seite wendet, und wenn er sich überzeugt, dass er nach der falschen Richtung blickte, so wendet er den Kopf geradeaus und dann nach der contralateralen Seite.

Schon am 7ten Tage beginnt der Hund, auf Schallreize von der con-tralateralen Seite ziemlich prompt zu reagiren.

Am 9ten Tage ist auch nicht der geringste Unterschied im Hörvermögen für beide Gehörorgane nachweisbar.

Die Resultate dieser Untersuchungen waren sowohl für den linken als für den rechten Schläfenlappen vollkommen übereinstimmende. Wir konnten auch nicht ein einziges Moment ausfindig machen, aus welchem für einen der beiden Schläfenlappen, soweit die bezeichneten Partien in Frage kommen, eine grössere Bedeutung gegenüber dem anderen hervorgehen würde. Liessen wir dem ersten Eingriffe die Abtragung der Rinde des zweiten Schläfenlappens folgen, so konnten wir folgende Beobachtungen anstellen:—Die Thiere zeigten durch 10-12 Tage keinerlei Reaction auf die intensivsten Schallreize, wobei die gleichen Hörprüfungsmethoden zur Anwendung gelangten, wie wir sie eben geschildert haben. Nach dieser Zeit konnte man constatiren, dass die Hunde auf die verschiedensten Geräusche und auf Zuruf nicht reagirten, wohl aber sehr lebhaft erschracken, wenn man plötzlich in ihrer Nähe einen sehr intensiven Schallreiz, z.B. ein Detonationsgeräusch oder starkes Hämmern auf einen Ofenschirm, erzeugte. Die Thiere fuhren erschreckt zusammen und blickten nach der Schallrichtung. Von Tag zu Tag konnten wir eine Besserung des Hörvermögens wahrnehmen, und zwar in der Weise, dass immer weniger intensive Geräusche erforderlich waren, um eine Hörreaction auszulösen.

So konnten wir nach 3-4 Tagen wahrnehmen, dass die Hunde stutzten, wenn man eine Radfahrglocke läutete oder mit einem Holzstab eine Glasglocke anschlug.

Schon am 20ten Tage merkten die Hunde Zuruf.

Der 24te Tag nach der Exstirpation des zweiten Schläfenlappens war der längste Termin, wo noch Spuren einer trägeren Reaction auf Schallreize nachweisbar waren.

Von da ab verhielten sich die Hunde ebenso empfindlich für jede Schalleinwirkung wie normal hörende Thiere.

Wir gelangen nun zu jenen Versuchen, welche darin bestanden, dass wir bei Hunden zunächst die Schnecke eines Gehörorgans in der geschilderten Weise zerstörten und sodann die Rinde des gleichseitigen Schläfenlappens exstirpirten (meist nach vier Wochen, mitunter auch unmittelbar im Anschlusse an den ersten Eingriff).

Die Thiere waren am Tage nach der Operation ganz munter, nur zeigten sie öfter Coordinationsstörungen, die wohl auf eine Mitverletzung der Bogengänge zu beziehen waren. (Der Kopf war nach der contralateralen Seite und nach unten gedreht, der Gang war unsicher, namentlich beim Wenden und Umkehren).

Bei Hörprüfungen erwiesen sich die Thiere durch mehrere Tage völlig taub für alle Schalleindrücke. Dieser Zustand hielt in einzelnen Fällen bis zum 5ten, in anderen bis zum 7ten Tage an. Von da ab konnte bei sehr intensiven, plötzlich einwirkenden Schallreizen in unmittelbarer Nähe der Thiere (Ratsche, Detonation) eine deutliche Hörreaction

nachgewiesen werden, die sich durch erschrecktes Zusammenfahren der
Thiere manifestirte.

In ganz analoger Weise, wie wir es oben für die beiderseitige
Exstirpation der Rinde des Schläfenlappens schilderten, steigerten sich
die Hörspuren von Tag zu Tag, so dass immer weniger intensive
Geräusche erförderlich waren, um von der contralateralen Seite her
percipirt zu werden. Spätestens am 12ten Tage waren wir zu der
Annahme berechtigt, dass das Hörvermögen für das contralaterale Ohr
ein vollständig normales war.

Die von MUNK an Hunden ausgeführten, eingangs erwähnten
Versuche bei denen durch partielle Exstirpation der Horsphäre ein
bestimmtes Centrum für die Perception hoher und tiefer Töne ermittelt
worden sein soll, haben wir einer Nachprüfung nicht unterzogen,
obwohl wir zu diesem Zwecke ein eigenes musikalisches Instrumentarium
bereit hielten.   Es erschien uns nämlich nach den Erfahrungen, die wir
bei unzähligen Hörprüfungen gewannen, ganz und gar ausgeschlossen,
diesbezüglich irgendwelche einwandfreie Resultate bei Hunden zu
gewinnen.   Wir müssen vielmehr annehmen, dass bei allen einschlägigen Beobachtungen manche Fehlerquellen von MUNK nicht eliminirt
wurden.

Wenn wir die aus unserer Arbeit sich ergebenden Thatsachen
hervorheben, so müssen wir zunächst betonen, dass die Ausfallser-
scheinungen nach Exstirpation der Horsphäre eines Schläfenlappens
vollkommen übereinstimmende sind, sowohl für den rechten als für den
linken Schläfenlappen, dass wir demnach, soweit die bezeichneten
Partien in Frage kommen, kein Moment ausfindig machen konnten,
welches einem der beiden Temporallappen gegenüber dem anderen eine
grössere Bedeutung vindiciren würde.   Wir müssen ferner hervorheben,
dass nach Exstirpation der Rinde eines Schläfenlappens, die Thiere in
den ersten 2 Tagen nach dem Eingriffe auf Schallreize von geringer
Intensität garnicht reagirten, wohl aber auf solche von grösserer
Intensität.

Die Analysirung der bestehenden Schwerhörigkeit ergab, dass nach
einseitiger Exstirpation beide Gehörorgane in Mitleidenschaft gezogen
werden, das gleichnamige Ohr in unbedeutendem Grade (die Schwerhörigkeit schwand nach 2 Tagen vollkommen), das contralaterale Ohr
in ungleich höherem Grade.

Die Ausfallserscheinungen, welche das contralaterale Gehörorgan
betreffen, konnten wir genau beobachten in der zunächst auftretenden
völligen Taubheit, die in der geschilderten Weise einer hochgradigen
Schwerhörigkeit Platz macht, um sich dann vollkommen zu verlieren,
so dass schon am 9ten Tage auch nicht der geringste Unterschied im
Hörvermögen für beide Gehörorgane nachweisbar ist.

Noch deutlicher manifestirt sich diese Beziehung, wenn man zunächst
die Zerstörung einer Schnecke ausführt und dieser die Exstirpation des

gleichnamigen Temporallappens folgen lässt. Auch bei diesen Versuchen folgt einem meist 4-6 tägigen Stadium completer Taubheit eine kurze Periode hochgradiger Schwerhörigkeit, die einem völlig normalen Hörvermögen für das contralaterale Ohr weicht.

Wenn wir die Rinde eines Schläfenlappens exstirpirten und 4 Wochen später denselben Eingriff am zweiten Temporallappen ausführten, traten die Erscheinungen am deutlichsten zu Tage. Durch 10-12 Tage erwiesen sich die Thiere als völlig taub, dann trat auch hier ein Stadium auf, in welchem man von Rindenschwerhörigkeit sprechen konnte, das Hörvermögen nahm von Tag zu Tag zu, so dass immer weniger intensive Geräusche erforderlich waren, um eine Hörreaction auszulösen.

Ob nach einseitiger Exstirpation eines Temporallappens die Restitution des Hörvermögens dadurch erfolgt, dass der andere Schläfenlappen die Function übernimmt, ob nach einseitiger Schneckenzerstörung und Exstirpation des gleichnamigen Temporallappens eine Stärkung der Verbindung zwischen dem contralateralen Gehörorgane und dem anderen Schläfenlappen eintritt, ob nach Exstirpation der Rinde beider Schläfenlappen die Wiederherstellung des Hörvermögens durch Regenerationsvorgänge, durch vicariirendes Eintreten unmittelbar angrenzender Rindenpartien oder durch functionelle Vermittlung untergeordneter Centren erfolgt, wollen wir nicht des Weiteren erörtern, zumal die Frage der Restitution auch für andere Rindencentren noch nicht genügend geklärt ist.

Die durch das Thierexperiment gewonnenen Thatsachen stimmen mit den durch anatomische Befunde verificirten klinischen Beobachtungen vollständig überein. Es ist jedoch selbstverständlich, dass entsprechend der ungleich höheren Werthigkeit der Rinde des menschlichen Gehirns nach beiderseitiger Schläfenlappenaffektion, dauernde, irreparable Taubheit beobachtet wurde. Dass in der Litteratur auch nicht ein einziger Fall vorliegt, in welchem nach einseitiger Läsion des corticalen Hörcentrums eine Herabsetzung des Gehörs beider Gehörorgane constatirt wurde, ist wohl darauf zurückzuführen, dass die Beeinträchtigung des gleichnamigen Gehörorgans eine nicht sehr hochgradige ist, und so rasch vorübergeht, dass die bestehende Schwerhörigkeit entweder übersehen oder aber als Somnolenz nach einem eventuell vorausgegangenen apoplektischen Insulte gedeutet wurde.

Die durch totale Zerstörung des corticalen Hörcentrums bedingte Taubheit, ist eine complete für alle Schallqualitäten, Sprache, Töne und Geräusche.

DE L'UNITÉ DE MENSURATION DE L'OUIE.
DR. BARATOUX, Paris.

Dans l'état actuel de nos connaissances, nous croyons que le tableau suivant est suffisant pour nous donner une idée exacte de la mesure de l'acuité auditive.

La partie supérieure de notre première page est destinée à recevoir les renseignements subjectifs ; la seconde partie renferme les résultats des diverses épreuves de l'ouïe.

Le tableau est divisé en trois colonnes : la première, PA, pour la perception aerienne, la dernière, PO, pour la perception ostéo-tympanique et une intermédiaire comprenant les diverses épreuves de Schwabach, S, de Weber, W, de Rinne, R, etc.

De chaque coté de ces colonnes, on inscrit les résultats, à droite pour l'oreille droite, à gauche, pour l'oreille gauche.

PERCEPTION AÉRIENNE, PA.

Diapasons.—Les diapasons dont nous nous servons pour l'examen ordinaire sont ceux de la série de Hartmann. Le résultat est indiqué comme le recommande le Prof. Bezold au moyen du tableau des coefficients dont la recherche est facile, si l'on se sert de la table que nous avons établie.* Les diapasons C, c^1, c^3 suffisent, en général.

Dans les cas qui nécessitent une étude plus approfondie, nous avons recours aux diapasons d'Appun, d'Edelman ou mieux de Kœnig quand nous voulons par ex., faire la recherche de la limite des sons.

Nous employons les signes suivants :

⊙ = diapason non entendu.

∞ = diapason entendu seulement un instant.

Montre ; h.—Nous indiquons entre parenthèses la distance à laquelle la montre est entendue normalement et nous inscrivons la distance à laquelle cette montre est perçue par le malade.

⊙ = montre non entendue.

c = „ entendue au contact.

Voix de la conversation V, et voix chuchotée, v,—Pour ces deux épreuves, nous mettons avant le—le résultat de l'examen avec les sifflantes et après ce—le résultat de l'examen avec les mots à tonalité grave. (On emploie pour parler l'air qui reste dans les poumons après une expiration naturelle, non forcée).

⊙ = voix non entendue.

∞ = „ entendue mais non comprise.

c = „ „ au voisinage de l'oreille.

Sifflet de Galton, Gal.—Nous notons en millièmes le résultat de l'examen avec cet instrument.

Diapason strié, Bon.—Le Dr. Bonnier a proposé de faire la recherche de l'acuité auditive au moyen d'un diapason de 100 vibrations doubles à la seconde. Le déplacement angulaire du diapason fait apparaitre dans son image une striation qui disparait à un moment donné de son extinction ; c'est ce moment assez court que l'on prend pour O, et à partir duquel les capacités auditives tant solidiennes qu'aériennes sont mesures de valeurs positives et négatives évaluées en secondes.

---

* J. Baratoux. De l'unification de la mesure de l'ouïe. Pratique médicale 1899, Nos. 2, 3, 5, and 6.

Le diapason est frappé fortement avec le bord cubital de la main. Une oreille normale l'entend environ pendant quatre minutes par la voie aérienne et l'image reste striée pendant trois minutes environ. Donc une oreille normale doit mesurer + 60 secondes d'audition aérienne.

Nous indiquons par les signes + ou - le résultat de cette épreuve suivant qu'il est supérieur ou inférieur au zéro.

Nous ne croyons pas que cette épreuve puisse remplacer celle de tous les diapasons.

PERCEPTION CRÂNIENNE, PO.

Diapasons.—Nous indiquons le résultat de l'expérience des diapasons comme précédemment. Au cas où la perception du diapason serait supérieure à la normale on l'indiquera par N + plus le nombre de secondes pendant lesquelles le diapason sera encore entendu.

Jusqu' à ce jour on plaçait le pied du diapason en avant de l'oreille, sur l'apophyse mastoïde, au dessus du pavillon ou sur le vertex. Récemment le Dr. Delsaux a proposé une méthode de topométrie crânio-acoumétrique à laquelle nous nous rattachons presque entièrement.

Les points de repère qu'il a choisis se trouvent presque tous dans le plan de la ligne biauriculaire passant sur la voute crânienne. Cette ligne est coupée par une série de perpendiculaires dont la première appelée ligne médiane, est dans le plan sagittal de la tête. La jonction de ces deux lignes, M, marque l'union du frontal avec les deux pariétaux. De là diffusion du son dans toute la tête.

Le deuxième point de jonction, œ, est à l'intersection de la ligne biauriculaire et de la ligne paraorbitaire partant de l'angle externe de l'orbite. Ce point est situé exclusivement sur le pariétal : les malades accusent nettement la latéralisation lorsque le diapason est appliqué en cet endroit.

Le troisième point, temporal, *t*, se trouve à l'union de la ligne biauriculaire avec celle partant encore de l'angle externe de l'orbite, mais se dirigeant horizontalement. Nous préférons choisir sur cette ligne le point, t, immédiatement en avant de l'oreille, près de l'union de l'écaille du temporal avec le pariétal, ce qui augmente encore la latéralisation du son. (Ce point est en dehors de la ligne biauriculaire).

Le quatrième point supra-auriculaire, *p*, est situé sur le temporal derrière la partie supérieure du pavillon.

Le cinquième, mastoïdien, *m*, en dehors de la ligne biauriculaire correspond à l'apophyse mastoïde ou mieux à l'antre.

Il suffit d'inscrire le résultat trouvé pour chaque diapason dans la colonne correspondante à chacune des lettres. Dans la pratique ordinaire, on se contente d'employer le C, c^1, et c^3.

Pour la perception crânienne, PO, nous indiquons le résultat de l'épreuve des diapasons comme précédemment. Toutefois si la perception du diapason est supérieure à la normale on marque N + le nombre de secondes pendant lesquelles l'instrument est encore entendu.

Montre, h.—Pour la montre, l'on sait que le maximum d'intensité de perception est situé sur la saillie du tragus, *t* ; et que le minimum de l'intensité en arrière est à la pointe de l'apophyse mastoïde, *m.*

La formule normale de la montre est

$$t > m$$

Si la perception est plus marquée à la mastoïde, on met

$$m > t$$

Y-a-t'il diminution du son on met le signe – devant t ou m.

La perception est-elle égale, on inscrit

$$t = m.$$

La perception est-elle nulle, on l'indique ainsi : $\odot$

Perception secondaire, PS.—Dans cette recherche, on se sert d'un diapason à tonalité moyenne, le $c^1 = 128$ vibrations doubles, que l'on place sur l'apophyse mastoïde ; dès que le son s'éteint on bouche l'oreille et le son reparait de nouveau.   Les signes suivants représentent :—

$$+ :—\text{l'existence.}$$
$$- :—\text{l'absence.}$$

Contre-audition, CA.—Dans cette épreuve, on emploie le diapason c^3 appliqué sur la mastoïde.   Normalement le son est mieux entendu du côté du diapason l'oreille étant ouverte, *o* ; il est même renforcé si l'on ferme cette oreille, *f.*   En bouchant l'oreille du côté opposé au diapason, *opp*, le son passe de ce côté, il y a contre-audition ; ferme-t'on l'autre oreille (les deux sont alors fermées) *2f*, la contre-audition disparait. Dans cette série d'épreuves, il suffit d'indiquer par les lettres d ou g le côté où le son est perçu.

Expériences de Schwabach, de Rinne, de Weber, de Gellé, etc.

Expérience de Schwabach, S.—On utilise le diapason c dont on inscrit la durée de perception entre parenthèses ; il faut autant que possible choisir un instrument qui donne de 16 à 18 secondes de durée vibratoire sur l'apophyse mastoïde.

$\pm$ } Indique que la durée de perception est normale.

$+$ qu'elle est prolongée.

$-$ „   „   diminuée.

$\odot$ que le diapason n'est pas entendu.

Expérience de Weber, W.—Elle se fait également avec le diapason c = 128 vibrations allem. On indique la latéralisation du son par une flèche :

$\longrightarrow$ à droite, si le son est latéralisé à droite.

$\longleftarrow$ à gauche, „   „   „   „ à gauche.

$\longleftarrow \quad \longrightarrow$ „   reste médian.

$\odot$ „   n'est pas perçu.

Avec un des signes   =,   -,   ou +, placé dans la colonne horizontale près de f, on indique les résultats suivants ;

= diapason-vertex également perçu les oreilles ouvertes ou fermées.

–   „   „   moins   „   „   „   fermées.
+   „   „   mieux   „   „   „   fermées.

Expérience de Rinne, R.—Avec le diapason C = 64 vibrations doubles dont on se sert pour cette épreuve, la perception aérienne excède la perception osseuse de 18 secondes.

+″ signifie que la perception aérienne l'emporte sur la perception osseuse de tant de secondes.

–″ que la perception osseuse excède l'aérienne de tant de secondes.

±? indique que la perception est égale par les deux voies.

Dans le cas de Rinne positif, il est bon d'inscrire d'abord le nombre de secondes pendant lesquelles le diapason est perçu par la voie osseuse puis de mettre le signe + et de noter ensuite le nombre de secondes pendant lesquelles le diapason est entendu par la voie aérienne.

Si le Rinne est –, on note le temps pendant lequel le son est entendu par la voie aérienne.

A la rigueur, on peut se contenter de la notation.

+ > pour indiquer que le Rinne + a une durée moindre.

– >   „   „   „   –   „   „

+δ veut dire que le diapason est seulement entendu par la voie aérienne.

–δ   ..   „   „   „
osseuse.

Diapason-trompe, c′ T.—Cette épreuve consiste à placer le diapason c′ devant les orifices du nez. On en indique les différents résultats de la façon suivante :

d, si le son est perçu à droite.
g „ „ „ „ „ „ gauche.
= „ „ „ „ „ également des deux côtés.
⊙ „ „ „ n'est pas entendu.

Diapason strié, Bon.—Nous plaçons ici le résultat de l'épreuve par la voie crânienne avec le diapason telle que la recommande le Dr. Bonnier. Le son du diapason de 100 vibrations doubles doit être perçu pendant une minute environ par la voie ostéo-tympanique, tandis que l'onde reste striée pendant trois minutes : l'oreille normale mesure donc – 120 secondes d'audition solidienne.

+″ indiquera que la perception est supérieure à la normale de tant de secondes ;

–″ signifiera qu'elle lui est inférieure de tant de secondes.

Le rapprochement des résultats fournis par les voies aériennes et osseuses en facilite leur comparaison ; nous avons déjà dit que M. Bonnier leur donnait la supériorité sur le Rinne.

Pressions centripètes, PC.—Ces pressions se font au moyen d'un ballon relié au conduit par un tube en caoutchouc et du diapason c′ =

256 vibrations allem., placé soit sur le tube (P C. par voie aérienne) ou sur l'apophyse mastoïde (PC. par voie crânienne). A chaque pression, rapide et légère, à l'état normal, le son s'atténue : le résultat est dit positif, +. Si la pression ne modifie pas le son, l'expérience est négative, −.

> indique qu'avec PC le son s'atténue.

=   „   „   „   „ n'est pas modifié.

δ „   „   „   „ disparait.

⊙   „   „   „   „ n'est pas entendu.

Les résultats de cette expérience étant inscrits sur une même ligne horizontale, on a soin de noter tout d'abord PC par voie aérienne, puis PC par voie crânienne, en les séparant par −.

RÉACTION DU NERF AUDITIF, NR.

Dans la deuxième partie de notre feuille, nous notons les résultats de la recherche de la réaction du nerf auditif à la fermeture de la cathode (pole −) fc, pendant la durée du courant, dc, et lors de son ouverture, oc. On en fait tout autant pour l'anode.

S = son fort.

s = son faible.

⊙ si l'on ne constate aucune manifestation.

Dans les pages suivantes, on inscrit en regard de chaque organe les lésions que l'on y constate et avec des crayons de couleur, il est facile d'établir des schémas qui nous rappellent ce que l'examen objectif nous a montré.

CASE OF EXTENSIVE PURULENT THROMBOSIS OF LATERAL SINUS— SEPTIC PNEUMONIA—PULMONARY ABSCESS AND GANGRENE CONSEQUENT UPON CHRONIC PURULENT OTITIS MEDIA. GRADUAL IMPROVEMENT AFTER CLEARING OUT THE LATERAL SINUS AND LIGATURING THE INTERNAL JUGULAR VEIN.

DR. THOMAS BARR, Glasgow.

On the 17th day of June, 1899, I was called to see David Dunn, aged 30, who had suffered from a discharge from the *left* ear, off and on, for 15 years. The disease was supposed to be excited by the impact of a snowball. He had for years been in the habit of syringing the ear and insufflating boracic powder. I was informed that for three weeks prior to my visit the patient had suffered from pain in the ear so intense as to prevent sleep ; that the left side of the head had been swollen for some days previously and had been extremely tender to touch, but that this swelling had now disappeared ; that there had been constant vomiting for several days with great thirst, and no appetite ; that the chief symptom, however, was the occurrence for a week past of frequent and most severe rigors, during which, as his sister expressed it, "the bed shook and the teeth rattled." His sister, who had attended him closely, believed that there had been at least twenty rigors, and that one had lasted 25 minutes, each of them being followed by very profuse perspiration. The temperatures taken by Dr. Alexander, the family physician showed typical pyæmic fluctuations, ranging from 100 to 105, according to the periods of the rigors. Anti-streptococcus serum had been injected twice during the previous week, without apparent effect.

On examination I found the auditory meatus filled with granulation tissue, and there was a profuse discharge of fetid pus. The pain, which had formerly been worse in the ear, was now felt with greatest intensity in the frontal and occipital regions, while on pressure behind the mastoid area pretty severe pain was elicited. Additional important and ominous symptoms had shown themselves during the previous 24 hours, namely, rapid breathing, pain in the right side of the chest, and rusty expectoration. On auscultation, crepitation was heard at the back of the *right* lung. Notwithstanding this grave complication, so unfavourable to the prospects of operation, it was thought right to give the patient a chance, and on the day following, he was removed by ambulance waggon to the Glasgow Ear Hospital, a distance of 20 miles.

Within an hour after his arrival at the hospital, I operated on the mastoid. There was no external evidence of mastoid mischief, but, on making a long incision and reflecting the auricle and cartilaginous meatus forward, the greater part of the postero-superior wall of the osseous meatus was found to be destroyed by caries ; from this sprouted the granulation tissue which filled the meatus. On further removal of bone a large cavity, packed with cholesteatomata, was found to extend back to the posterior fossa of the cranium, and the cholesteatomata covered the sigmoid part of the lateral sinus, which was exposed by the disease over a considerable part of its extent. The cholesteatomata, with cario-necrotic debris and granulation tissue, were thoroughly removed, and I was surprised to find the sinus and dura mater normal so far as colour, appearance, and touch were concerned. On that account it was not considered desirable to open the sinus, but to wait and see the effect of this operation. The large opening was therefore simply treated by iodoform packing.

For the next eleven days, while only one rigor was observed, the temperature had wide ranges extending from 97° to 106°. The respirations were rapid relatively to the pulse, ranging from 28 to 36 in the minute, and the pulmonary condition developed with consolidation. The question during these days was, were these pyæmic temperatures connected with pus formation in the lungs, or were they due to continued septic infection from the sinus ? I asked Dr. J. H. Nicoll to see the patient, and the question of ligaturing the internal jugular vein was seriously considered. I also consulted Dr. Finlayson (although he did not at this time see the case), but he was rather unfavourable to the proposal for ligaturing the vein in the presence of such a condition of the lung. However, the pyæmic temperature continuing, Dr. Nicoll and I agreed that the internal jugular should be tied and the sinus freely opened, so as to avoid, if possible, any further infection.

On the 29th of June, eleven days after the previous operation, Dr. Nicoll tied the left jugular at the level of the cricoid cartilage. The vein seemed collapsed and empty. Immediately after tying the internal jugular, Dr. Nicoll opened the sinus which was found occupied by purulent thrombi, and there was no blood stream. The bone over the sinus was snipped away as far as close to the torcular, a large amount of bone being in this way removed, and the sinus, which was somewhat rough on its outer surface, was clipped open with scissors and in almost its whole extent was found occupied by pus and thrombi. The patient bore these formidable operations well and distinct improvement soon followed as shown by lower temperatures, and much less violent fluctuations. The condition of the right lung was now the main source of anxiety; there was now purulent expectoration, but we were encouraged by the fact that Dr. Finlayson, who saw the patient at this stage, expressed a favourable opinion of the prospects.

On the 16th of July a fresh complication showed itself in the form of a large abscess over the sacrum—where no pain had been complained of—the swelling being first observed by Dr. Finlayson while examining the back of the lungs. On the same evening a large quantity of matter was evacuated from this abscess, and it did not give much further trouble. But the sufferings of the patient now became aggravated by bed-sores. Painful inflammation with ulceration affected the back of the shoulder and right haunch.

At the end of July, a fortnight after the evacuation of the sacral abscess, the breathing somewhat suddenly became much more embarrassed, with distressing cough and pain in the right side of the chest, while the purulent expectoration became very profuse, to the extent of a cupful in the course of a night. The pulmonary distress continued, and the condition at the beginning of August resembled the advanced stage of Phthisis Pulmonalis—rapid breathing, extreme emaciation, hollow cheeks, great paroxysms of coughing with most profuse purulent expectoration, also high temperature and profuse perspiration, but no rigors. In so far as the cranial condition was concerned, everything seemed satisfactory, the wound in the scalp had been sutured and was now quite healed; we were confident that there could be no fresh infection from the sinus or ear. It was clear, however, that there were purulent foci in the right lung, resulting from septic infarctions. The left lung, however, still remained apparently unaffected, and we hoped that his strength might enable him to survive the terrible complication in his right lung. At this time Dr. John Rowan made an ophthalmoscopic examination and found the "optic discs somewhat pale on the temporal sides and edges slightly indistinct, veins slightly full, fundi practically normal."

During the early part of the month of August, he remained in somewhat the same condition with the exception that the purulent expectoration, which continued copious, began to emit a gangrenous odour, during coughing, when, especially in certain positions of the body, a whiff of air having a gangrenous odour was perceived. Signs of cavity existed, yet as the month went on his general condition seemed to become no worse, but rather better. The temperature ranged from 99° to 102°, and the strength seemed to improve, with some diminution, though not great, in the purulent expectoration. The latter was examined bacteriologically and found to contain numerous chains of streptococci but no tubercle bacilli. Towards the end of August the improvement seemed to be such as to justify his removal to his home in the country ; partly with the hope that the change to the country air might be beneficial. He was removed on the 30th day of August, still expectorating pus, though in less quantity, but gaining in strength. The ear was entirely dry, and the extensive incisions were completely healed over, the large gap in the bone was also filled with firm material. The temperature for a week before leaving the hospital ranged from normal in the morning to 100° in the evening.

The change to the country proved beneficial, and he continued to improve. The temperature continued to be normal in the mornings, and from 99 to 100 in the evenings. On the 14th of October, Dr. Alexander, the family doctor, sent me the following notes : "David Dunn is now walking about daily, but is rather breathless on any exertion. He has practically no cough, except in the mornings. The expectoration has diminished gradually, and now there is only a little nummular spit in the mornings, and this is entirely devoid of any gangrenous odour. He is now putting on flesh rapidly, and I should think that he must have increased to the extent of at least a stone. The temperature has only been taken in the morning, when it was normal. The physical signs over the left lung are quite normal except that the respiratory murmur is rather puerile. Over the front of the right side there is no dulness, but on deep inspiration and on coughing there are still some crackling râles ; over the back the râles are also present on deep inspiration, but in the *lower half of the right lung there is a large cavity* with loud râles. The râles all over the right side are diminishing gradually, and the lung is evidently healing up."

The following points are worthy of emphasis in connection with this case. (1) The serious significance of rigors, high temperature, pain behind the mastoid, sickness and vomiting in connection with chronic purulent inflammation of the middle ear. (2) The vital importance in such cases of prompt and thorough removal of all sources of septic infection. (3) If the sinus be not opened at the time of the mastoid operation it should not be long delayed, in the event of rigors or of high temperature recurring afterwards, and *we must not hesitate to do this although the outer surface of the sinus appears normal.* (4) This case shows that even when there is evidence of pulmonary mischief, such operations as ligature of the jugular and opening of the sinus may be safely and with advantage carried out. There is no doubt that distinct amelioration took place after these operations and the patient owes his recovery, so far as that has taken place, to these operations in connection with the preceding mastoid one. (6) While the ligature of the internal jugular vein may, by some, be still regarded as a debatable point in such cases, it is a wise precaution, as it diminishes the chance of purulent debris making its way into the circulation. The operation is the more justifiable in as much as it is by no means a dangerous one in the hands of an experienced surgeon.

ACOUMETRIE.

DR. PIERRE BONNIER, Paris.

Je considère comme tout-à-fait impossible, quelque nombreuses et précises que puissent être les données acoumétriques fournies par l'examen clinique le plus consciencieux, d'établir et de formuler un diagnostic valable à l'aide de l'acoumétrie seule. On a avec raison multiplié et les procédés d'analyse et les points de vue physiologiques qui cernent du plus près possible le diagnostic et l'interprétation rationnelle du fait clinique étudié, mais il faut reconnaitre que peu de symptômes pourront revètir une interprétation légitime et indiscutable ; peu de signes même parmi les plus classiques et les plus autorisés, auront une réelle signification.

Dans ces conditions, le mieux est sans doute de ne pas s'encombrer— dans la pratique courante—d'un inventaire forcément incomplet, puisqu'on en peut à l'infini multiplier les termes, et de simplifier l'examen en le réduisant à quelques notations formelles et fondamentales dont il s'agira de savoir utiliser la substance. Tel signe, telle notation très utile dans un cas donné, n'aura aucune utilité dans un autre cas ; il en est peu qui seront toujours nécessaires ; sachons au moins les fixer en une formule pratique, nous réservant de noter, suivant chaque cas, les points les plus saillants de l'aspect clinique. Commençons par imiter les tailleurs, les gantiers et les bottiers, qui se préoccupent avant tout de ce qu'ils appellent la "pointure," quitte à compléter ce premier classement par des mensurations secondaires et indiquées par la nature apparente du sujet.

Réduite à sa formule scientifique la plus simple et au seul point de vue acoumétrique, l'oreille est un organe qui doit entendre *le plus possible au dehors et le moins possible au dedans.* En d'autres termes, l'audition par l'intermédiaire du milieu aérien est en quelque sorte en raison inverse de l'audition par contact de la source sonore sur le corps. Cette formule grossière, suffisamment exacte, nous sera d'une grande utilité dans la pratique. En effet, il nous suffira d'évaluer, pour chaque oreille, l'audition aérienne et l'audition solidienne, pour avoir, outre ces valeurs notées, un signe supérieur au Rinne, en les comparant l'une à l'autre. Il nous suffira de comparer la valeur de l'audition solidienne à droite et à gauche, pour obtenir un signe supérieur au Weber, outre que l'évaluation simple est elle-même supérieure à l'épreuve de Schwabach, etc. Des données précises, absolues, au lieu de rapports mal définis entre des grandeurs inconnues, des chiffres comparables d'un sujet à l'autre, d'une séance à l'autre, et surtout un procédé simple d'acoumétrie qui nous permette d'évaluer les deux formes d'audition, l'aérienne et la solidienne, en les rapportant à la même source sonore, ce que ne fait pas le Rinne, qui apprécie l'une avec le pied du diapason, et l'autre avec la partie libre de la branche,—voilà ce dont il faut nous occuper tout d'abord.

J'emploie pour ma part un diapason grave, de 100 vibrations doubles, ce qui ne choque aucun système musical, et ce qui convient parfaitement à l'audition par contact. Pour supprimer à la fois les harmoniques et les étaux ce diapason a des branches de largeur croissante de bas en haut. Une branche a 180 millimètres de hauteur, et 15 d'épaisseur ; la largeur au bas est de 5 millimètres et de 15 au sommet. Ce diapason a peu de sonorité aérienne, mais une grande pénétration sonore par contact du pied, double condition que je cherchais à réaliser.

Pour l'audition aérienne, je pose le pied du diapason sur le tube otoscopique engagé dans le conduit, à quelques centimètres du pavillon ; pour l'audition par contact, je le place soit sur la mastoïde, pour l'évaluation de la paracousie prochaine, et sur le genou, rotule ou tibia, pour celle de la paracousie lointaine. Les trois valeurs sont notées A, P, p, et inscrites dans un ordre invariable, comme les mesures des tailleurs.

L'évaluation acoumétrique se fait par la notation de la quantité sonore minima perçue. Or, le diapason étant mis en oscillation avec une force suffisante pour être entendu, je le laisse s'éteindre librement jusqu'a ce que le sujet ne l'entende plus, et après avoir fait renaître plusieurs fois la perception par de nouveaux contacts, je compte le moment qui va s'écouler entre le moment de la cessation de l'audition et un point fixe, le zéro de l'échelle acoumétrique, dont je dois dire un mot. A l'extrémité d'une des branches est fixée une petite tige rigide et légère ; si j'agite doucement, et dans le sens de l'oscillation vibratoire, tout le diapason, la combinaison du mouvement total que j'imprime à l'instrument et de la vibration de la branche portant l'aiguille va ajouter les mouvements de même sens et retrancher les mouvements de sens contraire. Les premiers seront donc accélérés, et l'aiguille sera moins visible, les seconds seront ralentis, et l'image se fixera momentanément à la vue. Je verrai donc une série de petites aiguilles juxtaposées, et cette striation de l'image disparaîtra à un moment donné, quand l'oscillation sera très faible, et le temps d'incertitude entre l'image striée et l'image lisse sera très court, et sensiblement le même pour beaucoup d'observateurs visuels. C'est ce point de disparition de l'image striée qui est le zéro.

Une oreille normale entend encore 30 secondes environ après la disparition de l'image striée ; elle vaut + 30 ; il est naturel qu'elle soit positive. Une mauvaise oreille cessera d'entendre plus ou moins longtemps avant la disparition du phénomène ; elle vaudra—n secondes. Ceci pour l'audition aérienne.

Pour la paracousie de Weber, ou audition au contact, l'oreille normale vaut environ –30 à –40 secondes ; elle est fortement négative, à l'apophyse mastoïde ; et bien plus fortement encore au genou, où mon diapason ne doit pas être entendu d'une oreille normale.

Quand par suite de troubles auriculaires, la formule physiologique est troublée, l'audition aérienne peut devenir très négative, la solidienne très positive, et dans beaucoup de cas la paracousie est bien plus manifeste, avec une latéralisation plus précise que dans le Weber, au genou que sur le crâne.

Prenons une "pointure" quelconque, l'oreille droite étant inscrite au dessus de la gauche, selon l'usage ; je transcris une de mes dernières observations, où il s'agit d'une fillette de neuf ans, sourde depuis quatre ans de l'oreille droite. Je trouve au premier examen :—

$$-60, \qquad -10, \qquad -45.$$
$$+35, \qquad -40, \qquad \text{manque.}$$

Je traduis : audition aérienne droite très négative, audition mastoïdienne droite très augmentée, audition très sensible au genou droit, et je remarque que la diapason placé sur le genou gauche se fait entendre nettement dans l'oreille droite. Les chiffres –60 (A) et –10 (P), m'en disent plus que " Rinne négatif " ; et ces autres chiffres –10 pour la mastoïde droite et –40 pour la gauche, m'en disent plus aussi que " Weber droit." De même le signe du genou est également précis, puisqu'il manque à gauche, et apparait à droite, quelque soit le genou touché par le diapason.

Après un mois de traitement par tractions élastiques sur le marteau au moyen de mon tympano-moteur, je trouve à droite.

$$-35 \qquad -25 \qquad -60.$$

L'audition a donc augmenté et la paracousie a diminué. Actuellement, j'ai

$$-35 \qquad -30 \qquad -60.$$

L'audition aérienne n'a pas varié depuis ces huit jours de froid, la mastoidienne a baissé, et le Weber qui n'existe plus au cràne est encore sensible aux genoux.

ON THE LOCAL APPLICATION OF REMEDIES IN THE TREATMENT OF NON-SUPPURATIVE CATARRH OF THE MIDDLE EAR.

DR. ADOLPH BRONNER, Bradford.

Non-suppurative Catarrh of the Middle Ear is primarily a disease of the mucous membrane. It is therefore only natural that in treating the many and various kinds of so-called non-suppurative catarrh we should try and treat the mucous membrane directly. The simple introduction of air by Politzer's Bag or the Eustachian Catheter affects the mucous membrane in many cases indirectly, but it is imperative that we should try and introduce remedies into the Eustachian Tube and Tympanum which will come into direct contact with the diseased mucous membrane.

All kinds of vapours, sprays, and injections have been suggested and used, with varying results.

I have recently tried a so-called comminuter or nebuliser. The solution to be injected is put into a bottle and driven, in the form of a fine powerful spray, against the sides of the bottle. It is thus broken up into such extremely fine particles that it has the appearance of vapour. It is then blown through an ordinary Eustachian Catheter into the Middle Ear. The spray should be used for one or several minutes according to the nature of the case. The solution thus comes into intimate contact with the whole of the surface of the mucous membrane and penetrates into the smallest cavities and recesses. We are also able to apply strong remedies, which, if injected in an ordinary solution, would cause great pain and discomfort.

The nature of the remedy used will of course depend on the character of the disease of the mucous membrane. Thus in middle ear disease due to Atrophic Rhinitis, I use Menthol, Formalin, Alkaline solutions. In cases of Catarrh with much secretion, Iodine, Eucalyptus, Creasote, Tincture of Benzoin. In cases of so-called Dry Catarrh: Camphor, Iodide of Ethyl, Chloroform. Any liquid solution can be used; if watery, some glycerine should be added. For the essential oils and for Chloroform, Iodine, Menthol, etc., the most useful solvent is a Hydrocarbon oil, such as Chrismaline, Paroleine. I use a large compressed air apparatus, which is filled by a hand pump or by water pressure. Any of the smaller nebulisers made by Allen and Hanbury, Oppenheimer, etc., can be used.

Of course the nebuliser can only be of some use in certain kinds of Otitis Media. In suitable cases I believe it is much more efficacious than Politzer's Bag or the Catheter. The air is blown into the tympanum at a definite pressure, easy to regulate and control, and can be applied for any length of time. It is also possible to bring various remedies into direct and thorough contact with the whole of the surface of the mucous membrane of the Eustachian Tube and Tympanum.

ADENO-CARCINOMA OF MEATUS WITH CHRONIC MIDDLE EAR SUPPURATION. OPERATION.

MR. ARTHUR H. CHEATLE, London.

Mary Rayner. This patient has been for several years under my care, coming originally for right chronic middle ear suppuration. She had been in the habit of putting a pin down the meatus in order to clean it. Towards the latter part of 1895, a white sessile swelling gradually appeared on the posterior wall of the cartilaginous meatus : it was removed through the meatus and found to be an adenoma. At the same period the old Schwartze operation was performed, and nothing much found. During 1896 the tumour gradually reappeared, and was removed by turning the auricle forwards, the posterior and superior walls of the meatus being excised. In May, 1898, an indefinite swelling gradually appeared ; and as it grew, involved the whole cartilaginous meatus. In August and September there was considerable pain and somewhat rapid extension, the concha beginning to be involved. In October, 1898, I removed the lower third of the auricle, including the tragus, lobule, and concha, and the whole of the meatus down to the middle ear. The meatus was found to be replaced by a white firm tumour. Sections show spaces lined with epithelium, the spaces being packed with cells in many parts. The Malleus and Incus were removed at the same time, the former having lost its handle. The posterior part of the auricle was then brought forward and stitched in position ; the lower posterior edge forming a kind of lobule. As this large wound healed, I found it impossible to keep a meatal passage, so in May last, in order to establish a permanent opening behind, I performed the Radical post aural operation, finding caries of the outer attic wall and of the superior antral wall with the commencement of an extra dural abscess in the middle fossa.

There has been no sign of recurrence of the tumour. At no time has there been glandular enlargement.

There is now a fairly large wound behind the auricle leading to the antrum and middle ear. Through this wound the watch (10ft.) is heard at two inches, and conversational voice at a yard. The meatus has entirely closed.

SARCOMA OF THE EXTERNAL AUDITORY CANAL.

(Photographs of patient and sections of tumour were shown at the Congress.)

DR. J. GALBRAITH CONNAL, Glasgow.

Malignant tumours of the ear are rarely met with. Of the two forms of malignant disease, Sarcoma of the ear is more uncommon than Carcinoma. On looking over the statistics of the Glasgow Ear Hospital for the past twelve years, I find that in an aggregate of nearly 15,000 cases, malignant disease is noted as occurring six times—once in 2,500 cases—four times epithelioma, and twice sarcoma. These figures nearly agree with those of Bürkner, which are often quoted. More recently Asch, in 1896, reporting a case of Sarcoma of the auricle, mentioned that he had found only ten cases of Sarcoma of the ear described in literature.

Of the two cases of Sarcoma which have occurred at the Glasgow Ear Hospital, one was reported by Dr. Barr in the *British Medical Journal*, for October,1897, the second is the case which I have the honour of submitting to-day.

These two cases were in marked contrast in the way they developed. In Dr. Barr's case, where the sarcomatous mass originated in the middle ear, there was no external growth, and the symptoms latterly pointed to some intracranial mischief suggesting temporosphenoidal abscess. In the present case, where the sarcoma originated in the external auditory canal, the development of the tumour was outwards, and gave rise to a large swelling in front of and behind the ear.

The patient was a girl six years of age. About eight weeks before she came to the Hospital her mother noticed a small growth—said to be quite painless—in the external auditory canal. A portion of this growth was removed by the family medical attendant, but it quickly recurred, and afterwards pain was persistent and severe. Facial paralysis set in seven days later and persisted. There was no history of purulent discharge from the ear.

Inspection showed a greyish-looking mass occupying the external meatus. It was exceedingly painful to the touch, and with the probe it was found adherent along the posterior wall of the canal. There was slight matting of the tissues in front of the ear over the parotid, and the gland at the angle of the jaw was enlarged. As already mentioned there was marked facial paralysis on the same side.

Under chloroform the whole mass was curetted from the wall of the canal. The tympanic membrane was found destroyed and the bone on the inner wall of the tympanum denuded of periosteum. This gave relief from pain, she slept well and put on flesh, but in about a month's time the growth recurred and rapidly involved the mastoid region and the tissues in front of the ear.

The patient died seven months after her first visit to the Hospital.

No post-mortem examination was allowed.

Sections of the tumour showed a spindle-celled Sarcoma with the sarcomatous growth extending along underneath the epidermis.

These malignant tumours of the ear, though rare, are very

interesting.   A point of practical importance lies in the diagnosis.   As we know, sarcoma is apt to manifest itself in the earlier years of life, at a time when we often meet with polypi and granulations in the external auditory canal, as the result of neglected purulent otitis media. Excessive pain should always excite suspicion of malignant mischief, and lead to a microscopical examination of the tissue.   So far as I have examined the literature on the subject, excessive pain is the prominent symptom.   If, in addition to pain there is marked and rapid recurrence of the growth, with glandular involvement, we have a group of symptoms which should make one careful as to the diagnosis and prognosis.

In the present case, the excessive pain and—what was very marked— the greyish look of the tumour, which was unlike ordinary granulations, the intimate adherence of the tumour to the posterior wall of the external auditory canal, the matting of the tissues in front of the ear, the glandular involvement and the facial paralysis, these—apart altogether from the history of the case—presented a clinical picture which at once arrested attention, and led to a microscopical examination of the tissue being made when the diagnosis of sarcoma was confirmed.

L'AUDITION CHEZ LES BEETLERS.

CONTRIBUTION À L'ÉTUDE DE LA SURDITÉ PROFESSIONELLE.

DR. E. COOSEMANS, Brussels.

L'influence néfaste, exercée sur l'organe de l'ouïe par certaines professions manuelles, s'accomplissant au milieu d'un bruit intense, est un fait connu depuis longtemps en Otologie.   Les "métiers bruyants" qui ont été le mieux étudiés à ce point de vue, sont ceux de chaudronnier, de riveur de chaudière, de conducteur de locomotives, de forgeron, de mécanicien, de tailleur de pierres, de meunier, d'arquebusier et de serrurier.   Je n'ai pas trouvé la profession de "Beetler," quoique s'accomplissant dans un tappage assourdissant, signalée parmi les métiers donnant lieu à la surdité professionelle.   C'est pourquoi il m'a paru doublement intéressant de vous exposer le résultat de mes recherches à cet égard, d'abord à cause de cette omission, ensuite parceque ce Congrès a lieu dans la Capitale du Royaume Uni, dans lequel l'industrie du lin a pris un si grand développement.

La "beetling machine," dont je fais circuler une photographie parmi l'assistance, est un appareil composé d'une vingtaine de marteaux métalliques qui, dans leur chute rapide et répétée, viennent frapper un rouleau de tissu de lin, à l'effet d'en applatir le fil et de lui donner cette finesse et ce brillant, tant recherchés par la clientèle.   Chaque marteau pèse 100 kilos et il frappe 400 coups par minute.   Sa force vive, évaluée au moment du contact, est de 333 kilos. L'atelier, dont j'ai examiné les ouvriers, renferme une vingtaine de ces machines ou d'autres semblables. Lorsque l'une d'elles est mise en marche, soudainement devant un spectateur non prévenu, celui-ci est saisi d'un brusque mouvement d'effroi et il recule vivement, d'une manière instinctive, tant le tapage produit, accompagné de tremblement, est considérable. Le bruit de toutes ces machines, travaillant ensemble est formidable, c'est un grondement *sourd* d'une puissance colossale, ébranlant à la fois l'atelier avec tout ce qu'il contient.

Les ouvriers examinés, au nombre de 17, travaillent au milieu de ce vacarme assourdissant, six jours par semaine depuis six heures du matin jusqu'à six heures du soir. Tous se plaignent d'entendre mal, au sortir de la fabrique, pendant 1 à 2 heures ; puis la finesse de l'ouïe revient insensiblement et le plus grand nombre d'entre eux, après le repos du Dimanche, reconnaissent entendre à peu près aussi bien qu'avant leur entrée au "beetle." Habermann, qui examina les ouvriers de 3 fabriques, immédiatement après le travail, constata la même particularité. Lorsqu'on passe dans cet atelier, on se demande comment il se peut que tous les ouvriers ne soient pas frappés de surdité absolue, et pourtant aucun d'eux n'est tout à fait sourd. Le plus gravement atteint (obs. v) entend la montre à 2 ctm. à gauche, et à 15 à droite (distance normale = 1 mètre) la voix haute à 2 m. et la voix basse à 75 ctm. ; par contre le sujet de l'obs. x, âgé de 61 ans travaillant au beetle depuis 39 ans, a une audition absolument normale pour son âge. On ne peut expliquer ce phénomène, en apparence paradoxal, que par la nature du bruit, au milieu duquel travaillent ces ouvriers ; ce bruit est très-violent, il est vrai, mais il est *sourd*, c'est à dire d'une tonalité très-basse ; en outre, il est *continü*, c'est un véritable roulement de tonnerre, dont les coups sont si rapprochés qu'ils se fondent en un tout uniforme. On peut estimer que les 20 beetling machines, travaillant en même temps, donnent 160,000 coups par minute. Or, si on compare ce bruit à celui d'autres professions, qu'on reconnut depuis longtemps comme nuisibles à l'oreille, p. ex. les forgerons, les riveurs de chaudière, les canonniers etc., on constate entre eux des différences fondamentales.

(a) Ce dernier bruit est d'une tonalité plus élevée.

(b) Il est intermittent : l'oreille fortement excitée au moment de la production du bruit, peut revenir à l'état de repos ou à peu près pendant la cessation de celui-ci : l'organe est donc soumis à des alternatives d'excitation violente et de repos relatif, alternatives qui, par leur répétition continuelle, doivent avoir pour effet de diminuer rapidement et d'abolir ensuite la finesse et la faculté même de l'ouïe.

Les observations, ci-après rapportées, peuvent se ranger en 2 groupes principaux :

(1°). Celui dans lequel une affection concommittante du nez, du pharynx, de l'oreille moyenne ou externe, soit l'habitude invétérée de

v

l'abus de l'alcool ou du tabac, expliquent la diminution de l'ouïe, du moins partiellement.

(2°). Celui où l'on ne remarque l'existence d'aucune cause semblable.

Dans le 1ᵉʳ *groupe* rentrent les observations I, III, IV, VI, VII, IX, X, XI, XII, XIII, XIV, XV, XVI, et XVII, donc 14 fois sur 17. Mes recherches confirment ainsi les résultats observés déjà par Boucheron et Garnault dans d'autres professions, à savoir que les lésions de la surdité professionelle se produisent de préférence chez les personnes qui y sont prédisposées par une affection concommittante des cavités annexes.

Quant à la *durée de travail* au beetle des ouvriers observés, elle va de 2 à 39 ans.

Les différentes *épreuves acoumétriques*, auxquelles ils ont été soumis, sont :

(1). La *Montre*—par voie aérienne—celle employée a un tic-tac tellement faible qu'une oreille normale ne le perçoit pas au delà d'un mètre de distance. Tous les sujets l'ont perçu à un éloignement variable de l'oreille, sauf le sujet de l'obs. VII, qui ne l'entendait qu'au contact pressé à G. et pas du tout à D., mais il avait les deux narines obstruées par des polypes muqueux tellement anciens, que leur enveloppe s'était quasi cutanisée et il est âgé de 68 ans.

(2). Le *Weber*—le diapason employé est le c_2 de 512 vibrations.

(3). Le *Rinne*—a été *positif* chez tous les sujets sauf chez celui de l'obs. XVII, atteint d'otite moyenne purulente chronique à D. et de catarrhe chronique sec à G. Il a été *raccourci*—par la voie osseuse et par la voie aérienne—dans une mesure plus ou moins forte chez tous les sujets, sauf chez celui de l'observation XVI, âgé de 18 ans seulement et ne travaillant au Beetle que depuis 2 ans, chez lequel il était normal.

(4). Le *Bing* a donné lieu à la récupération du son chez les 11 sujets chez lesquels l'expérience a été tentée.

(5). Le *Gellé* ou pressions centripèdes, a donné des résultats variables : Il y eut *diminution* ou *suppression* du son dans les obs. I, II, III, IV, VIII, XIV, XV, XVI,—*pas de changement* dans l'obs. XVII, et une *augmentation* dans les obs. V, VI, et XII. Ce dernier résultat doit être attribué, je pense, à un défaut d'attention de la part du sujet : en effet, lorsque le tuyau de caoutchouc de la poire à insufflation est introduit dans le conduit, celui-ci se trouve bouché, ce qui augmente le son, en empêchant les ondes sonores de se répandre au dehors (Mach, Politzer). Le sujet, s'en tenant à cette première impression, n'analyse plus celle qui se produit pendant la pression même.

(6). La *Voix*—haute et basse—la salle d'examen n'ayant que 4 mètres de long, il faut en tenir compte dans l'interprétation des résultats observés.

Il résulte de ces différentes épreuves que, la part faite aux lésions de la trompe et de la caisse, etc., dans certains cas, la diminution plus ou moins appréciable de l'ouïe est d'origine labyrinthique, à l'exclusion des canaux demi-circulaires, aucun sujet ne s'étant plaint de vertiges.

Conclusion. Il résúlte donc de mes observations : que

Tout métier bruyant n'est pas nécessairement nuisible à l'oreille. Il faut pour qu'il le soit :

(a). Que l'ouvrier soit prédisposé aux affections auriculaires par l'existence de lésions dans le nez ou le pharynx.

(b). Que le bruit soit intermittent.

(c). Qu'il soit d'une tonalité rélativement élevée.

———

Obs. I.—V. W......Adolphe, 34 ans, travaille au Beetle depuis 17 ans.

Jamais d'otorrhée, pas d'hérédité, habitudes alcooliques et tabagiques invétérées. Se plaint de bourdonnements ronflants et de diminution de l'ouïe à la conversation.

M. = 80 ctm. des 2 côtés.

W. = à gauche.

R. = positif bilatéral, légèrement raccourci.

Bing = récupération des 2 côtés.

Gellé = suppression des 2 côtés.

Voix haute = 4 mètres, voix basse = 2 mètres.

T. G. = blanc, légèrement opaque, déprimé, triangle raccourci, osselets mobiles.

T. D. = mêmes caractères.

Nez = hypertrophie des 2 cornets inférieurs, à G. contact avec la cloison ; à D., cornet moyen couvert d'exsudat muco-purulent.

Pharynx = granuleux.

Trompes = libres, pas de râles.

Obs. II.—De C......Joseph, 35 ans, travaille au Beetle depuis 19 ans.

Jamais d'otorrhée, pas d'hérédité. Se plaint de bourdonnements bilatéraux par un temps couvert, humide, non par un temps clair et sec.

M. = 50 ctm. à G., 80 à D.

W. = à G.

R. = positif bilatéral, légèrement raccourci à D., davantage à G.

B. = récupération des 2 côtés.

G. = diminution des 2 côtés.

V. haute = 4 m.

     basse = 1.50 m.

T. G. = légèrement déprimé, brillant, transparent, triangle en situation, osselets mobiles.

T. D. = légèrement dépoli, triangle en situation, osselets mobiles.

Nez = normal.

Pharynx = normal.

Trompes = perméables, sans râles.

Obs. III.—Dew...... Polydore, 35 ans, travaille au Beetle depuis 15 ans. Jamais d'otorrhée, pas d'hérédité. Entend bien la conversation quand l'interlocuteur est près de lui mais non quand il est p.ex. à 2m. de distance ; il entend alors mais il ne comprend pas. Se plaint en outre de sifflements continus à D. Habitudes alcooliques et tabagiques.

M. = 45 ctm. à G.

    40 ctm à D.

R. = positif bilatéral mais très-raccourci.

W. = à G. (?).

B. = récupération des 2 côtés.

G. = diminution des 2 côtés.

V. haute = 4 m.

  basse = 1.50 m.

T. G. = déprimé, légèrement opalescent, triangle déprimé, angle très aigu avec le manche, osselets peu mobiles.

T. D. = déprimé, triangle presqu'entièrement effacé, osselets moins mobiles que normalement.

Nez = normal.

Ph. = vernissé, atrophique.

Tr. = libres, pas de râles.

Obs. IV.—P......Jean, 22 ans, travaille au Beetle depuis 8 ans. Jamais d'otorrhée, pas d'hérédité. Il entend moins bien, dit il qu'un garçon de son âge, mais la finesse de l'ouïe revient quand il quitte l'atelier pendant un jour. Se plaint de ronflements bilatéraux.

M. à G. = 60 ctm.

  à D. = 35 ctm.

W. = à D.

R. = positif bilatéral, légèrement raccourci à G. davantage à D.

B. = récupération des 2 côtés.

G. = diminution bilatérale.

V. haute = 4m.

  basse = 2m.

Nez = rhinite sub-aigüe.

Ph. = granuleux.

Tr. = libres.

T. = normal des 2 côtés, osselets mobiles.

Obs. V.—Br......Henry, 56 ans, travaille au Beetle depuis 39 ans. Jamais d'otorrhée, pas d'hérédité. Se plaint de ronflements intermittents à G. et d'entendre mal la voix.

M. à G. = 2 ctm.

  à D. = 15 ctm.

W. = à D. (?).

R. = positif bilatéral, surtout raccourci à G.

B. = récupération à G., rien à D.

G. = augmentation (?) légère des deux côtés.

V. haute = 2 m.

  basse = 75 ctm.

Nez. = normal.

Ph. = normal.

Tr. = libres.

T. G. = sclérosé, opaque, triangle presqu' effacé, osselets mobiles.

T. D. = clair, brillant, transparent, triangle normal, osselets mobiles.

Obs. VI.—Deg...... François, 32 ans, travaille au Beetle depuis 13 ans. Jamais d'otorrhée, pas d'hérédité. Se plaint de ronflements dans les deux oreilles, n'entend pas la voix haute à 2 mètres, dit il.

M. à G. = 60 ctm.

  à D. = 80 ctm.

W. = à D. (?).

R. = positif bilatéral, légèrement raccourci à G,. presque pas à D.

B. = récupération des 2 côtés.

G. = renforcement des 2 côtés (?).

T. G. = opaque, sclérosé, conduit eczémateux, osselets mobiles.

T. D. = clair, transparent, triangle en situation, beaucoup moins d'écailles dans le conduit qu'à G., osselets mobiles.

Nez = rhinite hypertrophique bilatérale surtout prononcée à G., avec forte déviation de la cloison du même côté.

Ph. = normal.

Tr. = normales.

Obs. VII.—Tr......Guillaume, 68 ans, travaille au Beetle depuis 26 ans. Jamais d'otorrhée, pas d'hérédité. Il n'entend la voix haute, qu'à 1 mètre, dit il, et il ne peut pas prendre part à une conversation en groupe.

M. = à G. contact pressé.

à D. non perçue.

W. = à G.

R. = positif bilatéral, très raccourci à D, moins à G (?)

T. G. = blanc, sclérosé, triangle en situation, osselets mobiles.

T. D. = mêmes caractères.

Ph. = normal.

Nez = les deux narines sont obstruées par de nombreux polypes muqueux, très-anciens. Le sujet a *toujours* eu le nez bouché, dit il.

Obs. VIII.—Ann......François, 32 ans, travaille au Beetle depuis 11 ans. Jamais d'otorrhée, pas d'hérédité. Il a parfois des ronflements dans les oreilles, au sortir de l'atelier ; il entend mal la parole.

M. = 30 ctm. à G.

35 ctm. à D.

W. = à G.

R. = positif bilatéral mais légèrement raccourci.

T. G. = parfait, normal, osselets mobiles.

T. D. = mêmes caractères.

Nez = forte déviation de la cloison à G., rien à D.

Ph. = normal.

Tr. = perméables, pas de râles.

Obs. IX.—Tr...... Guillaume, 30 ans, travaille au Beetle depuis 14 ans. Jamais d'otorrhée, pas d'hérédité. Entend mal la parole.

M. = 65 ctm. des 2 côtés.

W. = à G.

R. = positif bilatéral mais raccourci surtout à G.

B. = récupération des 2 côtés.

G. = diminution des 2 côtés.

V. haute 4 m.

basse = 2 m.

T. = normaux, osselets mobiles.

Nez = normal.

Ph. = normal.

Tr. = perméables, pas de râles.

Obs. X.—Dequ...... Josse, 61 ans, travaille au Beetle depuis 39 ans.   Jamais
d'otorrhée, pas d'hérédité.   S'aperçoit d'une diminution de l'ouïe
depuis 1 an.

    M. = 65 ctm. à G.

          60 ctm. à D.

    W. ≃ central.

    R. = positif bilatéral, légèrement raccourci des 2 côtés.

    T. G. = blanc, opaque, déprimé, triangle effacé, osselets mobiles.

    T. D. = mêmes caractères.

    Nez = hypertrophie des deux cornets inférieurs, mais le nez est libre.

    Ph. = normal.

    Tr. = libres, pas de râles.

Obs. XI.—No...... François, 36 ans, travaille au Beetle depuis 19 ans.

    Jamais d'otorrhée, pas d'hérédité.   Se plaint d'entendre mal depuis 3
ans ; bourdonnements soufflants.

    Bouchon a G. = extraction.

    M. = 70 ctm. des 2 côtés.

    W. = central.

    R. = positif bilatéral, légèrement raccourci.

    T. G.= déprimé, opaque, triangle disparu, osselets mobiles.

    T. D. = mêmes caractères.

    Nez = normal.

    Ph. = normal.

    Tr. = perméables, sans râles.

Obs. XII.—Van H......J.B. 37 ans, travaille au Beetle depuis 18 ans.

    Jamais d'otorrhée, mais des furoncles du conduit D. et hématôme du
pavillon D.   Il entend bien la voix dans la conversation ordinaire.

    M. = 1m. de chaque côté.

    W. = Légèrement à G.

    R. = positif bilatéral, à peine raccourci.

    B. = récupération des 2 côtés.

    G. = augmentation des 2 côtés.

    T. G. = déprimé,   blanc,   sclérosé,   triangle diminué en hauteur,
presqu'effacé, osselets mobiles.

    T. D. = normal, triangle en situation, osselets mobiles.

    Nez = forte déviation de la cloison à D., hypertrophie localisée du
cornet inférieur gauche.

    Ph. = normal.

    Tr. = libres.

Obs. XIII.—T. D. P......Jules, 22 ans, travaille au Beetle depuis 6 ans.

    Jamais d'otorrhée, pas d'hérédité.   S'aperçoit depuis 1 an que l'ouïe
diminue, surtout à D. ; ne saisit pas bien la parole articulée surtout
au sortir de l'atelier.

    M. = 60 ctm. à G.

          40 à D.

    W. = à D.

    R. = positif bilatéral, très légèrement raccourci à G. davantage à D.

    T. D. = déprimé, dépoli, triangle réduit à un point, osselets mobiles.

    T. G. = déprimé, dépoli, triangle disparu, osselets mobiles.

    Nez = rhinite subaigüe bilatérale, forte déviation de la cloison à D.

Ph. = normal.

Tr. = libre à G., légers râles humides à D.

Obs. XIV.—De D......Jean, 35 ans, travaille au Beetle depuis 20 ans.

Jamais d'otorrhée, pas d'hérédité. Il n'entend pas bien la conversation éloignée, surtout à G.

Bouchon obturant à G. = extraction.

M. = 60 ctm. à G., 70 ctm. à D.

W. = à G.

R. = positif bilatéral, raccourci de moitié à G., presque pas à D.

B. = récupération des 2 côtés.

G. = diminution bilatérale.

Nez = normal.

Ph = id.

Tr =libres.

Obs. XV.—Su...... Tolie, 24 ans, travaille au Beetle depuis 7 ans.

Jamais d'otorrhée, pas d'hérédité. Il a eu des bouchons dans les deux oreilles, il y a 3 ans. Il en a encore, aujourd'hui : obturant à D., non-obturant à G. Il n'entend pas bien la conversation depuis 4 ans. Extraction des bouchons.

M. = 30 ctm. à G., contact à D.

W. = à D.

R. = positif bilatéral, légèrement raccourci à G., plus à D.

B. = récupération des 2 côtés.

G. = diminution des 2 côtés.

T. G. = normal, osselets mobiles.

T. D. = déprimé, triangle déformé en cercle, osselets mobiles.

Nez = forte déviation de la cloison à G., hypertrophie du cornet inférieur D.

Ph. = normal.

Tr. = libres, sans râles.

Obs. XVI.—Von. M......Jean, 18 ans, travaille au Beetle depuis 2 ans.

Jamais d'otorrhée, pas d'hérédité. Entend bien, ne se plaint pas de bourdonnements.

M. = 1m. de chaque côté.

W. = central.

R. = positif bilatéral, non raccourci.

T. G. = légèrement opalescent, triangle en situation, osselets mobiles.

T. D. = mêmes caractères.

Nez. = Rhinite hypertrophique à G., moins prononcé à D.

Ph. = granuleux.

Tr. = libres.

B. = récupération des deux côtés.

G. = diminution des 2 côtés.

Obs. XVII.—L......Emmanuel, 30 ans, travaille au Beetle depuis 14 ans. Otorrhée à D. depuis l'enfance, à eu plusieurs crachements de sang, pas d'hérédité otitique.

W. = à D. jusqu'à l'apophyse G.

M. = contact à D., 10 ctm. à G.

R. = négatif bilatéral.

B. = récupération des 2 côtés, surtout à D.

G. = pas de changement des 2 côtés.

T. G. = légèrement grisâtre, déprimé, manche très-saillant, triangle réduit à une ligne, osselets mobiles.

T.D. = conduit rempli de pus et d'écailles épidermiques, tympan disparu.

Nez. = déviation de la cloison à G. rhinite subaigüe chronique à D.

Ph. = normal.

Tr. = libre à G., râles nombreux à D. avec bruit de gorguillement.

BIBLIOGRAPHIE.

1. *Urbantschitsch, Politzer, Delstanche*, 66e, réunion des médecins allemands, 1894.

2. *Habermann.* Heidelberg 1889. Ueber die Schwerhörigkeit der Kesselschmiede.

3. *Bürckner.* Arch. für Ohrenheilkunde. Bd. XVII. S. 14.

4. *Gottstein* et *Kayser.* Breslauer ärtzlicher Zeitung. 1881. No. 18.

5. *Gradenigo.* Arch. für Ohrenheilkunde. Bd. XXVIII. S. 194.

6. *Bezold.* Zeitschrift für Ohrenheilkunde. Bd. XVII. S. 195.

7. *St. John Roosa.* Zeitschrift für Ohrenheilkunde. Bd. XIII. S. 102.

8. *Holz.* Arch. für Ohrenheilkunde. Bd. XX. S. 62.

9. *Gellé.* Dictionnaire de Jaccoud.

10. *Garnault.* Précis des maladies de l'oreille. P. 174.

11. *Boucheron.* Revue de Moure. Tome V. P. 250.

L'ÉTAT DES OREILLES, DU LARYNX, ET DU NEZ CHEZ LES VIEILLARDS.

DR. A. COSTINIU, Bucharest.

Le nombre des vieillards examinés par moi à l'Hôpital "Pantelimon" (dans le service du Dr. Turbure dont j'ai l'honneur d'être adjoint et dans le service du Prof. Dr. Marinesco), s'élève à 148, dont 89 hommes et 59 femmes.

J'ai partagé ces cas en plusieurs catégories,

1) Sénilité pure.

2) Sénilité avec hémiplégie.

3) Sénilité accompagnée de différentes maladies, comme l'ataxie, la maladie de Parkinson, la chorée chronique, la paraplégie spasmodique, la sclérose latente, amyotrophique, etc.

Leur âge varie entre 50 et 107 ans.

Dans le tableau ci-joint, j'ai divisé dans toutes ces catégories l'audition de la voix parlée à 5 mètres en : bonne, diminuée, et abolie, où il y est marqué tout ce que comporte l'oreille. J'ai procédé de même pour le nez, la cavité buccale et le larynx.

Ici je ne vous donne qu'un résumé en termes généraux. Ceux qui s'intéresse à cette question voudront bien consulter le tableau.

Ainsi tous les cas réunis, sans exception, m'ont donné 72 fois l'audition bonne, 59 fois l'audition diminuée, et 17 fois l'audition abolie.

Pour l'audition bonne (72 cas) j'ai trouvé :—Perception crânienne abolie des deux côtés 12 fois : Le signe de Weber positif à droite 34 fois, à gauche 33 fois ; négatif 23 fois à droite, 20 fois à gauche : Le signe de Rinne, je l'ai trouvé 4 fois négatif aux deux oreilles.

La membrane du tympan sclérosé à droite 32 fois, à gauche 19 fois ; opaque à droite 26 fois, à gauche 38 fois.

Dépôts calcaires à droite 7 fois, à gauche 6 fois.

Triangle lumineux disparu à droite 11 fois, à gauche 13 fois.

Le marteau prenant différentes formes à droite 8 fois, à gauche 11 fois.

Ankylose des osselets à droite 29 fois, à gauche 31 fois.

Le conduit auditif atrésié 31 fois à droite, 22 fois à gauche.

Cerumen à droite 3 fois.

Otorrhée 1 fois.

Dans 59 cas d'audition diminuée j'ai trouvé :—Perception crânienne abolie 27 fois, à droite 1 fois, à gauche 4 fois. Perception aérienne diminuée des deux côtés 8 fois ; abolie à gauche 3 fois, à droite 1 fois. Le signe de Weber positif 22 fois des deux côtés, négatif 17 fois aux deux oreilles. Le signe de Rinne négatif à droite 10 fois, à gauche 11 fois.

Bourdonnements doubles 1 fois, à droite 6 fois, à gauche 3 fois.

Conduit auditif atrésié à droite 12 fois, à gauche 11 fois.

Cerumen abondant aux deux oreilles 3 fois ; à droite 5 fois, à gauche 2 fois.

La membrane du tympan sclérosé à droite 21 fois, à gauche 23 fois ; opaque à droite 15 fois, à gauche 9 fois.

Dépôts calcaires 11 fois des deux côtés.

Perforation du tympan 8 fois dans les deux oreilles.

Triangle lumineux disparu à gauche 10 fois, à droite 4 fois.

Le marteau prenant différentes formes à droite 6 fois, à gauche 11 fois.

Les osselets ankylosés à droite 23 fois, à gauche 27 fois.

Otorrhée des deux côtés 5 fois.

Dans 17 cas d'audition abolie j'ai trouvé :—La perception crânienne abolie 11 fois, aérienne des deux côtés 9 fois, seulement à gauche 3 fois.

Rinne et Weber négatif, excepté 1 fois.

Le conduit auditif atrésié à gauche 3 fois, à droite 3 fois.

Cerumen 5 fois.

Le tympan droit sclérosé 11 fois, gauche 5 fois ; opaque à gauche 4 fois.

La membrane détruite complètement 2 fois.   Otorrhée double 2 fois.
Ankylose des osselets à droite 4 fois, à gauche 6 fois.

Pour les autres organes j'ai remarqué :—Les cornets du nez sont le plus souvent hypertrophiés.

J'ai trouvé des polypes muqueux dans 8 cas : La destruction de la cloison 9 fois : Le voile du palais, les piliers et la luette ont été trouvés congestionnés 40% : Varices de la base de la langue 28% : L'odorat abolie 27%, perverti 15% : Le gout diminué 15%, perverti 2½% : L'épiglotte prenant différentes formes dans la prononciation 34% : congestionnée 11% : Mouvements réduits à la respiration et prononciation 21% : Les cordes vocales jaunâtres et plus grosses que normalement 20%, diminuées de volume 16%.

Chez les vieillards hémiplégiques, j'ai trouvé notamment la parésie du voile du palais de même côté que l'hémiplégie ; 4 fois elle a été double, 5 fois adduction incomplète des cordes vocales.

Dans les cas compliqués d'ataxie locomotrice, 2 fois il y a eu tremblement fibrilaire des cordes vocales pendant la respiration.

Presque chez tous les vieillards, les amygdales palatines sont si atrophiées qu'il n'en existe plus même de traces.   Chez trois d'entre eux, nous avons trouvé les amygdales normales comme volume, mais transformées en un tissu fibreux, blanchâtre et dur.

Les dents manquent dans 70%.

Le réflexe pharyngien a été trouvé abolie dans tous les cas ; les vieillards se prêtent très bien à toutes les manoeuvres de l'examen, sans ressentir quelque chose de désagréable.

Nous avons trouvé une seule fois une tumeur maligne dans la fosse nasale gauche.   Dans un autre cas il y avait une soudure complète du voile du palais au pharynx, sans le moindre orifice de communication pharyngo-nasale ; la cause en était le syphilis.

L'examen microscopique fait au différentes organes nous a montré toujours des lésions banales de sclérose et ne présentant aucune particularité digne d'être particulièrement signalée.

Dans ce travail, j'ai été aidé par l'interne du service Goldring ; qu'il me soit permis de lui addresser ici tous mes remerciments.

SOME ASPECTS OF AURAL PRACTICE IN INDIA, ANCIENT AND MODERN, WITH SPECIAL REFERENCE TO BOMBAY.

DR. JEHANGIR J. CURSETJI, Bombay.

MR. PRESIDENT AND GENTLEMEN,

In contributing the present paper to the Congress, I regret I have nothing new or original to offer.   All that I have attempted is to lift the curtain somewhat from a strange land and its stranger methods, in the belief, that it might interest at least some of those present here

TOTAL 106 (64 HOMMES ET 42 FEMMES).

AUX DEUX OREILLES.

27 hommes.   16 femmes.

AUDITION BONNE.

À DROITE.   À GAUCHE.

AUDITION DIMINUÉE.

À DROITE.   À GAUCHE.

SIGNE WEBER.

SIGNE RINNE.

PERCEPTION.

LE MARTEAU.

TYMPAN DROIT.   TYMPAN GAUCHE.

MOUVEMENTS DES OSSELETS.

TRIANGLE LUMINEUX.

LE NEZ, FOSSES NASALES, CAVITÉ BUCCALE AVEC SÉNILITÉ PURE.

VOILE DU PALAIS.

PILIERS ANTÉRIEURS.   PILIERS POSTÉRIEURS.

DESTRUCTION DU CLOISON : 6 HOMMES ET 4 FEMMES; ULCÉRATIONS À GAUCHE ... 2 HOMMES ET UNE FEMME, FRACTURE DE CLOISON ... 2 HOMMES.

FOSSE NASALE DROITE.   FOSSE NASALE GAUCHE.

NEZ EN BEC DE F...

Observation : cicatrice versus avec attachement de plaque.

Chart A illustrating Dr. Cost...

VIEILLARDS AVEC HÉMIPLÉGIE

TOTAL 30 (14 HOMMES ET 16 FEMMES)

AUDITION DIMINUÉE | 5 HOMMES ET 9 FEMMES.

AUDITION BONNE | 9 HOMMES ET 7 FEMMES.

BASE DE LA LANGUE.

VARIÉT. DE. papillaire	CONSERVÉE. 3 hommes	
partie latérale 2 hommes		

ANTYGDALES LINGUALES.

HYPERTROPHIES. 9 hommes 5 femmes	ATROPHIES. 1 homme

LE GOÛT.

| | DIMINUÉ 7 hommes 9 femmes | PERVERTI 1 homme 2 femmes |

PHARYNX.

| | GRANULATION. 2 hommes 5 femmes | CONGESTION. 7 hommes |

VESTIBULE DU LARYNX.

HYPERTROPHIE. de gauche 1 homme	HYPERTROPHIÉ. de gauche 1 homme

ÉPIGLOTTE EN FORME, ETC.

| MUSEAU DE TANCHE 6 hommes 1 femme | CREVASSE. cicatrice 2 hommes | HYPERTROPHIES. 9 hommes 5 femmes |

ADDUCTION INCOMPLÈTE DOUBLE.

| | 4 hommes 2 femmes | PLUS GROSSIÉ, ET FAUXATRES. 10 hommes 11 femmes | MOUVEMENT RÉDUIT 14 hommes 8 femmes | GRANULATION. 1 hommes 3 femmes |

CORDES VOCALES.

DIMINUÉES ET AMINCIES.

| 2 hommes 13 femmes | | ANKYLOSÉE. 2 hommes |

LARYNX.

VESTIBULE DU LARYNX.

| THE BOUCHON. 3 hommes | ODIVE 3 hommes | CONSERVÉ. 1 homme 1 femme | | POLYPE. 2 hommes 1 femme | KYSTE. 2 hommes | ATROPHIÉ. 1 homme |

SIGNE WEBER.

| POSITIF. 8 hommes 3 femmes | NÉGATIF. 1 homme | NUL. 4 femmes |

TYMPAN GAUCHE.

| NORMAL. 3 hommes 3 femmes | DÉF. CALCAIRES. 1 homme 1 femme | OPAQUE. 2 hommes 1 femme |

SIGNE RINNE.

| POSITIF. 0 hommes 7 femmes | CRÂNIENNE AIGÜE de deux côtés 4 femmes | NÉGATIF. | EXANGLE. 2 hommes 4 femmes |

PERCEPTION.

| | CRÂNIENNE AIGÜE de deux côtés 4 femmes | AÉRIENNE diminuée 4 femmes |

TYMPAN DROIT.

| NORMAL 3 hommes 4 femmes | NÉGATIVE. 2 hommes 2 femmes | OPAQUE. 1 homme 2 femmes | DÉPOTS CALCAIRES. 1 homme 1 femme | PERFORÉ. 3 hommes 2 femmes |

AUDITION INCOMPLÈTE DOUBLE.

| 4 hommes 11 femmes |

SIGNE WEBER.

| POSITIF. 3 hommes 2 femmes | NÉGATIF. 3 femmes |

VESTIBULE.

| HYPERTROPHIÉ à gauche 1 femme |

LUETTE.

| LARGEUR SE. 1 homme | CONGESTION. 1 femme |

TYMPAN GAUCHE.

| NORMAL. 4 hommes 1 femme | SCLÉROSE. 1 homme 2 femmes | OPAQUE. 1 femme | DÉPOTS CALCAIRES. 4 femmes |

LARYNX.

| ADDUCTION incomplète à gauche 1 homme 1 femme | LANGUE. 1 homme 2 femmes |

BASE DE LANGUE.

| VARIÉTÉS. 3 femmes 3 femmes | CORSET INFÉRIEUR. hypertrophie 1 homme |

CORDES VOCALES.

| LOUGRAT. alódí 2 hommes 4 femmes | CORSET INFÉRIEUR. hypertrophie 1 homme | ADDUCTION incomplète 2 femmes |

C.

VIEILLARDS AVEC:—1.—ATAXIE LOCOMOTRICE. (3 HOMMES.)

[...]IMINUÉE. che ıme	SIGNE WEBER. positif 1 homme	négatif 1 homme	SIGNE RINNE. négatif 3 hommes	sclérosé 1 homme	TYMPAN DROIT. enfoncé 1 homme	congestionné 1 homme	Dép. calcaires 3 hommes	TYMPAN GAUCHE. Le marteau élevé 1 homme	Mouvem. ankilosés 3 hommes	FOSSE NASALE DROITE. CORNET SUPÉRIEUR. hypertrophié 1 homme	CLOISON bombé 1 homme	FOSSE NASALE GAUCHE. CORNET SUPÉR. hypertrophié 1 homme	éperon 1 homme	CLOISON. cicatrice 1 homme; polype 1 homme
[...]née	AMYGD. LINGUALES. atrophiées 1 homme		EPIGLOTTE. irrégulière 1 homme	congestionnée 2 hommes	VESTIBULE. congestionné 1 homme		grosses et jaunâtres 1 homme		diminuées et jaunâtres 1 homme	CORDES VOCALES. adduct. incomplète 1 homme		œdème 1 homme	congestionnées 2 hommes	tremblement fibrillaire 2 hommes

MALADIE DE PARKINSOHN. (1 HOMME ET 1 FEMME.)

TYMPANS. sclérose totale 1 homme	opaque total. 1 femme	FOSSE NASALE DROITE. CORNET MOYEN HYPERTROPHIÉ. 1 femme	CORNET SUPÉRIEUR HYPERTROPHIÉ. 1 femme	MUQUEUSE CONGESTIONNÉE. 1 homme	PILIERS POSTÉRIEURS. CONGESTIONNÉS. 1 femme.	EPIGLOTTE. MOUVEMENT RÉDUIT 1 homme et 1 femme.	CORDES VOCALES. ŒDEMAT. 1 femme

2.—CHORÉE CHRONIQUE. (1 HOMME.)

TYMPAN GAUCHE. congestionné 1 homme	TRIANGLE DROIT DISP. 1 homme	MARTEAU ÉLEVÉ. à gauche 1 homme	CLOISON GAUCHE. Tumeur 1 homme	VOILE DU PALAIS. hypertrophiée 1 homme	LUETTE. congestionnée 1 homme	AMYGDALES. hypertrophiées 1 homme

3.—PARAPLÉGIE SPASMODIQUE. (3 HOMMES.)

TYMPAN GAUCHE. sclérosé 1 homme	opaque 1 homme	LE MARTEAU. élevé à gauche 1 homme	MOUVEMENTS. ankilosés doubles 3 hommes	FOSSE NASALE DROITE. CORNET MOYEN. atrophié 1 homme	FOSSE NASALE GAUCHE. CORNET INFÉRIEUR. hypertrophié 1 homme	atrophié 2 hommes	CORNET SUPÉRIEUR. hypertrophié 1 homme	MUQUEUSE. anémiée 1 homme	CLOISON GAUCHE. bombé 1 homme	L'ODORAT. aboli 1 homme	perverti 1 homme
LUETTE longue 1 homme	BASE DE LANGUE. varices 1 homme	LE GOÛT. diminué 3 hommes	EPIGLOTTE EN FORME, &c. museau de tanche 1 homme	CARTILAGES ARYTENOÏDES. hypertrophiés 3 hommes	CORDES VOCALES. plus grosses 1 homme	diminuées et jaunâtres. 2 hommes					

4.—PARALYSIE INFANTILE. (1 HOMME.)

TRIANGLE. disp. à gauche 1 homme	LE MARTEAU. disp. à gauche 1 homme	FOSSE NASALE DROITE. CORNET MOYEN. hypertrophié 1 homme	FOSSES. obstruées 1 homme	MUQUEUSE. congestionnée 1 homme	PHARYNX. granulations 1 homme	LE GOÛT. diminué 1 homme	EPIGLOTTE. congestionnée 1 homme	VESTIBULE. congestionné 1 homme	CORDES VOCALES. congestionnées 1 homme

5.—SCLÉROSE LATERALE AMYOTROPHIQUE. (1 HOMME.)

TYMPAN GAUCHE. sclérosé total. 1 homme	FOSSE NASALE DROITE. cornet moyen hypertrophié 1 homme	VOILE DU PALAIS. hypertrophiée 1 homme	parésie à droite 1 homme	LUETTE. congestionée 1 homme	CORDES VOCALES. paresseuses 1 homme

6.—SOURD-MUET. (1 HOMME.)

Perceptions abolies	Les Tympans sclérosés total.

moins que l'autre qui n'est pas bouchée, et par Signe de Weber négatif, l'inverse.

Chart C illustrating Dr. Costiniu's paper on the Condition of the ears, larynx and nose in old age.

to know something of the peculiar ways and curious conditions, under which diseases of the ear have been'treated in India for ages past, and to contrast the practice of the olden times with what obtains at the present day. The contrast will show that the study and practice of Ear Diseases have not advanced much, if at all, at the present time, from what it was, say a thousand years ago. The native of India is just as fond of his itinerant medicine vendor, his Vaid (Hindoo Practitioner of Medicine), and his Hakim (Mahomedan ditto) now, as 2,000 years ago. The paper thus resolves itself, to some extent, into one more of anthropological interest than a study of any real scientific value. And I have been so fully conscious of this fact, that when your honoured President, under whom I had the pleasure and the privilege of learning my first lessons in Otology, and acquiring my first experiences of ear diseases, requested me to contribute a paper, it was with no little hesitation and diffidence that I consented, in the hope, that the defects and shortcomings of the paper would be condoned a good deal in one who hails from many thousand miles across the seas.

The subject matter of the paper may be divided into four sections. (1). A brief reference to the study and practice of Aural Diseases in India in the ancient times, and to the evidence obtainable of the knowledge of ear diseases, and their treatment. To this section is attached the appendix A, giving a list of the diseases of the ear, and their treatment, described in the oldest Sanscrit Works. (2). A description of the men who practise the art of medicine, including diseases of the ear, at the present day, and of some of their better known remedial measures, both medical and surgical, in the treatment of ear diseases. To this section is attached a tabulated list of the more important drugs, and a list of a few of the more reputed Indian recipes and prescriptions, said to be useful in ear diseases (appendix B). (3). Some remarks on the position of the present day practice of aural medicine in Bombay, according to western methods of treatment. (4). Types of ear diseases met with most frequently in ordinary private practice in Bombay, in their order of frequency.

SECTION 1.—India, or more properly speaking, Hindustàn, has been *par excellence*, a land of medicine from very remote antiquity. The most ancient treatise known amongst the Hindoos, on the science of medicine, was the Ayurvéda, written in the Sanscrit language, and said to be entirely composed in verse by the gods, for the benefit of mankind. The word, Ayurvéda, literally means the knowlege of living, or the science of medicine. Only a very few fragments of this great work still exist, the greater portion of the original, consisting of one hundred thousand Slokàs, or verses, having been lost. This work was originally divided into eight sections, describing a large number of diseases, in almost all departments of medicine and surgery, and their treatment, one section being specially devoted to diseases of the eye, nose, and ear (vide appendix A).

Dhanvantari, the founder of the Ancient Hindoo School of Medicine, finding the Ayurvéda too voluminous and erudite for ordinary intellects, advised one of his most celebrated disciples, Susruta, to abridge it. The treatise compiled by the latter is still extant, and in use at the present day, and is known as the Susruta, after his name. The Charaka and the Susruta, are the two Hindoo medical works of the highest authority and antiquity, and are mentioned in the Purànas, and the Máhábhárat. Like the Susruta, the Charaka is the work of another sage, after whose name it is called, and is said to be of a still older date. Prof. H. Wilson puts them down approximately, to the 9th or 10th century B.C., and some authorities even to 2,000 years B.C. The Charaka is celebrated as a medical work chiefly, and the Susruta more as a surgical and anatomical one. Evidence obtainable from these two great Sanscrit treatises conclusively shows that a large number of various surgical operations were performed in those olden days, and the author of the Susruta mentions as many as 101 Yantras, or surgical instruments for them, some of which were specially devised for the ear. It would also seem, that to the Hindoo of old is due the credit of having first practised plastic operations for the reparation not only of lost noses, but of cut or injured ears. Various diseases of the ear are mentioned, and their treatment is described in detail, in these two classical works—a list of some of these is given in Appendix A.

Turning to the Mahomedan writers on medicine, their works are of much more recent date, most of them dating from the 17th century. Their principal medical works, in which occasional references to ear diseases and their treatment are found, are the Tib-i-Akbari, Alfáz-el-Adwiyá, Magzàn-el-Adwiyá, Ibu Sinà, and Ibu Baitár. One of these, the Magzan-el-Adwiyá, is a very complete treatise on materia medica, and was compiled about the year 1771 A.D.

SECTION 2 may be conveniently sub-divided into (A), a description of the men who practise the act of medicine, including diseases of the ear, in India, at the present day, and (B), a description of some of their better known remedial measures, both medical and surgical. In this connection, I can speak with special reference to Bombay alone, to which city my experiences have been chiefly confined.

A. The practice of Aural Medicine in India at the present time, is unfortunately, like most other branches of medicine, largely, if not entirely, in the hands of the quack, pure and simple. The men who practise it are (a) the Hakims, (b) the Vaids, and (c) a mixed class of itinerant medicine vendors, known as the Khávois, the Gossáins, the Sadhoos, or Báwás, all mostly Hindoos, and the Mailvállás, mostly Mahomedans.

(a). The Hakims are the Mahomedan practitioners, who, unlike the Hindoo Vaids, practise according to the Unàni "Hakimá, or the Greek School of Medicine. They derive their knowledge of medicine by studying medical works in the Persian, Arabic, and Urdoo languages. They are mostly Indian Mahomedans, and although in former times, many of them were really learned men, as the word Hakim itself implies, a good many of them at the present day, are quacks and charlatans, and trade on the credulity and ignorance of the people by dabbling in charms, amulets, holy waters, and magical incantations, in addition to their drugs.

(b). The Vaids are the Hindoo prototypes of their Mahomedan *confrères*, so to say, and practise on similar lines, except that they ignore the Greek system altogether, and stick entirely to that of the Ayurvéda. The Hindoo physicians of the olden times were said to be far superior to the Vaids of the present generation, who entirely lack their scientific attainments. Some of these modern Vaids are hereditary practitioners of medicine, the practice descending from the father to the son in many families, and such families are also surnamed Vaids.

(c) Of the three classes of native practitioners, this is, generally speaking, the lowest in the scale, and proportionately ignorant. The Gossáins, the Sádhoos, and the Báwás are not regular practitioners of medicine in the strict sense of the word, but simply religious mendicants, who wander all over the various provinces of India, and very often live in the jungles for months. They thus mix with some of the wild tribes, and sometimes pick up some very useful remedies from them, which are occasionally found to be highly efficacious. The Khávois are a distinct class by themselves, who must have originally belonged to some wild Indian tribes. They are mostly denizens of the forest and the jungle, and living on the outskirts of civilisation, they migrate every year, during the cold season, into the nearest towns and villages, and there vend their heterogeneous stock of goods. They are a weird and wild-looking people, and both the males and the females "practise the profession." They are generally seen wandering about the streets and the bazaars of Bombay, shouting out the names of various drugs and medicines, and praising their efficacy in various diseases, in a peculiar nasal sing-song tone. Both males and females generally carry their stock of goods in two large saffron-coloured cloth bags, slung at each end of a bamboo pole, and balanced across the neck, or on either shoulder. Their stock is a very motley and curious collection, consisting of bits of dried twigs, bulbs, or roots, popularly known as "Jari Bootees," with a bogus reputation for high efficacy, bits of various minerals or coloured stones, of coral, mother-of-pearl, reduced ashes of various vegetables and minerals, known as "Khàk," various powders, collyria, oils and ear-drops, tiger's claws and fat, and the hair, nails, and even the excretions of rare and wild animals and birds. One oil

in particular, known as the "Sándhánoo Tél," extracted from a live animal, resembling a chameleon, has a high reputation as an external application for all kinds of pains, including ear-aches, and rheumatic and neuralgic pains. In fact, these saffron-coloured bags serve as a regular portable pharmacy for the jungle man, and there is in them a cure or an antidote for every imaginable disease or injury that flesh is heir to.

They also treat ear diseases, and it is possible their name Khávoi is a corruption of the original Kàna-Vaid, or ear doctor. They are to be seen squatting by the roadside, or under the shade of a tree, with all their goods spread out on the bare ground before them. They soon attract the passers-by, who are generally ignorant, illiterate, and very poor people, and begin to collect small coppers, never more than a farthing or a halfpenny in value, in exchange for their herbs and simples.

(d) .The Meilwállás form another unique class of "Ear Doctors" peculiar to India. They are generally Mahomedans, sometimes Chinese by nationality. It is no exaggeration to say that the people of India, especially the lower classes, have a sort of mania, so to speak, for getting their ears frequently cleaned of wax by these ear-cleaners, and thus the Meilwállás earn a fairly decent livelihood by plying this particular "profession." I have observed in my own private practice several cases of dry middle ear catarrh, with considerable hardness of hearing, and often with a sclerosed or highly congested tympanum, as a result of these frequent ear-cleaning operations. These Meilwállás generally carry their small stock of instruments and oils in their turbans, or in their broad waistbands. Their instruments consist of perhaps half a dozen or more thin long metal probes, like large hair-pins, some of them tipped with a little cotton wool at both ends. Three or four of these probes are generally carried like quill pens, behind the ears, and the Meilwállás are at once known amongst the people by this outward evidence of their special art. They also carry with them one or two fine pointed forceps, a small quantity of spare cotton wool, and some Til oil (oil expressed from Sesamum indicum, N.O. Pedalinæ), a little of which is poured into the ear after it has been cleaned of all wax.

Besides those mentioned, there is another local celebrity, all by himself, in Bombay, who has made quite a reputation as an Ear Doctor. He is a Chinaman, by name Àsàm Akào. He is quite an expert in the art of skilfully removing cerumen from the ear without the least pain, and is superior to the Mahomedan Meilwállás in this particular line. It was with some difficulty I succeeded, quite recently, in obtaining small quantities of his stock medicines, which are said to be very efficacious in rapidly relieving pain, and stopping recent or old standing purulent discharges, in otitis media, and even in improving the hearing. They consist chiefly of two substances, one a brownish watery liquid, with a little resinous deposit in it, and the other a dark greenish coloured powder, a combination of three other powders, one white and two greenish ones. In cases of acute and chronic suppurative catarrh of the middle ear, the auditory canal is thoroughly dried by him of all purulent matter, some of the resinous liquid, which has probably good antiseptic properties, is then brushed into the canal by means of a feather-tipped whalebone probe, and through an improvised paper funnel a little of the powder is poured into the ear. The results are said to be really very good in rapidly relieving the pain, and in stopping the purulent discharge. In cases of simple pain in the ear, of whatever nature, the white powder alone is blown in. I got the substances chemically analysed at the Government chemical laboratory, but failed to get anything out of it, except that one of the three powders was calomel. All the rest were organic resinous substances. For the inspection of members present, I forward small quantities of these substances, all that I have, along with some of the ear-cleaning instruments, *Fari Bootees*, etc., in a separate box. So much for the men of medicine in India.

Let us now consider the remedies they generally employ. For the relief of acute pain, or inflammation, actual cantery, blisters, leeches, dry-cupping, issues, poultices, and thick applications, in the form of a paste, known as Lép, and made out of various herbs, are used. Syringing out the ear is very little known, or practised, except by the regularly qualified practitioners, and the more intelligent classes. But I may mention a somewhat novel method of doing it, amongst the poor people, which I came to know of by a mere chance. I had once prescribed for a poor Hindoo child, suffering from a rather troublesome otorrhœa, some antiseptic lotion, with which to wash out the ear, asking the mother to buy a small ear-syringe for the purpose. At the end of a week, the child was brought to me, with the discharge all stopped. On enquiring how she had managed the syringing, I was shown her primitive method of doing it, which was to first cleanse the mouth by some plain water, then to take a mouthful of the antiseptic solution, and spurt it into the affected ear, and repeat the process till the prescribed quantity was finished, and then wipe the child's ear dry, and cleanse her own mouth with some more plain water!

The actual cautery, and the blister, are the two most favourite and common modes of treatment. The blister is very crude, and is generally produced by the application, over the mastoid or near the temple, of some irritant substance. That in most general use, is an oil of a brownish colour, obtained by heating the nut of Semi-Carpus Anacardium (N.O. Anacardiaceæ), and known in the Vernacular, as Bhiláwá, or Bibbá.

Dry-cupping, by means of what is known as Roomri, is also re-sorted to, as a counter-irritant, in pain and inflammation about the ear. This Roomri, is merely the small conical horn of a goat, or a sheep, or a bullock, hollowed out. It is also made of metal. The broad end is pressed firmly over the mastoid, or on the temple, and powerful suction is applied at the smaller end, by the mouth of the operator, and kept up for some time, till the skin is raised, and the horn fixed over it as with cupping glasses. The horn is also used for extracting live worms which, according to popular belief, exist in some diseased ears. It is also used to extract guinea-worms.

Leeches are largely used, usually about half a dozen or more, applied behind the ear, or over the temple, and generally repeated the next day, because there is a popular notion, that the first day's applica-tion is not enough, and even injurious, if not repeated the next day, in order to remove the " sour blood " set up in the leeched part, by the leech bites.

Issue behind the ear, or in the neck, or in one of the lobes of the ear, is also very popular, for the relief of constant or chronic pain and inflammation, and is generally done by inserting bits of rolled cloth or twine, dipped in some irritant medicine.

Metallic rings of lead, silver, gold, and other metals are also worn in the lobes of the ear, for persistent pain, and purulent discharges from it. Instillation of mother's milk, and warm cow's urine, and even ordinary Eau de Cologne, are other favourite modes.

Poultices, plasters, and external applications of various kinds, some of them very curious, and even disgusting in their composition, are also much in use for the relief of pain and inflammation. A very efficacious remedy for the relief of pain, especially of a neuralgic character, is the instillation of a few drops of a thickish liquid, obtained by rubbing the small conical root of the plant, known as Vachnág or Bachnág (also known in other parts of India as Bish or Bikh, Aconitum ferox, N.O. Ranunculaceæ) in some water or spirit, on a curry-stone. The effect of the instillation in rapidly relieving the agonising pain, is sometimes marvellous. I well remember the case of a highly neurotic and intelligent Parsee lady, who suffered from intense pains in one of her ears for several days, probably of a neuralgic character, and which everything that I tried failed to relieve. They were completely stopped within a few minutes, however, by a couple of instillations of these drops. Another very efficacious application, which I have also person-ally tried, in a good many cases with painful swellings about the ear, in inflammation and pain in the auditory canal, such as that produced by furunculosis, and in neuralgic conditions, is the expressed juice of the plant known as Kàli dàndi-chá-Daturà (Datura Fastuosa, N.O. Solanaceæ) or Datura with black or grey branches, as distinguished from the white variety, or Daturà Alba. If the pain is inside the ear, a few drops are also instilled into the canal.

Gugal. Boswellia Serrata (N.O. Burseraceæ) is another drug very commonly employed with good effect in painful or glandular swellings near the ear. This is applied over the painful swelling as a thickish emulsion, made up in milk or water.

Some plants belonging to the N.O. Liliaceæ, E.g. Tulsi or Tulas (Ocimum Sanctum), and Sabjá (Ocimum Basilicum), are also used to relieve pain and purulent discharges from the ear. The former is a plant sacred to the Hindoo God, Vishnu. Its dried and powdered leaves are also used as a snuff in ozæna.

An extremely common household remedy to relieve pain in the ear, is an oil prepared by boiling a few pieces of the bulb of Lashan, Allium Sativum (N.O. Liliaceæ) in Sesamum Oil, and a few drops of it instilled into the ear. The effects may be good in some cases, but when employed indiscriminately, I have found its use disastrous to the drum head.

There are various other plants and drugs used for the relief of pain and inflammation, and for acute and chronic suppurative inflammation of the middle ear, noises, and deafness. They are described in the appendix B.

SECTION 3.—Coming now to a description of the present day practice of aural medicine in Bombay, it is with extreme reluctance I am obliged to offer the following rather unpleasant but honest criticism. It may perhaps seem a little strange, that amongst nearly two hundred qualified private practitioners in this city, there are not more than three or four who practise as specialists in diseases of the ear, nose, and throat, by reason of their special knowledge and training, though specialists in eye diseases alone, may be counted by the dozen.

The causes of this backwardness are not far to seek. Up to within a very recent period, strange as it may appear, not a single lecture, much less a course of lectures, or clinical demonstrations, was ever given in diseases of ear, nose and throat, to the students of the only local centre of medical education that exists in this city, viz., the Grant Medical College, and the Jamsetjee Jeejeebhoy Hospital, both affiliated institutions. This was mostly due to the fact, that the exigencies of what is known in India, as the Indian Medical Service, a purely military service, subordinated all other considerations of medical science, and the proper education of students. What is still more deplorable is, that most, if not every one, of these appointments on the hospital and professorial staff, no matter whether they require any special qualifications or not, are made from the ranks of that department, for the grotesque reason of seniority in its regimental service, hardly ever *pour le Mérite*, or by open competition, outside it. This may seem an absurd anomaly, almost a scandal, in this advanced 19th century. It is none the less a lamentable fact. It is not surprising, under the circumstances, if the students who passed out of their hands, should also be very ignorant. I must say, however, that within the last

w

four or five years, a course of lectures and demonstrations in Aural Surgery has been instituted, and a good knowledge of ear-diseases is being imparted to the present students.

In offering these remarks, I need hardly explain, I have no wish to disparage or detract in the least from the merit of the work done by some men of the Indian Medical Service in other directions. For it will be readily seen, what I have criticised is the system of selection, and not the men. My chief object has been a desire to see some improvement in the present anomalous and injurious system of appointments, and the consequent imperfect teaching. The fact of there being a special chair in Ophthalmic Medicine and Surgery at the G. M. College, and none, not even a joint one, for ear, throat, or nose diseases, is significant, and suggestive of the direction in which improvement is most needed. It is also necessary, both in the interests of the general public, as well as of the local medical profession, that postgraduate courses of clinical lectures and demonstrations should be instituted as soon as possible.

Another cause of this backwardness and apparent lack of zeal in the local medical practitioners is the want of opportunities for surgical work in private aural practice. The native of India is, as a rule, somewhat averse to the European methods of treatment, and is a great believer in the efficacy of drugs, as I have already mentioned. It is only in the last resort, that he avails himself of the former. Besides, the poorer classes are really too poor to be able to pay for skilled medical advice, and are, therefore, content to completely neglect all treatment, except their own homely remedies, till they go from bad to worse. The opportunities for purely surgical work in ear-diseases for a duly qualified medical practitioner are thus somewhat limited.

SECTION 4.—Taking for convenient reference statistical tables of about four thousand ear-cases, given in Macnaughton Jones and Stewart's Diseases of the Ear, and comparing them with a fairly large number of cases that have by now accumulated in my own private note-books, I find that the order and percentage of frequency is about the same here, as in England, except in one or two minor divisions. Cases of middle ear disease, and the consequent troubles of one kind or another, largely preponderate here, as in England. I believe the climatic conditions of Bombay greatly contribute to this result. The atmosphere is more or less moist and humid, and charged at all times and seasons of the year with a large amount of watery vapour, much more so during the months of heavy rain, from June to September, locally known as the S.W. Monsoons. I have often seen cases, which have resisted all treatment in Bombay, improve very rapidly and permanently in the dry atmosphere of the hill-stations, under almost identical lines of treatment.

Another very frequent cause of chronic suppurative otitis media is

the complete neglect of a large number of cases of middle ear inflammation, following specially on measles and small pox. Want of cleanliness
and absence of all treatment, when it is most needed, frequently end in
mastoid inflammation, and often in caries and necrosis, with their
attendant complications.

Next in the order of frequency, come the diseases of the external
ear, including the meatus. And in this class, I have several times come
across cases of eczematous, and even erysipelatous inflammation of the
auricle, and the skin over the mastoid, due to a special cause unknown
in Europe. It may, perhaps, surprise those present here to know, that
a very large proportion of the natives of India, especially the Hindoos,
have the peculiar custom of having the helix, the lobule, the concha,
and the nose of children and even of adults of both sexes, pierced in one
or more places, and the ear, sometimes in as many as half a dozen, in
order to wear ear-rings and large and heavy ear-ornaments. This
piercing operation is generally done by the village goldsmith, with a
pointed piece of iron, or a silver probe, without any antiseptic precautions
whatever. The hole thus made, is generally kept patent by thin wire
rings at first, and then a bit of bristle, or a rough piece of wood, or a
thin dirty roll of paper. And as a result, in many cases, the holes in-
flame, suppurate, and ulcerate, sometimes leading to very severe reaction
and considerable erysipelatous or eczematous inflammation. So frequently
is this mischief set up, that in the classification of ear-diseases, given in
the old Sanscrit Standard Work, by Susruta, prominence is given to it
as a special disease.

Cerumen in the ear forms another large class of cases, which come
under observation indirectly. The dirty habits of the poorer classes,
and the favourite practice of instilling very frequently all sorts of oils
into their own ears and those of their children, from infancy upwards,
contribute largely to a dense accumulation of dirt and cerumen. And
sometimes it is a rather difficult matter, and very puzzling for the
novice, to treat the chalky and almost stony deposits which thus form
in the ear-canal.

Furunculosis and abscesses, near the auditory meatus, are also
frequent. Amongst fungus growths in the ear, Aspergillus Nigricans
is rather frequent. But most cases generally go unrecognised by the
ordinary medical practitioner and are usually taken to be cases of
suppurative otitis media, or an eczematous condition of the auditory
canal. That this form of otomycosis is more frequent than in Europe,
may be due to the favourite practice already mentioned, of frequently
dropping oils and other greasy substances into the ear, which afford a
good nidus for its development.

I have only come across four cases of exostosis of the meatus, never
more than one in each ear. Of these, two were really not the true
eburnated variety, or the ivory exostosis. Of the other two cases,

one was in a very old gentleman, in whom both the meatus were quite closed by the encroachment of the growths, and the patient was almost stone deaf.   The other was the case of a young Parsee lady, belonging to a wealthy family, aged about nineteen years, in whom there were small rounded growths of the true ivory type in each meatus auditorius externus, probably congenital and leading to a considerable narrowing of the lumen of the meatus.   They caused a moderate amount of deafness, and troublesome noises in the ears.

Of aural polypi I have had several cases, generally single, in two cases only multiple, and occasionally with several granulations, filling a large portion of the canal.   They need no special mention.

True Ménière's disease is a very rare affection with us, and I have come across two cases only, both males.

Turning to the nasopharyngeal passages, I have observed several cases of adenoid growths in the nasopharynx, within the last few years, ever since my attention was drawn to them by the observations of Meyer, of Copenhagen, and of Guye, and Löwenberg.   ·I have observed them mostly in thin, scrofulous-looking, weakly children, mostly boys, between the ages of six and fifteen, with all the typical signs and symptoms.   I find that I meet with such cases rather frequently, ever since I have come to recognise this diseased condition.   I particularly recall to mind the case of a young Parsee lad, of about fifteen years of age, who, except for frequent frontal head-aches, a defective memory, some backwardness in school studies, a slight difficulty in breathing through the nose, and frequent attacks of profuse epistaxis, which always seemed to relieve his troubles temporarily, was in every way in good, one might almost say, robust health.   When I put my finger into his naso-pharynx I did so more with the object of ascertaining any other possible cause but the adenoids.   But to my surprise I found soft velvety masses of adenoid growths, partially filling both the posterior nares.   Their complete removal by the finger nail, at two separate sittings, cured the patient of all his troubles.

It may, perhaps, interest the members present to know something of the nature of ear complications in cases of Bubonic Plague, which has been raging as a most virulent epidemic in Bombay for the last three years.   From the information I have been able to gather through the courtesy of the chief Physicians of the Arthur Road Plague Hospital, and the Parsee Fever Hospital, and from my own private practice, and that of other medical men of whom I have made enquiries, I find that about the only ear complications observed are acute Otitis Media, generally ending in suppuration, and deafness, which is central, and not due to local causes.   The former is found in about two per cent. of the cases treated at the hospitals, and is noticed as a concurrent complication (hardly ever as a sequel), mostly in cases of Bubonic Plague, with parotid, cervical, or submaxillary buboes, in the ratio of about 20, 15, and 10 per cent. respectively, as compared with its presence in the other varieties of buboes. It has never been noticed in any other forms of plague except in the Bubonic type. The course is a very rapid and acute one, owing to the intensity of the blood poison, often ending in meningitic symptoms and death, in about 70 per cent. of cases. Only one ear, as a rule, is affected. The character of the discharge in most cases is found to be thin, scanty, and serous or sero-sanguineous, in the beginning, and later, sero-purulent. No plague bacilli are found in these discharges under the microscope. If the case improves, the discharge soon ceases, the defect in hearing rapidly improves, and the ear is restored to its normal state in about a fortnight or three weeks' time. No case has been noticed to end in severe mastoid inflammation, terminating in necrosis. Occasionally however, the parotid bubo suppurates, and makes its way out gradually through the external meatus, and the pus is found to contain the specific bacilli.

Of mastoid inflammation I have had several cases. They are rather frequent, because the people of India are, unfortunately, averse as a rule to all surgical treatment, and I have, hence, known of cases of mastoid inflammation, ending in necrosis, meningitic inflammation and death, which might have been most surely saved by a timely interference of the surgeon, but for the great dread, and consequent obstinate refusal of all operative interference by the patient, and more especially by the relatives.

It was my original intention, to have given brief notes of a few interesting cases, from my note-books. But as the paper has expanded a great deal more than I had anticipated, I have dropped the idea altogether. There is one case, however, which I have operated upon recently, detailed notes of which I am induced to give here, as it is somewhat interesting from the fact that it was a case of mastoid inflammation of more than five months' duration, which eventually ended in necrosis and suppuration, and in which I had to operate without chloroform, owing to the greatly exhausted condition of the patient and his feeble heart's action, and to use instead, subcutaneous injections of a weak solution of cocaine, and ethyl chloride spray, for the purposes of anæsthesia, with very satisfactory results.

Mr. P. J. S., a Parsee gentleman, aged 45 years, was brought up to my consultation rooms, on the 22nd December, 1898, for severe, and more or less constant, throbbing pains in the right ear.

History : More than five months ago, the patient caught a chill while out on a bicycle, on a somewhat wet morning. One night, three or four days later, he woke up in bed with an intense throbbing pain in the right ear. To relieve this, he instilled a few drops of Eau de Cologne. This however, greatly increased the pain for a while, till he fell asleep exhausted, and woke up the next morning with a profuse, somewhat thickish, purulent discharge from the ear. The discharge ceased within three or four days, but the pain continued with varying intensity. A few days later he began to notice noises in the ear, more or less constant, like the blowing of a conch, and these have continued ever since. No history of any venereal disease. He was variously treated for more than five months, by several qualified medical men, as well as quacks, but his condition gradually grew worse, till, when I saw him for the first time, he was greatly exhausted, owing to the intense pains in the ear, and several successive sleepless nights. General health indifferent of late.

On examination a somewhat brawny, diffused, and painful swelling, somewhat tender to the touch, was noticed over the right mastoid, extending upwards and outwards over the parietal and occipital regions. Patient unable to open his mouth freely, or masticate any solid food without much pain. Pharyngeal mucous membrane and the tonsils slightly congested. The right auditory canal somewhat tender to the introduction of the speculum, but not affected otherwise. The membrana tympani slightly congested at its periphery, and along the handle of the malleus, and somewhat dull and opaque, but not bulging. Watch faintly heard, only on contact Left ear normal. Heart sounds feeble, the first sound faint, and partly lost in an ill-defined mitral regurgitant bruit. Temperature 99.6°, pulse 96, full and regular.

Half-a-dozen leeches were at once ordered over the mastoid, to be repeated the next day, and to be followed by the constant application of an ice bag. Internally, a dose of calomel, followed by a saline mixture, with digitalis and strychnine in small doses, and an opiate at bed time. This line of treatment seemed to relieve the patient somewhat for a while, the pain and swelling subsiding considerably, and he was able to sleep fairly well for the two or three nights following.

On the 26th December, however, the pain again became much worse. The right membrana tympani appeared more deeply injected, and slightly bulging, and a longish incision was therefore made in the posterior quadrant, behind the handle of the malleus, from below upwards, with the usual antiseptic precautions. The ear was then carefully inflated with Polizer's bag, and bandaged. Politzerisation was repeated the next two days, but there was no escape of air, or any serous or purulent discharge whatever, at the time of the operation or subsequently. The operation, however, seemed to relieve the patient very considerably for another two or three days, and the patient was able to sleep for several hours immediately after it, without any opiate. The ice-bag, becoming very irksome to the patient, was discontinued soon after the operation. But the pain and the swelling again gradually increased, till the latter spread as a diffused inflammation, over almost the whole of the right side of the head, and the face became puffy and œdematous. Notwithstanding the re-application of the ice-bag, and all other remedies that could be thought of, the pain became much worse, till, on my visit late on the evening of the 30th December, indistinct fluctuation could be felt on deep pressure, at a spot about five inches above the tip of the mastoid, and over the right parietal region. The temperature was 100.5°, and the pulse 86. The patient felt a little chilly, and became somewhat drowsy, and disinclined to talk, and all the symptoms pointed to suppuration, and impending meningitis.

An operation was at once decided upon, and on the morning of the 31st, it was performed under strict antiseptic precautions, with the valuable help of my friend, Dr. D. B. Master. In view of the cardiac complication, and the greatly exhausted condition of the patient, chloroform was not administered. Coryl not being obtainable, about four grammes of chloride of ethyl was sprayed on, and a weak solution of cocaine (prepared after Schleich's method, viz : one part of cocaine in 1,000 parts of a 0.2 p.c. solution of sodium chloride), was slowly injected, deep into the subcutaneous and muscular tissues, at half a dozen different points round the area of operation. Some more ethyl chloride was then sprayed on, till the parts became completely deadened. The usual curved incision, recommended by Wilde, was then made from the tip of the mastoid process, upwards, for about $3\frac{1}{2}$ inches, cutting perpendicularly deep down to the bone, and the periosteum completely divided, but no pus came up. The left fore-finger was then passed into the wound, and the periosteum, which was firmly adherent at the upper part of the incision, stretched by the retractors, and gradually separated and torn with the point of a director, till the finger entered a superficial cavity, under the scalp, and about an ounce of thick but perfectly inodorous pus, which had been imprisoned by the thick mass of inflamed tissues, suddenly welled out of the opening. On passing the director further up, it entered a large, superficial, and rough cavity, indicating superficial necrosis, just underneath the swelling over the parietal bone. It was then withdrawn, and passed in different directions. In passing it a little downwards and inwards, over the mastoid process, it appeared to slide over the digastric fossa, into a very small rough bony cavity, about a third of an inch deep. Two small necrosed pieces of bone were carefully removed, the cavity thoroughly scraped and curetted, by Volkmann's spoons, the whole wound douched with some carbolic lotion, and the wound thoroughly dried, and bound up with bandages, over several layers of boric cotton-wool, and iodoform gauze. Very little blood was lost, and no vessel of any importance cut. The patient bore the operation very well, and did not feel the least pain throughout, except when the bone was being scraped, and this was deadened by spraying over it a little more of the ethyl chloride. The dressings were changed daily, for the first few days, and the parts thoroughly washed with either iodine or carbolic lotion. The wound was allowed to heal slowly from below upwards, the edges being separated by a probe when necessary. No drainage was employed, and the wound was kept dry as much as possible, and dressed with powdered boracic acid and iodoform. It healed up completely in about three weeks, and would have healed up quicker, but for a small abscess, which formed about ten days after the operation, under the cellular tissue, about half an inch below the lower angle of the wound. The hearing of the right ear also became normal by the end of the month.

The points of interest in this case are (a), the great length of time before the mastoid inflammation ended in suppuration ; (b), the complete anesthesia produced by the combined use of weak cocaine injections and the ethyl chloride spray, allowing of considerable manipulations right down to the bone and into it, and (c), the complete restoration of the patient's hearing, and entire cessation of the noises.

Appendix A.

As already mentioned in the body of the paper, the *Charaka* and the *Susruta*, are the two oldest medical works in existence in India, and perhaps in the world. The former mentions four, and the latter about twenty-eight diseases of the ear, of which the following are the more important, the rest being mere sub-divisions. These are des-cribed under special names in Sanscrit, but I have simply classified them as follows, without giving the names in the Vernacular, to avoid being tedious.

A. *Diseases of the external ear:* 1, Simple inflammation of the external ear. 2, Inflammation of the lobule and the pinna, due to injury. 3, Inflammation of the helix, due to hard rubbing, or wearing heavy ear ornaments. 4, Piercing the helix in a wrong place, causing inflam-mation and swelling of the lower lobe, with ulcerating pimples and pustular eruptions. The treatment recommended for these inflamma-tions is for 1, extraction of blood from the inflamed parts, followed by soothing and emollient applications ; for 2 and 3, cold evaporating lotions ; for 4, applications of sandal wood rubbed in goat's urine, and cowdung poultices.

B. *Diseases of the auditory canal and the middle ear:* 1, Otalgia. 2, Noises in the ear. 3, Deafness. 4, Itching in the ear. 5, Discharges from the ear, other than purulent. 6, Simple Otorrhœa. 7, Otorrhœa with maggots. 8, Otorrhœa, with very fetid discharges. 9, Ulcerations inside the auricle, and extending into the auditory canal. 10, Swellings near the meatus, which burst after a very long time, and discharge pus or blood. 11, Small fleshy growths in the canal.

These diseases were treated in various ways, of which instillation of oils and expressed juices of plants, form the chief modes of treatment. Some of these recipes are given in the appendix B.

Surgery of the ear was, of course, very little practised in the olden times. Still, in the Susruta, allusion is found to the removal of aural granulations or polypi by instruments. There is also a detailed description of the method of restoring portions of the ear, which may have been accidentally or intentionally cut off, by fixing and uniting the freshly cut portions by means of stitches. Cutting off of portions of the ear, or even of the entire auricle, was a very common form of punishment in India before the advent of British rule, and is occasionally practised even at the present day. In the very serious religious riots which have taken place in the Travancore district, in the Madras Presidency, during this month, and which are still going on unabated, tearing of the lobules and cutting off of entire ears of unfortun-ate women and children, both out of pure revenge, as well as to get at their ear ornaments, have been very freely resorted to by the rioters. Careful directions are also given as regards boring holes in the cartilages of the ears of children for wearing ornaments.

N.B.—For much useful information in the appendices A and B, as as well as for considerable help in collecting, identifying, and preparing pressed specimens of indigenous botanical plants, exhibited in the album, I am greatly indebted to my friend, Dr. L. B. Dhargalkar, a well-known botanist of this city. I am also indebted to Dr. Popat P.

Vaid, for information of a similar nature. He is the son of a well-known Vaid of this city, Mr. Prabhúram Vaid, whose photo appears on the first page of the album, and being a qualified medical man, assists his father in lecturing at what is called the Ayurvédic school of medicine, founded by him quite recently in this city, with the special object of imparting instruction in the Hindoo system of medicine. Similar schools have been founded of late, in some of the other larger cities of India.

Appendix B.—(A List of Drugs.)

	Botanical Name.	Natural Order.	Vernacular Name.	Part of the Plant Used.	Uses.
1	Gossypium stocksii	Malvaceæ	Kapàsi	Leaves	Warm juice, to relieve deafness and otorrhœa.
2	Cleome viscosa	Capprideæ	Kánphuti	Ditto	Juice of the leaves mixed with Sessamum oil, for purulent discharges.
3	Feronia elephantum	Rutaceæ	Kavitha	Fruit	For otorrhœa.
4	Raphanus sativus	Cruciferæ	Mulà	Leaves	To relieve pain in the ear.
5	Cratæva religiosa	Capparideæ	Vàya-varna	Seeds	To relieve pain in the ear, and also external inflammation of the auricle, and of the auditory canal. The seeds are coarsely powered mixed with water, warmed, and applied.
6	Asparagus racemosus	Liliaceæ	Satmuli	Juice of the fresh root	Ditto.
7	Acorus calamus	Aroideæ	Vékhand	Juice of the fresh rhizome	For otorrhœa and pain.
8	Careya arborea	Myrtaceæ	Kumbha	Calices of the flowers	Ditto.

Botanical Name.	Natural Order.	Vernacular Name.	Part of the Plant Used.	Uses.
9 Bassia latifolia	Sapotaceæ	Mohà, or Mohwrá	Juice of flowers & seeds	For otorrhœa and pain.
10 Eugenia jambolana	Myrtaceæ	Jàmbul	Juice of the ripe leaves	Ditto
11 Piper longum	Piperaceæ	Pipli	Seeds	To destroy maggots in the ear, and dry up purulent discharges.
12 Piper nigrum	Ditto	Káli-miri	Ditto	Ditto
13 Aegle marmelos	Rutaceæ	Bél	Fruit	For deafness.
14 Mangifera indica	Anacar-diaceæ	Ámbà	Juice of leaves, & fruit	Otorrhœa.
15 Butea frondosa	Leguminosæ	Pàlas or Khákhro	Root	Chew the root, and also the root of Valeriana Hardwickii by the teeth, collect the saliva, and put a drop of it into the ear, to destroy maggots and flies that may have entered it.
16 Pongamia glabra	Ditto	Karanj		
17				
18 Moringa pterygo-sperma	Moringæ	Shégat	Root	For pain in the ear, and to destroy maggots.
19 Momordica charantia	Cucurbita-ceæ	Kàrlà	Juice of fruit	For deafness and noises.
20 Plumbago rosea	Plumbagi-neæ	Lál-chitrá	Root	Ditto.
21 Melia azadir-achta	Meliaceæ	Nimb	Leaves	Juice instilled to relieve pain, and purulent discharges.

Botanical Name	Natural Order.	Vernacular Name.	Part of the Plant Used.	Uses.
22 Calotropis gigantea	Asclepiadeæ	Ákrà	Ditto	For deafness and purulent dischar-ges, the juice is in-stilled in the way mentioned in one of the recipes given in this appendix.
23 Tagetes patula	Compositæ	Shend	Juice of the flowers.	Ditto.
24 Eclipta alba	Ditto	Màkà, or Bhàngrà	Leaves and stem	For deafness and noises of the ear.
25 Vitex Nigundo	Verbenaceæ	Lingur	Leaves and root	Ditto.
26 Ocimum sanctum	Labiatæ	Tulas	Leaves	For pain and puru-lent discharges.
27 Trigonella frænum græcum	Leguminosæ	Méthi	Seeds	Ditto.
28 Achyranthes aspera	Amaranta-ceæ	Aghàdà	The juice of the flower-ing spike and leaves	Ditto
29 Jasminum auriculatum	Oleaceæ	Jái	Leaves and flowers	Ditto.
30 Ficus religiosa	Urticaceæ	Pipal	Powdered root-bark	Ditto.
31 Ficus bengalensis	Ditto	Vad	Juice of leaves	For Otorrhœa, with very fetid dis-charges.
32 Musa sapientum	Scitamina-ceæ	Kél	Ditto	For relief of pain in the ear.
33 Calendula officinale	Compositæ	Hajarigal	Leaves	For noises, purulent discharges, and pain in the ear.
34 Allium cepa	Liliaceæ	Kàndo	Bulb	Heat the juice with equal parts of the oil of Brassica Campestris, gently over the fire, and instil a few drops, when cooled, to relieve pain, and as a germicide.

Botanical Name.	Natural Order.	Vernacular Name	Part of the Plant Used.	Uses
35 Zingiber officinale	Zingibera- ceæ	Ádoo	Juice of the fresh rhizome	Mixed as above, and instilled for noises in the ear, and itching and irritation.
36 Citrus medica	Aurantia- ceæ	Bijoroon	Juice of the fruit	The juice, mixed with a little commercial carbonate of soda, and instilled, to relieve otorrhæa, and pain.
37 Ocimum basilicum	Labiateæ	Sahjo	Juice of leaves	To relieve pain and purulent discharges.
38 Aconitum Ferox	Ranun- culaceæ	Bachnag, Bish, or Bikh	Root	To relieve severe pain in the ear.
39 Datura fastuosa	Solanaceæ	Kàli-dán- dichà- Dhatura	Juice of leaves and stalks	To relieve pain, swelling, and inflammation in the auditory canal, and over the auricle.
40 Cannabis sativa	Urticaceæ	Bhàng	Ditto	Ditto.
41 Saussurea Lappa	Compositæ	Ouplaite	Root	To relieve pain, and purulent discharges.

APPENDIX B.—(RECIPES).

The following are some well-known recipes, used by the natives of India, in certain diseases of the ear. Many of these are mentioned in that ancient Sanscrit Medical Work, the Susruta.

(1). For Otalgia (neuralgic, or otherwise):

(a)   Juice of fresh ginger, zingiber officinale, Vern :—Ádoo.
       Honey.
       Sindhav (a natural rock-salt, consisting of impure chloride of sodium and magnesium).
       Black Mustard Oil (Brassica Campestris), N. O. Cruciferæ, Vern : Sarsu Tél.
       The above are well-mixed, and boiled over the fire, and dropped into the ear, in small quantities, after cooling.

(b) The bulb of Allium Sativum (N. O. Liliaceæ), Vern: Lahsan.
Juice of fresh ginger.

The root of Moringa pterygosperma (N. O. Moringae), Vern:
Shégat.

The seeds of Cratæva religiosa (N. O. Capparideæ), Vern:
Váyavarna.

The juice of Raphanus Sativus (N. O. Cruciferæ), Vern: Mulà.

The leaves of Musa Sapientum (N. O. Scitaminaceæ), Vern:
Kél.

The expressed juices of the above are mixed, warmed over the
fire, and instilled into the ear.

(c) Juice of Cannabis Sativa (N. O. Urticaceæ).

Ditto of fresh ginger.

Liquid extract of opium.

Oil expressed from Allium Sativum, Vern: Lahsan.

Ditto from Allium Sipa (N. O. Liliaceæ), Vern: Kándó.

The above are also instilled separately, for the relief of pain
in the ear.

(d) A little clarified butter is spread over a leaf of Calotropis
Gigantea (N. O. Asclepiadeæ), Vern: Ákrà, and the leaf
warmed over the fire. The juice is then pressed out of the
leaf, and a few drops instilled, warm, into the ear.

(e) The following three substances are digested in some oil expressed from Brassica Campestris (N. O. Cruciferæ), Vern:
Sarsu Tél, and some of it instilled, to relieve intense pain.

Sindhav (Rock-Salt).

Ferula alliacea (N. O. Umbelliferæ), Vern: Vaghárni.

Dry ginger.

(2). For Otorrhœa (Simple).

(a) The shell of the Cuttle-fish, burnt in an oven, reduced to
powder, and a little of the calcined powder blown in, after
the ear is thoroughly cleaned.

(b) Juice of the fruit of Gossypium herbaceum (N. O. Malvaceæ),
Vern: Kàpsi.

Powder of the bark of Shorea robusta (N. O. Dipte-
rocarpeæ), Vern: Sál.

Honey.

The above mixed, and instilled into the ear.

(c) Oil expressed from Saussurea Lappa (N. O. Compositæ),
Vern: Ouplaite.

Assafætida.

The bulb of Acerus Calamus (N. O. Aroideæ), Vern: Vékhand.

The wood of Cedrus Deodara (N. O. Coniferæ), Vern: Deodar.

The juice of Asparagus racemosus (N. O. Liliaceæ), Vern:
Satmuli.

Dry ginger.

Sindhav (Rock-Salt).

The above are mixed with sheep's urine, and a few drops instilled.

(d) An. oil prepared from the expressed juices of the ripe leaves of Eugenia Jambolana (N. O. Myrtaceæ), Vern: Jàmbul.

Mangifera indica (N. O. Anacardiaceæ), Vern : Amba.

Fruit of Feronia elephantum (N. O. Rutaceæ), Vern : Kavitha.

Gossypium herbaceum.

Juice of the leaves of Melia azadirachta (N. O. Meliaceæ), Vern : Nimb.

Oil expressed from Pongamia glabra (N. O. Leguminosæ), Vern : Karanj.

The above are well mixed, and instilled into the ear.

(e) The expressed juices of the following are also instilled individually.

Tagetes erecta (N. O. Compositæ), Vern : Galgotá.

Ruta Graveolens (N.O. Rutaceæ), Vern : Sitáb.

Jasminum Auriculatum (N. O. Oleaceæ), Vern : Jái.

Helecteres Isora (N. O. Sterculiaceæ), Vern : Murádsingh.

Oil expressed from the seeds of Oroxylum indicum (N. O. Bignoniaceæ), Vern : Phalphurá.

(f) After cleaning the ear thoroughly dry, a few drops of the common lime juice are instilled into the discharging ear, and then a small quantity of finely-powdered Sepia officinalis (Mollusca, Cephalopodia) is insufflated. This is considered a very efficacious remedy for chronic purulent discharges. Sometimes powdered borax is blown in after the lime juice instillation.

(g) Take about a drachm by weight, of each of the following, powder them coarsely, and boil in about an ounce and a half of Sessamum oil, and i istil a few drops daily into the ear, to relieve pain, and purulent discharges.

Anacyclus Pyrethrum (N. O. Compositæ), Vern : Akalkaro.

Caryophyllus aromaticus (N. O. Myrtaceæ), Vern : Laving.

Ptychotis Ajván (N. O. Umbelliferæ), Vern: Ajmo.

Symplocos Racemosus (N. O. Styraceæ), Vern : Lodar.

Saussurea Lappa (N. O. Compositæ), Vern : Ouplaite.

(3).   For Otorrhœa, with a fetid discharge.

(a) Oil expressed from Mangifera indica (N. O. Anacardiaceæ), Vern : Ámbà.

Eugenia Jambolana (N. O. Myrtaceæ), Vern : Jàmbul.

Ficus bengalensis (N. O. Urticaceæ), Vern : Vad.

Bassia latifolia (N. O. Sapotaceæ), Vern : Mohà.

Oil expressed from Sessamum indicum (N. O. Pedalineæ), Vern : Til.

Mix the above, and instil a few drops into the ear.

(b) Instillation of a few drops of the oil expressed from Jasminum auriculatum, Vern : Jái.

(4)   For Deafness.

(a) Expressed juice of the fruit of ægle marmalos (N. O. Rutaceæ), Vern : Bael, ground in cow's urine.

Goat's milk.

Sessamum oil.

Water.

Boil the above, and instil a few drops.

(b) Vitex Negundo (N. O. Verbenaceæ), Vern : Lingur.

Jasminum auriculatum.

Calotropis Gigantea (N. O. Asclepiadeæ), Vern : Ákrà, or Rui.

Eclipta alba (N. O. Compositæ), Vern : Bhàngrà.

Allium Sativum (N. O. Liliaceæ), Vern : Lahsan.

Musa Sapientum (N. O. Scitaminaceæ), Vern : Kél.

Gossypium herbaceum.

Morynga pterygosperma.

Zingiber officinale.

Ocimum Sanctum (N. O. Labiatæ), Vern : Tulas.

Momordica Charantia (N. O. Cucurbitaceæ), Vern : Kàrlà.

Aconitum Ferox (N. O. Ranunculaceæ), Vern : Bachnáb, Bish, or Bikh.

The above formidable combination is a sort of a general panacea for all ear diseases, and is said to be useful in deafness, noises in the ear, maggots in the ear, pain, and purulent discharges.

(5).   For Maggots in the ear.

(a) Juices of Eclipta alba (N. O. Compositæ), Vern : Màkà, Morynga pterygosperma.

Bulb of Gloriosa Superba (N. O. Liliaceæ), Vern : Nágkaria.

The juices of the above are instilled into the ear, also,

Dry ginger.

Piper Nigrum (N. O. Piperaceæ), Vern : Kàlimiri.

Piper longum (N. O. Ditto), Vern : Pipli.

The last three powdered, and blown into the ear.

(6).   For Noises in the ear.

(a) Lemon juice.

Piper longum.

Honey.

The above mixed together, and instilled into the ear.

(b) A salt, as well as a decoction in Sessamum oil, of Achyranthes aspera (N. O. Amarantaceæ) : Vern : Aghádá.

THE VARIOUS DOMESTIC REMEDIES WITH THEIR EFFECTS USED BY
THE PEOPLE OF INDIA FOR CERTAIN DISEASES OF THE EAR.

Dr. H. J. DADYSETT, Bombay.

Diseases of the ear are not so common in India as in cold countries.
There are however certain complaints from which people of India,
whether rich or poor, do suffer, due in most cases to their habit of sleep-
ing with their beds close to the windows which are generally kept open,
and thus exposing themselves to draughts. Again, poor people and
domestic servants sleep on open verandahs, and are thus exposed to cold
draughts and chilly winds. The diseases due to this cause are
Myringitis and Furuncles in the Meatus auditorius externus. In my
practice for the last seven years, as an Aural-Surgeon in Bombay,
I have had to treat a large number of patients suffering from the
above complaints, and on enquiry I found that before they came to
me they had tried various domestic remedies, consisting of various
simple or medicated oils, juices of plants, powders, &c. Once my
attention was drawn to this subject, I began collecting information in
connection with it, and the following notes, I hope, will be found interesting to the learned members of the 6th International Otological
Congress :—

I.—The Bulb of Allium Sativum (*Garlic*):—It is boiled with salad
oil, and the oil when cooled is dropped into the ears for relieving the
pain due to Myringitis or Furuncles. I believe it has a temporary
soothing effect in some cases. But in others I have observed that it
does more harm than good.

II.—Sesamum Oil or Tull-Tella:—It has been used mostly by people
belonging to the "Ghatty" caste to soften the cerumen when there is
much gathering in the ears. I think it has the same effect as the
ordinary olive oil.

III.—Oil of Andropogon Citratus and Dhuprel Oil (consisting of
various bland oils with a number of aromatics used as hair-oil) :—

These oils have been largely used by the Parsees for deafness and
noises in the ears. The noises in the ears do sometimes disappear under
this treatment, due I believe, to the oil having the power to soften
cerumen. The ear is generally syringed with water after the oil has
been dropped into it.

IV.—Sweet-Oil Boiled with Ptychotis Ajvan:—It is used mostly
by the Mahomedans for noises in the ears under the belief that it relieves
the congestion of the middle ear. I think it has some effect in relieving
the noises.

V.—The Juice of the petals of the Marigold Flowers (Calendula
Officinalis) known as gulgotta :—It is used in catarrhal deafness ; but I
have never seen a single case of recovery under this treatment.

VI.—The juice of the leaves of Ruta Graveolens called by the natives *sitab* :—It has been used for relieving ear-ache. I have seen some patients benefited by this juice.

VII.—The juice of the leaves of Anona Squamosa known in India as "*Andoos* or *Sitaful*" :—It has been used by Wagri women in India in ear-ache arising from various causes. They first pour the juice into the ear, and then with a hollow copper or brass tube suck out worm-like bodies from the canal. This, of course, is a trick practised upon ignorant and credulous people. The worm-like bodies are simply pieces of vermicelli. This practice of what they call removing worms from the ears is rather common in India, and these Wagri women make their living by it.

VIII.—The Juice of Pansupari :—It is syringed into the ears by ignorant Hindoos belonging to the "Ghatty" caste for relieving ear-ache. The Juice is produced by chewing together "Areca-nut" known as Betel-nut *(sopari)*, and the leaves of "Chavikạ-Betel" *(pan)*. It is a common practice in India to offer pansupari to a friend on a visit just as a European would offer cigarettes in Europe. I have never seen a single case benefited by its use.

IX.—Ginger and Onions :—The fresh juice of Zingiber Officinale known as "*Adoo*" or of "Allium Cepa" known as *Kanda* is dropped into the ears for relieving ear-ache. This is a favourite remedy with Parsee women for very young children. It has some effect in relieving ear-ache.

X.—The juice of the leaves of "Ocimum Sanctum" known as *Toolsi* :—It is used by the "Ghatties" for ear-ache with some benefit.

XI.—The juice of the Mint *(Mentha Sativa)* known as "Phu-dina" :—It is used for dry catarrh of the ear without any benefit.

XII.—The juice of the leaves or flowers of "Jasminum Grandi-florum" known as *Chumpeli* :—It is boiled with sweet-oil and used in acute suppurative inflammation of the middle ear. I have seen only one case in which it was used without any good result.

XIII.—The fruit of "Tricosanthes Palmata" known as *Kaundala* :—It is boiled with cocoa-nut oil and used for stopping fœtid discharges from the ears. I have never seen a single case in which it has done any good.

XIV.—The juice expressed from the leaves of "Cleome Viscosa" and known as *Tilvun* :—It is used for otorrhœa and deafness in the Concans, mostly by the Hindoos, without any benefit.

XV.—The juice of the leaves of Datura Alba and also that of the Lily:—These are used for relieving ear-ache by women of the "Ghatty" caste in India with temporary relief.

XVI.—Tea :—Warm infusion of tea is syringed into the ear in cases of pain due to furuncles. It has a temporary soothing effect similar to that obtained by syringing the ears with warm water. The tannin contained in the tea however, acts as a mild astringent.

x

XVII.—The leg of Peacock :—It is boiled with ground-nut oil, and used in chronic catarrhal deafness. This remedy is recommended mostly by *bawas* and *jogis*, a set of Hindoo *Hermits* or *Ascetics*, who are supposed to be well versed in jungle medicines. I have never come across a single case either cured or relieved of the deafness by this remedy.

XVIII.—Cat's Urine and Urine of Newly Born Babies :—It is poured into the ear in otorrhœa to reduce the discharge. It has however in many cases caused tympanic and mastoid abscesses which had to be opened. I have never seen or come across a single case of cure under its use.

XIX.—Dead Scorpions:—These are boiled in sweet-oil and put into the ear by Madrasee women in India to relieve ear-ache. I have never seen any good effect from it.

XX.—The Gall-Bladder of the young sheep :—It is boiled with sweet oil, and the oil is then filtered and dropped into the ear slightly warmed. It is used in deafness, brought on by dry catarrh of the ear. I know of two cases in which the oil was used by a Borah hakim without any benefit. On the contrary, the deafness increased and the patient had to consult me for treatment.

XXI.—Honey *(Apis Mellifica)* :—It is used by old women for otorrhœa. For this purpose a plug of cotton-wool or cloth is smeared with honey and introduced into the meatus, but it gives no permanent relief.

XXII.—Milk, specially of a primipara :—It has been dropped into the ears to relieve ear-ache in children. I have seen some good result from its use.

XXIII.—Eau de Cologne :—It has been poured into the ears for relieving ear-ache. It is commonly used by the people of India, and I have seen many cases in which bad results have followed its use, such as meningitis, mastoid abscesses, otorrhœa, &c.

XXIV.—The Otto de Rose and the Essence of Jasemine :—These are commonly dropped into the ears for catarrhal deafness and ear-ache mostly by Bhatias and Khojas. I have seen some temporary benefit from their use.

XXV.—Assafœtida :—A small piece is introduced into the ear for relieving ear-ache without the least benefit.

XXVI.—Powder made of " Sepia Officinalis " known as "*Summudarfin*" and found on the sea-shore in India :—A powder of it is insufflated into the ear in otorrhœa. This powder has some effect in drying up secretions. It is commonly employed by the Hindoos.

XXVII.—The red dry powder known as " Kunkun " (red powder obtained from the rhizome of *Curcuma Longa).* It is used by the Hindoos for decorating the foreheads with a mark known as tila and also used by the Parsees on birthdays of their children as a mark of good omen. This powder is insufflated into the ear for otorrhœa through a quill-pen. In 1896, I saw four cases in which this powder had been used and had brought on mastoid abscesses which had to be opened.

XXVIII.—" Mellwallas " or " Ear-Cleaners " :—They are a class of quack-aurists. They are generally Mahomedans or Chinese by nationality, and go about from street to street hawking aloud their arrival. They remove the wax from the ears by means of two thin pointed probes, and many a time they perforate the tympanum under a mistaken notion that they are removing thin epidermal scales from it. They generally use sweet-oil mixed with Tinctura Lavandulæ Co., 1 in 4, as drops for softening the cerumen before beginning the operation. I have had to treat a number of cases with perforations caused by these ignorant mell-wallas.

THE RADICAL CURE OF CHRONIC PURULENT OTORRHŒA BY ANTRECTOMY AND ATTICO-ANTRECTOMY. BASED ON THE RESULTS OF 26 OPERATIONS.

MR. PHILIP R. W. DE SANTI, London.

The present paper gives the results obtained by me in the years 1896 and 1897 in the treatment of chronic purulent inflammation of the middle ear by means of the operations of Antrectomy and Attico-Antrectomy, the so-called Radical Cure through the mastoid.

The number of patients operated on amounted to eighteen, and the number of operations performed to twenty-six.

In every case systematic and long-continued treatment through the external auditory meatus and Eustachian tube was carefully carried out prior to operation.

In regard to age and sex the youngest was 5 years and the oldest 50 years : ten were females, eight were males.

With regard to the duration of the purulent mischief the shortest was 6 months, and the others ranged between one year and 15 years.

6 months	...	...	1	8 years	...	...	1
1 year	...	...	3	9 „	...	...	3
3 years	...	...	2	11 „	...	...	1
5 „	...	...	2	12 „	...	...	2
6 „	...	...	1	15 „	...	...	1
7 „	...	..	1				

In eight cases the left ear was operated on, in three cases the right, and in seven cases both sides.

Method of Operation.—In twenty cases I performed Antrectomy, and in six cases Attico-Antrectomy.

The following is a brief description of the method of operating I employ :

Preliminary thorough cleansing of the skin and shaving of the hair; as thorough cleansing of the external auditory canal and tympanum as possible. I then make a free incision parallel with the attachment of the auricle and just behind it from the top to the bottom of the mastoid process. Any hæmorrhage is checked by pressure forceps or hot sponge pressure. I then bare the bone by raising the periosteum on either side of the incision with a periosteal elevator : the bone being well exposed and the ear held well forwards by a retractor I note the condition and appearance of the mastoid, and proceed to carefully define Macewen's triangle. If any soft or carious spot or sinus is seen I follow it up with a small gouge. Otherwise I proceed to open up the mastoid antrum through Macewen's triangle.

In a certain number of cases I used a small trephine to open the antrum but have discarded this instrument in favour of small sharp gouges or a chisel and mallet.

Personally I am anxious to try the globular dental burs so well spoken of by Dr. Macewen but we have not yet got them at the Westminster Hospital. With whatever instrument I elect to use for opening the antrum the bone is carefully and gradually removed in layers, the direction of the opening being downwards and forwards and absolutely parallel with the course of the external auditory canal. As I get deeper and deeper the cavity is sounded with a probe until eventually the probe is found to enter the antrum. In several of my cases on entering the antrum thus, there has been very free venous hæmorrhage. This has always been easy to check.

As soon as I have penetrated into the antrum the opening is carefully enlarged, a strong light cast into it and the cavity dried with aseptic cotton wool mops so as to be able to see the condition of the interior of the antrum.

I next proceed to carefully remove any débris from the cavities partly with small blunt spoons and partly with cotton wool mops. I make a point at this stage of having a good electric light thrown into the area operated on. I next cleanse the deep external meatus and then proceed to syringe through the mastoid antrum, the solution, generally warm boracic lotion, issuing freely through the external meatus. The whole of the parts are now thoroughly dried with cotton wool mops, iodoform and boracic powder insufflated into the dried cavities and an iodoform gauze plug passed through the antrum and out if possible at the external meatus. The skin wound except at its lower angle is then united with horse-hair sutures and the whole of the parts covered carefully with a double cyanide gauze and wool dressing.

In several of my cases I have used a pewter drainage tube instead of iodoform gauze plug, but I have recently given up the former and now use the gauze plug. I have found that after a time the pewter tube irritates the parts a good deal and when prolonged drainage is required and the patient has left the hospital, it is apt to be left out.

The above description applies to my method of performing Antrectomy ; *Attico-Antrectomy* which I performed six times is a more difficult operation to carry out satisfactorily : The ear has to be carefully detached from its insertion and for this purpose a nearly semi-circular incision has to be made $\frac{1}{3}$ of an inch behind its line of attachment and extending from near the tip of the mastoid process to the anterior point of the insertion of the Helix. The soft parts have to be separated sufficiently to expose the posterior superior edge of the bony meatus and the membranous meatus has to be separated from its posterior superior insertion and drawn downwards and forwards.

In this way the surface of the mastoid process and posterior superior wall of the deep bony meatus are exposed. I now open the antrum in the usual way and pass a small bent probe from it along the aditus into the tympanum. This acts as a guide and a protector. The next step is to remove the posterior superior wall of the meatus with either chisel or gouge. I have always found this the most anxious and difficult part of the operation and it is no use being in a hurry over its performance. It is at this stage that there is so much danger of wounding the facial nerve and careful watch should be kept by the anæsthetist for any twitching of the face and the operator should employ a good light to see exactly where he is going.

The object of removing the greater part of the posterior superior wall of the meatus is to throw the antrum, attic, and tympanum into one large cavity. All débris should be removed with blunt spoons also any carious ossicles or polypi.

The parts having been thoroughly cleansed and dried should be packed with iodoform and iodoform gauze, the auricle then replaced, a drainage tube inserted into the meatus, and the skin wound closed except at its lower angle.

The whole area operated on must then be covered with an efficient antiseptic dressing. I have never had occasion to "paper" the parts. It has been my experience and I have had occasion to perform several similar operations besides those just recorded (in 1898 and this year), that no two mastoid operations are the same. Many variations are found in the density of the bone, in the size and situation of the antrum, and proximity of the lateral sinus : in three cases though the antrum was opened in the usual place and way, I exposed the lateral sinus ; in no case with any ulterior harm.

In one case I wounded the facial nerve (No. 12), and the result has been partial facial paralysis permanent. This accident occurred whilst chiselling the posterior superior wall of the meatus ; a piece was fractured and facial paralysis resulted.

After-Treatment.—Unless very careful attention be given to the after-treatment the results will be found unsatisfactory. To begin with it is wise to warn the patient or the patient's parents that the after treatment may extend over several months before actual cure is obtained.

Out of my series of twenty-six operations I note that the after-treatment ranged between one month and eighteen months. The objects of the operation are to remove the sources that are keeping up the suppuration and to allow of free and efficient drainage. It is therefore essential that the drainage should be kept up until all suppuration has ceased.

I at one time tried the dry treatment as advocated by Dr. Macewen, leaving on the dressing applied immediately after the operation for a week. In each case where I tried this method, I found it unsatisfactory; the dressings when taken off were found to be infected, and in one or two cases a rise of temperature was the result.

I, therefore, invariably change the dressings the second or third day after operation, thoroughly syringe the parts out and through, dry them and repack with gauze and powder. This after-treatment consisting of daily careful dressing and cleanliness has given in my cases very satisfactory results.

I usually employ one of the following solutions for after-syringing : Boracic lotion (1 in 8), Peroxide of Hydrogen (10 vols.), Corrosive Sublimate (1 in 4000): for insufflation after drying, Boric powder 4 parts, Iodoform 1 part. Iodoform alone, in my experience, is apt to cause too much irritation, and the formation of excessive granulation tissue. If there is any excess of granulation tissue it must be destroyed, and I usually employ for the purpose Chromic Acid fused on a probe.

Results.—Out of eighteen patients operated on in the two years 1896 and 1897, and all of whom were suffering from intractable purulent Otorrhœa, an eventual cure of the condition was obtained in seventeen.

Taking the actual number of the operations and their nature I find out of twenty Antrectomies I performed, the following results :

Discharged cured	17 cases.
Marked benefit (occasional moisture) ...	2 „
*Failure	1 case.

Out of six Attico-Antrectomies :

Discharged cured	5 cases.
*Failure	1 case.

The longest period, which has elapsed since the cessation of the discharge has been three years, and the shortest duration two years.

The most instructive case of the eighteen and one which up to the hilt proves my contention for the necessity of these operations is case No. 1. This boy, aged 7, came under my observation in April, 1896, with Right

* The same patient, May 1899.

Otorrhœa of five years duration. ·I performed Antrectomy and subsequent drainage with the result that all discharge ceased within three months. This boy I eventually lost sight of until October, 1898, when he was brought up to my out-patient department suffering from Left Suppurative Otorrhœa of, according to the mother, quite short duration.

He was very ill and had symptoms pointing to intracranial mischief. He was admitted, and I opened up his left antrum, exposed his lateral sinus, which contained a septic thrombus, ligatured his internal jugular vein and evacuated a cerebellar abscess of left side.

He died a fortnight afterwards and I obtained P.M., both temporal bones: these specimens I hand round and you will see that on the right side the antrum and tympanum are dry and healthy whereas on the left side there are well-marked inflammatory changes. Now I hold that this case most excellently illustrates the beneficial effect of the operation performed two and a half years' previous to the boy's trouble on the left side : it shows moreover, that the operation remained a successful one, and in all probability was the means of preventing intracranial mischief on the right side.

I have already noted that the after-treatment in these cases has varied in my hospital patients from a period of one month to eighteen months.

When I have had to perform these operations on private patients I have always found the after-treatment much less lengthy : as a rule under two months. This I ascribe to the much better surroundings and to the greater care that can be bestowed on asepsis

It is impossible, in hospital patients to keep them in for any very lengthy after-treatment and as out-patients they cannot get the individual attention they should, nor do they keep their dressings clean.

With regard to the artificial opening, in only one of my cases has it remained permanently open, and in this particular case, the discharge has not ceased, there are tubercle bacilli in the pus, and facial paralysis resulted from the operation.

It is the only case of failure I have to record out of the eighteen patients.

I have not found in any case resulting deformity. In regard to the hearing powers of the patients I find *considerably improved*, i.e., from Watch on contact only to distances ranging from 15 to 30 inches, nine cases.

Not noted ... ... 5 cases.
Not improved ... ... 4 „

In conclusion I think it is only necessary for me to mention the conditions which I hold justify the employment of these operations on the mastoid, always presupposing of course that we have to deal with genuinely chronic affections which have lasted a long while, and which have not given rise to any alarming symptoms.

1.	Simple chronic purulent inflammation of the middle ear, which has resisted prolonged treatment through the external meatus and Eustachian tubes.

2.	The same condition when accompanied by the formation of granulations and polypi which recur after removal and in which carious bone is diagnosed.

3.	Attic suppuration in which carious ossicles if present have been removed, and counter drainage in the membrane made and intra-tympanic syringing carried out, but without success.

4.	Cholesteatomata in the tympanum and mastoid antrum.

5.	Constant pain in the mastoid pointing to sclerosis ; the relief obtained is analogous to linear osteotomy in chronic periostitis of the tibia or femur.

6.	Great narrowing or closure of the external meatus from chronic inflammation or hyperostosis or exostosis.

7.	In cases with sinus leading from the mastoid or deep external meatus.

Case.	Sex.	Age.	History.	Method of Operation.	Date of Operation.	Operator.	Result of Operation.	Last Seen or Heard of
1	M.	7	Right otorrhœa 5 years, following measles; admitted with Mastoid Abscess.	Abscess opened by Wilde's incision; 2oz. fœtid pus between bone and periosteum. Antrectomy with gouge; cheesy fœtid pus evacuated; drainage with pewter tube.	April 29, 1896.	Mr. de Santi	Discharge ceased in about 3 months. *Cured.*	Was brought up to my Out-Patients in Oct 1898, with symptoms of Lateral Sinus Pyæmia, due to otitis media suppurativa of left side. Rt. Ear had remained perfectly well since operation in 1896. I opened skull and found Lateral sinus Pyæmia and cerebellar Abscess. Jugular vein ligatured. Clot in Sinus scooped out and cerebellar Abscess drained. Death 15 days lar. P.M. Right E. quite healthy. Left M. Ear clean. After operation: large ragged cerebellar abscess left side, and pus in jugular vein to level of ligature.
2	M.	11	Sc. Fever at 2. Rt. otitis media supp. ever since. Mastoid Abscess at 2½ and 5. (Operated on by Mr. Jacobson). Left otorrhœa 3 years. O.P. 2½ years. No benefit.	Right Attico-Antrectomy. Bone much sclerosed; antrum small, deep-seated, and filled with foul cholesteatomatous mass. Pewter drainage tube.	May 5, 1896		Discharge ceased 2 months later. *Cured.*	October, 1897.
3	F.	13	Measles as a baby; double perforative otorrhœa ever since. Severe eczema both ext. aud. meatus. O.P. for 18 months. No benefit.	Double Antrectomy with trephine and gouge. Both antra contained unhealthy granulation tissue. Pewter tube drainage.	June 11, 1896		Discharge right side ceased by Nov. 1896. Occasional clear moisture left. Hearing before operation: W. on contact. March, 1898: Rt. 2ft. Lft. 13in. *Cured*	March, 1898.

Case.	Sex.	Age.	History.	Method of Operation.	Date of Operation.	Operator.	Result of Operation.	Last Seen or Heard of.
4	M.	12	Sc. Fever at 5. Discharge from both ears on and off ever since. Under treatment fairly continuously last 5 years. Discharge recently more profuse.	Double Antrectomy. Curetted granulations. Drainage.	Sept. 9, 1896	Mr. de Santi.	Discharge Right Ear ceased G. 1896. L. E. 3 wks later. W. before. faintly on contact. Now, R. E. 16 inches. L. E. 30 ,, Cured.	March, 1898.
5	F.	14	Double perforative otorrhœa 11 years. Last 2 years fœtid; increasing deafness. Both Ex. Aud. Meatus nearly closed from chronic inflammation. W.O. on contact. Three months O.P. treatment.	Double Antrectomy. Drainage.	Sept. 15, 1896		March 17, 1897. R. E. sound. L. E. very slight discharge. Cured.	June, 1898. Watch, 6-7 inches. Rt. well. Left well for 3 months. Watch, 2-3 inches.
6	F.	13	Double perforative otorrhœa 6 years. Long course of O.P. treatment, but discharge has remained profuse for last year. W. only on contact.	Double Attico - Antrectomy. Drainage.	Sept. 19, 1896		Dec.1896 both ears dry. June, 1898 W. left E., 13in., Rt. 12in. Cured.	June, 1898.
7	F.	20	Sc. Fever at 5. Discharge left E. probably ever since Recurrent polypi. Had good medical treatment at home. Now large polypus in middle ear.	Antrectomy. Drainage, with Iodoform Gauze plug.	Dec, 9, 1896		Benefitted at first, but relapsed; operation repeated; discharge ceased Dec., 1898.	April, 1899. Remains well. Hearing good.
8	M.	14	Left otorrhœa 3 years. Now very foul. Left Facial Paralysis three weeks. O.P. treatment some months.	Attico-Antrectomy. Lateral Sinus abnormal and exposed at operation. Gauze plug.	Jan 18, 1897		Aug., 1897. Quite well; E, dry and Facial Paralysis quite gone Hearing not improved.	August, 1897. When written to in 1898 no answer.
9	F.	22	Constant left otorrhœa 9 years. Attended O.P.'s King's and London; no benefit. Now polypus notch of Rivini. Mastoid tenderness; parietal headache.	Left Attico-Antrectomy. Lateral Sinus exposed.	Feb. 8, 1897		Cured. Drained for 2 months.	December, 1897.
10	M.	16	Rt. post scarlat. otorrhœa since 13. Nov., 1892, polypi removed. Later adenoids and tonsils. Discharge persisted and polypi recurred. 1896. Polypi notch of Rivini, darkish brown discharge, also perf. in ant. inf. quadrant of membrane.	Antrectomy. Removal of polypi and ossicles.	Feb, 18. 1897		Cured. Drained for 5 months.	January, 1899. Watch, 12 inches, previously 1¼ inches.

No.	Sex	Age	History	Operation	Date		Result	Follow-up
11	M	12	Continuous left otorrhœa 13 months. Polypi. Removal of polypi; continuance of discharge.	Antrectomy. Lateral Sinus exposed.	March 11, 1897	Mr. de Santi.	*Partially cured.* Discharge ceased for 6 weeks (Oct., 1897).	March, 1899. But little discharge. Facial Paralysis less.
12	F.	11	Left post scarlat. otorrhœa 8 years. O.P. 6 months. Tubercle Bacilli in pus.	1. Antrectomy. 2. Attico-Antrectomy.	March 15, 1897 May 21, 1897	,,	*Failure.* The second operation was followed by Partial Facial Paralysis	October, 1898. Hearing in statu quo.
13	F.	19	Congenital Syphilitic double otorrhœa. Constant Mastoid pain. Five months previously Mr. Ballance operated on both Mastoids, bone much sclerosed. Done to relieve pain. Relief for short time.	Double Antrectomy. Both antra were enlarged, and with oily pus inside.	Aug. 18, 1897	,,	Cure left side ; benefit right side. All pain relieved.	
14	M.	14	Double purulent otorrhœa as long as he can remember. Often very fœtid. Occasional pain and giddiness. Enlarged glands.	Double Antrectomy.	Sept. 19, 1897	,,	*Cured.*	
15	M.	14	Double otorrhœa 9 years. O.P. 9 months.	Double Antrectomy. antrum very small. Left	Sept. 15, 1897	,,	*Cured.*	April, 1898.
16	F.	5	Left otorrhœa 20 months. O.P. most of time.	Antrectomy.	Sept. 23, 1897	,,	*Cured.*	June, 1898. Occasional moisture. Hearing much improved.
17	F.	50	Left fœtid otorrhœa 5 years. Syphilis.	Antrectomy.	Sept. 30, 1897	,,	*Cured.* Discharge ceased in 1 month.	June, 1898.
18	F.	25	Sinus back of left ear discharging pus. No perforation. Six months history.	Antrectomy. Antrum dilated; cheesy pus	July 11, 1897	,,	*Cured.* Discharge ceased July 30, 1897.	December, 1898. W. from on contact only, to 20 inches.

Chart illustrating Mr. Philip De Santi's paper on the Radical cure of chronic purulent otorrhœa by Antrectomy and Attico-Antrectomy.

Some Cases Illustrating the Intracranial Complications of Neglected Otorrhœa.

Mr. Philip de Santi. London.

MASTOID ABSCESS. PERFORATION OF TEGMEN, EXPLORATION OF ANTRUM, LATERAL SINUS, AND TEMPORO-SPHENOIDAL LOBE. DEATH.

Case 1. A man, aged 35, applied at my Out-Patient Clinic, March 2nd, 1896. He stated that he had pricked the drum of the left ear with a hairpin whilst cleaning out the orifice, a little before Christmas, 1895.

This was followed by pain and deafness within three hours. He had continuous pain in left ear for some six weeks, when pain became easier, and a swelling formed over the mastoid process. Never noticed any aural discharge.

On examination I found a large perforation in left M. T. : ossicles gone : over left mastoid process was a large fluctuating swelling with tenderness, redness, and oedema. Temperature 101. Refused admission. Came to Hospital on March 5th, as pain and swelling had increased. Temperature was 101. He felt sick and there was redness and oedema of left eyelid, tenderness over left parietal region and internal jugular vein. He was admitted, and on March 6th, I made a free incision into the mastoid abscess letting out much foetid pus. The mastoid process was bare, and there was a small soft spot over the mastoid antrum, this I followed up. The sinus led to the tegmen antri which was perforated ; there was no pus in the antrum or mastoid cells. The lateral sinus and temporo-sphenoidal convolution were exposed, but with negative results.

Subsequent to the operation the patient's symptoms got worse, he developed typical signs of meningo-encephalitis, and died on March 9th.

Post-mortem. General purulent cerebro-spinal meningitis ; both tympana full of pus ; ossicles gone left side ; dura not especially affected at sites of operation.

Trephine apertures :—(1) At base of mastoid. (2) Over lateral sinus. (3) Over third left inf. temp. sphenoid. convolution, no abscess of brain or cerebellum.

SYMPTOMS OF INTRACRANIAL ABSCESS. EXPLORATION OF MASTOID, CEREBRUM, AND CEREBELLUM. NEGATIVE RESULTS. RECURRENCE OF SYMPTOMS ONE YEAR LATER. OPERATION. EVACUATION OF EXTRA-DURAL ABSCESS. RECOVERY.

Case 2. A woman, aged 21, was admitted under me on February 7th, 1896, with symptoms of intracranial mischief of otitic origin.

There was a history of more or less continuous discharge from both ears from the age of 7½. She had been treated for some six years previously to my seeing her, and had had adenoids and tonsils removed and exploration of both mastoids for persistent pain in 1894.

When seen by me on February 6th, 1896, her condition was as follows : persistent giddiness with tendency to fall, persistent headache on right side which had for two weeks been getting worse ; latterly apathy, stupidity, and drowsiness. On admission she lay on her right side supporting the right side of her head with her hand. Occasional sharp attacks of pain in right mastoid and parietal regions. Much pain on pressure and percussion over these regions. Temperature 99·4° F. Pulse regular, 70. Nausea but no actual vomiting. Bowels very constipated.

No paralysis, or paresis, slowness of speech, or aphasia ; sensation and reflexes normal, optic discs normal.

Had emaciated very much during the last two weeks. Profuse foetid discharge from right ear. Whole of M. T. and ossicles destroyed. Watch only on firm contact. She was well purged and watched.

The pain especially over the mastoid continued, the pulse became slower (65), and drowsiness more marked, and the sense of vomiting remained.

I decided to explore for pus.

On February 14th, I opened the right mastoid antrum with a gouge and trephine. The bone was very sclerosed, no pus was found, there was no fistulous track or carious bone to be seen.

I next trephined one inch behind and above centre of external auditory meatus, and explored the temporo-sphenoidal lobe ; the result was negative. I next explored the area corresponding to the tegmen antri et tympani but with again negative results.

On February 18th, the symptoms continuing, I explored the cerebellum on the right side, but nothing abnormal was noted.

By the 24th, though nothing had been found at the two operations, all drowsiness and giddiness had disappeared, there was no pain in the mastoid or head, and the operation wounds had healed by first intention.

On March 4th, she went to a Convalescent Home.

I saw her frequently on her return ; the discharge had almost disappeared from the ear and she remained well until the third week of December, 1896, when she began to complain of pain over the right parietal region ; she later developed similar symptoms to those she had in February, 1896, and she was therefore readmitted February, 1897. In bed, she lay curled up on her right side, and was very drowsy. Occasional cerebral vomiting. Facial expression, except when she had a sharp attack of pain, that of marked apathy. As she was becoming semi-unconsious I, on February 26th, 1897, explored the temporal bone over the site of the former trephine apertures. A sinus was discovered extending through the substance of the temporal bone, about midway between the two old trephine apertures made a year before. I removed a disc of bone corresponding to the sinus and came across foetid pus, situated between the dura mater and the posterior aspect of the petrous portion of the temporal bone, and in the bone itself. I evacuated about $9\frac{1}{2}$ drachms of pus ; the walls of the lateral sinus were much thickened and covered with granulations, the sinus however was patent ; there was carious erosion of the posterior aspect of the petrous portion of the temporal bone, and this I carefully scraped, and made an opening communicating with the middle ear and external auditory meatus. She was discharged on May 6th, with the wound quite healed, and the discharge from the ear stopped. Her temperature never rose above 100° F., but on March 23rd she developed right facial paralysis.

I have seen this patient frequently since, she has had no return of her old symptoms, and she has but very slight facial paralysis ; she has however occasional discharge of pus from both ears.

She is able to hear a watch at 5in. on the right, and 4½in. on the left side.

———

MASTOID ABSCESS. LATERAL SINUS PYÆMIA. ALSO OF SUPERIOR LONGITUDINAL SINUS AND INTERNAL JUGULAR VEIN. NECROSIS OF TEMPORAL BONE. EXPLORATION. DEATH.

CASE 3. A boy was admitted from my Out-Patients, November 2nd, 1898, with a fluctuating swelling over the left mastoid, extending up to temporal ridge and to just below the ear, and posteriorly almost as far as occipital protuberance. Left otorrhœa, one year. Swelling over ear, pain, and giddiness when walking ten days. Temperature 102°.

November 3rd. My colleague, Mr. Stonham, incised the swelling over mastoid, also in posterior occipital region, and let out much pus. Pus evacuated from mastoid antrum with chisel and hammer. Patient progressed fairly well until November 9th, when temperature began to rise. November 12th, temperature 103·2 ; November 14th, 105·6 ; November 16th, 106·2. Rigor. Pulse varied between 100 and 153. Respirations 20-25. No optic neuritis.

Mr. Stonham examined the wound : there was retention of pus ; this was evacuated. Between November 16th and 21st, temperature varied between 102 and 105·5 ; there was an occasional rigor. Patient lay quietly in bed looking very pallid but complaining of nothing ; took food badly ; mental condition unimpaired.

On November 21st I was sent for, the boy being very ill indeed. I laid original wound bare, enlarged it downwards and backwards 1½ inches. Retained pus evacuated, granulations scraped away, pus evacuated between lateral sinus and groove. Sinus not thrombosed. Iodoform gauze plug in antrum, and drainage tube in lower angle of wound. Temperature fell to 98·4, but later rose to 103·6.

November 23rd. Rigor, temperature 105 : from 23rd to 25th rigors daily and gradual failure of strength.

December 15th. Mr. Stonham trephined posterior inferior angle of parietal bone. Dura bulged, and no pulsation visible. Dura opened and brain explored : negative.

Lateral sinus examined, but no pus found, though bubbles of air appeared in the wound. The boy gradually got weaker, and died December 23rd.

Post-mortem. Septic thrombosis of left lateral sinus and superior longitudinal sinus, also of left internal jugular vein. Necrosis of temporal bone. No meningitis. Turbid fluid in both pleuræ. Abscesses in lungs and spleen.

RIGHT TEMPORO-SPHENOIDAL ABSCESS. LEPTO-MENINGITIS. DEATH.

CASE 4. Harry H..., 21, attended my Out-Patients in October, 1897, for double otorrhœa of sixteen years duration. On the 19th, I removed a large polypus from the right ear. He did not again attend the Out-Patients' department.

I subsequently heard from his medical attendant, Dr. Hardwicke, that two days after the removal of the polypus the patient had an attack of middle ear inflammation which yielded to treatment. He went on well until November 3rd, when he developed great pain in occipital region ; no other symptoms until November 7th, when the temperature rose to 101, the pulse became irregular, the tongue foul, the bowels constipated, and there was sickness. On admission under me November 8th, he had marked symptoms of lepto-meningitis, and died on November 10th.

At no time were there physical signs of any sort in the eyes, face, mastoids, trunk, or limbs.

Post-mortem. Brain 53 ounces : convolutions flattened : veins of pia full. In sub-arachnoid region of base, copious exudation of thick yellow pus ; also down the spinal cord. Right temporo-sphenoidal lobe a sphenoidal abscess with thick wall and dirty greenish foetid contents, partly purulent, partly necrotic. Abscess =

half a golf ball, and has reached to wall of lateral ventricle which contains dirty green purulent fluid.

The abcess is in the middle of the lobe, and in direct communication with the tympanum, by a perforation in the roof and covering dura. Left petrosal bone normal. The pus from the abscess contained two organisms—(1) Staphylococcus, (2) Another bacillus in size and shape resembling Bacillus of Diphtheria.

LATERAL SINUS PYÆMIA.   CEREBELLAR ABSCESS.   EXPLORATION.   LIGATURE OF
INTERNAL JUGULAR.   EVACUATION OF CEREBELLAR ABSCESS.   DEATH.

CASE 5. C. F..., aged 9, admitted under me October 16th, 1898, with symptoms of lateral sinus pyæmia.

In April, 1896, I operated on this boy for obstinate chronic otorrhœa on the right side. The mastoid was opened and drained, and though the otorrhœa had been in existence five years, he was cured in three months.

I lost sight of him until October, 1898, when he came to the Out-Patients' department for the *left* ear. The right side had remained well. On admission he had delirium, tremors, constipation, retching, and a high temperature. There was œdema over the left mastoid, parietal and frontal headache, and tenderness in the neck along the left internal jugular vein. Eyes normal.

I opened up the mastoid antrum, evacuated some pus, explored the lateral sinus which was thrombosed, tied the internal jugular vein opposite the cricoid cartilage, and washed out the clot from the sigmoid sinus. On further exploration, I found a cerebellar abscess which was opened and drained; the whole operation lasted about three-quarters of an hour. At first the boy improved, but later had several rigors ; pus kept coming away from the cerebellar abscess, and the patient became weaker, and he died seventeen days subsequent to the operation. He was conscious to the last, and lost all his headache and pain.

Post-mortem. An abscess found involving left lower-half of the cerebellum ; foetid pus. Middle ear and parts adjacent and posteriorly had been removed by surgical operation ; no general meningitis.

Left jugular vein tied opposite the cricoid ; upper part full of pus as far as the lateral sinus.

Right middle ear, previous operation, and quite healthy.

The two temporal bones and the cerebellum from this case are in the Museum.

The case illustrates fully the results of the Radical Cure on the right side to stop discharge and prevent intracranial complications, and the result of neglect on the left side ending in death from intracranial complications.

MOBILIZZAZIONE PRECOCE DELLA CATENA DEGLI OSSICINI NEL PERIODO SUB-ACUTO DI ALCUNE OTITI MEDIE NON SUPPURATIVE.

Prof. GIUSEPPE FARACI, Palermo.

Studiando il complesso sintomatico ed il decorso clinico delle varie otiti medie acute non suppurative che capitano spesso all'osservazione, un fatto principalmente richiama la nostra attenzione, la sproporzione, cioè, chè talune volte si osserva tra le alterazioni funzionali ed acustiche dell'orecchio ammalato rispetto ai disturbi subbiettivi ed alle alterazioni anatomo-patologiche otoscopicamente diagnosticabili. Infatti, si osservano spesso dei casi in cui ad un imponente corredo di fenomeni acuti dolorosi insopportabili con accentuati fatti infiammatorii locali, corrisponde invece lieve alterazione nella facoltà uditiva dell'organo leso, poco eccitamento nelle diramazioni cocleari e vestibolari dell'acustico, mentre in altri casi, ad una grave sordità con significanti disturbi paracustici e disordine nell'equilibrio fa riscontro una relativa mitezza di fenomeni dolorosi ed infiammatorî dell'orecchio.

Tale differenza che accompagna l'efflorescenza del processo flogistico locale si riscontra anche nell'esito definitivo della malattia. Infatti, mentre nella prima categoria di casi avviene una guarigione completa ed abbastanza soddisfacente, nelle altre forme morbose rimane, invece, costantemente un perturbamento grave nell'udito, gravissime paracusie spesso insopportabili, e qualche volta anche dei transitori fenomeni di vertigine, e questi disturbi presentano una tenacità tale che le cure locali più razionali che comunemente si praticano non riescono a portare la guarigione o almeno un positivo miglioramento nelle sofferenze dell'infermo.

È facile conoscere la ragione di questa apparente paradossale differenza se per poco si considera quanto diversa è l'importanza fisiologica delle singole parti della cavità timpanica. È evidente che, se un processo infiammatorio attacca di preferenza quelle parti destinate alla trasmissione dell'onda sonora, la funzione acustica ne deve maggiormente soffrire.

Cosi nelle epitimpaniti acute avviene, sia per il rigonfiarsi della capsula articolare incudo-malleare, sia per l'essudazione che si stabilisce attorno questa articolazione, che gravi ostácoli nascono all'oscillazione di questi ossicini e quindi una perdita grave dell'udito.

Lo stesso succede quando una flogosi attacca le vicinanze delle finestre labirintiche e degli essudati si depositano nella fossetta ovale immobilizzando la staffa. Mentre, se un processo flogistico acuto, anche intenso, interessa di preferenza le altre parti della cavità timpanica, la funzione acustica rimane poco compromessa.

Si comprende adesso la ragione per cui le otiti medie acute non suppurative che per la loro sede hanno portato gravi dissesti funzionali, lasciano traccie permanenti nella funzione dell'organo affetto anche quando il processo infiammatorio è completamente spento e l'orecchio è stato oggetto di razionali cure da parte del medico.

Gli elementi giovani di neoformazione che nel primo periodo della malattia formano assieme a cellule di epitelio, a cellule di muco, a qualche corpuscolo rosso, ad una sostanza intercellulare ialina, quell'essudazione gelatinosa densa che si riscontra principalmente nella fossetta ovale ed è causa di sordità, a lungo andare subiscono la fase evolutiva dei tessuti embrionali e si trasformano in connettivo compatto sia sotto forma di briglie che di membrane le quali legano allora in una maniera stabile la catena degli ossicini e si rendono causa permanente di disturbo funzionale ed acustico dell'orecchio affetto.

*
* *

Ciò posto, sorge spontanea una domanda : Perchè dobbiamo intervenire quando, essendo avvenuta la trasformazione in connettivo compatto degli elementi cellulari neoformati, l'operazione debba essere più complicata ed i risultati più scarsi, mentre invece la rimozione di questi prodotti infiammatorii nel primo tempo della loro formazione è assai più facile e più completa ?   Perchè aspettare che l'apparato meccanico della trasmissione sonora e quello di percezione subiscano a lungo andare delle alterazioni secondarie indelebili ?

Non sarebbe più razionale ed assai più vantaggioso per la funzione acustica del paziente intervenire quando la *vis neoformativa* ed *essudativa* essendo appena spenta, non rimane nell'orecchio che i prodotti di un processo morboso, esclusiva ragione di permanenti e gravi disturbi funzionali ed acustici ?

Quanto più completi non sarebbero allora i vantaggi conseguibili dall'oto-chirurgia, quanto maggiore la fiducia che i pazienti nutrirebbero per noi ?

Tali considerazioni mi spinsero a studiare con cura questo interessante capitolo e sin dal primo momento ho compreso che due erano le difficoltà che bisognava risolvere : la prima riguardava il timore che un intervento chirurgico in un orecchio in cui la *vis flogistica* non era ancora del tutto spenta o per lo meno di recente scomparsa potesse ridestare un'infiammazione possibilmente di natura suppurativa, in secondo luogo, quali criterî devono guidare l'otologo nello scegliere i casi adatti all'operazione e come stabilire il momento opportuno della medesima.

*
* *

Ho ritenuto invero la prima di queste difficoltà più immaginaria che reale, specialmente per quanto riguarda la possibilità di destare una flogosi purulenta nell'orecchio.

É vero che, mutate le condizioni di resistenza e modificato il terreno di cultura di un tessuto in mezzo a cui dei germi piogeni sono rimasti per tanto tempo innocui, questi allora si ridestano alla loro attività e dànno luogo ad una infiammazione purulenta, però è vero altresì, che se nuovi germi noi non abbiamo trasportato con l'operazione, questo pericolo non è temibile, dappoichè non è logico supporre che mentre agenti patogeni non si svilupparono prima nella efflorescenza del processo flogistico dell'otite media non suppurativa, abbiano a farlo dopo che una leggera flogosi reattiva segua il traumatismo chirurgico.

Infatti, come risulta dalle mie esperienze, operando con le più scrupolose cautele antisettiche, io non ho avuto mai in alcuno dei miei ammalati alcuna flogosi purulenta consecutiva.

La difficoltà invece riguardante la scelta del soggetto e quella del momento favorevole all'operazione sono meritevoli di considerazione ed accurato studio se si vogliono evitare inutili tentativi chirurgici e sconfortanti disillusioni nell'infermo.

*
* *

La sordità è il sintomo cardinale da cui bisogna lasciarsi guidare nella scelta dei casi, tutte le volte che questa sordità non possa mettersi in rapporto a precedenti alterazioni nell'orecchio e non possa essere spiegata da fatti locali otoscopicamente diagnosticabili, come sarebbe la presenza di un versamento intratimpanico, la coesistenza di uno spasmo del tensore timpanico, l'infiammazione dell'attico timpanico o infine gravi alterazioni flogistiche in tutto l'orecchio medio.

Allora, non potendo spiegarla per l'imbibizione del foglietto mucoso della membrana timpanica, per cui questa ha perduto gran parte del suo potere fisiologico nella trasmissione del suono, o per la diminuita elasticità di tutta la catena degli ossicini dovuta al rigonfiamento della mucosa che aumenta i punti di contatto ed irrigidisce le articolazioni, e molto meno attribuirla alla concomitante chiusura della tromba d'Eustachio, come crede il Bonnafont, avendo io trovato in qualche caso mancare tale ostruzione nonostante la grave dissecia riscontrata nel paziente, bisogna necessariamente ammettere l'esistenza d'altri fatti morbosi e precisamente o un'essudazione plastica nella fossetta ovale solamente o in questa e nella rotonda insieme in modo da rimanere immobilizzata la staffa.

Stante il numero esiguo di esperimenti da me fatti non posso sin da ora stabilire con precisione il perturbamento acustico qualitativo e quantitativo che subiscono i pazienti affetti da queste essudazioni nelle finestre labirintiche, essendo ciò subordinato alla intensità o meno delle alterazioni; posso solo affermare che negli ammalati da me operati l'udito per l'orologio oscillava tra il contatto e 0,10 ; per la voce afona la minima diminuzione riscontrata è stata 0,10 e per quella parlata si ebbe una diminuzione massima di 0,20 e minima di 2 metri.

Riguardo poi al momento opportuno d'intervenire non si può *a priori* stabilire, essendo ciò subordinato ad un complesso di circostanze che possono influire sia anticipando che ritardando l'intervento. È risaputo infatti che il periodo acuto di una flogosi dell'orecchio medio può essere più o meno lungo a seconda la natura del processo, l'età, la resistenza organica, il regime di vita e le abitudini dell'individuo.

V'influisce pure moltissimo le condizioni della mucosa nasale e naso-faringea. Se questa è sede di un processo catarrale diffuso alla mucosa della tromba, la risoluzione dell'otopatia avverrà più tardivamente.

In generale non bisogna mai lasciarsi guidare dalla durata della malattia nello stabilire l'epoca dell'intervento chirurgico, ma invece avere di mira i sintomi subbiettivi e l'immagine otoscopica della membrana timpanica e della mucosa della cassa. Allorchè l'ammalato non avverte più dolore forte, pulsante nell'orecchio, ma solo una leggerissima sensazione dolorosa che ritorna ad intervalli, accompagnata ad un senso di pienezza dell'orecchio, è segno che la flogosi acuta comincia a regredire. Caratteristica è allora l'immagine otoscopica della membrana timpanica. Questa non è più arrossata, lucente e sporgente all'esterno come nel primo tempo della malattia, ma invece floscia, retratta all'indentro, opaca, a superficie spesse volte ineguale, con punti cioè più infossati ed altri meno. L'opacamento della membrana non è uniforme ma a chiazze, si vedono delle piccole zone ancora trasparenti attraverso le quali è facile distinguere la mucosa della cassa la quale è ancora iperemica.

Si osservano altresi i vasi lungo il manico del martello fortemente iniettati ed una leggera iniezione è ancora visibile lunghesso l'anulo' timpanico.

Interessante è allora il fatto che nonostante la regressione dei fenomeni acustici, la perdita dell'udito come i disturbi subbiettivi, vertigine, rumori, persistono immutati o solo hanno subito lievissime oscillazioni.

Stabilito con questi criteri tanto la scelta del soggetto che quella dell'intervento chirurgico si passa all'operazione. Non parlo qui dei preliminari da me altrove descritti per rendere completamente asettico il campo operativo : mi limiterò solamente a descrivere per sommi capi la tecnica operativa che viene da me seguìta.

**

Due sono i tempi dell'operazione : formazione del lembo timpanico, estrazione dell'essudato.

Riguardo alla prima parte eseguo il processo classico del Prof. De Rossi di Roma. Incido con un ago lanceolare la membrana nel suo centro rasente il bordo posteriore del manico del martello e con un coltellino retto e smusso prolungo l'incisione in alto, costeggiando sempre l'ossicino. Passo indi immediatamente al disotto della piega posteriore, fino ad arrivare al livello del punto di partenza formando cosi un lembo *en charnière* che tiro in fuori verso il condotto.

Scoperta in tal modo l'articolazione incudo-stapedale e la lunga branca dell'incudine, con una pinzetta a branche sottili e terminanti in due piccolissimi cucchiai, la cui larghezza non supera ½ mm., prendo l'essudato che riempie la nicchia della fossetta ovale e con delicate manovre lo distacco dalle leggere aderenze contratte e lo porto via di un sol pezzo, liberando cosi completamente la staffa da ogni ostacolo al suo normale funzionamento.

Questo essudato si presenta molle come la gelatina, di colorito leggermente giallastro, ed osservato al microscopio si trova costituito essenzialmente da cellule linfatiche, da qualche corpuscolo sanguigno, da cellule epiteliali deformate con nucleo granuloso, da qualche corpuscolo di muco e da una sostanza intercellulare ialina.

Fatto ciò, eseguo l'esame acustico e se i risultati sono soddisfacenti rimetto il lembo a posto e medico : diversamente prolungo il lembo in basso e scopro la nicchia della finestra rotonda per vedere se anche in questa vi si trovi dell'essudato che allora porto via.

Eseguo, infine, tutti quei piccoli atti operativi conducenti allo scopo di mobilzzare completamente la catena degli ossicini. Finita l'operazione chiudo il condotto uditivo con un batuffoletto di cotone inzuppato in una soluzione di borogliceride. La guarigione procede rapidamente senza nessuna complicazione ed in meno di otto giorni la membrana è completamente cicatrizzata, la facoltà uditiva del tutto ripristinata.

*
* *

Il trattamento consecutivo consiste in giornaliere irrigazioni tiepide di una soluzione borica nel condotto uditivo per migliorare, mediante il caldo umido, la nutrizione della membrana, favorendo il riassorbimento degli elementi cellulari infiltrati nella trama della medesima, e nel cateterismo dell'orecchio o processo Politzer per ridare alla catena degli ossicini la loro normale funzionabilità.

Con questo trattamento la guarigione sia dal punto di vista acustico che funzionale è completa e gli ammalati rimangono oltremodo soddisfatti.

Quando l'ammalato si presenta in una fase non molto inoltrata della malattia, in maniera da potere escludere che l'essudato peristapedale abbia contratto solide aderenze e si sia in parte organizzato, e la membrana timpanica dell'orecchio da operarsi si presenta rilasciata, allora mi limito semplicemente nel primo tempo dell'operazione a praticare un lungo taglio parallelamente al bordo posteriore del martello ed attraverso quest'apertura introduco la pinza spingendola delicatamente nel solco prismatico peristapedale e procedo quindi all'estrazione del l'essudato secondo è stato descritto. Qualche ammalato è stato da me operato in tal maniera con ottimo risultato.

Esposto così quanto riguarda la diagnosi e la tecnica operativa passo a dire brevemente dei casi da me operati.

Caso I.—Giuseppe Santoro fu Salvatore, di anni 39, da Palermo, da 15 giorni, in seguito ad influenza, cominciò a soffrire forti dolori all'orecchio sinistro, con abbassamento considerevole dell'udito e fortissimo rumore, paragonabile a quello della corrente di un fiume. Da due giorni i dolori sono diminuiti, però i ronzì e la sordità persistono immutati. L'ammalato avverte pure il fenomeno dell'autofonia. Per lo passato è stato sempre bene. Nulla di ereditario.

Esame funzionale.—O. S. Orologio a contatto ; Ut $^{10}/_{50}$; Ut^r $^{20}/_{50}$; Voce afona 0 ; Voce parlata m. 1 ; Rinne negativo ; Galton 3,5 ; Weber a sinistra.

Esame obbiettivo.—Membrana timpanica molto opacata ed infossata, di colore rosso-scuro, ha perduto la sua lucentezza e trasparenza. Mancante il triangolo luminoso.

Il manico del martello, retratto in dentro, ha seguito pure lo spostamento del timpano. Iniettati soltanto i vasi lungo il manico del martello.

Diagnosi.—Otite media nel periodo sub-acuto, rigidità della catena degli ossicini, stenosi tubaria da catarro naso-fàringeo.

Operazione.—O. S. 20 febbraio 1899. Incido longitudinalmente due terzi superiori del segmento posteriore della membrana lungo il manico del martello. Introduco tra le labbra della ferita la descritta pinzetta e spingendola nella vicinanza della staffa, riesco a prendere ed asportare un pezzetto di essudato denso, della grossezza di una piccola lente, di color giallastro. Nessun inconveniente durante l'operazione. Medicatura al solito.

Risultato immediato è stato il seguente : Or. $^{10}/_{200}$; Voce afona 0,30 ; Voce parlata m. 2.

2 marzo. Cicatrizzata completamente la membrana timpanica, scomparsi i disturbi subbiettivi, migliorato considerevolmente l'udito. Or. $^{100}/_{200}$; Voce afona m. 3 ; Galton normale.

15 giugno. Avendo riosservato l'orecchio, l'ho trovato perfettamente guarito e con la funzione acustica uguale all'orecchio sano. Non ha avuto più rumori.

CASO II.—Rabbito Vincenzo fu Vincenzo, di anni 35, da Palermo. Dodici giorni addietro, essendo sofferente di catarro nasale, avvertì, nel soffiarsi forte il naso, dolore acuto ed insopportabile all'orecchio destro. Contemporaneamente ha notato una diminuzione notevole nell'udito ed un susurro continuo come il soffiare del vento. Da due giorne il dolore è molto diminuito. In precedenza l'orecchio era buono. Nulla di ereditario.

Esame funzionale.—O. D. Or. $^{10}/_{100}$; Ut. $^{15}/_{50}$; Ut^{t} $^{25}/_{50}$; Rinne negativo ; Weber a destra ; Galton, 3,6 ; Voce afona 0,10 ; Voce parlata m. 2.

Esame obiettivo.—Membrana timpanica poco arrossata lungo il manico del martello i cui vasi sono iniettati, nel resto della superficie è opaca, con un riflesso rosso-cupo. Scomparso il triangolo luminoso. Manico del martello leggermente spostato indentro assieme al timpano. Non visibili gli organi intratimpanici.

Diagnosi.—Otite media nel periodo sub-acuto, con rigidità della catena degli ossicini da rinite catarrale.

Operazione.—O. D. 25 febbraio 1899. Essendo insufficiente il solo taglio longitudinale come nel caso precedente, eseguo la miringectomia classica. Scoperta la regione della staffa, mi è facile vedere in questo sito una discreta quantità di essudato giallastro, denso, che porto via di un pezzo mediante la pinzetta. Ripristinato completamente l'udito, non sento il bisogno di fare altre ricerche, per cui rimetto il lembo e medico al solito.

5 marzo. Dopo dieci giorni il timpano era completamente cicatrizzato e la facoltà uditiva molto migliorata, come pure i ronzì. Seguito a curare l'ammalato con il metodo da me usato e dopo un mese di cura ottenni la quasi scomparsa dei rumori, i quali si facevano sentire un poco soltanto la sera, ed un grande miglioramento dell'udito, che si mantiene tuttora. Infatti l'esame acustico practicato il 1° giugno è stato : Or. $^{150}/_{200}$; Voce afona m. 4 ; Galton normale ; Weber appena lateralizzato a destra ; Rinne positivo.

CASO III.—Rosalia Pavone di Giovanni, di anni 32, da Palermo. Da 15 giorni soffre dolori intensi a sinistra, nella metà corrispondente della testa. Contemporaneamente ha notato sordità e fortissimi ronzì, paragonabili a quelli dell'acqua in ebollizione ed inoltre grave confusione alla testa ed accessi intercorrenti di vertigine. Da quattro giorni i dolori sono molto diminuiti, però gli altri disturbi persistono immutati. Nulla di ereditario. Per l'addietro è stata sempre bene.

Esame funzionale.—O. S. Or. $^{5}/_{200}$; Ut. $^{20}/_{50}$; Galton normale ; Voce afona a contatto ; Voce parlata m. 1,50.

Esame obbiettivo.—Leggiera iniezione vasale lungo il manico del martello e perifericamente all'anulo timpanico. La membrana timpanica è di aspetto secco, opaco, molto rilasciata ed infossata. La sua superficie non è uniformemente concava, ma in alcuni punti è più sollevata, in altri infossata. Scomparso il triangolo luminoso. Manico del martello spostato in dentro. Non visibile la branca verticale dell'incudine (Otite media nel periodo sub-acuto, con rigidità della catena degli ossicini. Stenosi tubaria).

Operazione.—10 maggio. O. S. Incisione longitudinale nei due terzi superiori del segmento posteriore del timpano lungo il manico del martello, introduzione delle branche della pinzetta attraverso le labbra della ferita ed estrazione dalla regione peristapedale di un globetto di essudato denso, giallastro, della grossezza di una lente.

Ritornata in gran parte la facoltà uditiva, eseguo la medicatura dell'orecchio, senza fare altre ricerche nella cassa timpanica. L'operazione procedette senza alcuna complicazione ed è stata benissimo tollerata dall'inferma.

18 marzo. Cicatrizzata del tutto la membrana timpanica. Or $^{80}/_{200}$; Ut $^{30}/_{50}$; Ut^t $^{40}/_{50}$; Voce afona m. 2 ; Galton normale ; Rinne positivo ; Weber a sinistra. Cessata completamente la confusione alla testa. Non vi sono stati più accessi di vertigine. Molto diminuiti i susurri.

Assoggetto sistematicamente l'inferma alla cura locale consecutiva e dopo un mese la lascio completamente guarita da tutti i disturbi subbiettivi e con la facoltà uditiva quasi normale, dappoichè è in grado di sentire l'orologio a $^{160}/_{200}$ e la voce afona a più di 4 metri. Non soffre più nè vertigini, nè rumori all'orecchio.

CASO IV.—Salvatore Raneli fu Benedetto, di anni 46, da Palermo. Venti giorni addietro, in seguito ad influenza, notò dolore violento all'orecchio sinistro, irradiantesi alla regione temporale dello stesso lato e notevole diminuzione dell'udito, con accessi intercorrenti di vertigine e gravissimo susurro, paragonabile al soffiar del vento. Da tre giorni i dolori sono diminuiti, però i rumori, la sordità e la vertigine sono aumentati. Nulla di ereditario. L'orecchio era precedentemente normale.

Esame funzionale.—O. S. Orologio a contatto ; Ut $^5/_{50}$; Ut^t $^{10}/_{50}$; Galton 3,5 ; Voce afona 0 ; Voce parlata 0,20 ; Rinne negativo ; Weber a sinistra.

Esame obbiettivo.—O. S. Membrana leggermente arrossata, principalmente lungo il manico del martello e nel quadrante postero-superiore, ove si presenta un po' sollevata e convessa all'interno. Anteriormente invece è infossata. In tutta la sua superficie è opaca in modo da non lasciar vedere gli organi intratimpanici. Mancante il triangolo luminoso. Manico del martello non spostato all'interno.

Diagnosi.—Otite media sub-acuta ; rigidità della catena degli ossicini da influenza.

Operazione.—O. S. 20 aprile. Formazione del lembo timpanico e scopertura della regione peristapedale. Osservasi la staffa quasi del tutto coperta da un essudato tenace, giallastro e copioso. La mucosa del promontorio nelle vicinanze è arrossata e gonfia. Asportazione dell'essudato e mobilizzazione completa della staffa. Quest'atto operativo è stato molto laborioso ed ha procacciato una discreta emorragia.

Avendo osservato che la facoltà uditiva era in gran parte ritornata, rimetto il lembo a posto e medico come di consueto.

Il processo di guarigione andò benissimo e dopo quindici giorni il timpano era cicatrizzato.

30 aprile. Non vi è stato più alcun accesso di vertigine ; sono diminuiti molto i susurri all'orecchio. Or. $^{80}/_{200}$; Ut $^{30}/_{50}$; Ut^t $^{40}/_{50}$; Voce afona m. 2 ; Galton 2,0 ; Rinne positivo ; Weber a sinistra.

30 maggio. Avendo sottoposto l'ammalato alla cura consecutiva ottenni un maggiore miglioramento nella funzione acustica. Or. $^{120}/_{200}$: Voce afona m. 3. Non più ritornate le vertigini. Appena sensibili i rumori.

I risultati di queste poche operazioni sono abbastanza incoraggianti e dimostrativi e credo che giustifichino appieno la mia proposta di operare i casi di otite media acuta non suppurativa con grave sordità appena il processo flogistico sarà spento, prima cioè che l'organizzazione degli essudati renda l'operazione più difficile ed i risultati più scarsi.

Ora se facciamo un parallelo tra i vantaggi che ci offre una precoce mobilizzazione della staffa rispetto alla tardiva risalta a prima vista la grande superiorità della prima.

Anzitutto in questa il processo di guarigione è assai breve. Ordinariamente in dieci giorni circa si è conseguita la guarigione e solo nei casi in cui è necessaria una cura consecutiva il processo di guarigione può durare un mese. Invece nella tardiva mobilizzazione, le cure consecutive sono sempre indispensabili e per poco che durino richiedono sempre più di un mese di tempo per completarle.

In secondo luogo i vantaggi acustici sono di gran lunga superiori.

Infatti, mentre nella tardiva mobilizzazione io non ho ottenuto mai un udito per l'orologio superiore a m. 1 e per la voce afona maggiore a m. 3 senza parlare delle altre prove acustiche, con la precoce mobilizzazione della staffa invece il minimo risultato ottenuto è stato m. 1,20 per l'orologio ; m. 3 per la voce susurrata : il massimo quello di riportare la funzione acustica alle condizioni normali antecedenti alla malattia.

I disturbi paracustici sono in entrambi i processi ugualmente influenzati, con la differenza che mentre nella precoce mobilizzazione la loro guarigione è la regola, nelle tardive invece costituisce l'eccezione. Solo per i disturbi dell'equilibrio non troviamo una vera differenza, dappoichè la mobilizzazione della staffa in qualunque periodo della malattia venga eseguita ha sempre per effetto di far cessare l'otopiesi, causa esclusiva della vertigine e della confusione di testa.

Riepilogando quindi, sia dal punto di vista funzionale che acustico, la precoce mobilizzazione della staffa è sempre preferibile alla tardiva, ed io mi auguro che tale argomento venga preso in considerazione dai colleghi, in maniera che col loro contributo si possa meglio definire la forma nosografica dell'otopatia in cui l'intervento precoce debba essere indicato.

IMPORTANZA ACUSTICA E FUNZIONALE DELLA MOBILIZZAZIONE DELLA STAFFA.

(Risultati di una nuova serie di operazioni).

Prof. GIUSEPPE FARACI, Palermo.

Tre anni oramai sono trascorsi da che con vivo interesse procedo in questo genere di studi, e ognora più sento affermarsi la mia convinzione e rinsaldarsi la mia fede sulla utilità della mobilizzazione della staffa per combattere non solo la sordità, ma anche gli altri disturbi subbiettivi.

E così giustificata mi sembra questa mia fiducia che non posso nascondere un senso di stupore quando vedo qualche illustre otologo combattere tale operazione e sostituirla con quei vecchi mezzi di cura che, passati oramai per le mani di tutti, si sono mostrati veramente impotenti a ridare alla catena degli ossicini quella mobilità che un processo di sclerosi o di neoformazione connettivale ha stabilmente distrutto.

Quando mi capita fra le mani qualche monografia di questi fautori della cura medica locale, mi viene subito fatto di pensare che costoro o non hanno mai praticato la mobilizzazione della staffa o sono stati molto disgraziati nella scelta dei casi, o inesperti nelle manovre chirurgiche, non hanno saputo riuscire allo scopo.

Oramai gli sforzi degli otologi devono essere rivolti non più a discutere l'operazione, la quale ha preso già il suo stabile posto nel campo della chirurgia otoiatrica, ma a perfezionare la tecnica operativa, a studiare meglio i casi in cui essa sarebbe di un indiscutibile vantaggio, a conoscere infine i limiti del miglioramento che può darsi in rapporto alle condizioni anatomo-patologiche dell'orecchio leso, in maniera di potere *a priori* conoscere quanto sarebbe il vantaggio acustico sperabile dal paziente, quanta probabilità questo avrebbe nel guarire dei susurri e della vertigine.

Il giorno in cui tale perfezionamento verrà raggiunto avremo segnato un gran passo nel progresso scientifico e non ci troveremo più nella infelice condizione di doverci stringere nelle spalle o dare delle risposte evasive quando un paziente ci domanda se con la mobilizzazione della staffa guarirà dei suoi rumori endottici.

Ora io sono convinto che non è tanto lo studio accurato delle alterazioni istologiche che avvengono nell'apparecchio di trasmissione del suono, non è ancora l'analisi delle conoscenze fisiologiche dell'orecchio e dell'influenza che le lesioni esercitano sull'eccitamento delle fibre cocleari e vestibolari del nervo acustico, quanto lo studio dei risultati clinici, in rapporto alla natura ed all'estensione delle alterazioni dell'orecchio curato chirurgicamente, che si possa arrivare alla desiderata meta.

Per questo credo giustificato non solo, ma necessario, pubblicare i risultati conseguiti con l'operazione, affinchè dall'analisi dei casi isolati si possa assurgere al concetto generale delle leggi che governano la fisiopatologia dell'organo ammalato.

È per questo che io, per sommi capi, mi permetto communicare i risultati delle mie operazione sulla mobilizzazione della catena degli ossicini.

CASO I.—Alfonso Marsiglia fu Carlo, di anni 54, da Campobello di Mazzara.

Storia.—Da molti anni suppurazione cronica intermittente a destra, con sordità progressiva, rumori continui, molesti ed accessi intercorrenti di vertigine.

Esame funzionale.—O. D. Orologio a contatto ; Ut $^5/_{50}$; Ut ^{1} $^{15}/_{50}$; Galton 3,0; Rinne negativo ; Weber a destra ; Voce afona 0,10 ; Voce parlata m. 1,50.

Esame obbiettivo.—O. D. Un residuo di membrana molto ispessita ed iperplastica rimane ancora attaccata in alto al manico del martello, il quale è retratto in dentro.

Mancante il rimanente del timpano. Mucosa della cassa arrossata e segregante.

Si vede poco la finestra ovale e pochissimo la staffa, la quale rimane nascosta in alto dietro l'orlo timpanico postero-superiore.

Diagnosi.—Otite media purulenta cronica, carie delle pareti dell'attico timpanico, rigidità della catena degli ossicini.

Operazione.—29 agosto 1898. Escissione del martello. Asportazione delle vegetazioni e delle briglie cicatriziali dalla nicchia della finestra ovale. Mobilizzazione della staffa.

Niente vertigine. Nessuna complicazione.

Risultato.—Orologio 0,05 ; Voce afona 0,20 ; Voce parlata m. 2 $^1/_2$; Galton 3,0.

15 novembre. Continua un po' di suppurazione. Persiste il miglioramento uditivo.

17 dicembre.—Cessata la suppurazione. La membrana comincia a rigenerarsi. La mucosa della cassa un poco umida e leggermente iperemica. Diminuiti i rumori. Cessata la vertigine. Or. a contatto ; Voce afona 0,10 ; Voce parlata m. 2,0.

1° giugno 1899.—Nessun cambiamento dall'ultimo esame.

CASO II.—Rainoni Annina di Francesco, di anni 19, da Palermo.

Storia.—Sin da bambina suppurazione cronica ad ambo i lati. Da un anno lo scolo marcioso è cessato. Sordità progressiva. Non ha sofferto mai vertigini. Solo ronzî intermittenti.

Esame funzionale.—O. S. Or. 0,30 ; Ut $^{10}/_{50}$; Ut^1 $^{20}/_{50}$; Galton 1,7 ; Weber a sinistra ; Rinne negativo ; Voce afona a contatto ; Voce parlata 0, 30.

Esame elettrico.—O. S. Ka. Ch. S. con 6 M. A. ; Ka. Ap. O. An. Ch. S. con 6 M. A. ; An. Ap. Reazione leggera di breve durata sotto forma di sibilo.

Esame obbiettivo.—O. S. Perforazione nel quadrante antero-inferiore del timpano. Resto della membrana molto sclerosata. Anteriormente e posteriormente al manico del martello si vedono delle macchie d'infiltrazione calcarea. La mucosa della cassa cicatriziale. Immobilità completa della membrana timpanica, tranne un piccolo segmento posteriormente ed in alto in vicinanza dell'anulo timpanico.

Diagnosi.—Esiti di otite media purulenta cronica, rigidità della catena degli ossicini, sinechia del timpano.

Operazione.—9 novembre 1898. O. S. Escissione delle macchie di infiltramento calcareo ; distacco della membrana dal promontorio e dalla branca verticale dell'incudine ; mobilizzazione della staffa. Nessun inconveniente.

Risultato immediato.—Or. 0,05 ; Ut $^{15}/_{50}$; Voce afona 0,20 ; Voce parlata m. 1,50.

24 dicembre 1898. Or. 0,70 ; Ut $^{20}/_{50}$; Voce afona 0,30 ; Voce parlata m. 2 ; Weber a sinistra ; Rinne negativo. Niente vertigini. Continuano i rumori come prima dell'operazione. Si vede una vasta perforazione nel quadrante posteroinferiore. Immobile il manico del martello con il resto della membrana.

30 maggio 1899.—Persiste immutato il miglioramento uditivo.

CASO III.—Marcianò Angela di Salvatore, di anni 18, da Carini.

Storia.—All'età di sette anni ebbe una suppurazione cronica bilaterale ed intermittente alle orecchio. Dopo pochi anni cessò la suppurazione, rimase però un grave abbassamento dell'udito, che andava sempre aggravandosi. Sin da quell'epoca cominciò ad avvertire rumori continui alle orecchie ed a lunghi intervalli qualche lieve dolore a trafittura. Nulla di ereditario. Non ha avuto vertigine, nè altre malattie.

Esame funzionale.—O. S. Or. 0,20 ; Voce afona 0,15 ; Voce parlata m. 1,0 ; Galton 2,0 ; Ut $^{20}/_{50}$; Ut^1 $^{25}/_{50}$; Rinne negativo ; Weber al vertice.

Esame obbiettivo.—O. S. Membrana di color roseo, molto ispessita, infossata ed aderente in tutte le sue parti al promontorio. Manico del martello retratto in dentro, sembra nascosto nello spessore del timpano. Vasi leggermente iniettati. L'orecchio destro è nelle stesse condizioni del sinistro (Otite media iperplastica secondaria ; sinechi del timpano ; anchilosi della catena degli ossicini da otite media purulenta).

Operazione.—1° dicembre 1898. Sinechiotomia del timpano. Vuotamento della cassa da un tessuto di neo-formazione, ancora sufficientemente vascolarizzato. Mobilizzazione della staffa. Operazione laboriosa. Nessun inconveniente, tranne un po' di emorragia.

Risultato immediato.—Or. 0,50 ; Voce afona 0,50 ; Voce parlata m. 3.

20 dicembre 1899.—Cicatrizzazione del timpano Funzione acustica migliora ta.

26 dicembre 1898. Or. 0,60 ; Ut $^{30}/_{50}$; Galton 1,8 ; Voce afona m. 2 $^1/_2$. Diminuiti i rumori. Assenza di vertigine.

25 giugno 1899. Continua il miglioramento uditivo. Molto diminuiti i rumori nel lato operato.

CASO IV.—Taccone Dorotea di Ignazio, di anni 18, da Palermo.

Storia.—Da cinque anni suppurazione continua all'orecchio sinistro con lievi intermittenze. Pochi susurri. Soffre continue vertigini, specie nel piegarsi o nel voltarsi.

Esame funzionale.—Or. 0,70 ; Ut $^{20}/_{50}$; Ut^1 $^{25}/_{50}$; Voce afona 0,15 ; Voce parlata m. 2 ; Galton 2,8.

Esame obbiettivo.—Vasta perforazione nel quadrante antero-inferiore, ove si vede la mucosa della cassa leggermente granulante ed umida. Il timpano, di aspetto sclerotico in alcuni punti ed atrofico in altri, si trova assieme al manico del martello infossato ed aderente in tutta l'estensione alla parete interna della cassa.

Diagnosi.—Otite media purulenta cronica, sinechia del timpano, anchilosi della catena degli ossicini.

Operazione.—20 dicembre 1898. Sinechiotomia del timpano. Mobilizzazione della staffa. Nessun inconveniente.

Resultato immediato.—Or. 0,80 ; Voce afona 0,50 ; Voce parlata m. 4,50. Scompare la vertigine.

20 gennaio 1899. Cessata completamente la suppurazione, migliorato ancora l'udito.

28 aprile 1899. Non ha avuto più nè vertigine, nè rumori. Si sente assai bene. Or. 0,80 ; Voce afona m. 1,50 ; Voce parlata m. 3 ; Ut $^{25}/_{50}$; Weber a sinistra; Rinne negativo ; Galton 2, 3. Persiste la perforazione come prima.

10 giugno 1899. Continua il miglioramento acustico come nell'ultimo esame ; guarita dalle vertigini e dai rumori.

CASO V.—Francesca Terzo di Vincenzo, di anni 21, da Palermo.

Storia.— Da cinque anni suppurazione continua all'orecchio sinistro, con abbassamento progressivo dell'udito. Contemporaneamente continui e fortissimi rumori, con accessi intercorrenti di vertigine, fino al punto di farla cadere e ciò specialmente nei movimenti laterali del capo.

Esame funzionale.—Or. 0,05 ; Ut $^{10}/_{50}$; Ut^1 $^{15}/_{50}$; Voce afona, 0 ; Voce parlata 0,30 ; Rinne negativo ; Weber a sinistra ; 'Galton normale.

Esame obbiettivo.—Rimane solo un piccolo residuo della membrana attaccata in alto al manico del martello. Quest'ultimo retratto in dentro ed aderente al promontorio. Manca la incudine. Mucosa della cassa enormemente ispessita, arrossata e segregante scorrevole sul promontorio. La regione della staffa coperta da un tessuto di neo-formazione.

Diagnosi.—Otite media purulenta cronica, carie delle pareti dell'*aditus ad antrum*, rigidità della staffa.

Operazione. —1° dicembre 1897. Asportazione del martello cariato con i residui della membrana, causticazione e raschiamento dell'attico timpanico e dell'*aditus ad antrum*. Escissione di tutta la mucosa del promontorio, essendo enormemente ispessita ed arrossata. Vuotamento della nicchia della finestra ovale. Mobilizzazione della staffa. Nessun inconveniente.

Risultato immediato.—Or. 0,10 ; Voce afona 0.05 ; Voce media m. 1 ½.

Un po' di reazione infiammatoria nell'orecchio medio, con abassamento della facoltà uditiva.

30 gennaio 1898. Persiste il miglioramento acustico, diminuita l'infiammazione purulenta dell'orecchio medio.

1° marzo. Cessata la suppurazione. Il promontorio è rivestito da un tessuto sottile, pallido, coperto di epitelio. Una parziale rigenerazione della membrana attorno l'annulo nasconde la regione della staffa. Or. 0,30 ; Rinne negativo ; Ut $^{10}/_{50}$; Ut^1 $^{15}/_{50}$; Galton normale ; Voce afona 0,40 ; Voce parlata m. 3. Cessate le vertigini gravi ed i rumori che soffriva.

1° maggio. Or. 0,30 ; Ut $^{20}/_{50}$; Rinne negativo ; Weber a sinistra ; Galton normale ; Voce afona m. 1 ; Voce parlata m. 4.

1° luglio 1899. Continua il miglioramento come nell'ultimo esame.

CASO VI.—Suora Eleonora Lo Presti, di anni 25, da Palermo.

Storia.—Da bambina ebbe suppurazione cronica all'orecchio sinistro, che dopo parecchi anni cessò completamente e non si è più riprodotta. Da poco tempo dice di avvertire confusione alla testa ed un po' di rumore.

Esame funzionale.—O. S. Or. 0,90 ; Voce afona m. 2.

Esame obbiettivo.—Membrana sottile ed atrofica, presenta una vasta perforazione nel quadrante postero-inferiore, il cui bordo superiore trovasi a livello dell'articolazione incudo stapedale. Mucosa della cassa pallida. Vuota la nicchia della finestra ovale e rotonda. Il timpano aderente alla branca verticale dell'incudine ed alla testa della staffa.

Diagnosi.—Esiti di otite media purulenta cronica, rigidità della catena degli ossicini.

Operazione.—13 dicembre 1898. Mobilizzazione della staffa, sinechiotomia del timpano.

Risultato immediato.—Or. 0,90 ; Voce afona m. 3. Aumentato l'udito per la voce.

18 gennaio 1899. Or. m. 1 ; Voce afona m. 3. Dopo l'operazione non ha avvertito più l'impaccio di prima, è rimasto solo un po' di rumore, il quale si fa sentire a lunghi intervalli.

Ho osservato che bagnando la membrana il rumore cessava.

30 giugno 1899. Continua il miglioramento dell'udito. Cessata la confusione ed i rumori.

CASO VII.—Adelina Franchina di Vincenzo, di anni 21, da Palermo.

Storia.—Sin ba bambina suppurazione cronica intermittente a sinistra con progressivo abbassamento dell'udito. Soffre pure di continui ronzi. Nulla di ereditario.

Esame funzionale.—O. S. Or. 0,40 ; Ut $^{10}/_{50}$; Ut^1 $^{20}/_{50}$; Galton normale ; Voce afona 0,30 ; Voce parlata m. 2 ½.

Esame obbiettivo.—Membrana in gran parte distrutta. Rimane solo un residuo attaccato in alto al manico del martello. Quest'ultimo retratto in dentro è fissato al promontorio. Visibile la staffa, la quale è poco mobile per una membrana di nuova formazione che ricopre la fossetta ovale e si fissa alle sue branche. Nascosta l'incudine. Delle granulazioni fuoriescono dall'antro mastoideo.

Diagnosi.—Otite media purulenta cronica. Carie delle pareti dell'antro mastoideo. Rigidità della staffa.

Operazione.—18 gennaio 1899. Estrazione del martello e causticazione delle pareti dell'antro mastoideo. Mobilizzazione della staffa. La finestra rotonda viene liberata da una membrana di neo-formazione molto vascolarizzata che la ricopriva. Nessun inconveniente.

Risultato immediato.—Or. 0,80 ; Voce afona m. 2.

24 gennaio. Continua la suppurazione, diminuito il potere uditivo.

10 febbraio. Diminuita la suppurazione ; l'udito minore che subito dopo l'operazione.

5 maggio. Guarita dal processo suppurativo. Diminuiti i rumori. Or. 0,40 ; Voce afona 0,60 ; parlata m. 3.

20 giugno. Funzione acustica come nell'ultimo esame.

5 luglio. Nulla di nuovo.

CASO VIII.—Bruno Saverio di Francesco, di anni 30, da Monreale.

Storia.—Quindici anni addietro, in seguito a suppurazione cronica della durata di parecchi mesi, cominciò a notare considerevole abbassamento dell'udito. Non ha avuto vertigine, soffre pochi rumori.

Esame funzionale.—O. D. Or. a contatto ; Ut. 0 ; Ut^1 $^{10}/_{50}$; Ut^2 $^{20}/_{50}$; Weber a destra ; Galton 3.1 ; Voce afona 0 ; Voce parlata 0,10.

Esame obbiettivo.—O. D. Nella metà superiore la membrana è ispessita, sclerotica, ed aderente alla parete laberintica. Una linea sottile, bianca indica ancora la presenza del manico del martello, il quale è retratto in dentro.

Posteriormente osservasi una lunga macchia d'infiltramento calcareo.

Nella metà inferiore la membrana è atrofica ed aderente al promontorio.

Non si vede la regione stapedale.

Diagnosi.—Esiti di otite media purulenta cronica. Infiltramento calcareo del timpano. Anchilosi della catena degli ossicini.

Operazione.—14 gennaio 1899. Escissione dell'infiltramento calcareo. Asportazione del martello ch'era fortemente attaccato al promontorio e circondato nell'attico da connettivo fibroso. La staffa, profondamente nascosta dietro la parete ossea del condotto, non si potè scoprire che incompletamente e quindi la mobilizzazione non potè essere fatta bene. Non si ebbe alcun inconveniente.

Risultato immediato.—Or. 0,10 ; Voce afona 0,15 ; Voce parlata 0,60.

1° febbraio. La guarigione avvenne senza suppurazione.

30 marzo. Persistenza del potere uditivo ricuperato ; nessuna influenza nei rumori.

27 giugno. Continua come nell'ultimo esame.

CASO IX.—Ignazia Culotta di Vincenzo, di anni 26, da Palermo.

Storia.—Dall'età di 13 anni cominciò a notare abbassamento progressivo dell'udito bilaterale, specialmente a sinistra. Contemporaneamente ha avvertito dei rumori molto forti. Non ha avuto mai dolori, suppurazioni e vertigini. Afferma che nell'orecchio sinistro ha notato un lieve miglioramento nell'udito in seguito al processo Politzer, che ha fatto per molto tempo. È stata operata molti anni addietro di vegetazioni adenoidi del cavo naso faringeo.

Esame funzionale.—Or. a contatto ; Ut $^5/_{50}$; Ut^1, Ut^2, Ut^3, Ut^4 vengono sentiti progressivamente sempre meglio. Rinne negativo ; Galton 4,0 (la scala di Galton presenta un'interruzione al 5,0 solamente, nel resto è positiva) ; Voce afona a contatto ; Voce parlata 0,10.

Esame obbiettivo..—O. S. Membrana leggermente ispessita ed opacata non lascia vedere per trasparenza la mucosa della cassa e gli organi in essa contenuti. Vasi del martello poco visibili. La membrana è mobile in tutte le sue parti e non infossata.

Diagnosi.—Otite media sclerosante ; rigidità della catena degli ossicini ; parziale e limitata lesione secondaria dell'acustico.

Operazione.—12 dicembre 1898. Mobilizzazione della staffa secondo il processo classico. L'operazione fu tollerata benissimo senza alcun inconveniente.

Risultato immediato.—Or. 10 ; Voce afona 0,20 ; Voce parlata m. 1.

20 gennaio 1899. Cicatrizzazione completa del timpano. Dal momento che si chiuse l'apertura della membrana cessò il miglioramento acustico ottenuto con l'operazione e l'ammalata ritornò nelle condizioni di prima.

1° febbraio. Si rifà l'operazione con la resezione del segmento postero-superiore dell'annulo timpanico. Si moblizza bene la staffa. L'udito ritorna meglio di prima. Or. 0,30 ; Voce afona 0,50 ; Voce parlata m. 2.

10 marzo. Non v'è stata alcuna reazione nell'orecchio. L'apertura timpanica si mantiene sufficientemente aperta. Continua il miglioramento acustico.

10 luglio. Si mantiene immutato il potere acustico come nell'ultimo esame ; solo i rumori rimasero quali erano prima dell'operazione.

Caso X.—Bracco Michele di Giuseppe, di anni 38, da Palermo.

Storia.—Da circa 30 anni abbassamento progressivo dell'udito a sinistra, con rumori forti e continui. Soffre ad intervalli di vertigine. Da qualche anno sordità quasi completa.

Esame funzionale.—O. S. Or. a contatto ; Ut 0 ; Ut^1 $^5/_{50}$; Ut^2 $^{10}/_{50}$; Rinne negativo ; Weber a sinistra ; Galton normale ; Voce afona 0 ; Voce parlata a contatto.

Esame elettrico.—O. S. Ka. Ch. S. con 23 M. A. Ripetendo l'esame si ottiene reazione anche con 3 M. A. Alla chiusura del catode la durata della sensazione dura 25″ con 7 M. A. e 40″ con 20 M. A. An. Ch. S. dapprima con 33 M. A. in seguito con 6 M. A. Nessuna reazione all'apertura del catode e dell'anode.

Esame obbiettivo.—Membrana bianca, opaca, ispessita, mediocremente infossata e con riflesso leggermente bluastro. Non si vede per trasparenza l'incudine.

Diagnosi.—Otite media sclerosante, anchilosi della catena degli ossicini.

Operazione.—3 gennaio 1898. O. S. Mobilizzazione della staffa secondo il processo solito, resezione del segmento postero-superiore dell'annulo timpanico. Nessun inconveniente nè durante, nè dopo l'operazione. L'ammalato andò via senza accusare fenomeni di vertigine.

Risultato immediato.—Or. a contatto ; Galton normale ; Ut $^{10}/_{50}$; Ut^1 $^{20}/_{50}$; Ut^2 $^{30}/_{50}$; Voce afona a contatto ; Voce parlata m. 1 ; Weber a sinistra.

30 gennaio. Nessuna infiammazione locale. La guarigione procede benissimo. Or. 0,50 ; Voce afona a contatto ; Voce media m. 1 ; Galton normale. Cessate le vertigini.

8 luglio 1899. Continua il miglioramento acustico. Guarito completamente dalle vertigini. Persistono solo i rumori, però meno intensi di prima. La membrana timpanica si mantiene perforata.

CASO XI.—Cristina Lombardo fu Ignazio, di anni 23, da Palermo.

Storia.—Nove anni addietro diminuzione progressiva dell'udito a destra. Cinque anni or sono sopravvenne un'otite media purulenta acuta, della durata di un mese circa, dopo la quale perdette completamente l'udito. Contemporaneamente ha sofferto accessi intermittenti di vertigine, specialmente nei movimenti laterali del capo e nel piegarsi a terra. Ronzii intermittenti sotto forma di sibilo.

Esame funzionale.—Or. 0,03 ; Ut $^{10}/_{50}$; Galton 2,2 ; Voce afona 0,05 ; Voce parlata 0,50.

Esame elettrico.—Ka. Ch. S. con 20 M. A. An. Ch. S. con 20 M. A.

Esame obbiettivo.—O. D. La metà anteriore del timpano ispessita ed opaca, la metà posteriore molto atrofica si modella sul promontorio, a cui trovasi aderente, assieme al martello, il quale è retratto in dentro. Si vede la testa della staffa, la quale è ricoperta dalla porzione atrofica del timpano. Mancante il solco prismatico triangolare della fossetta ovale, essendo ripieno da un tessuto fibroso di nuova formazione. Mancante l'incudine.

Diagnosi.—Esiti di otite media purulenta cronica ; anchilosi della staffa.

Operazione.—7 febbraio 1898. Mobilizzazione della staffa, escidendo il tessuto fibroso che ne circondava la base. Non fu tagliato il tendine dello stapedio. Nessun inconveniente nè durante, nè dopo l'operazione.

Risultato immediato.—Orologio 0,10 ; Ut $^{20}/_{50}$; Voce afona 0,20 ; Voce parlata m. 2.

15 febbraio. Cessate le vertigini, diminuti i rumori, l'udito si mantiene come dopo l'operazione.

7 luglio 1899. Or. 0,10 ; Voce afona 0,30 ; Voce parlata m. 2½ ; Galton 2,2. Cessate le vertigini, diminuiti i rumori.

CASO XII.—Lucrezia Gianfrida, di anni 27, da Floridia.

Storia.—Da dieci anni accusa sordità progressiva a destra con ronzî intollerabili ed accessi intercorrenti di vertigine, che taluni giorni sono così gravi da dar luogo a confusione intensa di testa e ad uno stato vertiginoso permanente. La sordità da qualche anno è completa. Nulla d'ereditario.

Esame funzionale.—O. D. Or. 0 ; Rinne negativo ; Weber a sinistra ; Ut 0 ; Ut^1 $^5/_{50}$; Ut^2 $^{10}/_{50}$; Ut^3 $^{10}/_{50}$; Ut^4 $^5/_{50}$; F^4 0 ; Galton 3,7 ; Voce afona 0, parlata 0.

Esame obbiettivo.—Membrana opaca, di aspetto sclerotico ed un po' infossata. Non si vedono per trasparenza gli organi intratimpanici. Mancante il triangolo luminoso ; vasi del martello poco visibili.

Diagnosi.—Otite media sclerosante ; anchilosi della staffa ; lesioni secondarie nell'acustico.

Operazione.—2 marzo 1898. O. D. Mobilizzazione della staffa. Ho trovato delle briglie connettivali, che a guisa di ponte passavano al disopra del solco prismatico peristapedale, legando le branche della staffa al bordo della finestra ovale.

Resultato immediato.—Or. a contatto ; Voce afona 0,20 ; Voce parlata m. ½ ; Galton 3,7 ; Ut $^{15}/_{50}$ Durante l'operazione ebbe qualche accesso di vertigine e vomiti di pocadurata.

1° marzo. Cicatrizzato il timpano, la guarigione procedette benissimo. Sono scomparse le vertigini. diminuiti molto i ronzî, ridotta un po la funzione acustica acquistata. Or. 0 ; Ut $^5/_{50}$; Galton 3,7 ; Voce afona a contatto ; Voce parlata 0,50.

28 giugno. Continua come fu trovata nell'ultimo esame, guarita cioè dalle vertigini, migliorati i rumori e l'udito.

CASO XIII.—Vittorio Pellara fu Salvatore, di anni 37, da Palermo.

Storia.—Cinque anni addietro soffrì un'otite media purulenta acuta a sinistra, della durata di un mese circa. Da allora sordità progressiva. Non ha sofferto nè rumori nè vertigini.

Esame funzionale.—O. S. Or. 0 ; Ut, Ut' 0 ; Ut² ⁵/₅₀ ; Rinne negativo ; Weber a destra ; Galton 5,0 ; Voce afona 0 ; Voce parlata 0,30.

Esame elettrico.—O. S. Ka. Ch. S. con 18 M. A. ; An. Ch. S. con 18 M. A.

La reazione acustica sotto forma di fischietto dura 15″. Nessuna reazione all'apertura, sia del catode che dell'anode.

Esame obbiettivo.—O. S. Cicatrice atrofica nella metà posteriore del timpano ed aderente al promontorio. La metà anteriore è invece molto ispessita e con infiltrazione calcarea. Manico del martello retratto in dentro e aderente al promontorio. Vasi del martello assottigliati. Non si vede l'incudine. Con lo speculo pneumatico notasi immobilità completa del timpano, meno un piccolo segmento atrofico postero-superiore, che si sposta. Lo stesso ottiensi col cateterismo.

Diagnosi.—Esiti di otite media purulenta cronica ; anchilosi della catena degli ossicini.

Operazione.—15 marzo 1898. Sinechiotomia totale del timpano ed asportazione del medesimo assieme al manico del martello. Non si trova l'incudine. La nicchia della finestra ovale piena di tessuto fibroso. Staffa immobile. Sinechiotomia delle branche di quest'ossicino, vuotamento della finestra ovale, mobilizzazione completa della staffa. Nessun inconveniente durante e dopo l'operazione.

Risultato immediato.—Orologio 0,05 ; Ut 0 ; Ut ' ²⁰/₅₀ ; Galton 4,0 ; Voce afona a contatto ; Voce parlata m. 1.

18 marzo. Dovetti partire ed abbandonare l'inferno.

5 maggio. Avendolo riveduto trovo Or. 0,10 ; Ut 10,50 ; Ut' ²⁰/₄₀ ; Voce afona 0,10 ; Voce parlata m. 2 ; Galton 3,5.

4 luglio 1899. Continua il miglioramento come nell'ultimo esame.

CASO XIV.—Vivona Gaetano, di anni 23, da Palermo.

Storia.—Da 18 anni suppurazione continua all'orecchio destro con intensi rumori ed accessi intercorrenti di vertigine, i quali disturbi da circa tre anni si sono così gravemente accentuati da impedire qualsiasi occupazione. Diminuzione progressiva dell'udito fino alla sordità completa. Nulla di ereditario.

Esame funzionale.—O. D. Or. 0,50 ; Ut ²⁰/₅₀ ; Ut' ²⁵/₅₀ ; Galton 1,8 ; Voce afona 0 ; Voce parlata 0,25 ; Rinne negativo ; Weber a destra.

Esame obbiettivo.—O. D. Vasta distruzione nel segmento postero-superiore della membrana, ove si vede la mucosa della cassa granulante e coperta da essudato. Visibile l'articolazione incudo-stapedale. Il resto della membrana opacata, ispessita ed infossata, fino a venire a contatto con la parete labirintica. Manico del martello raccorciato in prospettiva e aderente al promontorio. La nicchia della finestra ovale scomparsa, essendo occupata da un tessuto di nuova formazione.

Diagnosi.—Otite media purulenta cronica. Carie delle pareti dell'*aditus ad antrum mastoideo*. Anchilosi della catena degli ossicini.

Operazione.—3 marzo 1898. O. D. Escissione del martello e della incudine anchilosati. Dell'incudine esisteva solo una piccola parte del corpo corrispondente alla superficie articolare, mancava tutto il resto, come pure la piccola apofisi. La testa del martello era pure in gran parte distrutta, e furono raschiate e causticate le pareti dell'antro mastoideo e dell'attico timpanico. Mobilizzazione della staffa.

Risultato immediato.—Or. 0,50 ; Voce afona m. 1 ; Voce parlata m. 3.

14 novembre.   Or. 0,25 ; Ut $^{30}/_{50}$; Ut^{1} $^{40}/_{50}$; Galton 1,8 ; Weber a destra ; Rinne negativo ; Voce afona 0,30 ; Voce parlata m. 2.   Continua la suppurazione.

8 marzo 1899.   La suppurazione molto diminuita.   Cessate le vertigini.   Migliorati i rumori.   Or. 0,10 ; Voce afona 0,10 ; Voce parlata m. 1.

7 luglio 1899.   Guarito dal processo suppurativo.   La funzione acustica come nell'ultimo esame.

Caso XV.—D'Amico Irene di Giovanni, di anni 15, da Palermo.

Storia.—Da tre anni suppurazione continua all'orecchio destro, con abbassamento progressivo dell'udito.

Esame funzionale.—O. D. Or. 0,15 ; Ut 0 ; Ut^{1} $^{10}/_{50}$; Ut^{2} ; Ut^{3} $^{30}/_{50}$; Rinne negativo : Weber a destra ; Galton normale ; Voce afona 0 ; Voce parlata 0,40. O. S. normale.

Esame elettrico.—Ka. Ch. S., An. Ap. S. con 5 M. A. Avverte come un sibilo che dura pochi secondi.

Esame obbiettivo.—Assenza del timpano, di cui rimane un piccolo segmento in alto attaccato ad un residuo del martello.   Quest'ultimo spostato in dentro occupa una posizione orizzontale.   Mucosa della cassa, molto arrossata ed ispessita, scorre sul promontorio.   Non vedesi la branca verticale dell'incudine.   Al posto della fossetta ovale osservasi un tessuto di neo-formazione, che la riempie completamente. Naso e faringe normali.

Diagnosi.—Otite media purulenta cronica ; carie degli ossicini e delle pareti dell'attico, rigidità della staffa.

Operazione.—15 aprile 1898.   O. D. Asportazione del residuo della membrana con il martello, la cui testa è cariata, raschiamento delle pareti dell'attico timpanico pieno di granulazioni.   Rimuovendo il tessuto di neo-formazione, che riempiva la fossetta ovale si scopre la staffa, la quale è immobile.   Con un po' di difficoltà riesco a liberare la base dell'ossicino da questo tessuto connettivale ed a mobilizzarlo completamente.

L'operazione non fu seguita da alcun inconveniente.

Risultato immediato.—Or. 0,25 ; Ut $^{5}/_{50}$; Ut^{1} $^{15}/_{50}$; Voce afona 0,30 ; Voce parlata m. 1. Cessata la suppurazione.

15 maggio.   Una sottile membrana di neo-formazione sostituisce il timpano mancante.   Essa presenta un piccolo orificio anteriormente ed in basso.   Or. 0,30 ; Voce afona 0,60 ; Ut $^{30}/_{50}$; Ut^{1}, Ut^{2} $^{40}/_{50}$.

4 luglio.   Or. 0,90 ; Ut $^{30}/_{50}$; Ut^{1} $^{25}/_{50}$; Voce afona m. 2 ; Voce parlata m. 4, Galton normale.

20 novembre.   Or. m. 1 ; Ut^{1} $^{35}/_{50}$; Voce afona m. 3.   Membrana timpanica presenta ancora il piccolissimo orifizio sopra notato.   Non ha sofferto nè rumori ; nè vertigine.

4 luglio 1899.   Lo stesso che nell'ultimo esame.

Caso XVI.—Masnada Salvatore fu Francesco Paolo, di anni 19, da Palermo.

Storia.—Sin da bambino suppurazione continua a destra, con abbassamento progressivo dell'udito.   Niente vertigini e rumori.

Esame funzionale.—O. D. Or. 0 ; Ut, Ut^{1}, Ut^{2}, 0 ; Ut^{3} $^{5}/_{50}$; Rinne negativo ; Weber a destra ; Galton normale ; Voce afona 0 ; Voce media 0,10. O. S. normale.

Esame elettrico.—Ka. Ch. S. con 3 M. A. ; An. Ch. S. con 3 M. A. L'eccitazione elettrica del nervo dà la sensazione di un fischietto.   Nessuna reazione si ottiene all'apertura sia dell'anode che del catode.

Esame obbiettivo.—Nella metà anteriore la membrana è ispessita ed opaca, di aspetto sclerotico, posteriormente atrofica, aderente alla parete labirintica. L'atrofia è talmente pronunziata da ridurre la membrana ad un sottilissimo strato epidermico. Manico del martello retratto in dentro ed aderente al promontorio. Nel segmento postero-superiore si osservano due piccole vegetazioni rosee sanguinanti. Rinite cronica iperplastica. Prolasso dell'ugola.

Diagnosi.—Otite media purulenta cronica ; carie delle pareti dell'attico timpanico e dell'antro mastoideo ; anchilosi della catena degli ossicini.

Operazione.— 16 maggio 1898. Sinechiotomia totale del timpano, distacco del martello dal promontorio, tenotomia del tensore. Raschiamento delle pareti dell'antro mastoideo, essendo stato impossibile vedere la regione della staffa, pratico la resezione del segmento postero-superiore dell'annulo timpanico. Nonostante questa operazione la scoperta della staffa riesce incompleta e la mobilizzazione non sufficiente. Nessun incidente durante e dopo l'operazione.

Risultato immediato.--Or. a contatto ; Ut $^5/_{50}$; Voce afona 0 ; Voce parlata 0,60 ; Galton normale ; Weber a destra ; Rinne negativo.

22 maggio. Lieve suppurazione all'orecchio, senza dolori, nè vertigini. Funzione acustica come dopo l'operazione.

30 dicembre. Continua la suppurazione, sebbene diminuita. L'udito un po'peggiorato rispetto all'ultimo esame, Or. 0 ; Voce afona 0 ; Voce parlata 0,40.

3 luglio 1899. Guarito dalla suppurazione. Funzione acustica la stessa. Non ci sono stati nè vertigini, nè rumori.

CASO XVII. —Romano Rosina di Antonio, di anni 12, da Palermo.

Storia.—Sin da bambina suppurazione continua a destra, con abbassamento progressivo dell'udito. Non ha sofferto mai nè vertigini, nè rumori.

Esame funzionale.—O. D. Or. 0,05 ; Ut $^2/_{50}$; Ut^1 $^{10}/_{50}$; Rinne negativo ; Weber a destra ; Galton 3,0 ; Voce afona a contatto ; Voce parlata 0,30.

Esame obbiettivo. Vasta perforazione, a forma di cuore, del timpano. Martello fortemente retratto in dentro ed aderente al promontorio. Mucosa della cassa coperta di granulazioni.

Diagnosi.—Otite media purulenta cronica, carie delle pareti dell'antro mastoideo ; rigidità della catena degli ossicini.

Operazione.—5 maggio 1898. Escissione dei residui della membrana e del martello, raschiamento delle granulazioni, causticazione delle pareti dell'antro mastoideo. Mobilizzazione della staffa.

Risultato immediato.—Or. 0,05 ; Voce afona 0,05 ; Voce parlata 0,50.

20 maggio. Guarita dalla suppurazione. Udito come dopo l'operazione.

5 luglio. Or. m. 1 $^1/_2$; Ut $^{25}/_{50}$; Ut^1 $^{30}/_{50}$; Voce afona m. 1,20 ; Voce parlata m. 3 ; Galton 1,7.

30 giugno 1899. Nulla di nuovo. Funzione acustica come nell'ultimo esame.

CASO XVIII.—Lo Forte Rosaria di Pasquale, di anni 22, da Palermo.

Storia.—Da molti anni accusa indebolimento dell'udito a sinistra. Da tre anni sordità completa da questo lato e diminuzione a destra. Da bambina ebbe suppurazione a sinistra, che durò alcuni mesi senza veruna conseguenza. Soffre ad intervalli dei rumori. Ha inoltre accessi intercorrenti di vertigine, specie nei movimenti subitanei del capo.

Esame funzionale.—Or. 0,03 ; Ut, Ut^1 0 ; Ut^2, Ut^3 $^5/_{50}$; Galton 2,6 ; Rinne negativo ; Weber a destra ; Voce afona e parlata 0.

Esame elettrico.—O. S. Ka. Ch. S. con 25 M. A. Reazione acustica, leggiera e di breve durata, sensazione molto dolorosa. An. Ch.;—An. Ap.;—Ka. Ch.—con 25 M. A. Non ho aumentato l'intensità della corrente, perchè mal tollerata dalla paziente.

Esame obbiettivo.—O. S. Timpano ispessito, bianco, sclerosato e molto infossato. Trovasi molto aderente al promontorio. Manico del martello retratto in dentro. Quest'ultimo si vede assottigliato e quasi come nascosto nello spessore del timpano. *Operazione.*—7 maggio 1898. Sinechiotomia del timpano, tenotomia del tensore. Per scoprire la staffa dovetti fare la resezione di una porzione dell'annulo timpanico posteriore. Nessun inconveniente.

Risultato immediato.—Or. 0,30 ; Voce afona a contatto ; Voce parlata 0,60 ; Ut 0 ; Ut^1 $^5/_{50}$; Galton 2,6.

2 giugno. Completamente guarita dall'operazione. Rimase una perforazione nel segmento posteriore del timpano ; Orologio 0,60 ; Ut $^{10}/_{50}$; Galton normale ; Voce afona 0,40 ; Voce parlata m. 1 ½. Diminuiti i rumori e cessate completamente le vertigini.

22 giugno 1899. Continua lo stesso come fu osservato nell'ultimo esame.

Caso XIX.—Branda Giuseppa di Emanuele, di anni 20, da Palermo.

Storia.—Da bambina suppurazione intermittente a sinistra, con abbassamento progressivo dell'udito, vertigini e rumori. Da un anno la suppurazione è cessata, però gli altri disturbi continuano.

Esame funzionale.—O. S. Or. 0 ; Ut 0 ; Ut$_t$ $^{10}/_{50}$; Voce afona 0 ; Voce parlata 0,20 ; Galton normale ; Weber a sinistra ; Rinne negativo.

Esame obbiettivo.—Distruzione completa della membrana. Il martello, retratto in dentro ed aderente al promontorio, trovasi nella metà superiore impigliato in un tessuto fibroso, compatto, il quale riempie completamente la fossetta ovale. Non si vede l'incudine.

Diagnosi.—Esiti di otite media purulenta cronica. Anchilosi della catena degli ossicini.

Operazione.—20 maggio 1899. O. S. Asportazione del martello. Mobilizzazione della staffa. Nessun inconveniente nè durante, nè dopo l'operazione.

Risultato immediato.—Or. 0,20 ; Ut $^{10}/_{50}$; Ut^1 $^{20}/_{50}$; Rinne negativo ; Weber a sinistra ; Voce afona 0,30 ; Voce parlata m. 1$^1/_2$; Galton normale.

30 maggio. Cessata ogni reazione locale. Guarita dalla vertigine. Diminuiti i rumori. Or. 0,40 ; Voce afona 0,30 : Voce parlata m. 2.

15 luglio. Continua il miglioramento come nell'ultimo esame.

Caso XX.—De Clario Elvira di Domenico, di anni 28, da Palermo.

Storia.—Da 13 anni suppurazione intermittente all'orecchio sinistro, con abbassamento progressivo dell'udito. Negli intervalli di guarigione ha avvertito dei rumori. Niente vertigine.

Esame funzionale.—O. S. Orologio a contatto ; Ut $^{15}/_{50}$; Ut^1 $^{20}/_{50}$; Ut^2 $^{30}/_{50}$; Voce afona 0 ; Voce parlata a contatto ; Galton 3,7 ; Rinne negativo ; Weber a sinistra.

Esame elettrico.—O. S. Ka. Ch. S. con 3 M. A. (reazione molto forte [Trombetta]). An. Ap. S. con 5 M. A. (reazione più debole) paragonata dall'inferma al suono del flauto. Nessuna reazione alla chiusura dell'anode ed all'apertura del catode.

Esame obbiettivo.—O. S. Membrana mancante nel quadrante postero-superiore e nella metà inferiore. La porzione che rimane è molto ispessita, sclerosata ed aderente assieme al martello sulla parete laberintica. Non si vede nè la incudine, nè la staffa, La fossetta ovale, letteralmente coperta da un tessuto fibroso, compatto, di nuova formazione. In corrispondenza dell'*aditus ad antrum* mastoideo si vede una granulazione coperta da essudato.

Diagnosi.—Otite media purulenta cronica, aderenza del martello. Anchilosi della staffa.

Operazione —25 giugno 1898. O. S. Asportazione delle vegetazioni, raschiamento e causticazione dell'antro mastoideo. Vuotamento della fossetta ovale del tessuto fibroso che la riempiva completamente. Mobilizzazione della staffa, sinechiotomia del martello e rimozione di questo ossicino. L'operazione avvenne senza inconvenienti di sorta, solo l'inferma avvertiva delle scosse di vertigine transitoria nei tentativi di mobilizzazione.

Risultato immediato.—Or. 0,10 ; Voce afona m. 1 ; Voce parlata m. 3 ; Ut $^{20}/_{50}$; Ut$_t$ $^{30}/_{50}$.

25 luglio 1898. Cessata la suppurazione. Mucosa della cassa asciutta, si vede bene la finestra rotonda. La nicchia della finestra ovale vuota, la staffa mobile. Orologio 0,35 ; Ut $^{30}/_{50}$; Voce afona m. 1 ; Voce parlata m. 3 ; Galton 2,7. Diminuiti i ronzî.

7 luglio 1899. Continua immutato il miglioramento conseguito.

Aggiungendo a questi 20 casi altri 8, pubblicati nel fasc. 2 del vol. VII dell'*Archivo italiano di Otologia* ed altri due, pure pubblicati nel fasc. 4 dello stesso volume, e dei quali avendo controllato i risultati fino al presente non ho trovato serie differenze da quelli già pubblicati, si ha un totale di 30 casi che, a seconda la natura del processo morboso, possiamo ripartire in 3 categorie. La 1ᵃ costituita dalle *otite secche*, sia sclerosanti che iperplastiche, comprende 11 casi. La 2ᵃ formata dagli esiti di otite media purulenta cronica, racchiude 9 casi, ed infine la 3ᵃ, rappresentata da processi cronici purulenti, comprende gli ultimi 10 casi.

Degli ammalati appartenenti alla 1ᵃ categoria 5 ebbero un miglioramento positivo per l'orologio, rappresentato da una minima differenza di contatto a 0,05 e da una massima di 0,03 a 0,60 ; per gli altri 6 la forza uditiva per l'orologio restò o la stessa o di poco migliorata.

Per la voce afona 6 se ne avvantaggiarono molto, presentando una minima differenza di 0 a 0,20 ed una massima di 0 ad 1½ m. Negli altri 5 il miglioramento è stato lievissimo.

Per la voce parlata invece 7 acquistarono un potere acustico grande con una minima differenza di contatto a m. 1 ed una massima di 0,30 a m. 3.

In nessun ammalato si ebbe peggioramento. Interessante è rilevare inoltre la maniera di comportarsi della funzione acustica di questi ammalati, sia subito dopo l'operazione che ad un'epoca remota. In 7 l'udito si è, coll'andare del tempo, migliorato, in modo che il risultato finale è stato superiore all'immediato ; in 4 invece è avvenuto il contrario. La ragione del peggioramento in questi ultimi è stata in 3 la rigenerazione della membrana timpanica ed in uno lo sviluppo di otite suppurativa di lunga durata per cui ebbero luogo nuovi processi iperplastici che ristabilirono in parte le condizioni anatomo-patologiche rimosse con l'operazione. In questi ammalati inoltre l'udito, tanto per il diapason che per i suoni acutissimi del fischietto di Galton, generalmente migliorò, solo in pochi rimase qual era prima.

Per quanto riguarda i disturbi subbiettivi vi è da osservare che il fenomeno della vertigine è stato con l'operazione guarito completamente, mentre i ronzî, meno che in pòchi in cui diminuirono un po', rimasero immutati.

Il processo morboso rimontava ad un'epoca non inferiore a 5 anni e non maggiore di 30 anni. Meno che in 2, in cui i risultati furono controllati per la durata di 3 a 6 mesi, negli altri la durata dell'osservazione è stata da un anno a due anni e mezzo.

Concludendo, possiamo quindi affermare :

1° Che nelle otiti medie secche, tanto a forma iperplastica che sclerosante, la mobilizzazione della staffa, purchè l'apparecchio di percezione del suono sia in ottime condizioni, e si ha cura di evitare una flogosi purulenta consecutiva di lunga durata, dà sempre buoni risultati, per quanto riguarda la sordità e la vertigine, pochissimi o nulli per rapporto ai rumori.

La natura dei suoni che meglio vengono intesi secondo l'ordine decrescente è la seguente : la voce parlata, la susurrata, l'orologio, il diapason, il fischietto.

2° Meno che rare eccezioni, i buoni risultati si hanno quando rimane aperta l'apertura timpanica e per questo è necessario praticare in tutti gli ammalati affetti da questo genere di otopatia la resezione della porzione postero-superiore dell'annulo timpanico.

3° Con l'operazione non si hanno mai inconvenienti o complicazioni di sorta.

* *

I risultati acustici negli esiti delle otiti medie purulenti croniche sono ancora più confortanti. Dei 9 ammalati appartenenti a questa categoria solo in uno l'udito per l'orologio rimase immutato, negli altri 8 invece si conseguì un miglioramento variabile tra una differenza minima di contatto a 0,05, ad una massima di 0 a 0,40 ; per la voce afona solo in uno il guadagno è stato lieve, negli altri 8 si ebbe un vantaggio minimo da 0 a 0,15 e grande da 0,15 a m. 2. Per la voce parlata invece tutti 8 ne furono avvantaggiati in una estensione variabile tra un minimo di 0,05 a 0,50 ed un massimo tra 0,40 a 3 m. La percezione dei suoni bassi del diapason subì in tutti un miglioramento, quella degli acuti del fischietto di Galton in pochi rimase immutata, nella maggior parte fu migliorata.

È interessante far notare che il potere uditivo conseguito dagli ammalati di questa categoria è stato sempre progressivo, di guisa che l'esito, definitivo è stato migliore di quello immediato. In questi ammalati ordinariamente rimase una perforazione timpanica.

A differenza che nelle forme secche, i disturbi subbiettivi vennero in questa specie di otopatie meglio curati, pochè si è notato in qualcuno la guarigione quasi completa dei susurri, in tutti gli altri un positivo miglioramento. Le vertigini poi guarirono sempre.

In questi casi l'affezione auricolare rimontava ad un'epoca non inferiore ai 5 anni, e non superiore ai 30, ed il controllo dei risultati è durato solamente in uno 3 mesi, negli altri ha variato tra i 6 mesi e i 2 anni e mezzo.

Concludendo, quindi abbiamo :

1° Negli esiti di otite media purulenta cronica, purchè non vi sia lesione dell'acustico, la mobilizzazione della staffa, qualunque sia la durata della malattia dà sempre un positivo miglioramento uditivo sia per l'orologio, che per la voce afona e susurrata, come pure per i suoni bassi ed acuti.

2° L'operazione guarisce costantemente la vertigine, qualche volta i susurri ; sempre però questi ultimi vengono scemati.

3° Nessuna dannosa conseguenza è temibile con la stessa.

La mobilizzazione della staffa eseguita nel periodo di una suppurazione cronica dell'orecchio, contemporaneamente a quegli atti operativi che mirano a combattere la causa della malattia ci dà pure degli utili ammaestramenti che è utile rilevare.

Il numero degli ammalati appartenenti alla 3ª categoria e da me operati ascendono a 10. In tutti io ottenni un miglioramento acustico per l'orologio variabile da una minima differenza di 0,05 a 0,10, ad una massima di 0,05 a m. 1½. Soltanto in uno, coll'andare del tempo, si perdette il miglioramento conseguito e l'udito per l'orologio ritornò nelle primitive condizioni.

Lo stesso può dirsi per la voce afona. Tutti conseguirono un grande miglioramento costituito da una differenza minima di 0 a 0,10 e da una massima di 0 a m. 3. Solo in uno di questi ammalati avvenne la perdita di tale miglioramento ; invece per la voce parlata tutti se ne avvantaggiarono e si ebbe un guadagno minimo di 0,10 a 0,40 ed uno massimo di 0,40 a più di m. 4.

L'udito si avvantaggiò pure in tutti per i suoni bassi, la scala degli acuti non subì variazione in alcuni, negli altri invece migliorò.

In questa categoria di operati è avvenuto il seguente fatto : in cinque di essi*, nei quali il processo suppurativo si protrasse ancora per molti mesi, il risultato acustico che si ottenne con l'operazione, andò poco per volta a diminuire, però non si perdette mai completamente.

Negli altri invece in cui guarì subito il processo suppurativo, avvenne il contrario, la facoltà uditiva andò cioè sempre più migliorando.

L'influenza spiegata dall'operazione sui disturbi subbiettivi è stata ottima, dappoichè le vertigini sono sempre guarite, i susurri in qualche caso sono scomparsi, generalmente però sono migliorati.

L'affezione auricolare in questi ammalati rimontava ad un tempo non inferiore ai tre anni e non superiore ai 15, ed i risultati furono controllati per un tempo corrente da 6 a 25 mesi.

* Tra questi è compreso uno dei casi da me pubblicato nel fasc. 2°, vol. VII, dell'*Archivio italiano di Otologia*, in cui essendo riapparso e durato a lungo il processo suppurativo, la facoltà uditiva andò man mano indebolendosi.

Concludendo abbiamo :

1° La mobilizzazione della staffa nel corso di processi cronici purulenti dà pure ottimi risultati tutte le volte che la malattia guarisce subito, diversamente il miglioramento conseguito si va mano mano perdendo, fino ad arrivare quasi alle condizioni primitive, e ciò per la rigenerazione di quegli ostacoli che sono conseguenza del processo suppurativo, e ch'erano stati rimossi con l'operazione.

2° Nei disturbi subbiettivi in questa categoria di ammalati si hanno gli stessi risultati che negli esiti di otite media purulenta cronica.

3° L'operazione non dà luogo ad alcuna conseguenza spiacevole.

* * *

Riepilogando abbiamo :

1° La mobilizzazione della staffa qualunque sia la lesione per la quale s'interviene, purchè l'apparecchio di percezione del suono sia normale o pochissimo compromesso e purchè si eviti una flogosi post-operativa li lunga durata, dà sempre buoni risultati acustici ; però sono *migliori* quelli che si hanno nel corso di processi cronici purulenti, purchè, però si riesca a guarire subito la malattia principale ; *buoni* i risultati negli esiti di processi suppurativi e *mediocri* nelle otiti secche, a condizione che in queste ultime forme morbose si abbia cura d'impedire la rigenerazione della membrana timpanica.

2° Le vertigini sono i disturbi subbiettivi che meglio guariscono, qualunque sia la forma dell'otopatia (esclusa sempre ogni lesione dell'orecchio interno).

3° I rumori invece rare volte guariscono ; questo è solo sperabile nel corso di processi cronici purulenti o negli esiti di questa affezione, poche volte migliorano, spesso rimangono inalterati.

4° Nessuna complicazione ed inconveniente è da temersi con l'operazione.

THE AMPLIFIED BIBLIOGRAPHICAL OTOLOGICAL NOTATION, ACCORD-
ING TO THE DECIMAL SYSTEM OF MELVIL DEWEY.

PROF. G. GRADENIGO, Turin.

The bibliographical problem is at present everywhere a subject of discussion : this must also be the case in Otology, and I believe that one of the chief functions of the great International Congresses is to treat of such universal questions. I will not insist here on the necessity for a rational classification of the always increasing scientific publications, and I maintain the great advantages which Dewey's decimal method offers.

In Dewey's system Otology is a branch of Surgery, and bears the number 617.8, in this manner :—   '

> 6   Applied sciences.
> 61   Medical sciences in general.
> 617   Surgery.
> 617.8 Otology.

I have amplified and completed the decimal Tables in regard to Otology, and I have tried to put them in accord in the best manner with the actual conditions of our science.*

I found it necessary only to modify the primary classification of Dewey, for group 617.81 (diseases of the external ear), because these diseases are included—even according to that classification—in the groups 617.82 (diseases of the Auricle), and 617.83 (diseases of the external auditory canal).

The classification, which I propose, is the following :—

617.80   Otology in general.
617.81   Diseases common to two or more segments of the ear (Congenital Malformations, New Growths, Tuberculosis, Syphilis, Foreign Bodies, Wounds and other injuries, Necrosis, etc.).
617.82   Auricle.
617.83   External auditory canal.
617.84   Membrana tympani. .
617.85   Tympanic cavity.
617.86   Eustachian tube.
617.87   Mastoid.
617.88   Labyrinth and acoustic nerve.
617.89   Complications of ear diseases.

The following specimen will give an idea of the system :—

617.8 Otologia Generale.
617.80.1   Statistica, frequenza, gravità delle malattie dell'orecchio in generale.
    80.101 Frequenza in rapporto al sesso.
    80.102 Frequenza in rapporto all'età.
    80.103 Frequenza in rapporto al lato colpito.
    80.104 Frequenza in rapporto ai segmenti dell'orecchio.
617.80.11 Etiologia.
    80.111 Ereditarietà.
    80.112 Età, sesso.
    80.113 Professione.
    80.114 Ambiente, clima.
    80.115 Malattie generali quali causa di malattie di orecchio (vedasi anche 617.80.19).
617.80.12 Esame funzionale dell'orecchio.

---

*I have done the same for Laryngology and Rhinology.

80.121 Voce.
80.12.11 Voce afona.
80.12.12 Voce di conversazione.
80.12.13 Voce gridata.
80.12.2 Orologio.
80.12.3 Acumetri.
80.12.31 Acumetro di Politzer.
80.12.32 Acumetri elettro-telefonici.
80.12.33 Altri acumetri.
80.12.4 Diapason.
80.12.41 Serie completa dei diapason.
80.12.42 Esperimento di Rinne.
80.12.43 Esperimento di Weber.
80.12.44 Esperimento di Schwabach.
80.12.49 Altri esperimenti.
80.12.5 Altri strumenti sonori.
80.12.6 Esame elettrico dell'acustico.
80.12.7 Esame del senso statico.
617.80.13 Esame obiettivo.
80.13.1 Otoscopia.
80.13.11 Luce per l'esame.
80.13.12 Specchi, speculi ed altri strumenti per l'esame.
80.13.2 Ascoltazione dell'orecchio.   .
80.13.21 Cateterismo.
80.13.22 Esperimento di Valsalva.
80.13.23 Esperimento di Politzer.
80.13.29 Altri procedimenti.
617.80.14 Sintomatologia delle malattie dell'orecchio.
80.141 Modificazioni nel potere uditivo.
80.14.11 Diminuzione di udito.   Sordità.
80.14.12 Iperacusia funzionale.
80.14.13 Iperacusia dolorosa.
80.14.14 Autofonia.
80.14.15 Paracusia di Willis.
80.14.16 Diplacusia.
80.14.17 Audizione colorata.
80.14.19 Altre particolarità della audizione.
80.14.2 Rumori di orecchio.
80.14.21 Rumori entotici.
80.14.22 Rumori subiettivi propriamenti detti.
80.14.3 Vertigini, disturbi di equilibrio, vomito.
80.14.4 Dolori di orecchio.
80.14.5 Otorrea.
80.14.6 Otorragia.
80.14.7 Paralisi facciale otitica.

80.14.71 Paralisi facciale nelle otiti purulente.

80.14.72 Paralisi facciale nelle otiti secche.

80.14.8 Disturbi vasomotori e trofici.

80.14.9 Azioni reflesse originate dall'orecchio.

80.14.91 Azione reflessa sugli organi dei sensi.

80.14.92 Sulle condizioni psichiche.

80.14.93 Sul sistema simpatico.

80.14.94 Sull'apparecchio motore.

617.80.15 Anatomia ed istologia patologica dell'osso temporale.

80.15.1 Alterazioni anatomo patologiche diffuse del temporale.

80.15.2 Batteriologia nelle affezioni dell'osso temporale. (La anatomia patologica e la batteriologia delle singole parti costituenti l'organo dell'udito vanno comprese nei singoli capitoli che trattano delle affezioni di tali parti nel riguardo clinico).

617.80.16 Medicina legale dell'orecchio.

80.16.1 Docimasia auricolare.

80.16.2 Simulazione e dissimulazione della affezione dell'orecchio.

80.16.3 Influenza delle malattie dell'orecchio sull'attitudine al servizio militare.

80.16.4 Influenza delle malattie dell'orecchio nel determinare azioni criminose.

80.16.5 Affezioni dell'orecchio in rapporto alle Compagnie di Assicurazioni.

617.80.17 Trattamento delle malattie di orecchio.

80.17.1 Trattamento generale.

80.17.11 Cura medicamentosa.

80.17.12 Azioni termiche.

80.17.13 Elettroterapia.

80.17.14 Deplezioni sanguigne.

80.17.15 Cura climatica.

80.17.16 Cura dietetica.

617.80.17.2 Trattamento locale.

80.17.21 Applicazioni locali medicamentose.

80.17.22 Cure chirurgiche.

17.22.1 Antisepsi.

17.22.2 Anestesia locale generale.

17.22.3 Strumentario.

17.22.4 Tecnica operativa.

80.17.23 Azioni meccaniche.

17.23.1 Lavacri.

17.23.2 Pulitura a secco.

17.23.3 Compressione e rarefazione dell'aria.

17.23.4 Massaggio.

80.17.24 Applicazioni elettriche locali.

80.17.25 Azioni termiche locali.

80.17.26 Sanguissugio locale.

80.17.27 Protesi ed apparecchi di protezione.

    17.27.1 Miringoplastica.

    17.27.2 Timpani artificiali.

617.80.18 Rapporti tra le malattie dell'orecchio e le intossicazioni.

80.18.1 Intossicazione da chinino e da salicilati.

80.18.2 Idem da alcool.

80.18.3 Idem da tabacco.

80.18.9 Intossicazione da cause diverse.

617.80.19 Rapporti tra le malattie dell'orecchio ed altre malattie.

80.19.1 Malattie della rino-faringe, del naso, della regione periauricolare.

80.19.2 Malattie infettive acute generali.

    19.21 Influenza.

    19.22 Pneumonite.

    19.23 Morbillo.

    19.24 Scarlattina, difterite.

    19.25 Parotite.

    19.26 Tifo addominale.

    19.27 Eresipela.

    19.28 Piemia.

    19.29 Altre malattie di infezione acute (febbre ricorrente, vaiuolo, ec.).

80.19.3 Malattie infettive croniche.

    19.31 Tubercolosi.

    19.32 Sifilide costituzionale.

80.19.4 Malattie del ricambio.

    19.41 Diabete.

    19.42 Reumatismo, gotta.

    19.43 Rachitide.

    19.44 Anemia, clorosi, anemia perniciosa.

    19.45 Leucemia.

    19.46 Porpora emorragica.

80.19.5 Malattie dell'apparecchio di circolazione.

    19.51 Endocardite.

    19.52 Ateromasia.

80.19.6 Malattie dell'apparecchio uro-genitale.

    19.61 Nefrite.

    19.62 Gravidanza, puerperio, allattamento.

80.19.7 Nevrosi.

    19.71 Isterismo.

    19.72 Nevrastenia.

    19.73 Epilessia.

    19.74 Corea.

80.19.8 Malattie del cervello, midollo spinale e meningi.

19.81 Tabe dorsale.

19.82 Pachimeningite emorragica.

19.83 Leptomeningite.

19.84 Tumori cerebrali.

19.85 Malattie mentali.

80.19.9 Malattie della pelle.

617.80.2 Trattati di Otologia.

617.80.3 Atlanti.

617.80.4 Rendiconti di Cliniche, di Ospedali. Conferenze.

617.80.5 Periodici concernenti la Otologia.

617.80.5 (42) Inghilterra.

617.80.5 (43) Germania.

617.80.5 (436) Austria.

617.80.5 (44) Francia.

617.80.5 (45) Italia.

617.80.6 Rendiconto di Congressi di Riunioni, di Società scientifiche.

617.80.7 Insegnamento della Otologia. Cliniche, Ospedali.

617.80.8 Raccolta di memorie concernenti la Otologia in genere.

617.80.9 Storia della Otologia.

80.91 Fino al principio del XVI° secolo.

80.92 Periodo dal 1500 al 1821 (Itard).

80.93 Periodo dal 1821 ai nostri giorni.

617.81 Affezioni comuni a due o più segmenti dell'orecchio.

617.81.1 Cattiva conformazione congenita dell'osso temporale.

617.81.2 Neoplasmi.

81.21 Neoplasmi benigni.

81.22 Neoplasmi maligni.

617.81.3 Tubercolosi, lupus dell'orecchio.

617.81.4 Sifilide.

617.81.5 Corpi stranieri.

81.51 Nel Condotto uditivo esterno.

81.52 Corpi stranieri nell'orecchio medio.

81.53 Corpi stranieri nella tromba di Eustachio.

617.81.6 Traumi ed altre lesioni violente dell'orecchio.

81.61 Esplosioni.

81.62 Ferite di arma da fuoco.

81.63 Ferite di corpi taglienti e contundenti.

617.81.7 Nevrosi dell'orecchio.

81.71 Nevrosi di senso.

81.71.1 Anestesia, ipoestesia, iperestesia acustica.

81.71.2 Anestesia, ipoestesia, iperestesia tattile della cute del padiglione e del condotto uditivo esterno.

81.72 Nevrosi di motilità.

617.81.8 Varia.

617.82 Malattie del padiglione dell'orecchio.

617.82.1 Iperemia, esantemi.

617.82.2 Eczema, erpete.

617.82.3 Otematoma.

617.82.4 Pericondrite del padiglione.

617.82.5 Cancrena del padiglione.

617.82.6 Ustioni e congelazioni.

617.83 Condotto uditivo esterno.

617.83.1 Otite esterna diffusa.

    83.11 Otite eczematosa e desquamativa.

    83.12 Otite esterna difterica.

    83.13 Otite esterna sifilitica.

617.83.2 Otite esterna circoscritta (foruncolosi).

    83.3 Otomicosi.

617.83.4 Raccolte di cerume.

617.83.5 Parassiti; corpi stranieri.

617.83.6 Stenosi del condotto.

617.83.7 Iperostosi ed esostosi.

617.84 Membrana timpanica.

617.84.1 Miringite acuta.

617.84.2 Miringite cronica.

617.85 Cavità timpanica.

617.85.1 Otite media acuta catarrale.

617.85.2 Otite media acuta purulenta.

617.85.3 Otite media catarrale cronica.

617.85.4 Sclerosi dell'orecchio medio con diffusione all'orecchio interno.

617.85.5 Otite media purulenta cronica.

    85.51 Carie delle ossicina e della pareti della cassa.

    85.52 Polipi.

    85.53 Affezioni dell'epitimpano.

617.85.6 Esiti di otite media purulenta cronica.

617.85.7 Otalgia.

617.86 Tromba di Eustachio.

617.86.1 Stenosi catarrale acuta.

617.86.2 Stenosi catarrale cronica.

617.87 Apofisi mastoide.

617.87.1 Periostite e flemone retroauricolare.

617.87.2 Empiema mastoideo acuto.

617.87.3 Mastoiditi croniche.

    87.31 Empiema mastoideo cronico, carie.

    87.32 Colesteatoma.

617.87.4 Mastoidite di Bezold.

617.87.5 Sclerosi della mastoide.

617.87.6 Mastoidalgia.

617.88 Affezioni dell'apparecchio di percezione del suono (orecchio interno e nervo acustico).

617.88.1 Modificazioni nella circolazione e nella pressione endolabirintica.

617.88.2 Lesioni infettive del labirinto eccetto che la sifilide (Vedasi 617.81.4).

    88.21 Panotite.

    88.22 Leucemia.

    88.23 Anemia perniciosa.

617.88.3 Lesioni labirintiche reumatiche e gottose.

617.88.4 Lesioni labirintiche per azione dei suoni.

    88.41 Acutamente sviluppantisi.

    88.42 Lentamente sviluppantisi.

617.88.5 Lesioni labirintiche senili.

617.88.6 Affezioni purulente del labirinto.

    88.61 Panotite.

    88.62 Necrosi labirintica.

617.88.7 Nevroabirintite da meningite, specialmente da meningite cerebro-spinale (Ve dasi anche 617.80.19.83).

617.88.8 Lesioni dell'acustico e del labirinto da neoplasmi endocranici.

617.89 Complicazioni delle malattie dell'orecchio.

617.89.1 Ascesso estradurale e pachimeningite.

617.89.2 Leptomeningite otitica.

617.89.3 Trombosi infettiva dei seni della dura madre.

617.89.4 Ascesso cerebrale.

617.89.5 Ascessi cerebellari.

617.89.6 Complicazioni al collo.

617.89.7 Piemia otitica senza trombosi.

617.89.8 Altre infezioni generali derivanti dall'orecchio.

617.89.9 Emorragia grave dall'orecchio.

    89.91 Per arrosione dell'arteria carotide interna.

    89.92 Per lesione del bulbo della giugulare.

SUI MEZZI PIÙ OPPORTUNI PER PROMUOVERE UN CONVENIENTE INCREMENTO DEGLI STUDI OTOLOGICI NELLE UNIVERSITÀ E NELLA LEGISLAZIONE SOCIALE.

PROF. G. GRADENIGO, Turin.

Nel campo pratico la Otologia, malgrado i progressi recentemente realizzati, non ha ancora certamente il posto che le spetta. Le cattedre Universitarie sono poche di numero e per lo più insufficientemente dotate, anche nei pæsi più colti di Europa; nell'ordinamento degli studi medici l'esame non è obbligatorio; nell'enorme produzione letteraria otologica manca da parte autorizzata quel controllo, che valga a distinguere i lavori scientifici serii e di valore da quelli che non hanno importanza. Se tale stato di cose è di ostacolo ai progressi scientifici, esso torna in alto grado dannoso nella pratica ; i falsi specialisti colla loro imperizia e coi loro errori destano sfiducia nel pubblico e contribuiscono a mantenere anche nel ceto medico in generale quella sfavorevole opinione sul valore della Specialità, la quale in parte poteva esser giustificata solo nella prima metà del corrente secolo.

Ad eliminare per quanto è possibile tali inconvenienti è necessario che venga diffusa nel pubblico—(e nel nostro caso vanno compresi nel pubblico la maggioranza dei medici pratici)—la nozione che la Otologia odierna è qualche cosa di fondamentalmente diverso da quella della prima metà del secolo, che essa esige in chi la coltiva una buona preparazione di medicina e di chirurgia generale, che, come la Oculistica, essa, per la importanza dell'organo studiato e per i metodi proprii di ricerca e di trattamento, tiene un posto a sè tra le altre discipline mediche. La Otologia deve perciò venir convenientemente rappresentata nelle Università, negli Ospedali, nei rapporti sociali. Siccome altrettanto si può ripetere per la Rinologia e la Laringologia,—le quali sono pure così strettamente connesse colla Otologia, e le quali sono oggi ancora relativamente poco considerate,—ragioni di opportunità pratica consigliano a riunire in uno solo lo studio di queste tre discipline, come si pratica ormai generalmente in Europa, mentre la Oculistica tiene un posto a sè.

I Congressi Internazionali come il nostro rappresentano una grande esplicazione della forza intellettuale del mondo moderno ; facciamo in modo che questa forza non vada perduta in discussioni di dettaglio, ma che affermi l'importanza ormai raggiunta dalla Specialità e reclami per essa i provvedimenti che ormai si impongono nell'ordinamento della Società.

Si deve far voti per ciò :

1°. Che nelle Università sia stabilito un insegnamento ufficiale obbligatorio con Cliniche per malati degenti. Perchè l'insegnamento abbia una sanzione, è necessario che gli esami sieno obbligatori. D'altra parte tenuto conto della grande quantità di insegnamenti che aggravano lo studente negli ultimi anni del Corso Universitario, è opportuno che l'insegnamento delle nostre Specialità non occupi in via generale più di un semestre e sia rivolto soltanto ad illustrare le parti che offrono un interesse pratico diretto.

2°. Che negli Ospedali sieno destinati Reparti speciali diretti da personale idoneo alla cura delle malattie che rientrano nel quadro delle nostre discipline, come si fà da tempo per le malattie degli occhi.

3° Che presso le Scuole, gli Istituti di Educazione, e più specialmente presso gli Istituti dei Sordomuti, nelle grandi Società e intrapprese industriali, nelle Società di Assicurazioni, nell'Esercito, nella Marina la trattazione delle molteplici questioni che si riferiscono al buon funzionamento e all'igiene delle prime vie aeree e degli orecchi sia affidata a cultori autorizzati delle Spécialità.

Per quanto concerne poi il titolo di Specialista in Oto rino-laringologia si deve notare che i requisiti necessari per divenire buon specialista non si possono ottenere oggi, coll'ordinamento moderno, nelle Università. D'altra parte non si può impedire ad un medico regolarmente laureato l'esercizio pratico della Specialità anche se egli non abbia studiate tali malattie nel corso Universitario.

A limitare l'esercizio pratico delle Specialità per parte di chi non possiede i requisiti necessari e a combattere l'abuso del titolo di Specialista, si potrebbe chiedere al Governo che volesse stabilire degli esami per il conferimento ufficiale di tale titolo, come fà già adesso in alcuni paesi per il conferimento di speciali attribuzioni mediche.

DIMINISHED BONE-CONDUCTION AS A CONTRA-INDICATION FOR OSSICULECTOMY.

DR. DUNDAS GRANT, London.

With very few exceptions, all authorities in otology are agreed that under certain circumstances the malleus, incus, and membrana tympani, whether whole or incomplete, cease to be of use for the transmission of sonorous vibrations to the stapes, and even offer an obstruction to that transmission. Under such circumstances the question of their removal may be usefully considered, quite apart from the major operations required for the saving of life, and, indeed, the performance of ossiculectomy becomes a duty. Do such circumstances arise? Undoubtedly, as the result of adhesions arising from inflammatory changes either of purulent or non-purulent nature. In the former it is unusual for the malleus and incus to be rendered immobile without the stapes being rendered even more so, if we leave out of account the ankylosis of the malleus to the outer wall of the attic as the result of exhausted attic inflammation. The removal of the outer ossicles is not likely, then, to offer hope of much improvement in chronic non-suppurative inflammation, especially in view of the fact that, in addition to fixation of the stapes, there is in the worst cases an involvement of the contiguous parts of the internal ear.

The conditions following suppuration of the middle ear are more favourable, and we may have absolute immobility of the outer ossicles—or, at least, of the malleus—while the stapes is mobile in the highest degree, and even to an inconvenient extent. For instance, in a case under my care in which a radical mastoid operation has been performed without removal of the ossicles, the malleus is quite fixed and the incus has probably disappeared, but the stapes is perfectly accessible to sight and touch, so that its mobility can be affirmed. An artificial drum applied over it increases the distance for hearing the whispered voice from 5 inches to 5 feet. In this instance, were the malleus to interfere with hearing either by favouring the heaping up of débris or by preventing the application of an artificial drum, I should feel called upon to remove it.

If the outer ossicles are fixed, and hamper the movements of a presumably or possibly mobile stapes, their removal is indicated on account of the hearing-power, apart from other and even weightier considerations. Of course, we must not remove ossicles if our so doing is at all likely to make the hearing worse—that is to say, if these ossicles are of functional value. How are we to decide on this point? Professor Politzer has laid down the valuable practical rule that if the hearing is sufficient for the perception of the whispered voice at the distance of 1 metre there is a fair presumption that the ossicular apparatus is acting, and the ossicles should not be removed. Hearing the whisper at the distance of 1 metre is, then, a very strong contra-indication against ossiculectomy. If the deafness is entirely or to a great extent due to concomitant disease of the internal ear or auditory nerve, it is obvious that the results, quâ hearing, obtainable from ossiculectomy can be of little or no value. Diminished bone-conduction is therefore considered a contra-indication. As a general rule, this may be accepted without demur, particularly by those who are inclined to perform ossiculectomy in non-suppurative cases, because it argues a degree of fixation of the stapes and of involvement of the auditory nerve which removal of the larger ossicles cannot touch. In suppurative cases also, diminished bone-conduction suggests a labyrinthine complication, and, it may be, a tuberculous affection of the petrous bone, as without this the tendency is for the tympanic changes to bring about an increase of conduction through the bones.

The arguments are therefore very strong in favour of the rule laid down by Politzer as to diminished bone-conduction being a contra-indication even in post-suppurative cases. While subscribing most heartily to this view in the main, I hope to show that the rule is not without exceptions. In some instances the line between hearing sufficient and not sufficient for business is a very fine one, and a very slight improvement may make the difference which renders the sufferer fit to follow his avocation : and when the difference is on the wrong side of the line a breach of the above-stated rule becomes highly justifiable if it offers the chance of even a slight increase of hearing-power.

If we allow that the ossicles may hamper the conduction to the extent of 10 per cent., then their removal, restoring this 10 per cent., may make the difference between, say, 20 and 30 per cent. of hearing-power, whether the auditory nerve be answerable for some of the wanting 70 per cent. of hearing or not.

The following cases illustrate the attainment of improvement of hearing in post-suppurative cases after the removal of the ossicles, although there was diminished bone-conduction :

CASE OF POST-SUPPURATIVE DEAFNESS, WITH DIMINISHED BONE-CONDUCTION, IMPROVED BY OSSICULECTOMY.

Mr. G. M..., aged thirty-four, lecturer, came under my care in June, 1897, complaining of dulness of hearing in both ears, which in the right had lasted twenty-five years. In spite of treatment at the hands of a skilled aurist, no improvement had taken place, and the patient felt himself face to face with the necessity of resigning his appointment.

The right ear had been deaf for twenty-five years, but the left one was fairly good until February 1, 1897, when on waking up he found the ear to be almost entirely deaf. There was no nervous shock to account for this, no hemianæsthesia, no diminution of pharyngeal reflex, or other sign of hysteria. He had a trace of sugar in the urine, the patellar reflex was almost absent, and he could not stand so well on the left foot alone as on the right one. On the right side the watch was not heard in contact. The whispered voice was not heard at all. Rinne's test was " negative reversed," and there was a distinct diminution of bone-conduction on the mastoid.

On the left side the watch could be heard at 2 inches. The whispered voice was heard at 1 foot. Rinne was " negative reversed," and on this side also there was a diminution of bone-conduction. The tuning-fork on the vertex was heard louder in the better ear.

On inspection, the major portion of the right membrane was destroyed, especially the antero-inferior segment. In the left ear there was a perforation of moderate size in the lower half of the membrane. He was treated with boracic and spirit drops, and after a couple of weeks his hearing-power was found to be more equable and somewhat better for class purposes.

He was slightly improved when an artificial drum was introduced, and pushed under the edge of the perforation up towards the right stapes.

I then considered that, with a view to facilitate the application of the artificial drum, it would be right to remove the ossicles, more especially as the patient complained of a fulness in the head, especially on the right side. The operation was performed, and for the moment the hearing in the right side was distinctly improved, to the extent that he could hear the whispered voice at 3 inches, and the fulness in the head disappeared ; but the hearing-power afterwards diminished to some extent, remaining, however, better than it was at first.

The small supplement of hearing derived from the operation on the right ear appeared to increase his total hearing-power to such an extent that he was able to carry on his classes instead of retiring, and at the end of the session he reported that he had had comparatively little difficulty in performing his work. In this case the trifling improvement seemed to be sufficient to make the difference between his following his avocation and giving it up, and so far to justify the exceptional use of the operation of ossiculectomy.

A confusion in the head from which he previously suffered entirely disappeared after the removal of the ossicles, and it may be that the improvement in the hearing was more or less directly the result of this.

I am indebted to Mr. MacLeod Yearsley for notes of the following case in which he performed ossiculectomy with beneficial results, in spite of the presence of diminished bone-conduction.

CASE OF DEAFNESS FOLLOWING SUPPURATIVE OTITIS IMPROVED BY OSSICULECTOMY, ALTHOUGH THERE WAS DIMINUTION OF BONE-CONDUCTION.

J. B..., a female aged forty, was first seen by Mr. Yearsley on July 8, 1898. She had been deaf to some extent since childhood, the left side being the worse. As a child she had discharge from both ears, but this ceased " some years ago." On the right side she was able to hear a watch at 3 inches instead of 60, and on the left side she could not hear it at all. In the left ear there was a large kidney-shaped perforation occupying the whole of the posterior and inferior quadrants. The ossicles were found to be fixed both to massage by the pneumatic speculum and to the probe. Ossiculectomy was performed on July 16, 1898. Previous to the operation the hearing had never been tested with the tuning-fork, owing to accidental circumstances.

On July 22 the bone-conduction on the left side was found diminished to the extent of about 10 per cent. Instead of not hearing the watch at all on the left side, she now heard it at a distance of 11½ inches. A month later she could hear the watch on the left side at a distance of about 4 inches, and she stated that she could now hear conversation with greater ease than formerly.

In conclusion, I would summarize as follows :

The presence of the ossicles may interfere with the hearing-power in post-suppurative cases in the following ways :

1. By being fixed themselves, and thereby making the stapes immobile.

2. By favouring the accumulation and retention of desquamative and exudative products which impede the movements of the stapes.

3. By preventing the application of a cotton-wool drum to the stapes.

Their removal is under these circumstances justifiable and desirable, if the hearing-power is less than for the whispered voice at 1 metre and the bone-conduction is good.

Even if the bone-conduction is diminished to some extent, a slight improvement in hearing may follow the operation of ossiculectomy. A very slight improvement in hearing may make the difference to the patient of being able to follow his employment.

Therefore, when hearing is so bad that the patient is unable to follow his employment it is justifiable to remove the outer ossicles and remains of the membrane, even though there is some diminution of bone-conduction.

A CASE OF TUMOUR OF THE MEDULLA AND PONS, CAUSING DEAF-
NESS AND OTHER REMARKABLE SYMPTOMS.

DR. ALBERT A. GRAY, Glasgow.

The following case is of interest on account of the remarkable series of symptoms produced by a lesion, which proved to be very small in extent. The patient was admitted into Dr. Samson Gemmell's ward in the Western Infirmary, Glasgow, and it is owing to his kindness that I am enabled to relate the case here.

J. K., aet. 22, a butcher, was admitted on the 7th of December, 1895, complaining of difficulty in swallowing and giddiness of a month's duration ; and " paralysis of the face," and deafness in the left ear of a fortnight's duration.

Family History—his father is alive and well, his mother died at the age of thirty-nine, but the patient does not know the cause of her death, though he knows that she was not ill for long. He has two brothers and two sisters, these are all alive and well.

The previous history of the patient is very good. He has never at any time suffered from illness, except from measles when a boy. There is no history of syphilis or diphtheria.

He is a butcher, and works in a draughty shop, but he noticed no extra chilliness before the commencement of this illness. For a fortnight before the paralysis appeared he was troubled with a choking feeling when swallowing. At this time also a cough, associated with expectoration, made its appearance and is still present. The cough is worse after he takes food ; the expectoration is scanty, though it looks abundant from admixture with what are apparently stomach contents.

His head feels light and giddy, so much so that he cannot walk without support ; but there has not been the slightest headache at any time, and no intellectual disturbance. During the whole of last week he had double vision, mostly in the morning, but also during the day ; this now appears to be absent.

He says that his speech is not so distinct as it used to be ; it has a nasal quality, and the articulation is somewhat impaired, due to the paralysis of the lips and tongue.

The condition of the ear and the throat is reported by Dr. Albert Gray, as follows :—

Before the present attack the patient had not anything wrong with his ears, neither is there any family history of deafness, beyond the fact that his father suffers slightly in that respect ; this, however, may well be attributed to an accident to the head.

Simultaneously with the onset of the deafness there occurred a subjective sensation of noises in the ear, these are of a singing quality. There has been no pain in the ear or head, nor is any discharge present.

On testing with the whispered voice, the right ear is found to be unaffected ; the watch however is not heard so well, being heard at a distance of one yard, while a normal ear hears it at three yards distance. The left ear on the other hand, is very deaf to the whispered voice, hearing it only at a distance of two inches ; the watch is unheard by this ear, except on contact.

Tuning-fork Tests. Weber's :—On placing the fork on the middle line of the head it is heard best in the right ear. This test was carried out several times, and with forks varying in pitch from a_1 to a_2, and the results were constantly the same.

Rinne's. In the right ear the fork is heard thirty-five seconds longer by air-conduction than by bone-conduction. In the left ear, the same fork is heard seven seconds longer by bone-conduction than by air-conduction.

The membrana tympani of the right side is normal in appearance ; that of the left side is indrawn. There is no secretion in the left middle ear however, and no evidence of disease in that cavity, except in so far as Rinne's test was negative.

On examining the throat, the left side of the palate is paralysed, and the uvula is drawn up to the right. There is a considerable amount of anæsthesia over the soft palate. The larynx shows signs of slight laryngitis, due probably to foreign substances finding entrance.

The left vocal cord is absolutely fixed in the middle line, even during deep inspiration. On phonation, this cord still remains perfectly motionless, while the right one comes up to meet it. The movements of the right cord are unaffected both during respiration and phonation.

The left eye is bloodshot, and both pupils are contracted, but the left more so than the right. The left eye is kept open to about half the normal extent; he can shut both eyes. The right pupil responds to light, but not to accommodation, while the left pupil gives no reaction to either. He can read with the right eye, but only with difficulty, and with the left he cannot read at all. The colour-sense for both eyes is good for red and blue, but he is not decided about the green.

Examination of the eyes with the ophthalmoscope reveals no change in the right eye. As regards the left eye, the examination is unsatisfactory on account of the anæsthesia and consequent muddiness of the cornea, but so far as can be judged there is no evidence of pressure.

The patient's mouth is drawn somewhat to the right, the naso-labial fold on the left side is obliterated, and saliva runs out of his mouth on this side. The lower jaw is stiff, he cannot open his mouth far and does so more on the right side than on the left. He states that he can chew his food quite well, but that it gets between his cheek and gums on the left side. He cannot protrude his tongue far ; it is turned towards the right and rounded at the extremity. On trying to whistle the air escapes at the left angle of the mouth. The buccinator on the right side is much more powerful than that on the left.

Tests as to the sense of taste can only be applied to the anterior part of the tongue, as the patient cannot open his mouth properly, or protrude the tongue far. It is found that on the left side the sense of taste is abolished ; it was tried with acetic acid, quinine, and saccharine solution.

He has a good grip with both hands. Plantar and knee-jerk reflexes are stronger on the left side than on the right : ankle-clonus could not be produced on either side.

The right leg and occasionally the right hand feel cold. On the left side of the body, face, and limbs, he could tell the difference between hot and cold tubes, while on the right side he could tell no difference at some parts, and as regards others he seemed to be guessing. On the left side of the body and left limbs, he felt and could tell the difference between the touch of a finger and a pin, while on the left side of the face and on the right side of the body and right limbs he could not tell the difference between the finger and the pin, except on his fingers ; and even of these his little finger was unable to convey any difference of sensation.

On testing sensation with pair of compasses, it is found that the minimum distance at which two points can be perceived as such, is as follows :—

Right hand, $6\frac{1}{4}$ mm.   Left hand, $3\frac{1}{4}$ mm.
Right leg, 125 mm.   Left leg, 50 mm.
Right foot, plantar surface, 12 mm.   Left foot, 12 mm.

On palpation behind and below the ears, it is found that the mastoid process on the left side is more massive than that on the right, but the difference is not so great as to be considered morbid.

The lungs and heart appear to be normal. He perspires very much. The amount of urine passed in twenty-four hours was 52 ozs., the specific gravity was 1025, and the reaction slightly acid. A pinkish deposit was present, but the urine itself was the normal amber colour, and there was no albumen. Microscopic examination shows amorphous urates and stellate crystals.

December 24th, 1895. During the first few days of residence in hospital there was little change in the patient's symptoms. On the evening of the 13th, however, the temperature rose to 100°, and subsequently his case has gone steadily downward.

His various symptoms were intensified, and hiccough, which had only been present for brief periods previously, became more distressing ; there was but slight cessation of this symptom, and he obtained little sleep at night ; various measures were taken, but only temporary relief could be obtained.

The condition of the left eye became worse, and an ulcer formed on the hazy cornea. Speech became more difficult, and the paralytic condition of the left vocal cord found expression in a hoarse incomplete cough. Swallowing also became more impaired, and fits of painful coughing followed the attempt. Paresis of the left arm became pronounced, and the grip of the hand weaker. There was no complaint of headache, but the patient was quite unable to walk on account of extreme giddiness. Coincident with the persistent hiccough a gnawing pain developed in the epigastrium. The bladder and rectum were not affected.

At six o'clock in the evening of the 17th, the temperature stood at 102° F., rising at midnight to 103·6° F. This was not preceded by rigor or even chilliness, but was accompanied by a good deal of perspiration. During the following day the pyrexia abated somewhat, but at six p.m. the register was 102·6°, and 101·4° at nine p.m. From the 20th to the 23rd the records of the temperature did not show any rise above 100°. At twelve noon on the 23rd the pyrexia again asserted itself, 104·4° being noted, and to-day (24th) at noon 103·2° was reached, and by three p.m. it had dropped to 102.8°.

During the early part of the day (24th) it was evident that the lad was sinking fast. The emaciation which had been in progress was more obvious, and the face became livid. The pulse was rapid, and the respiration was hurried and often very irregular. During the evening he had several convulsive movements, both sides of the body being affected, but the left more especially. The arms were flexed at the elbow in a jerky fashion, and there was subsultus at the wrist, and occasionally a definite flexion of the hand to the radial side of the wrist. The head was turned distinctly to the left, being approximated to the shoulder of that side. The legs were for the most part kept in a rigidly extended position, and the chest was thrust forward and kept fixed in that position for a few seconds. The breathing at such times was noisy, and as the seizure passed off, ceased for a short time.

At 4.30 p.m. the lividity became more marked, but there was no chilliness of the extremities. The pulse ran at 120 per minute, and was full and soft. Another seizure, similar to that just described, came on, and continued for a few minutes. As this seizure passed off, and the muscles gradually relaxed, the pulse suddenly fell to under 60 per minute, the respirations became shallow and infrequent, and at 4.50 p.m. he expired quietly.

During the twenty minutes before his death he recognised no one, and did not seem to hear words spoken to him. No change in the condition of the pupil was noted.

Death occurred seventeen days after his admission to hospital, and thirty-one days after the first symptom of illness.

Treatment was for the most part palliative, though iodide of potassium was also tried but found to be of no avail.

Dr. Lewis Sutherland performed the post-mortem examination, which took place on the .27th :—" There is found to be some slight œdema of the soft membranes of the brain, and both lateral ventricles contain a small amount of blood-stained fluid. The cerebrum and cerebellum appear quite normal ; the part to be described being the only affected portion of the encephalon.

There is a lesion occupying the left half of the medulla and floor of the fourth ventricle. This portion of the medulla is swollen, and its tissue softer than that of the opposite side. The swelling involves the entire half, and may be traced into the floor of the fourth ventricle, where it gradually shades off. It involves an area measuring 4 cm. × 1·3 cm. It touches the middle line. but does not cross it.

As viewed from the fourth ventricle, and particularly as seen on transverse section, the affected area has a distinctly mottled appearance, irregular areas of hæmorrhage, alternating with areas of an opaque yellow colour.

The bones of the skull and upper cervical vertebrae are normal. There is no disease of the middle or internal ear.

The left lung is loosely adherent throughout, and is hyperaemic on section. The right lung is non-adherent, but otherwise normal. Both the larger bronchi contain a frothy yellow fluid, and their mucous membrane is hyperaemic. The spleen shows moderate hyperaemia. The kidneys are distinctly hyperaemic, but otherwise normal. The adrenals are normal. The liver, stomach, intestines, pancreas, œsophagus, trachea, etc., are all normal. There is no glandular enlargement."

After prolonged hardening in Müller's fluid, a series of sections was made, including the cord, medulla, and pons, by Dr. Mackenzie Anderson.

"The inferior limit of the lesion, corresponds with the decussation of the pyramids. It becomes progressively more pronounced in successive sections, attaining its maximum development in the posterior part of the pons. Here it occupies an area measuring 1·7 cm. in diameter ; it is confined to the left side, and involving the upper portion of the pons, it appears in the floor of the fourth ventricle. The anterior limit of the lesion corresponds roughly with the middle of the floor of the fourth ventricle. The lesion presents the appearance of a glio-sarcoma, with minute hæmorrhages into its substances."

The case described presents interest from several points of view, and from the circumscribed nature of the lesion, and the absence of pressure, has the value of a physiological experiment, without the wound and injury which the latter entails.

In regard to the deafness in the left ear, this was of course brought about by the destruction of the auditory nuclei, and the fibres of the nerve within the medulla. The contradictory results which were given by Weber's and Rinne's tests, are remarkable at first sight, but on consideration they are quite explicable and rather interesting. The result of Weber's test pointed in the direction of an affection of the nervous apparatus for the perception of sound, which was clearly enough correct. But when we examine the result of Rinne's test the matter is more involved, for as described above, it was negative in the left ear by seven seconds. The explanation of this fact is no doubt to be found in the condition of the membrana tympani which was, as noted above, indrawn.

Thus, although properly speaking there was no actual disease of the middle ear, yet there was a condition of increased tension in the membrane, which no doubt increased somewhat the deafness for sounds conducted by the air, but lessened it for sounds conducted by the bones.

The sequence of events which brought about the indrawn condition of the membrane is also interesting. In the report it will be noted, that almost the first symptom of illness was the difficulty in swallowing, due to paralysis of the muscles involved in that act. When therefore these muscles could no longer perform their function the Eustachian tube would no longer be opened during swallowing, and hence a partial vacuum would be created in the middle ear, with the inevitable result, an indrawn membrane.

The occurrence of subjective noises, is also of interest in this case. According to Siebenmann (Ueber d. Central. Hörbahn. Zeitschr. f. Ohrenh. Bd. xxix. s. 78), this symptom occurs in a small minority of cases of tumours in these regions.

In the two cases related by Politzer (Dis. of Ear, trans. by Dodd, 1894, p. 692), and Moos (Urich. Arch. Bd. lxviii.) respectively, this symptom was present at first, but disappeared as the tumour increased.

The median position of the vocal cord is worthy of remark, and should be taken in conjunction with the experiments and observations of Horsley, Semon, Grabower, Onodi, and others, in regard to the functions of the recurrent laryngeal nerve.

The paralysis of motion on the same side as the lesion, and of sensation on the opposite side, is very remarkable, though it is of course in keeping with the results of physiological experiments upon the course of the nerve-fibres in the cord and medulla.

Other points of interest are the persistent hiccough, the fluctuations of temperature, and the profuse perspiration.

UEBER EINEN FALL VON HIRNTUMOR BEI ACUTER MITTELOHREITE-RUNG UND UEBER DIE DIFFERENTIALDIAGNOSE ZWISCHEN HIRNTUMOR, HIRNABSCESS UND HYDROCEPHALUS INTERNUS.

Prof. HESSLER, Halle, a/S.

Ein viel bearbeitetes Thema der Gegenwart ist dasjenige von den intrakraniellen Komplikationen der Mittelohreiterung, sowohl in Diagnose als in Therapie. Ist auch die Diagnose in den typischen Fällen der häufigsten Komplikationen leicht, wie bei der Sinusphlebitis, der Meningitis, dem Hirnabscess, so ist sie schon schwer bei weniger deutlich gezeichnetem Krankheitsverlaufe, und noch schwieriger, wenn gleichzeitig mehrere Komplikationen vorhanden sind. In vielen Fällen ist der Hirnabscess infolge seines latenten Verlaufs in vita überhaupt nicht geahnt, und erst bei der Sektion auch bei grosser Ausdehnung desselben zur grossen Ueberraschung gefunden worden. Dieser graduelleUnterschied in der Diagnose ist natürlich von grossem Einflusse auf die Therapie. Je sicherer die Art und der Ort der Komplikationen diagnosticirt werden kann, desto eklatanter der sofortige Erfolg der Therapie. Bei unsicherer Diagnose muss die intrakranielle Nachbarschaft des erkrankten Ohres nach einer bestimmten Reihenfolge, die je nach der Diagnose eine verschiedene sein wird, durch chirurgische Eingriffe blossgelegt und auf ihre sekundäre Mitbetheiligung untersucht werden. Heute möchte ich die Aufmerksamkeit auf eine andere, von der Mittelohreiterung unabhängige Komplikation derselben, auf den Hirntumor lenken, und im Anschluss an einem Fall von mir die Literatur kurz citiren und die Differentialdiagnose zwischen Hirntumor, Hirnabscess, und Hydrocephalus internus besprechen. Der Fall ist folgender :

Bei einem zwölfjährigen, kräftig entwickelten Mädchen, war am 5ten Tage nach Ablauf von Scharlach plötzlich linksseitige Ohreiterung entstanden. Es fand sich rechts absolute Taubheit für Sprache und cranio-tympanale Leitung bei negativem Trommelfellbefunde, die seit Jahren schon erkannt war, und mit dem bisher normalen linken Ohr wurde nur Umgangssprache dicht am Ohre gehört ; das linke Trommelfell war stark serös durchfeuchtet, hinten oben vorgetrieben, und nach der Paracentese entleerte sich eitriges Serum. Keine Erleichterung. Raschzunehmende Schwellung am Warzenfortsatze erforderte 2 Tage später die Aufmeisslung desselben ; der Knochen war aussen hart, frisch durchfeuchtet, nach innen zu mehr schwärzlich verfärbt ; aus Antrum quoll förmlich der dünne Eiter heraus, seine Knochenwandungen frisch cariös arrodirt ; die ersten 4 Tage wechselndes Fieber, dann normale Temperatur, die Sekretion bald so profus, dass die ersten 8 Tage 2 Mal täglich zuerst trocken verbunden, dann mit Borsäurelösung ausgespült werden müsste ; beim gelegentlichen Blasen mit dem Politzer'schen Ballon kamen aus Antrum Eiter und Foetor leicht heraus ; es bestanden hierbei absolute Appetitlosigkeit, Apathie und mehrmaliges Erbrechen. Gegen die Scharlach-Albuminurie Schwitzbäder und Diuretin. Plötzlich Nachts des 18ten Tages nach der Aufmeisslung Erbrechen, 3 Stunden später Zuckungen, zuerst in der linken Hand, dann im gleichseitigen Bein, dann im linken Gesicht, weiter in gleicher Reihenfolge auf der rechten Körperhälfte, Augen nach links aussen verdreht, 5-6 Mal wiederholt, ½-1 Minute andauernd, nach 3 Stunden Bewusstsein zurückgekehrt, und mit gutem, alten Appetite kräftig gegessen und getrunken. Nachmittags Rückkehr der Krämpfe, Steigerung der Temperatur rasch auf 38,8 und 40,1, beiderseitige Pupillenerweiterung, Puls 160, beginnende motorische und sensible Parese der ganzen linken Körperhälfte, keine Gesichtslähmung. Diagnosticirt wurde per exclusionem Hirnabscess. Trepanation direkt auf Schläfenlappen : Dura stark gespannt, nicht pulsirend wird incidirt ; Gehirn drängt sich stark vor ; venös hyperämisch ; 6 Punktionen mit Troikart nach verschiedener Richtung und in wechselnde Tiefe resultatlos. Collaps. Am folgenden Tage Sensorium frei, Appetit wieder der gute alte ; nun weiter normaler Verlauf. Plötzlich in der Nacht des 13ten Tages heftiges Aufschreien, Schmerzen im linken Ohr, fast sofort Verfallen in Koma, dass bis zum Tode unverändert anhält ; linke Pupille ganz erweitert, rechte stark verengt. Wiedereröffnung der Trepanationswunde. Gehirn kirschengross vorgestülpt, ganz oberflächlich necrotisch ; bei Wegtupfen dieser Partien spritzt im starken continuirlichen Strahle von Taubenfederdicke wasserklar Flüssigkeit, ungefähr 2 Esslöffel heraus, offenbar von einem Ventrikelhydrops stammend ; durch die klaffende Fistel kommt man mit der Sonde in mehr als apfelgrosse, weichwandige Höhle, besonders weit nach hinten innen. Steigerung der Temperatur auf 40,8, des Pulses auf 120-160. Tod nach vier Tagen, Ende der 7ten Krankheitswoche.

Sektion ergab ein im gangränösen Zerfall begriffenes Sarkom des linken Schläfenlappens, das nach der microscopischen Untersuchung grosszellig war, mit punktförmigen Hämorrhagien in der erweichten Umgebung, bis dicht an den Seitenventrikel heranreichend, der bedeutend erweitert ist ; im linken Lateralsinus ein frischer adhärenter, theilweise verfärbter Thrombus, keine Meningitis, Lungenödem, parenchymatöse Nephritis.

Der Fall bietet verschiedene sehr interessante Eigenthümlichkeiten. Es bestand bei negativem Befunde am Trommelfelle und in der Paukenhöhle rechts absolute Taubheit für alle Stimmgabeln und die Sprache. Ob dieselbe mehr von einer Labyrintherkrankung als von einer Affektion des linksseitigen Gehörcentrums abzuleiten ist, ist nicht zu entscheiden, da eine Untersuchung des Schläfenbeins verweigert wurde. Die Reizungs und die darauffolgenden Lähmungserscheinungen am Körper begannen linkerseits, also gleichseitig mit dem Schläfenlappensarkom und theilten sich erst später der contralateralen Körperhälfte mit. Es fehlte ferner jede Spur von Aphasie, freilich war Patientin mehr linkshändig. Ich will hier nicht weiter auf die anatomische Möglichkeit eingehen, dass in diesem Falle die normale Kreuzung der Hirnfasern in den Pyramiden nicht stattgefunden hat. Aber dann konnte die rechtsseitige Taubheit nicht Folge einer Ausschaltung des linken Hörcentrums sein, sondern müsste als Folge einer Labyrintherkrankung gedeutet werden.

Ich hatte per exclusionem am wahrscheinlichsten einen Hirnabscess angenommen, aber auch eine tuberkulöse und seröse Meningitis zumal als Nachkrankheit des Scharlachs für möglich gehalten. Anstatt des Abscesses ergab die Sektion ein im gangränösen Zerfall begriffenes Sarkom des Schläfenlappens. Der Zerfall des Sarkoms, der so selten bei dieser Tumorart vorkommt, ist als Folge einer Selbstinfektion nach der acuten Mittelohr-Warzenfortsatzeiterung aufzufassen und eine Infektion desselben bei den verschiedentlichen Gehirnpunctionen abzuweisen. Die Anamnese hatte ergeben, dass Patientin in der Kindheit einmal auf den Kopf gefallen war, ohne aber das Bewusstsein verloren zu haben, öfters an migräneartigen Kopfschmerzen gelitten und eine Zeitlang beim Kämmen des Kopfes am linken Hinterkopf Schmerzen geäussert hatte. Perkussionsempfindlichkeit des Schädels war aber weder früher noch jetzt von mir nachzuweisen gewesen. Es sind niemals anhaltende Kopfschmerzen noch Schwindel, Pulsverlangsamung, noch andere Symptome von Hirntumor beobachtet worden. Deshalb ist auch von mir nicht einmal an die Möglichkeit eines

Hirntumors als Komplikation der Mittelohreiterung gedacht worden. Leider hat keine Untersuchung des Augenhintergrundes und auf Hemianopsie stattgefunden. Am auffallendsten ist die einseitige Erweiterung des Hirnseitenventrikels durch einen enorm grossen Hydrocephalus internus. Hydrops der Seitenventrikel findet sich besonders bei Tumoren des Kleinhirns und der Vierhügelgegend; derselbe ist dann doppelseitig und erklärt sich genügend infolge Stauung im Gebiete der V. magna Galeni vom Druck des Tumors. Ein einseitiger Hydrocephalus internus kommt nur zu Stande durch einseitige Stauung in dem Plexus choroideus und gleichseitigen Verschluss des Foramen Monroi.

Soweit mir die Literatur zu Gebote stand, habe ich weitere 18 Fälle von Mittelohreiterung complicirt mit Hirntumor gefunden und zusammen stellen können.

1. Abercrombie, Untersuchungen über die Krankheiten des Gehirns und Rückenmarks. Deutsch von v. d. Busch 1829. S. 227.

2. Arbuckle, Glasgow Medical Journal, July, 1876.

3. Robert, Le Progrès Médical, 1876. S. 454.

4. Friedenreich, Kliniske Foredrag over Nervesygdomne, 1882.

5. Matthieu, Le Progrès Médical, 1882. S. 186.

6. Bruns, Neurolog. Centralbl. 1886. S. 151.

7. Mills und Bodamer, Journal of Nervous and Mental Diseases, 1887. S. 716.

8. Schwartze, Archiv. für Ohrenheilkunde, 33. 1895. S. 292.

9 & 10. Passow, Berlin. Klin. Wochenschr. 1895. No. 44.

11. Dinkler, Deutsche Zeitschrift für Nervenheilkunde. 1895. VI.

12. Gesselewitsch und Wannach, Botkin'sche Hospitalzeitung, 1895. No. 7.

13. Donath, Wien. Med. Wochenschr. 1896. No. 29 und 30, und Pesth. med. chirurg. Presse 1896. No. 5.

14. Poli, Zeitschrift für Ohrenheilkunde, 1897. S. 385.

15. Jaffé, Deutsche Med. Wochenschr. 1897. Vereinsbeilage 4. S. 24.

16. Oppenheim, Deutsche Med. Wochenschrift. 1898. No. 10. S. 155. und Neurolog. Centralblatt, 1898. S. 136.

17. Handford, The British Med. Journ. 1898. S. 1585.

18. Nonne, Verhandlung d. deutsch. Naturf. und Aerzte Versammlung, Düsseldorf, 1898. S. 260.

Die Patienten waren dem Geschlecht nach, in 14 Fällen, 9 Mal männlich, und 5 Mal weiblich; dem Alter nach, 3 Mal im 1. Decennium, 5 Mal im 2., je 2 Mal im 3. und 5. und je 1 Mal im 4. und 6. Decennium. Hiernach findet sich der Hirntumor wesentlich häufiger im 1. und 2. Decennium, während der otogene Hirnabscess besonders häufig im 3. und 4. Decennium vorkommt. Die Otorrhöe war 8 Mal links, 5 Mal rechts, und 6 Mal doppelseitig. Ueber die Seite des Hirntumors waren die Angaben zu ungenau, als dass sie des Zählens werth gewesen wären.   Die Tumoren waren 11 Mal Sarkom, 5 Mal Tuberkel und je 1 Mal Carcinom, Gliom, und als Tumor überhaupt bezeichnet.   Der Sitz derselben war 8 Mal im Grosshirn, 4 Mal im Kleinhirn und je 1 Mal im Gross- und Kleinhirn, Vierhügel, Corpus callosum, Hirnschenkel, Brücke und innerer Kapsel.   Es war diagnosticirt worden: 7 Mal Hirnabscess in den Fällen von Friedenreich, Matthieu, Passow, Gesselewitsch und Wannach, Poli, Nonne, und mir: 4 Mal Hirntumor in den Fällen von Dinkler, Donath, Jaffé und Oppenheim; und je 1 Mal richtig Hirntuberkel von Bruns, Tumor oder Hirnabscess von Mills und Bodamer, Tuberkel oder Abscess von Schwartze, wahrscheinlich Hirnabscess von Passow, und tuberkulöse Meningitis von Robert, wo sich Solitärfollikel daneben fanden.   In 12 Fällen war der Augenhintergrund untersucht und 10 Mal Stauungspapille und Neuroretinitis gefunden worden, und 2 Mal in den Fällen von Arbuckle und Friedenreich normaler Befund vorhanden.   Dieses Ergebniss würde mit der Angabe von Oppenheim übereinstimmen, der in 82% Stauungspapille bei Hirntumor fand.

Die Zusammenstellung der Operationsangabe ergibt folgende Tabelle: 8 Mal war trepanirt worden, mit negativem Erfolge in den Fällen von Schwartze, Passow, Gesselewitsch und Wannach, Poli, Jaffé, Oppenheim, Nonne und mir; 5 Mal durch Aufmeisslung des Warzenfortsatzes Eiter im Antrum mastoideum gefunden worden in den Fällen von Schwartze, Passow, Poli, Oppenheim und mir; je 2 Mal war Ventrikelserum entleert in den Fällen von Nonne und mir, und die Lumbalpunction von Dinkler und Oppenheim gemacht worden; und 1 Mal in dem Falle von Nonne war das Antrum eröffnet worden ohne Eiter darin zu finden.   Der Tod war 3 Mal in den Fällen von Arbuckle, Donath und mir nach plötzlichem Koma plötzlich erfolgt, und 2 Mal in den Fällen von Passow und Oppenheim infolge Chloroformnarkose und Stillstand der Respiration unter noch einige Zeit fortdauernder Herzthätigkeit.   Bei der Sektion fand sich Hydrocephalus internus 6 Mal hochgradig in den Fällen von Abercrombie, Robert, Schwartze, Dinkler, Donath und Nonne; und 4 Mal nicht vorhanden in den Fällen von Gesselewitsch und Wannach, Poli, Oppenheim und Handford; je 1 Mal fanden sich bei Matthieu beide Hirnseitenventrikel erweitert, und der gleichseitige rechts um das 3 fache, und bei mir der gleichseitige Seitenventrikel allein durch kolossalen Hydrops erweitert.

Ich komme zur Diagnose.

Griesinger* hebt 1860 folgende Punkte als wichtig für die Differentialdiagnose zwischen Hirntumor und Hirnabscess hervor:—

1.   Wenn bei einem Hirnleiden mit Herdsymptomen traumatische Ursachen, Stösse, Schläge auf den Kopf und dergleichen voraufgegangen sind, so scheinen diese wohl viel mehr für Abscess zu sprechen.

*Griesinger.   "Diagnostische Bemerkungen über Hirnkrankheiten."   Archiv für Heilkunde 1860.   S.   54.

2. Wenn bei einer Hirnkrankheit Otorrhoe vorauf ging, und Caries des inneren Ohres anzunehmen ist, so ist bei schweren Herd-symptomen immer ein Abscess (gewöhnlich mit lokaler Meningitis, oft auch, aber durchaus nicht immer mit Blutcoagulation in dem Sinus) bei weitem am wahrscheinlichsten.

3. Der Kopfschmerz ist im Allgemeinen bei den Tumoren viel stärker als bei den Abscessen.

4. Krämpfe mögen bei den Hirnabscessen etwas häufiger als bei den Tumoren sein.

5. Die Dauer des Leidens ist im Grossen und Ganzen betrachtet bei den Tumoren länger als bei den Abscessen.

6. Die wichtigsten Momente der Unterscheidung aber liegen in den Verlaufsweisen beider.

Fast 20 Jahre später sagt Huguenin* über denselben Punkt der Diagnose :—1. Im Verlauf und Gruppirung der Symptome haben Hirnabscess und Hirntumor viel Aehnlichkeit; beide üben Druck aus, kommen verschieden lange zur Ruhe, machen entzündliche Störungen in der Nachbarschaft, haben denselben Sitz, machen demzufolge oft keine Herdsymptome, oft nur Allgemeinsymptome. Die *Aetiologie* ist verschieden : bei Tumor Trauma, bei Abscess Otorrhœ häufiger. 2. *Verlauf* mit Remissionen bei Hirntumor häufiger, bei Abscess höchstens 1-3 Mal Besserung vorübergehend; bei Tumor werden die Symptome später stärker, zu Kopfschmerzen kommen motorische und sensible Lähmung, manche Fälle verlaufen auch ohne Remissionen. 3. Am untauglichsten für die Differentialdiagnose sind die Symptome; es können nur die Reihenfolge und Gruppirung herangezogen werden. Psychische Schwäche langsam zunehmend spricht mehr für Tumor als Abscess; Kopfschmerzen sind bei beiden Affektionen gleich, machen beide Intermissionen. steigern sich bei Tumor stetig bis in das Somno-lenzstadium hinein ; Fieber, Schüttelfröste sprechen für Abscess, Sen-sibilitätsstörungen für Tumor ; Lähmungen sind bei gleichem Sitze bei Tumor häufiger ; Konvulsionen kommen bei beiden Erkrankungen gleich häufig vor ; auch epileptische Anfälle sind nicht zu verwerthen, ebenso wenig spricht Lähmung nach einem solchen Anfall für Abscess. 4. Das terminale Stadium ist ohne diagnostische Bedeutung. Ein rascher apoplektiformer Tod spricht für Durchbruch eines Abscesses in den Hirnventrikel. Das Ende ist bei Tumor gewöhnlich steigend in Koma, bei Abscess acut steigend zu meningitischen Symptomen bei Durchbruch. Huguenin schliesst diesen meisterhaft ausgearbeiteten Abschnitt seines Buchs mit der nicht genug beherzigenswerthen Bemerkung S. 823: "Wir haben Fälle gehabt, wo die Diagnose schwankte zwischen Meningitis tuberculosa, einfacher Meningitis der Basis, multiplem Hirntumor, Meningitis der Convexität, terminalem Ende eines Hirnabscesses und multipler Embolie der Hirnarterien."

*Huguenin. Gehirnkrankheiten in Nothnagel, Handbuch der speziellen Pathologie und Therapie 1873 S. 819.

In demselben Buche, S. 277, macht *Obernier* darauf aufmerksam, dass langebestehendes Kopfweh, stürmisches Erbrechen, Sehstörung, spät auftretende epileptoide Anfälle eine Täuschung mit Hi rntumor begünstigen, er verlangt deshalb, wie neuerdings Oppenheim* wiederholt, dass Herz, Urin und Augenhintergrund vor jeder Diagnose auf Hirntumor untersucht werden müssen.

Zu diesen diagnostischen Hauptsätzen habe ich auf Grund der in der Literatur gefundenen Beobachtungen nur wenig hinzu zu fügen. Wir wollen hier zwischen den einzelnen Symptomen und dem Verlaufe derselben unterscheiden.   Ohne Zweifel, sind beim Hirnabscess die Hirndruckerscheinungen nicht so stark, da er aus einer eitrigen Erweichung des Gehirngewebes direkt entsteht ; daher kommt es, dass derselbe häufig symptomlos und ohne jeden Hirndruck verläuft, damit* stimmt überein, dass Stauungspapille bei Hirntumor zumal bei Klein hirntumor viel häufiger beobachtet ist, als bei Hirnabscess nach Mittelohreiterung, wo er häufig nur auf der collateralen Seite nachzuweisen war.   Erkrankungen der von einander anatomisch verschieden entfernt gelegenen Hirnabschnitte und Nerven sprechen für Hirntumor. In dem oben citirten Falle Donath bestanden gleichzeitig Atrophie der N. optici, oculomotorius und trochlearis, und im Falle Handford war die beiderseitige Paralyse der N. abducens und facialis dadurch entstanden, dass ein wallnussgrosses Myxosarkom des Pons rechts den 6 & 7 Gehirnnerven eingeschlossen hatte.   Im Falle Oppenheim (16) hatte der Tumor beim Aufrichten des Körpers die Schläfenwindung belastet und dadurch ein Hinzutreten von Worttaubheit zur anamnestischen Aphasie und Paraphasie bedingt.

Brunst hält den Charakter der Kopfschmerzen für charakteristisch und entscheidend für Hirntumor ; derselbe ist nach ihm dumpf, tiefsitzend, manchmal bohrend, besonders dem Migränekopfschmerz vergleichbar, ebenfalls oft von Erbrechen und Uebelkeit begleitet, anfangs gering, stetig bis zum Unerträglichen steigend, bei Kindern geringer, da sich die Kopfnähte noch dehnen können, ständig vorhanden oder wechselnd mit tagelangen freien Pausen, bis mehrere Wochen ; oft des Morgens besonders heftig, veilleicht von Lymphstauung bei während des Schlafs vermindertem Hirndruck abhängig, gesteigert durch Stauung, kalte Füsse, Obstipation, Husten, Fahren und durch Fluxion, Alcohol, Erregung, diffus oder an Herdstelle besonders.

Eine gewisse Verschiedenheit der Symptome besteht bei den verschiedenen Hirntumoren, und es ist die Möglichkeit gegeben, aus der ersteren auf den Charakter der letzteren zu schliessen.   Die Gliome entstehen zumeist acut und nach einem Trauma, der Verlauf ist langsam fortschreitend und dabei wechselnd mit Intermissionen und Nachschüben, unterbrochen mit apoplektischen Anfällen wie bei Aneurysma, die zu einseitigen oder doppelseitigen epileptiformen Anfällen mit

---

*Oppenheim, Die Geschwülste des Gehirns, 1897. S. 197.   † Bruns, Die Geschwülste, 1905. S. 65 und 179.

verschiedengradigen Bewusstseinsstörungen führen können. Die Sarkome wachsen rascher, liegen mehr an der Hirnbasis und führen so mehr zu Lähmungen der basalen Hirnnerven, auch verlaufen sie viel seltener mit epileptiformen Anfällen und Bewusstseinsstörungen. Zumeist ist eine differentielle Diagnose zwischen Gliom und Sarkom nicht möglich. Die solitären Hirntuberkel kommen einfach und multipel vor, an jeder Stelle des Gehirns, besonders aber in der Hirnrinde, im Kleinhirn und in der Brücke ; die Folge ihres multiplen Vorkommens ist das Entstehen eines sehr verschiedenen Symptomencomplexes, der nicht von einem Herde aus abgeleitet werden kann, sie zeigen häufig langjährige Lähmung und finden sich zumal im Kindesalter sehr häufig neben Hirnabscess, nach Mittelohreiterung. Tuberkulöse Allgemeinerkrankungen in Lungen und Knochen, und Choroidaltuberkel sprechen für Hirntuberkel. Hirncarcinome entstehen fast immer als sekundäre Neubildungen.

Noch schwieriger ist endlich die Diagnose zwischen Hirntumor und chronischem Hydrocephalus internus. Beide kommen häufig, wie wir gesehen haben, zusammen vor, und hier wurde zumeist die Diagnose Hirntumor allein gestellt. Für den Hydrocephalus internus sprechen die sekundären Veränderungen des Schädels, wie sie auch bei jugendlichen Individuen zuerst beobachtet worden sind, der langsame, symptomenlose und remissionslose Verlauf ohne das Auftreten eines Herdsymptomes. Neuerdings hält Schmidt* das Auftreten von Symptomen intracranieller Drucksteigerung, besonders Erbrechen und Schwindel bei einer ganz bestimmten Seitenlage für charakteristisch für einen Tumor auf der der "Brechlage" gegenüberliegenden Seite, der nicht genau median gelagert ist, sondern von einer Kleinhirnhemisphäre ausgeht. Die Erscheinung kommt durch die einseitige Belastung und consekutive Kompression der V. Galeni magna zu Stande. Ein 2tes Symptom, das Fehlen des Patellarreflexes würde mehr für Kleinhirntumor als Hydrocephalus internus sprechen.

Diese beiden Symptome von Oppenheim und Schmidt, die genügend anatomisch begründet und klinisch erklärbar sind, müssen in der Zukunft in jedem einzelnen Falle von intracranieller Komplikation bei Mittelohreiterung berücksichtigt werden und dürften vielleicht ein wesentliches diagnostisches Symptom zwischen Hirnabscess und Hirntumor abgeben.

Der Hauptzweck meiner casuistischen Mittheilung ist, bei den Herrn Collegen Umfrage nach ähnlichen Fällen zu halten.

---

*Schmidt.—Zur genauen Lokalisation der Kleinhirntumoren und ihrer Differentialdiagnose gegenüber acquirirten chronischen Hydrocephalus internus. Wien. klinische Wochenschrift 1898. No. 51.

THE FORMATION OF A CIRCUMSCRIBED INTRA-DURAL ABSCESS AT
THE SITE OF THE SACCUS ENDOLYMPHATICUS.

DR. JOBSON HORNE, London.

This communication was based upon a dissected specimen of a temporal bone which had been removed, together with the dura-mater
lining it, from a boy, aged 19, who had died of lateral sinus thrombosis
and meningitis. The specimen demonstrated how pus, when it has
entered the labyrinth, may reach the cranial cavity along a route which
at times offers but little resistance; and form a circumscribed abscess
between the layers of the dura mater, covering the petrous bone on its
posterior aspect. The specimen was also of interest as showing how the
vestigium of an embryonal structure may be a source of danger to
life.

The patient, a wood carver, had had discharge from the right ear
and deafness since infancy. He had been in his usual health, which he
regarded as good, up to thirteen days before his death, when he felt
giddy, perspired profusely in the night, and awoke with a bad headache.
He became drowsy and slept badly. On the fourth day after the onset
of the symptoms, the temperature was 103·5° F., the headache persisted,
and pain was complained of in the back. The deafness increased, and
during the night of the fifth day he vomited three times. The following day he was admitted to St. Bartholomew's Hospital under the care
of Sir Dyce Duckworth. Herpes developed on the upper lip and chin.
He was fully conscious and rational, the head was retracted and the
neck somewhat rigid; the face and arms at times twitched. The pulse
was 100, regular, full volume, low tension, and slightly dicrotic. The
respirations 40 and tranquil. There was no facial paresis. The urine
contained a cloud of albumen.

On the ninth day, patient had a rigor lasting ten minutes, temperature rising to 105·4°. The ear continued to discharge freely. The following day the antrum was explored, and also the lateral sinus. The
temperature fell to 97°, and he passed a fairly good night. On the
eleventh day, patient had another rigor, temperature rising to 104·6°.
On the fourteenth day of the illness, the pulse was 184, temperature
105·6°, and death occurred. Temperature in the rectum immediately
after death was 108°.

Post-mortem, a slight amount of meningitis was found over the pons
and medulla, more marked over right than left side, and the serous
fluid beneath the tentorium was increased. In the neighbourhood of
the mastoid cells on the right side, beneath the dura mater, and almost
surrounding the lateral sinus, was a collection of pus—about three
quarters of a drachm. No pus was found beneath the dura mater over
the middle ear. In the lungs there was some old tubercle at both apices;
at the right apex there was one small cavity containing pus. Bacterio-

scopic examination of the pus from the middle and internal ear yielded a diplococcus as well as staphylococci and streptococci.

An examination of the temporal bone revealed the following. Upon removing the anterior meatal wall, the posterior wall was found eroded ; Shrapnell's membrane perforated, and the incus lost. There was considerable destruction of the outer attic wall up to the roof of the middle ear. In the middle fossa could be seen some localised pachy-meningitis over the roof of the middle ear, which was an irregular carious area and perforated. In the posterior fossa, immediately beneath the superior petrosal sinus, in the neighbourhood of the site of the saccus endolymphaticus, and stretching across the lateral sinus (as seen in the accompanying plate), was an abscess sac. The incision through the abscess [see photograph], shows that its walls are between the layers of the dura mater. The abscess has perforated in two directions ; there is a perforation (through which a bristle passes) into the posterior fossa, which caused posterior lepto-mening-itis, and on opening the lateral sinus, it was found that the abscess had perforated the wall, causing septic thrombosis of the sinus from that point downwards. On reflecting the dura mater from the internal auditory meatus, pus was found surrounding the seventh and eighth nerves. The labyrinth, as seen through the bone, looked yellow. The roof of the labyrinth was dissected out, and the internal ear was found to be occupied throughout its entire extent with dark brown pus. Infection had spread from the middle ear to the labyrinth, viâ the oval window ; and on stripping the dura mater from above downwards to the aquæductus vestibuli, it could be seen that pus had emerged along the aqueduct to the saccus endolymphaticus.

A question arises as to what part the saccus endolymphaticus can take in the formation of the walls of such an abscess. Was the abscess formed within the saccus itself by distension of its walls ; or was it formed between the two layers of dura mater, which originally received the saccus endolymphaticus ?

Dr. Jansen in an important paper in the Archiv. für Ohrenheil-kunde, Bd. 35, S. 290, " Zur Kenntniss der durch Labyrintheiterung inducirten, tiefen extraduralen Abscesse in der hinteren Schädelgrabe,' expresses the opinion, " der Saccus Endolymphaticus kann durch die Eitermenge sehr stark erweitert werden, zu Bohnengrosse und mehr."

Dr. Horne is inclined to the view that such an abscess is not formed within the saccus itself, but between the two layers of dura mater, which originally contained the saccus. These two layers are carried into the fissure immediately over the orifice of the aquæductus vestibuli ; and after foetal life and the disappearance of the saccus, may continue to form a potential cavity, communication with the internal ear being determined on complete closure of the fissure. It therefore follows that

DB

an abscess, such as the one described, is more likely to be met with in early life.

Dr. Horne, in conclusion, expressed his indebtedness to Sir Dyce Duckworth, through whose kindness he was able to record the case.

Cases of Mastoid and Intracranial Extension of Suppuration from the Tympanum, with Remarks and Queries respecting the Chronology of Complications, and its Bearing upon Treatment.

Mr. Hugh E. Jones, Liverpool.

Mr. President and Gentlemen,

The first four cases I am about to relate, make with two fatal cases,* previously reported and specimens from which are shown in the Museum, a series exhibiting the following facts :—

1st. That at no period in the course of suppurative otitis media is the cerebellar fossa free from the danger of invasion.

2nd. That the tympanic and mastoid affection may appear to get well without operation, while a focus of infection remains behind which may at any moment burst into activity.

3rd. That where the antrum is small and the mastoid diploëtic, the extension to the cerebellar fossa is practically without warning, and may for a time cause no alarming symptom.

4th. That occasionally a severe and extensive lesion may exist without giving rise to grave symptoms and so lead an unwary practitioner to suppose that the mere opening of a superficial abscess is sufficient.

5th. The truism that the earlier the complication is detected and attacked, the more surely and speedily the danger is averted.

CASE 1.—CHRONIC SUPPURATIVE OTITIS. SEPTIC THROMBOSIS OF THE LEFT SIG-
MOID AND LATERAL SINUSES. PROBABLE EXTENSION OF THE PHLEBITIS. OSCILLATING
TEMPERATURES FOR 10 WEEKS. OPERATIONS. ANTITOXIN. RECOVERY.

J. G., a strong and healthy miner, 23 years of age.

History. Otitis media purulenta of several years standing. Cessation or marked diminution of discharge for 3 weeks accompanied by pain over mastoid stiffness of neck, rigors but not vomiting.

Condition on admission. Both ears somewhat deaf. Slight offensive discharge from the left tympanum. Greater part of the membrana tympani and the ossicles destroyed. Bare bone in and about the "aditus." No swelling or redness over mastoid nor in the triangles of the neck, but all these points were very tender to pressure, and the muscles rigid. The chest was clear of physical signs and remained so. Pulse and respiration rate kept about the normal ratio to the temperature

----

* Cases of Septic Thrombosis of the lateral sinus which extended to the opposite sinus. Vide Catalogue of Sixth International Congress of Otology.

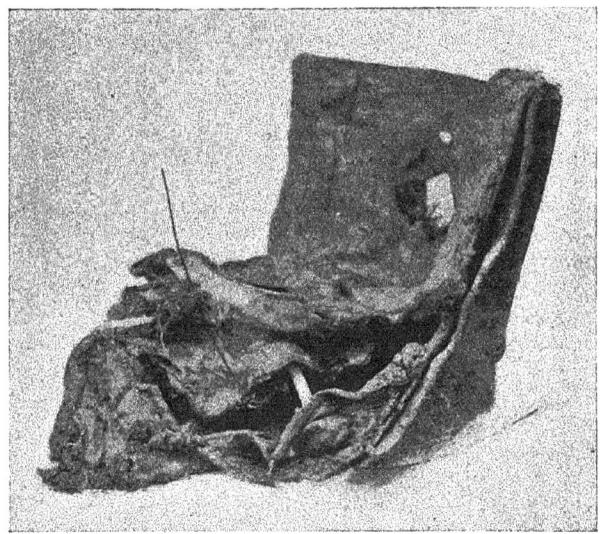

Photograph of posterior part of a right temporal bone to illustrate Dr. Jobson Horne's paper on "The Formation of a Circumscribed Intra-Dural Abscess at the Site of the Saccus Endolymphaticus." The lateral sinus is laid open in its entire extent. A white rod stretches across the sinus and lies within the abscess sac. A bristle passes through the perforation in the posterior wall of the sac through which pus escaped into the posterior fossa. Another white rod is placed in the internal auditory meatus.

though the oscillations in pulse and temperature charts were more marked than in the respiration chart. There appeared to be no serious disturbance of the functions of the brain, though there was a suspicion of optic neuritis. A marked feature of the case was constipation. A slight rigor occurred on the morning after admission while the temperature was 103·4.

September 6th. First operation.—On cutting down to the antrum the bone was found to be extremely hard. After penetrating about ¼ inch the cerebellar fossa was opened. The hollow of the sigmoid groove reaching to within a quarter of an inch of the meatal surface of the mastoid. No cells were found until the antrum was reached. This cavity was found to be small in diameter and opening posteriorly into the sigmoid groove. About a drachm of pus escaped from the antrum and an extradural abscess. The bridge between the antrum and tympanum was removed and the latter cavity was cleared out.

After this operation the temperature fell but rose again on the second day.

September 8th. Second operation.—Following up the opening into the antrum, bone was removed in the course of the sinus for 2″. The outer wall of the sinus had sloughed and a disintegrating clot was found and removed from the cavity, the sloughs being cut away with a pair of scissors. The whole cavity was then packed with iodoform gauze. Though the wound did not clean perfectly, marked general improvement followed until the 9th day when the symptoms returned and culminated in a rigor on the 11th day. On the 15th day after the second operation, *September 23rd*, a *third operation* was performed. Another inch of the sinus was laid bare and it was found that the clot at this point was suppurating. It was removed.

After this operation there was never any more trouble with the wound which was now nearly four inches long. A healthy granulating process set in.

As we were not sure that the recrudescence of the symptoms was due to the suppurating clot now removed, 5 c.c. of antistreptococcic serum were injected and 10 c.c. the following day. Unfortunately no bacteriological examination was made. It would be tedious to describe the course of the case in detail.

September 23rd to October 20th. During the next 27 days 10 rigors occurred and 40 c.c. serum was injected in doses of 5 or 10 c.c. There was no vomiting, and the appetite was good. The temperature fell every day to or below normal, and rose to 103°, 104°, and 105°. The bowels never acted without an enema until true convalescence set in. In spite of all this, the patient always said he was feeling better, and he was the only person concerned who took a cheerful view of the case.

After the period described the temperature improved considerably, only occasionally rising to 102° and once to 104°.

October 21st to November 7th. After sixteen days the right side of the neck (opposite to the original lesion) became slightly red, painful, and tender without obvious swelling, at first high up behind the jaw and travelling slowly down until the clavicle was reached, and the temperature rose to 103°. Antitoxin was again injected, and hot fomentations applied to the neck. The pulse rate also increased, but no physical signs of a heart lesion could be detected. This went on for ten days, culminating in a rigor.

November 7th to November 18th. After this last rigor the temperature became steady at or about normal, except for one sudden rise to 103°. Throughout the illness the patient's mind was clear, and though he was quiet and subdued during the greater part, he always gave one the impression of being perfectly composed and determined to get well.   He often asked to be allowed to get up and go home, and moreover had an excellent appetite.   When however he was allowed to get up he was quite unable to stand without ass'stance.   He was discharged on December 22nd, after a month's convalescence.   The wound was then firmly cicatrised with a small permanent opening into the antrum.

	R. 5″ (dry perfor.)		B. C. full. Rinne +
Hearing. W.		T. Fork.	
	L. nil.		B. C. full. Rinne neg.

No discharge, tinnitus, vertigo, or pain in either ear.

During the last five months he has been working down a coal pit, apparently in perfect health.

The points of interest in this case are :—

1.   Temporary facial paralysis, following use of Stacke's protector.

2   The absence of mastoid cells and the approximation of *the sulcus to the antrum and meatus externus.

3.   The creeping phlebitis (?) and symptoms of septic absorption, with oscil- ˙ lating temperature lasting ten weeks.

4.   The use of antitoxin.   Doubtful efficacy.

CASE 2.—RELIGHTING OF INFECTIVE FOCUS IN APEX OF MASTOID, RESULTING IN EXTRADURAL ABSCESS WITH IMPLICATION OF THE WALL OF THE SINUS.   OPERATION. RECOVERY.

S. F., a boy, aged 11 years.   Admitted to the Liverpool Eye and Ear Infirmary November 21st. 1898.

History.   Three years ago Scarlatina, enlarged cervical glands, but no hints of suppurative otitis media.   Twelve months ago had discharge from the left ear for *three days*.   This ear has been slightly deaf ever since.

One week ago the patient was boxed on the left ear by a schoolfellow.   Since then has suffered intense pain at the back of the ear, retching several days, actual vomiting yesterday and to-day.   Discharge from left ear four days ago.   Slight attack of shivering four days ago.

On admission.

	R. contact.		B. C. full. Rinne neg.
Hearing. W.		T. Fork.	
	L. nil.		B. C. full. Rinne neg.

No view of membrana tympani could be got.

Area of marked tenderness covering apex of posterior triangle, mastoid, and apex of anterior triangle.   No swelling.

Temperature 101°.6.   Pulse 140.

Operation.   November 21.   Outer wall of mastoid was sclerosed.   Softer bone was reached at the lower margin of the wound.   This bone was discoloured and following it up a greenish mass of caseous material was found in the mastoid pro-cess—old apical abscess.   This old abscess cavity had become continuous with the groove of the sigmoid sinus from which a quantity of pus escaped.   The antrum was high up and very small, and not in communication with the apical abscess or the cerebellar fossa.   About an inch of the sinus was next exposed and the greater part of the wall which appeared in the wound was covered with sloughy-looking grey lymph.   No clotting could be made out and fluid blood escaped on pricking the sinus.

The tympanum which did not appear to be much diseased was not cleared out, but gently irrigated.

No further symptoms of sinus infection arose.

On *December 12th*, nearly three weeks after admission, the wound not looking very healthy, it was decided to remove the ossicles. This was done with a good result.

On *December 30th*, the wound was freshened and the edges brought together by sutures in order to lessen the scarring. Healing took place, leaving a small permanent aperture leading to the antrum. A curious incident happened at the first operation. I was asked by the H. S. why I did not use Stacke's protector. I replied that it was because I was convinced that its introduction sometimes injured the facial. He then asked me to show him how the protector was applied. I did so, and immediately complete facial paralysis resulted. This was before the bone had been attacked *i.e.* directly after elevating the periosteum. The nerve ultimately recovered its function.

The points of interest in this case are :—

1. The temporary facial paralysis.

2. The existence of a dried up abscess in the apex of the mastoid for twelve months without causing symptoms. Its disturbance by a blow, causing it to communicate, not with the antrum but with the sulcus sigmoidalis.

3. The immediate cessation of the symptoms of septic phlebitis after operation.

CASE 3.—EXTRADURAL ABSCESS IN SIGMOID GROOVE, COMPLICATING ACUTE SUPPURATIVE OTITIS DUE TO SCARLET FEVER. OPERATION. RECOVERY WITH HEALED MEMBRANA TYMPANI AND PERFECT HEARING.

L. C., a girl, 12 years of age, was admitted into the Liverpool Eye and Ear Infirmary under my care on December 7th, 1898. Two days previously she had been discharged from the City Infectious Hospital—well.

Acute suppurative otitis had set in during the height of the attack but had apparently run a favourable course and when the patient was sent out the discharge had ceased. To avoid misapprehension I may say that the physicians of that Hospital pay careful attention to the cases with otitis media and keep them in the Hospital while the discharge lasts. The day following, pain and slight swelling appeared behind the left ear, and I was consulted by the parents.

Condition on admission. The child appeared to be quite well except for the slight pain. The posterior wall of the meatus dipped downwards and forwards considerably, hiding the greater part of the membrane. A small quantity of pus oozed from the tympanum.

The mastoid was tender, and there was a very slight swelling over the upper half which pitted on pressure.

On the day of admission this swelling was incised, no pus escaped.

On *December* 12th the pain in the mastoid had not subsided nor had the condition of the external meatus improved, but there was no constitutional disturbance. It was decided to open the antrum.

Operation. December 12th. The operation was commenced and proceeded with in the usual way through very dense bone until a cavity was opened and half a drachm of pus escaped. I thought at first that this was the antrum but on exploring with a probe, I found that I had opened the sigmoid groove. The bone separating the groove from the meatus was even thinner in this case than the first. The sinus was exposed for a short distance and its wall appeared very slightly thickened and velvetty but not sloughy. On searching the posterior surface of the petro-mastoid bone a small opening was found leading into the tympanum. The bone between this passage and the surface was then removed. The antrum, if it could be so called, was simply a slight extension backwards of the tympanic cavity. The ossicles and membrane were not interfered with. The patient made an uninterrupted recovery. No further discharge took place from the ear ; the hearing of that ear is quite as good as that of the right ear, which would be called normal and no perforation of the membrane can be detected.

The points of interest in this case are :—

1. The anatomical conditions found.
2. The absence of warning that an intracranial complication had arisen.
3. The occurrence of the complication in the early stage of suppurative otitis.
4. The likelihood of its being taken for an ordinary mastoid complication.
5. The rapid recovery with perfect hearing and healed tympanic membrane.

CASE 4.—CHRONIC SUPPURATIVE OTITIS, PROBABLY TUBERCULAR. LARGE SUB-PERIOSTEAL MASTOID ABSCESS EXTENDING TO ANTERIOR PART OF OCCIPITAL REGION ; EXTRADURAL ABSCESS ; SLOUGHING OF DURA OVER PART OF CERE-BELLUM ; SUB-DURAL ABSCESS ; CEREBELLUM EXPOSED. OPERATION. RECOVERY.

J. B., boy, aged 10 years.

History. Discharge from right ear at least 10 months. Has seemed stupid the last few days and has held his neck rigid. The ear has not been discharging as freely as usual lately. Stomach out of order. No rigors.

September 21st, 1898. Was seen at the Eye and Ear Infirmary by one of my colleagues. Pulse 100, temperature 99°. No optic neuritis. Advised to become an In-Patient.

September 28th. Discharge began again 6 days ago. No pain, no special tenderness on pressure. Has not been quite so dull in intellect. Pulse 128, temperature 99·4. A fortnight later he was admitted into Hospital under my care.

Condition on admission. October 12th.—Unhealthy-looking boy with enlarged glands along sterno-mastoid. Tubercular ?

Large superficial abscess over mastoid and extending backwards and down-wards for three inches. Free fluctuation. There was nothing to suggest a brain abscess or any other grave intracranial lesion.

Operation. October 12th.—Incision for antrectomy and another obliquely downwards and backwards so as to open abscess freely. Bone bare and granu-lating over anterior part of occipital bone below level of the sinus. Small opening leading obliquely forwards into cavity in mastoid in neighbourhood of antrum. On removal of the external shell of bone, this cavity was seen to occupy practically the whole of the mastoid. It was filled with granulations, pus, and debris of bone. This cavity extended backwards through an opening in the posterior wall of the mastoid and a probe could be passed behind the sigmoid sinus along the floor or external wall of the cerebellar fossa into an extradural abscess corresponding with the sub-periosteal one. Just external to the sinus the dura had become necrotic, and while granulations were being scraped out with the curette the dura broke away exposing a subdural abscess and a small portion of the laminæ of the cere-bellum. The sigmoid sinus itself was covered with granulations and raised up out of its groove ; as no symptoms of septic thrombosis existed, the sinus was not interfered with.

It was feared that the part of the occipital bone lying between the sub-periosteal and extradural abscesses would necrose. But the dura seemed to reapply itself very quickly and very little pus came from the intracranial abscesses after the first dressing. The external abscess caused more trouble and it was only after being laid open from end to end that it began to heal.

Patient left the Hospital November 8th. The condition of the tympanum improved so that the M. T. began to heal up.

The chief points of interest about this case are :—

1. The comparatively insidious way in which it progressed, absence of very grave symptoms.

2. The escape of the sigmoid sinus.

3. The recovery of much of the denuded bone.

To sum up the four preceding cases:—The first and last were genuine so-called chronic cases of suppurative otitis. The second was a case of mastoid disease which subsided without operation, only to break out again in a dangerous manner twelve months later. The third was a case of *acute* suppurative otitis complicating scarlatina, which, owing to the absence of mastoid cells, resulted directly in an extradural abscess.

The mastoid complications of influenza are so well known that I feel that I must apologize for referring very briefly to three cases which came under my notice three months ago. I relate them to show how early it may be necessary to operate in acute cases, especially if these are due to influenza.

The first—CASE 5—was that of a gouty gentleman of about 55 years of age recovering from an attack of influenza. He was suffering intense pain at the back of the ear and radiating from that situation to the parietal and temporal regions. He had not slept for several nights and demanded that something should be done to relieve him. The mastoid was very tender on pressure but not swollen. The meatus was a little reddened and there was some swelling of the posterior and inferior walls. The membrane was congested but I could not make out any perforation, though the physician, Dr. Wallace, thought there had been a slight discharge. My own feeling was that a delay of two or three days was advisable, but the patient and Dr. Wallace overruled this and it was decided to operate at once.

Nothing was found in the cells. In the antrum a granulation was found and some blood clot which appeared to be breaking down into pus. The wound next day was evidently infected from the antrum, the surface being covered with grey unhealthy looking lymph. The pain was not entirely relieved at first, but he soon began to sleep well and was able to get about in a fortnight.

The wound was not completely cicatrised until two months after the operation.

CASE 6. A gentleman, who had many years before suffered from suppurative otitis, and who had o·casional slight recurrence of the discharge, had, while away from home, what appeared to be a slight attack of influenza. A few days later a swelling appeared slightly behind and below the tip of the mastoid, while the whole mastoid became tender and painful ; a considerable amount of pus escaped from the ear which was very deaf. At this stage, I was asked to see him by his physician, Dr. Wilson, of Standish.

The swelling, which seemed to fluctuate, was situated in the upper part of the sterno-mastoid embracing the tip of the mastoid process and gave one the impression of an abscess associated with an apical mastoid abscess.

The patient being an extremely busy man, declined operation and unknown to us asked the opinion of an eminent surgeon in a neighbouring town. This gentleman confirmed our opinion and advised immediate operation.

The patient now yielded, and asked me to operate next day. After making the usual incision I pushed a director into the swelling in the body of the sterno-mastoid muscle, but found no pus. The muscular fibre seemed to be sodden, soft and of a very deep red colour.

The mastoid cells were then opened, but nothing was found until the antrum was reached, and here, as in the first case, we found granulations and breaking down blood clot.

Healing was rapid, the discharge from the meatus ceased from the day of operation and did not recur, and hearing soon returned to the same acuity, if not greater acuity than before this illness.

I frequently asked myself what would have happened in these two cases if they had been left alone and doubts arose in my mind whether the operations were not premature. But the following case occurred and re-assured me.

CASE 7.—INFLUENZA. SUPPURATIVE OTITIS, SEVERE MASTOID NEURALGIA, LOSS OF SLEEP, NO EXTERNAL SIGN OF MASTOIDITIS FOR FOUR MONTHS. SWELLING, OPERATION. COMPLETE RELIEF OF PAIN, CESSATION OF SUPPURATIVE OTITIS AND RECOVERY OF HEARING POWER.

The patient having an attack of suppurative otitis following influenza consulted an aural Surgeon in January of this year. This gentleman warned the patient of the possibility of a mastoid complication. The suppuration not subsiding quickly, an officious friend carried the patient off to a London quack. In May he was brought to me by Dr. Sanderson of Liscard, who had been hurriedly called in on account of sudden appearance of swelling over the mastoid. The patient declared that he had had pain in the mastoid for four months, that he had not a single good night's rest for three months and that the discharge from the ear was as profuse as ever.

I operated the following morning. There was a subperiosteal abscess and a newly formed fistula ; the whole of the mastoid was excavated up to the antrum and its posterior wall was so friable that the dura was exposed over a considerable area by the operation.

Recovery was rapid and uninterrupted. Neither pain in the mastoid nor discharge from the ear occurred after the operation. This is only one of a large number of similar cases upon which I have operated.

And now I wish to refer still more briefly to three other cases of chronic suppurative otitis in which operation was declined.

CASE 8.—J. T., a young maid-servant, 18 years of age.

Suppurative otitis of many years standing. Severe pain in right ear and all that side of the head for three days. Inferior and posterior wall of the tympanum covered with granulations. Three days later, patient reported giddiness and frequent vomiting. Pulse 100, regular. A few days later the pulse was irregular. Six weeks later although—under treatment—the condition of the tympanum had greatly improved, headache and vomiting recurred.

Six months later.—Discharge had quite ceased and patient appeared to be well until four days ago, when acute pain commenced again in the ear and temple.

Operation was steadily resisted. I think it is extremely likely that there is an intracranial lesion probably incipient brain abscess in this case.

CASE 9.—M. D., married woman, aged 30. Discharge from right ear for six years. Petit mal? Headache. Occasional attacks of giddiness and severe tinnitus. The suppuration which was chiefly in the attic was easily controlled by intratympanic irrigation, but the petit mal, attacks of giddiness and headache continue. Operation declined. I believe this to be a case of incipient intracranial extension.

CASE 10.—J. B., a man, aged 40. Attic disease. Operation declined. Discharge kept completely under control. Reported himself at intervals for three years and said he was practically well. After a longer absence than usual, I heard from outside sources, that the patient had been suddenly ill, convulsions, coma, and death.

Remarks.—1. I have endeavoured to show by means of cases in this and other communications* that meningitis and thrombosis of the sigmoid or lateral sinuses may occur within a very short time from the commencement of an acute suppurative otitis. Cases confirming this remark may be found scattered in large numbers through otological literature.

2. We cannot tell, in the present state of knowledge, at what particular moment in the history of a case of suppurative otitis media an abscess of the brain becomes an established fact. Many cases which have run an acute course have been reported, and the date of inception of these acute abscesses can be approximately fixed. But the majority of brain abscesses are " chronic," that is to say, when found post-mortem they have thick walls and their contents have undergone various changes. Sir William Gull wrote as far back as 50 years ago that the cause of death in a case of encysted brain abscess was not the mere existence of the abscess in the brain, but the occurrence of encephalitis around the old abscess. When are these old abscesses formed?

Much is written about osseous erosions of the tegmen and extra-dural abscess, and as if they only occurred after the suppurative otitis had gone on for many years. I have endeavoured to show that these occurrences may, and very frequently do take place within the first three or four weeks of acute suppurative otitis media. But even if erosions could not occur for months or years, they are not essential for the extension of the septic processes from the tympanum to the meninges or sinuses. Are they necessary for the formation of a brain abscess?

. The surgeon who could diagnose brain abscesses at their first inception would confer a great boon upon the science of Otology and brain surgery.

Although brain abscesses lie dormant for years without giving rise

* British Medical Journal. Vol. II., 1898. Liverpool Medico-Chirurgical Journal. Vol. I., 1899.

to recognizable symptoms, there must be symptoms especially at their inception by which, if our knowledge of them were sufficient, the abscess could be diagnosed.   I have included in this paper three cases which appear to me to present the kind of symptoms we must look for. Cases carefully recorded from the commencement of acute otitis to death from, or operation upon, abscesses of the brain after many years, are required.

3.   It follows from the foregoing remarks that in undertaking a prophylactic operation upon the attic or antrum of a case of chronic suppurative otitis we may be operating after the brain abscess has already been in existence for some time.

If so may we not unconsciously set up changes in the abscess wall or surrounding brain which will result in encephalitis ?

4.   The possibilities here mentioned and such cases as Nos. 2 and 3, suggest to me that the best time to operate upon the mastoid is at the period when suppuration has established itself in the tympanum and mastoid, and it is perfectly evident that rapid resolution is not going to take place.   I consider that this point of departure can be determined with a reasonable degree of certainty, and I have given the indications in the paper referred to (which is also abstracted in the Journal of Laryngology, Rhinology, and Otology for August, 1899).   I will try to illustrate and enforce my meaning by a reference to sympathetic ophthalmia.

No surgeon can say at what precise moment sympathetic ophthalmia becomes a certainty ; its evolution and appearance may be postponed for months or years.   All that he can say is that a certain injured eye is dangerous.

Occasionally an eye is excised too late, *although* at the time of excision absolutely no sign of sympathetic disease had arisen.

But here our analogy, if it may be so called, ends.   The wise ophthalmic surgeon who takes no risks and enucleates a dangerous eye promptly, makes a sacrifice which may be quite unnecessary and is sometimes in vain, and yet he is right.   But the Otologist who opens the antrum and cells in acute suppurative otitis—I say "opens the antrum and cells," not "performs a radical operation"—though he may occasionally find that his operation was not strictly speaking necessary, sacrifices *nothing*.   On the contrary, if it should turn out that extension had taken place to the mastoid, he has by his operation saved almost intact the organ of hearing (the discharge from the tympanum ceases almost immediately and almost perfect hearing is restored) and I can add with equal certainty he has saved his patient much pain and discomfort, and in some cases the patient's life.

POSTSCRIPT.—Symptoms re-appeared in case 8 three weeks ago, and the complete postaural operation has now been performed.   May 22, 1900.

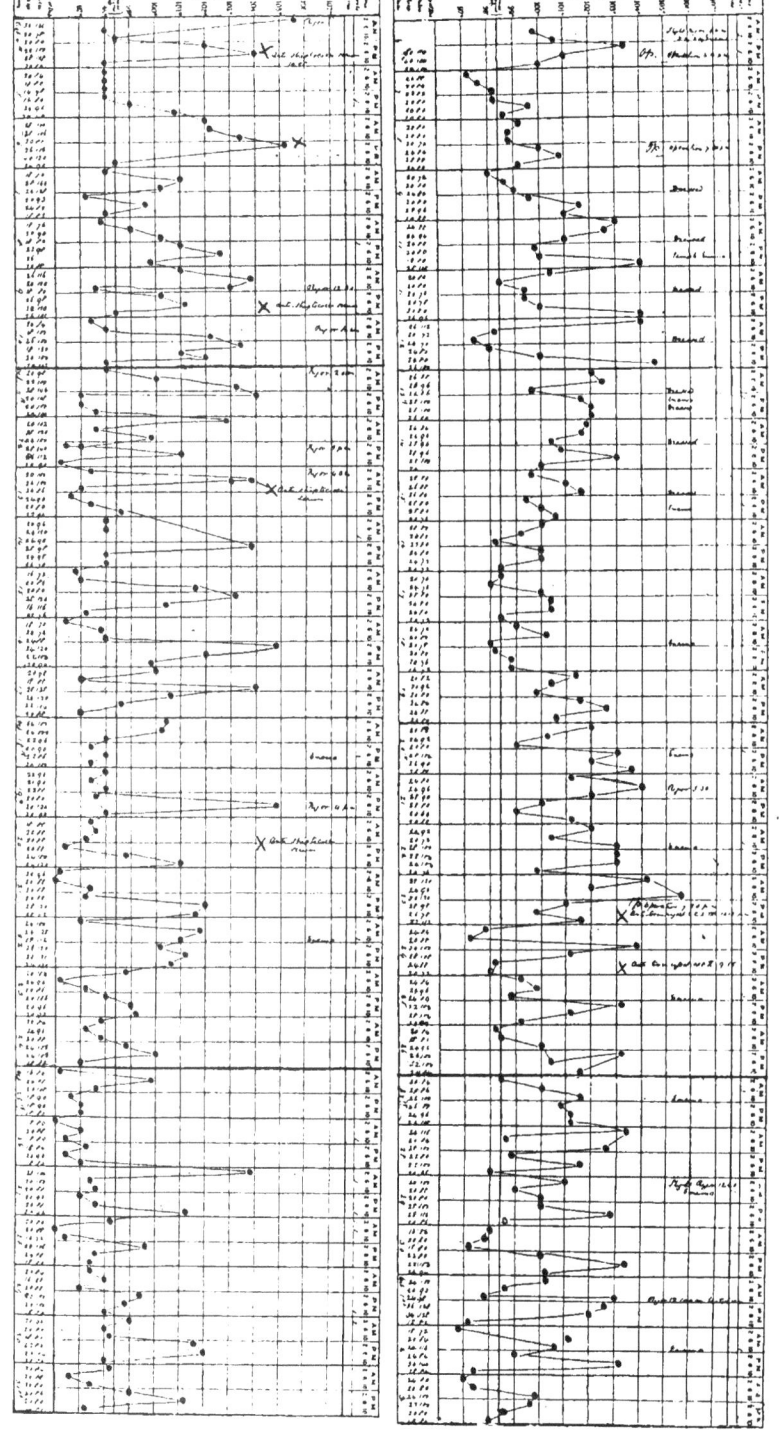

Admitted September 6th, 1898.

to give it a more natural position ; and secondly, to establish an opening into the Tympanum, with a view to improving the hearing. The Bone Conduction seemed sufficient to justify this attempt. An incision was made from the blind meatal orifice upwards, along the anterior border of the auricle, and continued down the posterior border nearly to the tip of the mastoid, then curved round and carried upwards and backwards for about 2½ inches. By this incision the upper two-thirds of the auricle was converted into a flap, and a reversed flap marked out on the mastoid.

On turning down the auricular flap, no external meatus could be found nor any tympanic ring, but in their place a dense mass of fibrous tissue. The mastoid flap was then raised and a hole cut at the usual site for Antrectomy ; at this part of the surface several small foramina were observed, but no supra-meatal spine. No air cells were met with until the antrum was reached, at a depth of half-an-inch from the surface. The bone was extremely hard.

The antrum was small, and communicated freely with the cavity of the Tympanum. In this cavity, apparently unattached, I found a dumbell-shaped ossicle about ⅓ inch long and $\frac{3}{16}$ inch thick. (This bone-let though carefully put aside was subsequently lost, without having been cut). We thought that it represented the heads of the malleus and incus, and that no articulation or processes had been developed.

The flaps described above were then transposed, the auricular flap over the mastoid and the mastoid flap brought to the front, and an attempt made to train the flap into the cavity in the bone by means of iodoform gauze packing. It was thought useless to attempt to establish an opening into the Tympanum by the natural route, and that the mastoid opening afforded some chance of success.

On the ninth day after operation a small quantity of mucus escaped from the Tympanum, and the gauze packing was replaced by a celluloid drainage tube. (This was directed backward, inwards, and upwards).

The tip of the skin flap within the artificial meatus was beginning to slough.

Four days later a little pus was mixed with the mucus from the meatus.

Fifteenth day : the flaps healed, stitches all removed. Tube did not reach quite to the bottom of the cavity.

The patient was kept in for a month longer (i.e., nearly seven weeks after operation), to ensure the artificial meatus being kept open.

As a result of the operation, there was little, if any improvement in aerial conduction of sound.

Three months later (nearly five months after first operation), patient was seen again and re-admitted. The meatus had quite closed up.

July 1st. A second plastic operation was undertaken with a view to re-opening the meatus and completing the transplantation backwards of the auricular mass.

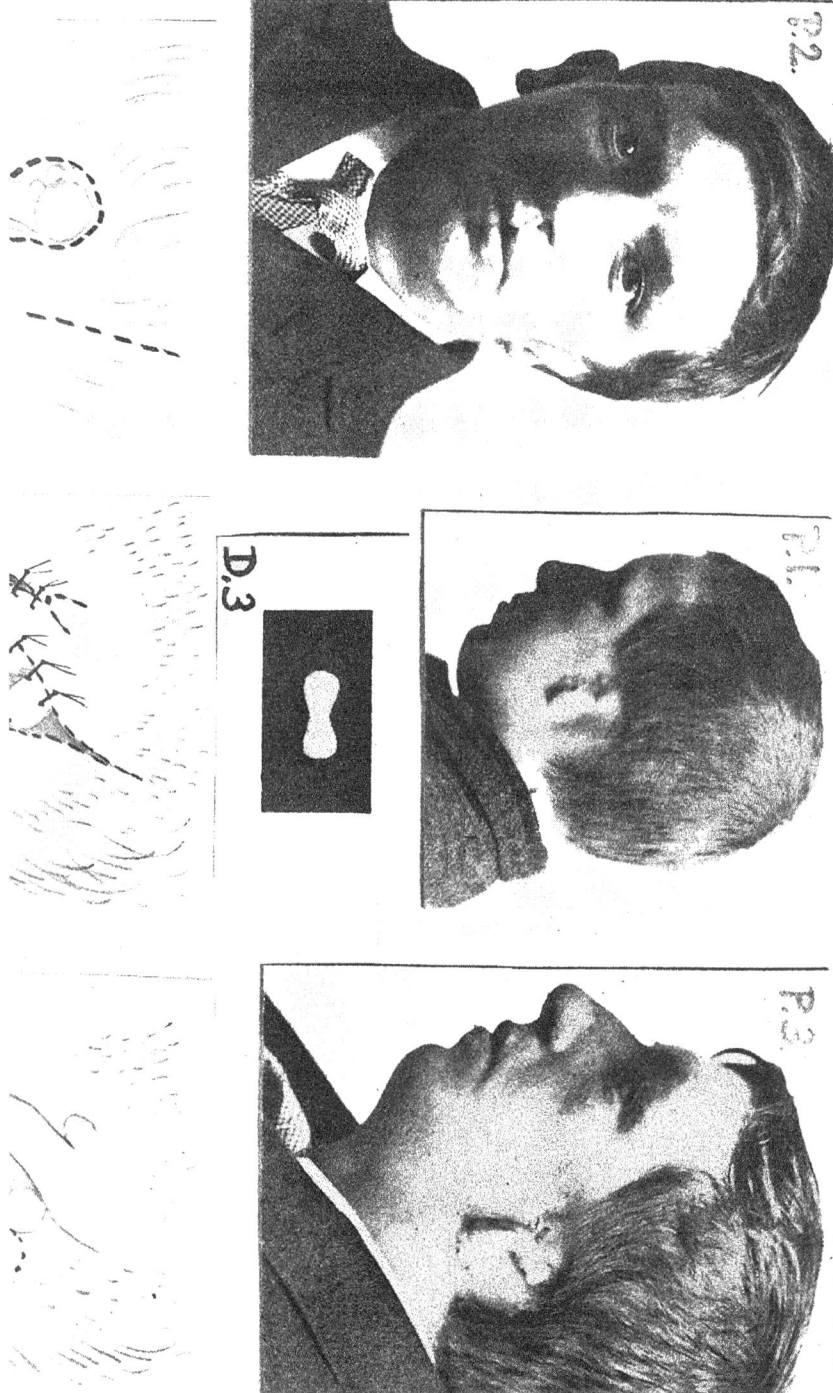

P.2.

D.3

P.3.

So far as the soft parts were concerned, the second operation was similar in character to the first, but referred to the lower third (or lobule) of the auricle, and the posterior skin flap was taken from behind the posterior flap of the first operation.

July 2nd. In the morning, the skin flap was cyanotic and apparently going to necrose, but recovered towards night.

July 10th. Retraction of cicatrix below anterior flap is dragging the lobule forward again.

July 12th. Three grafts were placed on granulating surface behind auricle, and on *July 22nd* two grafts placed in front of auricle after dissecting it back.

In spite of these various attempts the meatus closed up, and the lobule was dragged forwards to its old position, and the patient declining further operation was discharged. Parents were pleased with cosmetic result.

July, 1899. Patient came up, by request, for inspection and to be photographed.

Hearing was as follows :—

R. *Watch.* $\frac{4}{20}$, heard also on mastoid and Right frontal eminence.

T. F. B.C. $\frac{6}{6}$ Rinne +.

L. *Watch.* Nil.

T. F. B.C. $\frac{5}{6}$. A. C. nil.

Meatus completely closed.

Depression over bony meatus covered up.

Lobule pretty much in original position.

Generally speaking, appearance is improved.

Further operation declined.

Remarks. Incomplete though this communication may be, I trust that it may be of some interest and even of some use to surgeons who are interested in auricular malformations. The practical questions which arise are :—

1. Did the facts justify the attempt to improve the condition?

2. Was the method of operating the best that could be devised?

It seemed to me that the ugliness of the deformity, the normal appearance of the Eustachian orifice, and very fair bone-conduction, and also the alleged increase of deafness in recent years, justified the operation.

Judging by the result, I think it would have been better to have completely excised the rudimentary auricle and the fibrous cord leading to the Tympanum, because the bony opening made by operation lay behind the auricle in its new position, and this led to a great difficulty in keeping the new meatus open. An artificial auricle could have been worn to hide the hollow.

DESCRIPTION OF A SET OF MASTOID GOUGES.

DR. GEO. F. KEIPER, La Fayette, Indiana.

In the operating case of my former preceptor and esteemed friend, Dr. Geo. F. Beasley, of La Fayette, Ind., is an old gouge which has for many years served him well in operations upon the various long bones. We could not learn the name of the inventor. We were struck with its general design, and concluded that a set of various sizes would be as valuable in mastoid operations, as the large one which he has, has been in general surgery. Therefore the following set was made. The cutting edge of the smallest corresponding to the smallest cutting edge of the Schwartze set. The largest is just a size smaller than the old gouge referred to above. The other four are intermediate in size between the largest and smallest.

The gouges are each six inches long, with a knob on the end of the handle. This knob fits very snugly in the palm of the hand at the ball of the thumb, and is one of the features of the design in the gouge.

Two inches from the tip of the cutting edge the handle is bent to permit the index finger to find a lodging place for leverage. ·

The gutter of the largest gouge is $5/_{16}$ of an inch in the clear on the inside, and gradually tapers down to the cutting edge just as in the Schwartze's gouge. The gutter of the smallest size is $\frac{1}{8}$ of an inch across in the clear on the inside. The other four vary in size between the two.

It is believed that these will also prove a valuable adjunct to the armamentarium of the general surgeon. In operating upon the long bones gouges should be at least small enough to remove the smallest foci of caries.

UEBER COMBINATION VON OTITIS MEDIA "MIT RHINOGENEM GEHIRNABSCESS."

DR. KOEBEL, Stuttgart.

In dem Fall, den ich Mai d. J. beobachtete und zum Vortrag bringen möchte, handelte es sich um eine Otitis media purulenta mit Empyem des antrum mastoid., zugleich bestand eitriger Ausfluss aus der Nase in Folge von Stirnhöhlenempyem.

Ziemlich plötzlich traten Gehirnerscheinungen auf: neben den Allgemeinerscheinungen: Kopfschmerz, Erbrechen, Benommensein, Schwindel, noch 2 Herdsymptome: Lähmung des *Nervus hypoglossus und Zuckungen in der linken Hand und Arm.*

Die Gehirnerscheinungen wurden wegen der sehr abundanten Ohreiterung auf einen intracraniellen Eiterherd, sei es einen extraduralen oder cerebralen in der mittleren oder hinteren Schädelgrube bezogen.

Bei der Operation fand sich Eiter im antrum mastoid., aber kein Abscess im Schläfenlappen (die Suche nach einem Kleinhirnabscess sollte 1 oder 2 Tage später geschehen).

4 Stunden nach der Operation Exitus letalis.

Obduction: es fand sich *Eiter in beiden Stirnhöhlen, die hintere (cerebrale) Wand des rechten sinus frontalis war an 2 Stellen perforirt; im rechten Stirnlappen (an der Spitze und Basis gelegen) ein hühnereigrosser Abscess.*

Es ist bekannt, dass Abscesse im Frontallappen in der Regel gar keine Erscheinungen machen.

In meinem Falle sind, da ein makroskopischer Zusammenhang mit der vorderen Centralwindung nicht nachweisbar war, die bestehenden Herderscheinungen (Lähmung des Nervus Hypoglossus und Zuckungen im linken Arm und der linken Hand-Monoplegie und Monospasmen) als Fernwirkung anzusehen.

In der Literatur sind unter *18 Fällen* (die von Kuhnt und Dreyfuss gesammelten Fälle sind in der modificirten Tabelle von Dr. Hajek-Wien zusammengestellt) *von Exitus letalis nach Stirnhöhlenempyem* nur *6 wirkliche Frontallappenabscesse* erwähnt; ich fand dazu noch *einen* weiteren Fall von Heimann.

Diese sehr spärliche Casuistik wird durch meine Beobachtung um *einen Fall* bereichert.

Bis jetzt habe ich keinen weiteren Fall finden können, wo bei *Frontallappenabscessen eine Hypoglossus Lähmung* (Monoplegie) beobachtet worden wäre (gewöhnlich ist der nervus facialis befallen). So dürfte dieser Fall eine grosse Rarität sein.

EPILEPSIE AB AURE LAESA.

DR. M. LANNOIS, Lyons.

La tendance actuelle des neurologistes est de faire jouer aux intoxications un rôle de premier ordre dans la pathogénie de l'épilepsie. Malgré le bien fondé de cette opinion, il n'en reste pas moins nécessaire de laisser une place importante, dans la nosologie, à l'épilepsie réflexe.

Celle-ci, en dehors de l'observation des malades, repose sur des bases expérimentales indiscutables et, notamment, sur les expériences bien connues de Brown-Sequard, qui en coupant le sciatique ou la moitié de la moëlle chez des cobayes faisait apparaître chez eux les zônes épileptogènes et même une épilepsie transmissible aux rejetons. C'est là un procédé sùr pour produire l'épilepsie qui est couramment employé par les physiologistes dans les laboratoires.

Au point de vue clinique, on a rapporté de nombreux cas d'épilepsie réflexe due à des cicatrices cutanées, à des lésions de l'utérus, des reins, des dents et du tube digestif, etc. L'oreille ne pouvait manquer d'apporter son contingent d'observations.

De fait, depuis l'époque déjà fort lontaine où Fabrice de Hilden racontait l'histoire de Rose Chaperon qui fut guérie de crises epileptiques par l'ablation d'une perle de verre qu'elle portait dans l'oreille depuis huit ans, de nombreux exemples ont été rapportés par Itard, Maclagan, Moos, Gellé, Schurig, Steinbrugge, Trautmann, Noquet, Goris, Suarez de Mendoza, etc., etc., tendant à prouver la relation qui existe entre l'épilepsie et les maladies de l'oreille.   Boucheron qui s'est occupé plusieurs fois de cette question, a même essayé de différencier les épilepsies causées par l'excitation combinée des nerfs trijumeau, pneumogastrique et glosso-pharyngien dans les lésions du conduit ou de la caisse et les épilepsies par excitation localisée du nerf acoustique, dans l'otopiésis par exemple.

Mais en réalité cela paraît très théorique.   Si l'on s'en tient à la clinique, on ne peut manquer d'être frappé de la rareté de l'épilepsie ab aure laesa, étant donné d'une part que l'épilepsie est une maladie malheureusement trop commune et de l'autre que les porteurs d'affections d'oreilles sont légion.

D'un autre côté si on examine d'un peu près les cas publiés, on voit que peu d'entre eux résistent à une critique un peu serrée.   La primitive observation de Fabrice de Hilden, dont la malade avait des douleurs violentes de tête, une toux spasmodique, de violentes douleurs dans la moitié gauche du corps alternant avec de l'anesthésie, puis de l'atrophie du bras gauche, tous phénomènes qui disparurent rapidement et complètement, peut tout aussi bien s'appliquer à une hystérique.

Cette confusion avec l'hystérie, comme avec le vertige de Ménière, a du se produire plusieurs fois dans les anciennes observations et il n'est pas douteux qu'on ait eu une tendance trop marquée à étiqueter comme épileptiques quelques mouvements convulsifs de nature indéterminée, se passant dans les muscles du cou ou dans le menton du côté opposé, pendant les traitements appliqués à une oreille.

Dans d'autres cas encore la raison étiologique de l'épilepsie n'est pas suffisamment dégagée : ce seront par exemple des hérédo-syphilitiques porteurs d'otorrhée qui guériront sous l'influence combinée du traitement specifique et du traitement local.   Enfin il ne faut pas oublier que dans nombre de cas, la guérison de l'affection otique n'a pas fait disparaître l'épilepsie, de sorte qu'on est autorisé à penser à une simple coïncidence et non à une relation de cause à effet entre les deux maladies.

Pour ma part, j'ai à ma disposition dans mon service hospitalier un très grand nombre d'épileptiques (130 environ) et j'en vois beaucoup à ma consultation des maladies nerveuses.   L'examen systématique de ces malades m'a montré qu'il existait souvent chez eux des phénomènes auditifs en rapport avec les crises, et notamment des auras auditives sur lesquelles M. Gellé a attiré l'attention.   J'ai également vu la surdité plus ou moins passagère, comme M. Féré, à la suite des crises.* J'ai vu enfin coexister assez fréquemment les affections d'oreille et l'épilepsie sans pouvoir établir entre elles un lien de causalité.

J'avais donc conservé sur ce point un certain degré de scepticisme scientifique lorsque j'ai eu l'occasion de voir le cas suivant qui me démontra une fois de plus qu'en médecine il faut se garder des opinions absolues.

Hérédité tuberculeuse. Otorrhée double à l âge de 7 ans. Epilepsie à 13 ans. Disparition des crises après le traitement de l'otorrhée.

Le Né M., de Rive de Gier âgé de 26 ans, s'est présenté à moi le 16 avril 1897.

Le père est goutteux, non nerveux ; pas d'alcoolisme, ni de syphilis. La mère serait morte d'adénite (?) : elle paraît avoir été tuberculeuse. La grand'mère maternelle serait morte d'une pleurésie à 63 ans ; un oncle et une tante maternels sont morts tuberculeux et une autre tante est immobilisée au lit par une affection de la colonne vertébrale. Il n'y a pas d'affections nerveuses dans la famille.

Le malade est maigre, pâle, avec un gros crâne brachycéphale, des dents mauvaises, la voûte non ogivale, les oreilles en Wildermuth I avec solution de l'hélix à l'extrémité supérieure de la partie ascendante. Myopie assez forte. Sa force musculaire est faible, mais il dit se bien porter et affirme ne tousser jamais. On ne trouve absolument rien dans les viscères : il a au cou de cicatrices de glandes suppurées et il a eu récemment encore une petite fistule au côté gauche.

Il vient me consulter pour un écoulement de l'oreille droite. Les deux oreilles ont suppuré depuis l'âge de 7 ans, mais l'écoulement a cessé à gauche vers l'âge de 13 ans. Il persiste à droite, ce qui l'a fait réformer au conseil de révision.

Les deux tympans ont été complètement détruits : le manche est resté des deux côtés. A gauche il y a une cicatrice mince avec perforation persistante dans le quadrant postéro-supérieur : à droite la suppuration persiste d'ailleurs peu abondante accompagnée de nombreuses lamelles épidermiques : la cicatrisation est en voie de se produire et il existe seulement deux points ulcérés, rouges, en bas et en avant.

Pour la montre on a OD=contact osseux ; OG=4. Weber droit, mais difficile à faire préciser. L'expérience de Rinne est positive des deux côtés.

Le malade n'a pas de bourdonnements que lors des poussées aiguës qui se produisent du côté de l'otorrhée droite. Il ne paraît pas avoir de vertiges.

Il est épileptique. Les crises ont débuté à l'âge de 13 ans : d'abord espacées elles sont devenues très régulières et il ne se passe jamais six semaines sans qu'il s'en produise une. Elles sont très nettes et ont tous les caractères du mal comitial : cri initial, chute brusque (cicatrices sur le front et le nez), succession des phases tonique et clonique, écume à la bouche et morsure de la langue : les mictions involontaires sont rares. La grande majorité des crises sont nocturnes. La seule particularité qu'il y ait à noter dans celles de ces crises qui ont pu être observées pendant le jour, c'est qu'il a, au moment de la chute, un mouvement de gyration à droite et qu'il tombe sur le côté droit.

Le malade fut cathétérisé, mis au bromure de potassium et au traitement par l'acide borique pour l'oreille droite. Six semaines plus tard je notais une amélioration notable : l'oreille droite était sèche et percevait ma montre à 8 cm. : il n'avait pas pris de crise depuis plus de deux mois. Il ne veut plus prendre de bromure, dont il avait déjà absorbé de grandes quantités antérieurement et qui lui fatigue l'estomac.

---

*Le résultat de ces recherches sera consigné très prochainement dans la thèse d'un de mes élèves, M. Taillade.

Dix jours après, l'oreille droite se remit à couler et il eut une crise diurne violente le lendemain de cette suppuration renouvelée.

Le 31 août 1897, le malade n'avait repris qu'une nouvelle crise nocturne, et les oreilles étaient parfaitement sèches avec un petit trou seulement dans la cicatrice droite. Dans un certificat qu'il me demanda à ce moment pour l'administration où il est employé je disais que si on pouvait penser à une relation entre les crises et l'état des oreilles, il était impossible de l'affirmer.

A ce moment le malade fut perdu de vue, mais le 13 mars de la présente année il vient me faire une visite pour me dire que *ses crises avaient complètement disparu depuis que ses oreilles étaient définitivement sèches.* A vrai dire, il avait eu cependant deux vertiges ou crises très légères, l'une en février, l'autre en août 1898, mais il n'y attachait que peu d'importance en regard des crises violentes qui survenaient auparavant toutes les six semaines. L'aspect des tympans était le même, mais l'audition pour la montre avait très nettement augmenté, puisqu'on avait OD=20 à 25 et OG=10.

A noter que le malade n'avait jamais repris de bromure mais seulement, de temps à autre, du valérianate d'ammoniaque.

En résumé, il s'agit dans cette observation d'un homme prédisposé par son hérédité tuberculeuse à la dégénérescence nerveuse et à l'épilepsie (on sait que M. J. Voisin trouve l'hérédité tuberculeuse dans 28% des cas d'épilepsie), qui a une double otorrhée dès l'âge de 7 ans et qui devient épileptique à l'âge de la puberté. Sous l'influence du traitement dirigé presque exclusivement contre l'otite purulente, les crises s'espacent·et disparaissent même complètement lorsque l'oreille est guérie et que l'audition nulle au début est devenue moyenne. Au cours du traitement une récidive de l'otorrhée s'étant produite, le malade a eu une crise le lendemain.

Bien qu'on puisse faire à cette observation l'objection du " Post hoc, ergo propter hoc " et qu'on voie parfois des rémissions d'assez longue durée dans l'épilepsie, la relation de causalité me semble ici assez évidente. Il ne manque à cette observation pour être démonstrative que l'épreuve du temps, la guérison de l'épilepsie ne pouvant guère être tenue pour assurée que si plusieurs années se sont écoulées depuis la dernière crise. Il serait cependant désirable que les observations de ce genre fussent multipliées pour entrainer la conviction.

La conclusion qu'il importe surtout de tirer d'un cas de ce genre, c'est qu'il faut soigner systématiquement tous les épileptiques porteurs de lésions d'oreilles dans l'espoir de rencontrer parmi eux quelques cas aussi favorables.

On a Case of Nasal Hydrorrhœa.

Dr. Urbano Melzi, Milan.

We consider as a great rarity the continuous and copious secretion of a perfectly limpid liquid from the nostrils. I therefore think the description of a case of this nature which I have recently observed in my practice may be interesting. The case is one of a lady, aged 40, who does not present any symptoms of general disease, but who since a confinement six years ago has been affected with continuous and abundant discharge from the left nostril. The discharge is a perfectly colourless liquid, like water or the liquid of the pia mater, and is present in so great a quantity as to prevent the invalid from doing any work. It does not produce any excoriation of the vestibule of the nose or of the upper lip, over which it has been constantly running for so long a time. A handkerchief when drenched with it, if held before a fire and dried, remains unstiffened and without any mark, as if it had not been used. The liquid, odourless and colourless, is, according to the patient, also without taste.

The chemical and microscopic examination of the secretion made by Dr. Zenoni, of the Serotherapic Institute of Milan, gave the following result :—

Quantity of liquid : c.cm. 6·5.

Colour : slightly turbid, inclining to white, with a few very small whitish particles in suspension.

The liquid is very thin, fluid, watery, not viscous, odourless.

Specific gravity : 1009.

Reaction : slightly alkaline.

No precipitate with acetic acid :—absence of mucin.

No precipitate on heating :—absence of albumin.

Very slight turbidity on adding sulphate of ammonia, or a concentrated solution of NaCl., or absolute alcohol. The more important albuminoid seems to be a globulin, because if we let a drop of it fall into water we see a slight nubecula.

No turbidity on adding nitric acid in the cold.

No reaction with Fehling, no biuret reaction :—absence of sugar and peptone.

Copious milk-white precipitate on adding A_gNO_3 (after having acidulated the liquid with nitric acid).

On microscopic examination no morphological elements, numerous bacteria, some of which are disposed as zoogloea.

Water, 97·8%

Solids, 2·2% { Organic Substances, 0·8%
{ Inorganic „ 1·4%

The absence of reducing substances, the paucity of proteid substances, the slight turbidity as also some clinical considerations speak against the liquid being normal cerebro-spinal fluid. On the other hand the absence of mucin, the absence of morphological elements, the great quantity of inorganic substances are not characters corresponding to those of the liquid of nasal hydrorrhœa.

The liquid approaches lachrymal liquid in composition, having the same percentage of NaCl. However, I must say that a careful examination of the eyes made by Prof. Denti, of the Great Hospital of Milan, excluded every affection of the lachrymal apparatus.

The examination of the nose is almost impossible, because among the innumerable treatments tried by other specialists, general as well as local, there have been cauterizations which have left numerous synechiæ, closing the nostril almost completely. These synechiæ are perhaps in part due to the patient's treatment of herself, for the only method of obtaining even the slightest relief to her trouble she finds to be that of introducing deeply into the nostril plugs steeped in a saturated solution of cocain.

The sense of smell is preserved unchanged, relatively to the nasal stenosis which, according to the patient, did not exist before the disturbance began. Examination of the sinuses by transillumination gives negative results.

Vibratory massage of the nasal mucous membrane, undertaken by me through the little aperture which still remains in the nostril, at first relieved the trouble very much, but after a little while ceased to produce any benefit. It only remained for me to try the treatment, suggested by Lermoyez, with atropine internally and locally, and as a last resort the treatment recently suggested by Dr. Alexander of Berlin (Arch. f. Laryngol Bd. IX. H. 1) viz:—Massage of the nasal mucous membrane with plugs soaked in a 5% solution of protargol. By this means Dr. Alexander appears to have succeeded in curing an obstinate hydrorrhœa of long standing. I must confess that my hopes have been completely disappointed, because after a little improvement the patient returned in a few days in her previous condition.

In conclusion, from clinical and therapeutic considerations (the action of cocain) it is probable that this is a case of nasal hydrorrhœa, with a marked nervous element. The latter would explain in part the character of the liquid and the negative results of all treatments, whether general or local, suggested by the various authors.

On a Case of Endothelial Fibro-Angioma of the External Auditory Meatus.

Dr. Urbano Melzi, Milan.

I think it opportune to report this case to my colleagues, not so much for the position of the tumour—because although not very frequent, fibro-angiomata of the external auditory meatus are not very rare—as for its histological structure. The fact of the participation of endo- and perivascular endothelium in a connective-tissue neoplasm does not seem to me to be without interest.

The case is one of a girl of 22, of healthy and robust physical constitution, sent to me by one of my colleagues in the country that I might treat her for a polypus of the left ear. This, according to the doctor, was of some twelve month's standing, and caused an abundant secretion of pus from the ear. On examining the patient after careful cleansing, I found in the left external auditory meatus a tumour of the size of a bean, occupying all the lumen of the passage and giving exit to the pus that oozed from the deepest part. The tumour, of reddish-brown colour, of irregular and knotty surface, was movable, and took origin from the postero-superior wall of the meatus, so that I could easily take it away with a Wilde's polypus snare. On taking away the greater part of the tumour an abundant hæmorrhage took place, which I stopped with a very compact tampon of iodoform gauze. I immediately consigned the tumour to my colleague, Dr. Zenoni, for microscopical examination in order to learn the nature of the neoplasm, and so be guided in the treatment.

The result of the microscopic examination was as follows:—The tumour is of connective-endothelial nature, distinguishable from the real sarcomas, therefore of benign nature. The surface is covered with stratified pavement epithelium. Some parts are young, others older and more resistent. The former appear to be formed of a delicate stroma of fine, very loose, connective fibrils, among which are found rounded and polyhedral cellular elements with very evident nuclei. There are, besides, other cells with lamellated and slightly granular protoplasm, and a rather pale nucleus; sometimes two or three nuclei are present in one cell. The principal characteristic of the tumour consists of the numerous vessels that cross it in all directions, forming numerous anastomoses and sometimes disposed in groups presenting a plexiform aspect. These vessels are subject to special alterations, sometimes affecting the sheath, sometimes the endothelium of the internal membrane. The walls of the vessels appear for the most part thickened by proliferation, at the periphery, of the connective tissue, and of the endothelium. Where the fibrous network is thin and relaxed the vessels stand out clearly marked, but where the network is thicker and fasciculated the distinction is not so well marked. In the former positions the vessels are circular on section, in the latter positions the section is irregular and narrowed, owing to the compression produced by the tissue. At the same time owing to proliferation of the endothelial elements of the tunica intima, the calibre of the vessels is much reduced, and may even be obliterated. We can also observe an endothelial production of lamellated and star-shaped cells, which, by means of their processes, form a species of cellular network, both in the lumen of the vessels and round about them. From this, areas of endothelial connective tissue are formed, which soon lose the characteristics derived from their vascular origin, but retain the characters of the endothial elements. These areas in the older parts of the tumour are much poorer in cells, and are almost exclusively formed of bands of more or less compact, connective tissue, in which appear, here and there, either compressed blood-vessels or else blood-vessels with rather ample calibre. The fibrous connective tissue within the vessel walls is rich in young cells with rounded nuclei. It gradually undergoes fibrous transformation and produces connective tissue around the vessels. The endothelial elements of the perivascular lymphatics take part in this process : they present karyokinetic figures.

Gradually, as this proliferation increases, there is a decrease in the size of the fibrous intervascular areas, containing young cells, so that the intervals which separate the vessels from one another progressively diminish, and so that the vessels in the most compact parts become closely packed together.

The tumour, then, may be classed as an endothelial fibro-angioma.

In accordance with the microscopic examination I limited the further treatment of the tumour to a careful scraping of its base and to successive cauterizations, till the meatus presented a smooth and regular scar. After a short time the purulent secretion completely ceased, and the patient was dismissed cured.

On a Case of Retropharyngeal Abscess of Auricular Origin.

Dr. Urbano Melzi, Milan.

Among the different causes which may give rise to retropharyngeal abscess, one of the least frequent is doubtless old-standing or recent suppuration of the middle ear. In fact, in my researches into the literature of the subject I have only been able to find twenty-two cases cited. I therefore think that a case observed by me during May, 1898, is sufficiently interesting to be reported.

The case is one of a baby, two years old, who was put under my charge for suppuration of both ears. On otoscopic examination on either side I observed a large perforation of the tympanic membrane from which ran a considerable quantity of pus. After removal of the pus I saw the posterior wall of the tympanic cavity covered with granulations. After a few days of medication, consisting of washing with boric solution and instillation of alcohol with boric acid, the secretion of pus stopped completely in the left ear, persisted, however, in smaller quantity in the right, but after three weeks ceased completely. A month later the child had a bad attack of coryza and bronchitis, followed by pain and later by suppuration in both ears. I again began the washing and the instillation of alcohol with boric acid, and obtained marked improvement on the right side. After some days the child began to be feverish, and refused to take any food, complaining of pain in the throat, and her sleep was troubled and interrupted. She began also to snore. At the same time I observed a slight degree of stiff-neck, and a swelling and redness of the submaxillary region, whereas the mastoid region never presented any change.

Examination of the pharynx and of the nose showed marked congestion of the nasal and pharyngeal mucous membrane. I prescribed gargles, and insufflations in the nose, and a bladder of ice on the neck, but with little relief to the child. On the following day I heard from the relations that the child had refused all food, and during the night had had several attacks of suffocation. On examining the pharynx I discovered an enormous retropharyngeal abscess, which, on being opened, gave exit to a great quantity of pus. On examining with the probe I did not find any roughness of the vertebræ. Suspecting, therefore, that the cause of the abscess was the auricular suppuration, I made a bacteriological examination of the pus from the abscess, and that from the ear, and found the same bacteria in both. After a few days all tumefaction of the pharynx disappeared. The submaxillary swelling and the stiff neck also gradually passed off, and at the same time the discharge from the ear stopped.

When I saw the girl after three months' time, I found her in perfect health, with no disturbances on the part of the ear, the nose, or even the spinal column. This fact confirmed me in thinking that the cause of the retropharyngeal abscess was the auricular suppuration.

SUR LE TRAITEMENT DES OBSTRUCTIONS DE LA TROMPE D'EUSTACHE ET DE LA SURDITÉ CONSÉCUTIVE, PAR L'EMPLOI MÉTHODIQUE DES BOUGIES RÉGULIÈREMENT GRADUÉES.

DR. SUAREZ DE MENDOZA, Paris.

Depuis vingt ans je m'occupe d'une façon toute spéciale du traitement des obstructions de la trompe d'Eustache qui constitue comme on sait, une cause fréquente de la surdité.

Les besoins de chaque jour m'ont amené à créer quelques instruments qui ont été l'objet de plusieurs communications à diverses sociétés savantes. Aujourd'hui que la pratique me donne de plus en plus la conviction d'avoir été en cela, utile à mes malades, j'ai voulu soumettre mes instruments et ma méthode à votre savante et haute appréciation. D'autant plus que dans de récentes publications on a souvent oublié que j'ai été le premier à créer et à conseiller les bougies mathématiquement graduées (par dixièmes de millimètres) les seules qui permettent de mesurer exactement le calibre de la trompe et de franchir tout rétrécissement franchissable.

Voici, dans un ordre à la fois méthodique et chronologique les innovations et modifications que j'ai crû devoir apporter au traitement classique.

Dans les cas simples d'obstruction tubaire, lorsque l'insufflation pratiquée selon le procédé de Politzer ou à l'aide de la sonde d'Itard ne réussissait pas à faire pénétrer de l'air dans la caisse, je me suis bien trouvé du cathéterisme combiné, que je pratique depuis 1877. Je procède de la manière suivante : Le cathéter en place dans la trompe et mis en communication avec une poire à insufflation, je présente au malade un verre d'eau et un chalumeau en lui recommandant d'aspirer le liquide pendant que le ballon s'emplit d'air et d'avaler au moment précis où je presse la poire pour chasser l'air dans la caisse. Ce procédé m'a donné de bons résultats dans des cas où les moyens habituels d'insufflation restaient sans effet.

Contre les rétrécissements vrais ce moyen serait insuffisant et il me faut faire usage de mes instruments spéciaux, sondes et bougies.

Ces dernières sont, les unes en baleine, les autres en crin de Florence recouvert (boyau de ver à soie); certaines portent une armature métallique pour l'emploi de l'électricité. Elles forment trois séries, désignées suivant la forme de leur partie active, c'est à dire de leur extrémité pharyngienne : 1° bougies olivaires ; 2° cylindriques ; 3° cono-cylindriques. Chaque série se compose de onze bougies correspondant respectivement aux onze derniers numéros d'une filière que j'ai fait établir à cette fin et qui va progressivement d'un à quinze dixièmes de millimètres. Elles suivent ainsi une gradation très-douce et présentent en outre, l'avantage d'indiquer par leur numéro même, leur diamètre en dixièmes de millimètres. Je vais rapidement expliquer la destination et le mode d'emploi des unes et des autres.

Et d'abord, pour le diagnostic de l'obstruction, j'ai créé mes bougies olivaires en baleine. Ces bougies, *comme toutes celles en baleine deviennent, si on les met à baigner dans l'eau pendant au moins vingt-quatre heures, aussi souples que des bougies en gomme.* Ainsi préparées, elles acquièrent une grande souplesse, tout en conservant une rigidité suffisante pour vaincre la résistance lorsque le rétrécissement n'est pas tout à fait infranchissable pour le numéro employé.

Elles ont sur les bougies en celluloïd l'avantage de ne pas être fragiles et sur les bougies en argent celui d'être moins rigides et plus élastiques.

La bougie olivaire n'étant grâce à la saillie de son olive, en contact intime qu'avec un point du conduit, transmet des sensations très-nettes des actions que s'y produisent, et on perçoit très-bien soit la simple résistance, soit l'obstacle invincible, soit le franchissement de la portion rétrécie du canal.

On détermine le siège du rétrécissement au moyen d'une graduation faite ad hoc soit sur la partie libre de la bougie, c'est à dire non engagée dans le cathéter, soit sur une petite bande de bristol : en lisant sur cette graduation de combien, avant de s'arrêter, la bougie s'est avancée dans le cathéter, on voit de combien l'olive en dépasse le bout pharyngien, et par suite, quel point elle occupe dans la trompe ; c'est celui de la sténose.

Pour en connaître la longueur il faut avoir soin de noter le point où la bougie s'arrête dans sa marche, en avant de l'obstacle. Celui-ci franchi, on ramène l'olive en arrière jusqu'au dit obstacle ; on note ce nouveau point : alors l'écart existant entre ces deux indications donne, après déduction de la longueur de l'olive, l'étendue du rétrécissement.

Pour en apprecier le degré, il suffit, lorsque la bougie exploratrice s'est arrêtée, de choisir un numéro inférieur qui franchisse l'obstacle sans trop de frottement : le numéro de cette dernière bougie donne en dixièmes de millimètre, le calibre de la sténose, c'est à dire le degré de rétrécissement.

Pour le traitement j'ai fait établir deux séries de bougies, dont une série cylindrique en baleine, et l'autre en crin de Florence recouvert ; elles sont cylindro-coniques. Ces diverses bougies me servent d'abord pour la dilatation intermittente, conseillée par quelques auteurs, et qui suffit assez souvent dans les rétrécissements moyens, pour rétablir la perméabilité de la trompe ; en second lieu, pour pratiquer la dilatation progressive et continue, méthode que je préconise depuis onze ans contre les rétrécissements prononcés et qui m'a donné de nombreux succès. Mais si les mêmes bougies peuvent servir également contre les sténoses moyennes et les rétrécissements forts, leur mode d'emploi diffère absolument.

Pour ces derniers cas où la bougie dilatatrice doit rester plusieurs heures dans la trompe, j'ai dû, pour éviter au malade la gêne résultant de la présence d'un cathéter dans le nez, inventer la sonde gouttière à couvercle mobile. Cette sonde qui a encore pour but de faciliter la mise en place de la bougie dans la trompe présente dans toute sa longueur une fente assez large pour laisser sortir latéralement la dite bougie lorsqu'on l'expulsera de sa cannelure.

Je vais ici entrer dans quelques détails afin de bien faire saisir a simplicité extrême de mon procédé de mise en place et la facilité de la manœuvre. Tout d'abord, avant de glisser la bougie dans la sonde, je ferme préalablement la fente au moyen du couvercle qui s'ajuste à frottement doux contre la paroi interne de l'instrument et s'y maintient par le seul fait que son arc de courbure, c'est à dire, sa largeur, comprend un peu plus de la demi-circonférence intérieure de la sonde.

L'instrument armé de sa bougie je l'introduis dans la cavité nasale et engage son extrémité pharyngienne dans le pavillon de la trompe. Alors je pousse doucement la bougie dans ce canal. Quand elle a atteint la hauteur voulue, je retire le couvercle, puis à l'aide d'une tige cylindrique souple d'un diamètre égal au calibre de la sonde et que j'insinue entre sa paroi et la bougie, je déplace latéralement cette dernière et la fais sortir de l'instrument par sa fente longitudinale. Cela fait, je retire la sonde, coupe la bougie au niveau des narines, la fixe à l'aide d'un fil et d'un morceau de taffetas collé au voisinage du nez, puis la laisse à demeure le temps nécessaire—variant de deux à six heures—pour produire l'effet resolutif désiré. Les malades peuvent, pendant tout ce temps, vaquer à leurs occupations habituelles.

Pour certains cas très-rares qui résistaient à la dilatation simple et semblaient infranchissables, j'ai fait fabriquer des bougies métalliques à olive et armature en platine et recouvertes dans leur longueur d'une couche isolante, lesquelles me permettent d'employer l'action du courant continu. A l'aide de ces bougies conductrices et d'un faible courant galvanique d'un demi à un mille-ampère je suis arrivé à franchir des rétrécissements que l'emploi simple des diverses bougies n'avait pu vaincre.

Depuis près de vingt ans j'ai eu l'occasion de soigner plus de 360 cas de rétrécissement vrais, sur lesquels la dilatation progressive et continue soit simple, soit aidée du courant galvanique, ou de la galvano-caustique chimique m'a permis presque toujours de rétablir la perméabilité de la trompe et partant de guérir ou de soulager dans la mesure du possible, des malheureux voués au désespoir qui les conduit aux grandes interventions chirurgicales, qui dans l'espèce d'après une expérience de onze cas, n'augmentent pas *le résultat obtenu par l'emploi méthodique de la bougie.*

Je dis l'emploi méthodique de la bougie pour ne pas me servir du mot barbare de *bougirage* que je voudrais voir disparaître de notre littérature médicale.

DISEASES OF THE MASTOID, THEIR COURSE AND TREATMENT.

DR. FRANK S. MILBURY, Brooklyn, N.Y.

Before beginning the consideration of this paper, I wish to draw your attention for a few moments, to some of the anatomical features of the middle ear and mastoid.

It is in an air-containing space, lined throughout with mucous membrane, and continuous with the covering of the naso-pharynx and adjacent parts. Its divisions are the Eustachian tube, the tympanic cavity, and the mastoid cells. The first is the channel of connection between the pharynx and the tympanum, and consists of two portions, the cartilaginous and osseous; the widest opening being pharyngeal, and its narrowest point at the junction of the soft and the bony part. It is from one inch to one and one-third inches long, the osseous forming about one-third of its length, and the two portions meet at an obtuse angle. Its direction is obliquely outward, backward, and slightly upward. The tubal mucous membrane contains throughout a ciliated epithelium destitute of glands, the movements of the cilia being from the tympanic cavity, thus aiding in the drainage of the tympanum, and partially preventing its invasion by pathogenic organisms from the rhino-pharynx.

The tympanic cavity is an irregularly shaped pneumatic space with its longest diameters vertical and lateral, containing the ossicula, and consists of two portions, the atrium immediately behind the membrana tympani, and the attic which lies above the membrane. The communication between these two is quite narrow owing to the arrangement of the ossicles and folds of mucous membrane, and therefore a slight inflammation and swelling of the tissues may easily shut off the attic space, producing interference with its drainage, this being a serious factor in middle ear pathology. The mucous membrane lining the tympanic cavity is thin and delicate, and closely adherent with the underlying bone; its epithelium is usually tessélated, and may in places be ciliated, the latter being found most frequently in the vicinity of the Eustachian orifice. A little above, continuous and posterior to the attic, the mastoid antrum is situated, and is the only pneumatic space developed at birth, the others being formed subsequently. Not infrequently a second cell of considerable size is found at the tip of the process. The mastoid process, both externally and internally, varies greatly in its construction ; thus, we may have those which are entirely pneumatic, those which are pneumatic and diploetic, those which are wholly diploetic, and lastly, those which are altogether sclerotic excepting the antrum. Zuckerkandl, in the examination of 250 bones, found 36·8 per cent. completely pneumatic, while 42·8 per cent. were mixed diploetic and pneumatic, and 20·4 per cent. entirely diploetic or composed of dense osseous tissue throughout. These conditions are also found to vary on the two sides, one side being partly pneumatic and the other completely so. From such examinations it is evident that a sclerotic process does occur normally, as well as the result of inflammatory action. The position of the lateral sinus varies greatly in different individuals, sometimes being an inch or more posterior to the wall of the meatus, and, again, the bend of the sinus is so sharp, that it extends forward so near to the posterior wall of the meatus, that the opening of the antrum would be impossible without wounding this venous channel. To the operator, the position of the sinus and the middle cerebral fossa, is of special importance : and many efforts have been made, by the examination of specimens, measurements of the skull and its outward conformation, to determine the location of the sinus ; but all such researches have proved useless. Dr. Politzer states, that in 500 temporal bones which he examined, he found the position of the sinus most favourable when the mastoid process was strongly developed, and entirely filled with pneumatic cells. In these cases there is a broad space between the sigmoid sinus and the posterior wall of the external meatus ; which, in operating, permits access to the antrum without danger of wounding the sinus.   He found the relations less favourable in diploetic and compact mastoid processes.   How are we to know positively whether the process is diploetic or pneumatic ? Hence, for practical purposes these investigations prove as useless as others.

We will now take the individual mastoid diseases.

Primary mastoiditis is very rare, and when it does occur is usually the result of traumatism or exposure, but is sometimes without any traceable cause ; the latter is usually found in persons of a cachectic condition.   Only a few cases have been reported.

Secondary periostitis, however, is quite frequent, and is due to acute or chronic middle ear suppuration or necrosis ; the process extending outward from the tympanum, until the mastoid covering is reached.   It occurs oftener in adult than early life, owing to the much greater liability to ear disease.   In acute middle ear suppuration it is most frequent when free drainage is interfered with, as from a very small perforation badly placed, or from a possible pus retention by blocking up the opening with powders, such as acid boracic, alum, and some of the more adhesive new products.   The fluid must find exit, and will do so, at the point of least resistance.   This may be :—

1.   Through the external mastoid cortex, or into the external meatus ;

2.   Through the digastric fossa ;

3.   Through the roof of the antrum or the tympanic wall into the middle cranial fossa ;

4.   Into the posterior cranial fossa, by rupture usually, into the groove lodging the lateral sinus.

If the cranial cavity is invaded meningitis is induced and may be diffuse or circumscribed.   In the latter the limit appears to be caused by the formation of an epidural abscess ; the infectious material being walled in on all sides by adhesions between the dura and adjacent walls. Internal rupture may occur, or the free anastomosis between the blood-vessels and the dura and the pericranium may provide the channel through which the infectious material may pass to the brain, producing an intracranial abscess or a thrombosis of the lateral sinus.   Unfortunately these lesions often occur simultaneously, thus greatly increasing the danger to life.

Until within a comparatively recent period, the operation for acute disease of the mastoid was the principal surgical operation upon the ear.   It was near the end of the fifteen century that Piolanus proposed opening the mastoid cells ; later, about the year 1655, Sir Thomas Brown advised against such a procedure ; and it was not until 100 years later that the operation was first performed by Petit for the removal of secretions.   In 1776 Jassor performed the operation for necrosis of the bone with great success, but, after his decease, surgeons lost sight of the true indications for operating, and perforated the bone for various purposes, until the death of Bergen, a noted Danish surgeon, upon whom the operation was performed for the relief of deafness, and ended in fatal meningitis. This caused the procedure to fall into disrepute, and nearly a century elapsed before it was revived by Forget (1849), Follin, and Tröltsch (1859).

When there was inflammation, swelling, and tenderness over the mastoid, Tröltsch made an incision down to the bone to prevent necrosis, and if the symptoms indicated a deeper seat of the disease he perforated the bone with a blunt probe. To prevent injury to the brain or lateral sinus, he placed the instrument on a line with the meatus, and worked it forward and inward in a horizontal plane. If the cortex was thick, he used a small trephine. The sinus was kept open by means of a piece of gauze.

To Schwartze is due the credit of developing the operation; by 1883 he had reported 100 cases, which was the largest number reported up to that time.

Acute inflammation of the mastoid cells varies according to the stage in which the patient comes under observation. Acute otitis media without perforation is often accompanied by symptoms of mastoid irritation, which usually subside with slight antiphlogistic measures. In acute inflammation of the mastoid cells the prominent symptoms are (1) Intense continuous pain over the mastoid and radiating over the side of the head and into the neck, which is increased on pressure and percussion, redness, heat and œdema of the skin. When the abscess becomes localized the pain generally remains fixed at one point. (2) The membrana tympani appears strongly bulged forward before the pus perforates; following perforation a nipple-like projection is often found in the posterior-superior quadrant of the membrane, on the tip of which the perforation is situated. (3) A swelling and bulging of the posterior-superior wall of the canal, causing a narrowing of its lumen, and shutting from view all, or a part of the membrane. These two latter points are very indicative symptoms. Free discharge from the ear exists, which rarely ever ceases while the mastoid inflammation continues. However, the only absolutely positive sign of a mastoid abscess is pus found within its interior on opening it. The temperature usually ranges from 99·5° to 102°, but seldom higher.

The course of the affection varies considerably in different cases, in some running to a fatal termination in a few days, and in others occupying weeks and months and possibly years to indicate positive symptoms. In chronic otitis media purulenta the extension to the mastoid is often without characteristic symptoms. The quality and quantity of the discharge vary greatly, now very slight, now copious, according as to whether there is a narrow or free outlet for drainage from attic and antrum. A thickened cheesy pus may exist for a long time in the mastoid cells without indicating itself by any symptoms except a stubborn, fœtid otorrhœa, resisting cure in spite of thorough cleansing of the tympanic cavity. We may be almost sure of retention of pus in the antrum, provided caries of the external canal, ossicles or walls of the tympanic cavity can be excluded.

Inflammation of the mastoid process and fever only occur through traumatism or the retention of pus in the cells. They may subside only to reappear. Sharp pain on pressure, united with œdema, may have existed a long time without producing any perceptible change of periosteum and the bone surface. If the bone is greatly sclerosed and very dense, and the cortex much thickened, which may be congenital or occur as a result of chronic middle ear suppuration, such acute symptoms may never arise, even in a long course of the disease. However, the absence of the same cannot be looked upon favourably as a prognostic sign, for it is often just such cases that prove rapidly fatal through pyæmia. Zaufal and others have called attention to the frequent existence of optic neuritis, neuro-retinitis, and choked disc, in inflammation of the mastoid process, at times bilateral, at times unilateral, and not always on the affected side. The *course* of the morbid process in bone affection varies in different cases. Extension of the inflammation in an outward direction, with periostitis and abscess, is the most common course. Several such abscesses in more or less rapid succession, over the mastoid process, are indicative of disease of the bone. Occasionally the pus finds its way down the side of the neck, and forms a swelling of considerable size ; or it may pass forwards to the side of the pharynx, and downwards even as far as the pleura ; or, it may extend into the cranial cavity, and set up trouble in the lateral sinus, or involve the Fallopian aqueduct and the membranes of the brain.

Next to opening through the cortex of the mastoid, the most frequent point is through the posterior-superior wall of the external canal. If not recognised early it may cause such excessive bulging of the canal wall as to prevent free discharge. If seen at the proper time a generous opening followed by copious syringing may suffice to empty the mastoid process of all deleterious substances, such as pus, cholesteatoma, the cheesy exudate, epidermis masses, and even sequestra if very small. Bezold has well described those uncommon cases as mentioned above. When rupture takes place towards the digastric groove, or on the median surface of the mastoid process, owing to its deep position beneath the fascia, the pus easily finds its way into the deep sub-muscular tissues, and along the course of the large vessels, which causes the swelling in the side of the neck with abscess formation. In the early stages no perceptible difference may be seen between the sound and the diseased side. After the swelling beneath and on each side of the sterno-cleido-mastoid muscle has developed, deep pressure over the tip of the mastoid elicits acute pain. An early recognition of the condition is necessary, since from the consolidation of the parts invasion of the cranial cavity is likely to occur. In favourable cases the carious and necrotic portions are exfoliated, the granulation tissue is absorbed, and healing takes place. Several good recoveries have been reported, even after the whole of the mastoid process has been exfoliated. Again, only small portions of bone may be detached, and fistulous openings may remain indefinitely or until properly dealt with.

The prognosis in these cases of mastoid disease varies with the cause, extent, and severity of the affection, and with the general health of the patient. Following an acute otitis media, and promptly attended to, the prognosis is usually favourable, but in some such cases the advance may be so rapid as to baffle all our efforts to check it. It is unfavourable in tuberculosis, and in chronic purulent otitis with pent-up secretions, in cases that have been neglected, and in which there is a history of intermittent febrile attacks, and of several previous attacks referable to the mastoid region which have disappeared spontaneously or under palliative measures. The prognosis is always serious whenever there are symptoms of extension of inflammation to the membranes of the brain. Attacks of partial or complete unconsciousness, restlessness and feverishness, are of extremely grave import when occurring in a person suffering from disease of the mastoid process.

In the treatment, if the case is seen early, an attempt should be made to abort the attack by antiphlogistic measures. If the membrana tympani appears greatly congested, swollen and bulged outward, simultaneously with pain in the mastoid process, which is increased on pressure, a paracentesis of the membrana tympani should be made at once to permit the pus in the middle ear an opportunity of free exit ; and a spontaneous rupture, when not sufficiently large, must be enlarged. After free drainage has been obtained, frequent antiseptic irrigations should be instituted and carried out faithfully. A brisk purge should be administered. The application of cold to the mastoid by means of the icebag, iced cloths, or, what is better, the Leiter coil. The ear may be syringed with the apparatus in place. It is better to keep the coil in position continuously for 24 hours, and under no condition should it be kept on more than from 40 to 50 hours. Painting with iodine, blood-letting by means of leeches, and rest in bed. In influenza cases the Leiter coil does not appear very effectual in stopping the formation of abscesses. Cold is usually very soothing, and borne well. Often the pain will entirely disappear through these means while the patient is in bed and quiet, but on exertion in his duties they return. And thus it is said by some writers that if marked improvement has not occurred within 48 hours, operative treatment will be necessary subsequently, if not at once. If abortive measures have not been successful, then operative interference must be resorted to, and the following are symptoms as laid down by Politzer and others generally recognised as indicating the operation.

(1) Painful inflammatory infiltration of the covering of the mastoid process, especially if an accompanying narrowing of the meatus, or obstruction of the tympanum by granulations, renders it probable that a septic condition exists in the mastoid process. The operation becomes imperative when there is high fever and signs of meningeal irritation ; and when the symptoms in the mastoid process have repeatedly occurred and resisted all antiphlogistic treatment.

(2) Spontaneous pain in the mastoid process, increased by pressure, and accompanied by bulging of the posterior-superior wall of the meatus.

(3) Persistent or occasionally remittent pain in the mastoid process, with marked tenderness, even if there be no swelling of the external integument, and no apparent obstruction to the escape of discharge from the tympanic cavity.

(4) When cholesteatoma exists in the tympanic cavity and cannot be removed, or if after its extraction along with the malleus and incus the condition is not improved by careful irrigation.

(5) Fistulæ in the mastoid region and gravitation abscesses below it.

(6) Extensive caries and necrosis of the posterior osseous wall of the meatus.

(7) In all cases of middle ear suppuration, during which symptoms of meningeal irritation or of incipient sinus-phlebitis make their appearance.

(8) Continued septic suppuration in the attic, the symptoms remaining unchanged after removal of the malleus and incus and after several months energetic treatment, even if there are no general symptoms excepting an offensive otorrhœa.

(9) Pain in the mastoid process developing in certain rare cases of connective tissue hypertrophy, in osteo-sclerosis, and in osseous scars after the healing of a mastoid operation.

The Operation. A few hours before the operation the patient should be given a thorough bath ; the parts within a radius of three or four inches of the ear carefully shaved, and, if a man, the beard removed ; then the whole side of the head and neck energetically washed with soap and water, rinsed with sterilized water, and rubbed with ether to remove all oily substances. The ear is syringed with a solution of bichloride of mercury (1 to 1000) and a wet dressing of the same is applied over the entire field of operation until the patient is anæsthetized.

The antiseptic dressing is removed and the parts again cleansed with bichloride, and the ear tamponed. All instruments are sterilized by boiling, and the hands and dress of the operator and assistants should

receive the same careful attention as is demanded in all surgical operations. To some all these precautions may seem unnecessary, but when
doing a mastoid operation the surgeon never knows what he may be
compelled to do, as owing to anomalous position of the parts, or to
extensive necrosis, the cranial cavity may be entered, either accidentally,
or intentionally.

The incision through the soft parts should be made from the tip of the
mastoid and carried upward in a curved line $\frac{1}{4}$ of an inch posterior
to the insertion of the auricle and to its upper attachment. It is better
to make the cut, if possible, with one sweep of the knife. This is
practically what is known as Wilde's incision, and has been greatly
overestimated, as it is only admissible in children where the cortex is
very thin and may be opened by firm pressure of the knife, or sharp
curette, or pus may find an outlet. In the adult, however, experience
has taught all operators that it is not advisable to stop here, as the
cortex is too dense and non-permeable. It certainly is not wise to do
this and delay to ascertain what further may develop, and subject the
patient to a second anæsthetization and operation when both should
have been completed at first. Dench states that the division of the soft
parts within the meatus over the mastoid practically meets all the
indications of external incision. Next, elevate the periosteum, pushing
the entire anterior flap forward. The bleeding vessels should be taken
up with artery forceps or ligated. The parts are held back with
retractors, so that a good view of the posterior and superior margins
of the bony canal are distinctly seen, and the whole field of operation
laid bare. The bone should be carefully examined for fistulæ or carious
spots, which, if found, will serve as a guide for entrance into the bone.
If none is found, we proceed to open into the antrum, which is just
behind the posterior margin of the meatus, and just below its superior
margin. Until entrance has been gained to the antrum the opening
through the cortex should never extend above the superior wall of the
meatus, and should keep close to the posterior wall, thus avoiding the
middle cranial fossa and a possible wounding of the lateral sinus which
may be misplaced. The cortex is best removed with a broad chisel and
mallet, which is held parallel to the surface of the skull, and the bone
is cut away in thin, broad chips, the opening extending inward and
forward and gradually lessening in size until the antrum is reached.
This never lies less than half an inch below the surface, although large
pneumatic spaces may be found near the surface, which may lead us
astray unless we are cautious. To prove it, bend a probe at the tip and
pass it downward, forward and inward for a distance of $\frac{3}{4}$ of an inch or
more, at which depth it should pass into the tympanic cavity ; thus we
know that the antrum has been reached and passed through.

Having gained a free entrance to the antrum, any particles of bone,
cholesteatomatous masses or granulations, must be removed, and the

DD

opening to the middle ear freely curetted and enlarged to give sufficient drainage. We occasionally read of cases where, after penetrating to the extreme line of safety (about $\frac{5}{8}$ of an inch) no antrum is reached, and the operation is abandoned. This need never happen. After cutting to the usual depth without finding the cavity, the rule should be adopted to direct our canal more forward so as to bring its apex over the meatus, when we can easily chisel into the attic. The membranous meatus may be dislodged from the posterior wall and pushed forward or the entire cartilaginous meatus turned out, thereby making entrance to the attic quite easy. The latter method will apply to a sclerotic process. If, after entering the antrum, no pus is found, the large cell at the apex of mastoid must be particularly investigated, all carious and necrotic bone removed from mastoid, and its tip excised if carious.

The operation should be continued until sound bone is encountered in every direction. If the inner plate is diseased it may be removed with almost perfect safety, as an exposure of the dura is not a grave matter under proper precautions, whereas to leave carious bone at this point is very dangerous. Exposure or even a wound of the lateral sinus, either accidentally or intentionally, is not so serious a matter as it has heretofore been considered. It can be recognized by its bluish-grey colour. If the vessel is opened sharp hemorrhage ensues, which, if easy of access, may be readily controlled by a firm compress of iodoform gauze held by an assistant, and the operation is proceeded with as if this had not happened.

The good effects of opening the mastoid antrum and cleansing the middle ear are often manifested within a few hours of the operation. The pain and temperature are both diminished, alarming symptoms subside, while the state of the middle ear rapidly improves. Subsequent to the operation where the septic suppuration continues after weeks or months of careful treatment, there is probably a carious affection of the tympanic cavity or ossicula. If lumps of epidermis repeatedly appear in the irrigating fluid it is certain that there is a cholesteatoma in the attic, which indicates an operation on the tympanic cavity which will be described later.

Having completed the operation, dressing the wound is in order. I insert into the antrum a drainage tube, and pack loosely around it dry iodoform gauze, but not the external wound, merely keeping their edges separated by a strip of gauze. A tampon is placed in the meatus and the whole well covered with sterilized gauze and cotton. With a favourable course of healing it is sufficient to change the bandage every five or six days. If the temperature does not exceed 101° at any time during the first five or six days, or if it is not persistently elevated, there will be no necessity for changing the dressing. When the dressing is changed for the first time the wound and canal should be irrigated with a sublimate solution (1 in 8,000 or 10,000), and the wound cavity examined carefully for remaining granulations and roughness, which, if found, must be scraped away.

If there is a return of pain after the operation, increased temperature, and much septic discharge which would be indicated by a rapid soaking of the bandage and foetid odour, a daily change of dressing is indicated. So long as the secretion is ill-smelling I use sublimate solution in the strength indicated above. After the bad smell disappears, I use a one per cent. acid boracic solution. This must be continued until suppuration ceases. The proposition of Küster and Bergmann, that the syringing out of the operation cavity should be avoided, has not been sustained by the profession. So long as there is suppuration in the tympanic cavity the communication between it and the wound must be kept open for free drainage, and only when there is a certainty that suppuration has ceased may the wound be allowed to heal. Occasionally, there remains, after the most careful treatment, a sinus in the mastoid process connected with an abscess cavity which requires a second operation. The duration of after treatment varies from three or four weeks to one or two years before suppuration ceases. Sometimes the suppuration cannot be controlled no matter what is done.

It is wonderful what beneficial effect the operation often has upon the general system, which may be readily understood when we realize that before the operation the blood had been kept constantly in a more or less septic condition.

Since 1891 the mastoid operation described above was the typical one, but the collective experience in aural surgery for the last few years has shown that it proves insufficient in many cases, and so search for a more effectual process has developed several methods. In 1891, Stacke, of Erfurt, Germany, made known a new operation in chronic cases, based upon the surgical principles involved in the treatment of suppurations within rigid walled cavities ; namely, upon the complete and free laying open of the cavity, so that it can be curetted, tamponed, and treated surgically, and the operator not compelled to satisfy himself with a more or less imperfect irrigation. The method of Stacke is practically as follows : The cutaneous incision is made a little differently than has been described, the upper part being kept closer to the auricle and carried well around to the front. The lower end must also curve more forward and extend to the tip of the process, the cut, as it were, circumscribing the auricle. The bone being bared, the membranous meatus is separated from the posterior and superior walls, and its attachment internally being cut, is in its entirety shelled out of the osseous canal. With a small gouge or Dench's cutting forceps the most medial portion of the superior wall of the superior meatus (lower lateral wall of the attic) is cut away, and, if present, the malleus and incus removed. The superior wall is to be chiselled away near the drum insertion till a bent sound touching the tegmen tympani meets with no resistance on being drawn outward. The probe, as a guide, is then turned toward the antrum, and the posterior wall of the meatus chiselled away till that cavity is freely opened up. In this way Stacke converts attic, tympanum, antrum and meatus into one large cavity. After cleansing, the auricle is replaced, sutured, the lining membrane of osseous canal split and pressed as far back into the enlarged cavity as possible, by the iodoform gauze. All subsequent treatment is done through meatus.

This operation proving extremely difficult and unsatisfactory, other methods were suggested, and now what may be known as the Schwartze-Bergmann-Stacke operation has been quite generally adopted, and my experience has taught me that it is the ideal one in all chronic conditions, which have resisted cure after the ossicula have been removed. I now rarely perform any other, and am exceedingly happy with the results obtained. It is much quicker, easier and safer than the Stacke, and is done as follows: The incision over the mastoid and entrance to antrum is made as in the original mastoid operation. The membranous meatus is dislodged as in the Stacke and held well forward by a retractor. The operative field now shows the posterior-superior osseous canal, the antrum and a bridge of bone separating them. This bridge is now removed by rongeur forceps and chisel, the section being triangular in shape, the apex at the neck of the antrum. Thus the antrum, tympanum, and meatus will be converted into one large cavity. Care must be taken at this point not to wound the facial and semicircular canals which lie directly across from this point. As a protection, a sound is passed through the antrum into the middle ear, or, if not possible in that direction, from the middle ear as far as possible into the antrum, and if we confine our operating down to that, we will be within safe grounds. A wound to the external semicircular canal is more unlikely to occur than one to the facial nerve.

As much of the bone should be removed as is compatible with safety, so as to make the antrum and attic as accessible as possible from the external canal. There must, however, be a ridge between the meatus and the antrum (see Allen, p. 103). In this operation I find the dental engine a most useful adjunct. The posterior membranous canal is now split outwardly to the concha as in the Stacke, and pressed back as far as possible into the enlarged cavity and held in place by tamponing.

According to Stacke, the tamponing of the membranous meatus into the artificial opening has a double advantage: (1) It secures the formation of a persistant skin-covered communication between the antrum and the meatus. (2) It is a skin transplantation, from which the formation of epidermis over the entire cavity can take place. The better way, I believe, is to suture the wound over the mastoid and get primary union if possible, and do the entire treatment through the meatus.

If all goes well the dressings are to remain five or six days, after which daily tamponing must be most carefully followed out.

The granulations must be kept down and the cavity kept as freely accessible and of the same size as just after the operation. Even when the utmost care is taken, minute necrotic pieces of bone become surrounded by granulations, small fistulous canals are formed leading to these dead pieces, around which the suppuration continues even after it has entirely ceased elsewhere.

The duration of the after treatment varies in these cases also, but is, on an average, as experience has shown, several months shorter than by the old method, and the cure is much more permanent. The indications for this operation are about the same as for the ordinary mastoid operation.

Le vie nasali e auricolari dell'infezione endocranica.

Prof. Camillo Poli, Genoa.

Appena una quindicina d'anni fa uno studio che si proponesse di indagare i varii momenti eziologici dell'infezione endocranica, se poteva rispondere a un desiderio di indole puramente scientifica, non avrebbe potuto aspirare a quella alta importanza pratica alla quale oggi, dopo le mirabili risorse della chirurgia endocranica, ha veramente diritto. Si può anzi dire che pochi argomenti meritano in questo momento una ampia trattazione e hanno bisogno di contributi sperimentali e clinici come quelli che, ricercando le cause e studiando il decorso delle varie forme che può assumere l'infezione endocranica, facilitano nei singoli casi la diagnosi di natura e di sede e indicano a tempo al chirurgo quale debba essere il suo contegno.

Che se anzi si studia, come osservano Broca e Maubrac, l'evoluzione clinica delle lesioni intracraniche, a parte, s'intende, quelle in cui si è guidati da un segno fisico esterno visibile e tangibile, si arriva presto a convincersi che la diagnosi di esistenza, di natura e anche di sede di queste lesioni è generalmente subordinata alla nozione eziologica.

L'ovoide cranico, considerato dal punto di visto dalla sua resistenza, mentre presenta in corrispondenza della vòlta delle condizioni pressochè uniformi per la struttura e lo spessore delle ossa che lo compongono, offre in corrispondenza della base notevoli variazioni per il numero grande di fori e canali che lo attraversano ma sopratutto per l'esistenza di particolari cavità di varia grandezza e disposizione alcune delle quali sono separate dalla cavità cranica da pareti ossee sottilissime e talora incomplete. Si potrebbe pertanto dire che mentre il contenuto cranico è bene protetto superiormente e ai lati, è minato al di sotto per l'esistenza di cunicoli e di spazii cavi la cui presenza assume una vitale importanza ogni qualvolta si stabilisce in essi un processo suppurativo acuto o cronico *(vedi figura)*.

Di tali spazi, distribuiti sui vari segmenti della base, quelli in rapporto alle cavità nasali dominano particolarmente la fossa cranica anteriore, mentre quelli destinati a ricettare l'organo dell'udito sono in rapporto colle fosse craniche media e posteriore.

Appartengono al primo gruppo, oltre le cavità nasali propriamente dette, i seni da esse dipendenti, quali i seni frontali, etmoidali, sfenoidali e mascellari, mentre fanno parte del secondo gruppo la tuba e la cavità timpanica, il sistema delle cellule mastoidee e il labirinto.

Dai rapporti che tali cavità hanno coi diversi segmenti della base si può già pertanto fin d'ora arguire che l'infezione procedente dalle cavità nasali e seni annessi (eccettuato lo sfenoidale) prediligerà la fossa cranica anteriore e tenderà a localizzarsi nel lobo frontale, mentre l'infezione procedente dall'orecchio risiederà preferibilmente nelle fosse craniche media e posteriore, epperò rispettivamente nel lobo temporo-sfenoidale e nel cervelletto.

Le varie forme che riveste l'infezione endocranica sono la meningite, la trombosi infettiva e l'ascesso. Tali forme si presentano talvolta isolatamente, tal altra associate.

Le vie per le quali una infezione stabilitasi in una di tali cavità può raggiungere il contenuto endocranico possono essere rappresentate:

1.° da fori o canali preesistenti normali od anomali (deiscenze);

2.° da rapporti vascolari sanguigni o linfatici;

3.° da una morbosa distruzione delle loro pareti.

Si comprende pertanto come lo studio di tali vie sia connesso con ricordi anatomici, che occorre di rilevare, sia pure in modo sommario.

(A) FORI E CANALI PRESISTENTI NORMALI ED ANOMALI (DEISCENZE).

CAVITÀ NASALI.—L'intimità di rapporti esistenti fra le cavità nasali e la cavità endocranica si rileva sopratutto da ciò che, in corrispondenza del tratto orizzontale della vôlta, la dura madre da una parte e la mucosa nasale dall'altra, non sono divise che per l'intermezzo della lamina cribrosa dell'etmoide.

Ad onta però dell'esistenza di molteplici fori, non sembra questa la via abituale di diffusione di un processo suppurativo dalle cavità nasali al contenuto cranico. Solo in un caso descritto da Chiari, nel quale per una anomalia di formazione esisteva un difetto tra l'estremo anteriore della lamina cribrosa e la parte contigua dell'osso frontale, si verificò un ascesso del lobo frontale.

Più frequenti sembrano essere i difetti di formazione della lamina papiracea, per modo che attraverso ad essi è resa facile una comunicazione fra le cellule etmoidali e l'orbita e di quì alla cavità cranica. È molto probabile anzi che, come trovano una simile spiegazione i vari casi di enfisema dell'orbita sotto una violenta espirazione (Berlin), così debbano spiegarsi i casi più numerosi di flemmoni orbitali, seguiti spesso da una trombo-flebite oftalmica con diffusione al seno cavernoso e alle meningi (casi di Leber e di Vigla).

Il seno frontale, separato in condizioni normali dalla cavità cranica per mezzo della sua parete posteriore, e dall'orbita per la sua parete inferiore, può presentare, secondo le ricerche di Zuckerkandl, dei difetti tanto verso il cranio che verso l'orbita. Dei varii casi però di sinusite frontale, nei quali si è potuto accertare la via seguita dall'infezione, solo in due, descritti da Hoppe e da Gibson, si ebbe, per una lacuna preesistente nella parete posteriore, qualz complicazione intracranica, una meningite.

Anche il seno sfenoidale può, secondo Zuckerkandl, presentare delle deiscenze sotto forma di piccoli vani situati sulla parete laterale e conducenti nella fossa cranica media. Non sono però noti casi di infezione endocranica per tale via preesistenté.

Del seno mascellare non si conoscono altre vie di comunicazione oltre l'ostio per cui sta in rapporto colle fosse nasali. Possono però esistere, sempre sulla parete interna, degli ostii secondarii.

APPARATO UDITIVO.—La cavità timpanica è per molteplici vie in rapporto colla contigua cavità cranica.

A parte le deiscenze, fatte già conoscere da Hyrtl sul *tegmen tympani* e accertate 167 volte da Burkner su 765 crani, deiscenze attraverso alle quali però sono rari i casi bene accertati di una diffusione dell'infezione, il cavo timpanico è in rapporto diretto per la sua parete interna, mediante la finestra ovale e rotonda col labirinto e per esso col contenuto endocranico. Dal labirinto può infatti il pus raggiungere la cavità cranica o sulla guida dell'acustico verso il foro uditivo interno, o per l'acquedotto del vestibolo verso la fossa cranica posteriore (Rhoden e Kretschman) o per l'acquedotto della chiocciola, raggiungendo verso la faccia inferiore della rocca in corrispondenza del suo sbocco nella fossa giugulare, lo spazio subaracnoideo. È anzi probabile, osserva a questo proposito Körner, che alcuni casi di leptomeningiti, la cui origine auricolare resta nella sezione poco chiara, sieno derivati per quest'ultima via.

Un'altro mezzo di diffusione è rappresentato dal canale del facciale, e ciò specialmente in grazia dei rapporti che esso ha col cavo timpanico (eminentia pyramidalis : canalicolo della corda del timpano) e delle facili deiscenze che esso offre nel suo tratto intratimpanico. Sulla guida del canale di Faloppio può l'infezione raggiungere la fossa cerebrale posteriore per il *porus acusticus internus* o la fossa media per l'*hyatus Faloppii.*

Rapporti meno diretti ha il cavo timpanico cogli organi endocranici mediante la sua parete anteriore (canalicoli carotidei : cellule tubarie, *Urbantschitsch*) e la parete inferiore (deiscenza del pavimento timpanico).

Parlano in favore di tali vie di diffusione tre casi raccolti da E. Maier alla clinica di Schwartze nei quali un processo suppurativo auricolare terminò con una trombo-flebite del seno cavernoso propagatasi lungo il canale carotico.

In un caso osservato da Tröltsch la complicanza endocranica derivò dalla penetrazione del pus attraverso le cellule tubarie verso l'apice della rocca.

Che le deiscenze del pavimento timpanico possano favorire l'insorgenza di una trombosi del contiguo golfo della giugulare lo confermano i casi di Holst, Burkner, Iacobson e Körner. Quest'ultimo autore anzi osserva che tale trombo-flebite succede probabilmente molto più spesso di quanto lo lasci supporre la scarsa casuistica, e ciò per la ragione che molti di simili casi rimangono alle sezioni ignorati perchè raramente si porta l'attenzione sui rapporti tra il pavimento del timpano e la fossa giugulare.

La parete posteriore del cavo timpanico guida per l'*aditus ad antrum* al sistema mastoideo, costituito, come è noto, dall'antro e dalle cellule più o meno sviluppate. Nei casi di forte sviluppo non è raro trovare delle deiscenze vuoi in corrispondenza del tetto, epperò in rapporto alla fossa cerebrale media, vuoi in corrispondenza del solco sigmoideo nella fossa cerebrale posteriore. Che possa in simili contingenze trovare il pus una via preformata per l'invasione endocranica lo conferma il caso descritto da Gähde. Analoghe deiscenze del sistema aerifero mastoideo furono pure constatate da Körner in un punto che corrisponde alla parte più esterna del condotto uditivo nell'angolo che la parete laterale della fossa media fa col pavimento della fossa medesima.

(B) VASI SANGUIGNI E LINFATICI.

CAVITÀ NASALI.—Avuto riguardo al nostro scopo dobbiamo portare una speciale attenzione al sistema venoso. A parte la considerazione che la rete venosa, originando dai corpi cavernosi della mucosa nasale sta per reciproche anastomosi intimamente connessa, si può, secondo Zuckerkandl, suddividere tale sistema in varii gruppi dei quali noi dobbiamo sopratutto tener conto di due; l'uno, costituito dalle vene etmoidali e diretto in alto verso la cavità cranica ed orbitaria, l'altro rivolto in dietro e in alto verso la fossa pterigo-palatina.

Le vene dirette verso la cavità cranica si anastomzziano col plesso venoso della dura madre e con quello del seno falciforme superiore. Esiste poi un'altro rapporto più importante, sul quale particolarmente Zuckerkandl richiamò l'attenzione, fornito da una vena che accompagna una grossa branca dall'arteria etmoidale anteriore e che penetra nella fossa cranica anteriore attraverso la lamina cribrosa. Questa vena si inoscula sia col plesso venoso del tratto olfattivo sia con una grossa vena a livello del lobo orbitale ed è da ritenersi, secondo Zuckerkandl, che la corrente sanguigna in questa vena sia normalmente diretta verso il cervello. Verso questo gruppo venoso superiore confluiscono particolarmente le vene dei seni frontali e delle cellule etmoidali.

Per tali rapporti anatomici noi ci diamo ragione della relativa frequenza di una trombo-flebite del seno longitudinale o dei cavernosi per l'intermezzo della vena oftalmica, riscontrate nei casi di sinusite frontale. Tale era il rapporto anatomo-patologico in 3 dei 19 casi raccolti da Dreyfuss.

Il gruppo venoso postero-superiore, diretto verso il foro palatino e che raccoglie in gran parte il sangue refluo della mucosa dei turbinati medio e inferiore e dell seno mascellare, si anastomizza col plesso venoso della fossa pterigoidea. I rapporti anastomotici che tale plesso contrae colle vene orbitali spiegano la possibilità di propagarsi di una infezione verso il cranio per la fessura sfeno-orbitale.

Un caso assai caratteristico nel quale un empiema cronico del seno mascellare determinò per la descritta via venosa una trombo-flebite del seno cavernoso fu descritto da Foucher.

Il seno sfenoidale contrae tali intimi rapporti coi seni cavernoso e coronario che non fa meraviglia di rilevare come dei 13 casi raccolti da Dreyfuss in 7 sia segnalata una trombo-flebite di tali seni a cui spesso si associa una meningite. In tali casi la diffusione avvenne particolarmente per le vene diploiche, previo distacco della mucosa dall'osso per un processo di periostite.

Una diffusione per le vene diploiche, che specialmente viene in considerazione per il suo sfenoidale, in cui il fatto fu da Ostmann constatato microscopicamente su pezzi decalcificati, si può verificare anche per altri casi, e ciò specialmente, come vedremo, per le complicanze otitiche.

Per quanto riguarda i linfatici della mucosa nasale è da rilevarsi il fatto importante segnalato fino dal 1869 da Schwalbe dell'esistenza cioè di una unione fra i linfatici degli spazi subdurali e subaracnoideali con quelli della mucosa nasale.

Le ricerche successive di Axel Key e Retoius sugli animali confermarono tale fatto fino a mettere in evidenza l'esistenza di una comunicazione aperta, attraverso canalicoli speciali situati nell'epitelio della mucosa, fra la cavità sottoaracnoidea e sottodurale coll'aria esterna. Quantunque tali condizioni non siano state finora ampiamente confermate nell'uomo, resta però, per il fatto inconstatabile rilevato da Schwalbe, aperta la possibilità a una diffusione dell'infezione per la via linfatica. Non è pertanto improbabile che talune complicanze intracraniche, in casi specialmente di etmoiditi decorrenti in modo acuto e aventi per esito una meningite e nei quali non si è potuto alla sezione riconoscere alcuna lesione ossea (5 su 9 casi nella statistica di Dreyfuss) possano trovare la loro spiegazione in una diffusione per via linfatica.

APPARATO UDITIVO.—Una grande importanza nella diffusione dei processi suppurativi del cavo timpanico e mastoideo hanno particolarmente le vie vasali.

Se noi difatti teniamo conto dei numerosi seni venosi che costeggiano da ogni lato la rocca, il seno trasverso e il petroso inferiore posteriormente, il petroso superiore in alto, il cavernoso verso l'apice, il golfo della giugulare al di sotto, noi possiamo immaginarci la rocca come immersa in un lago di sangue. Se ora si considera che in tali seni confluiscono numerosi vasi dal temporale da una parte e dalle meningi dall'altra, noi comprendiamo quanto numerose siano le vie aperte al trasporto di germi infettivi nei casi di suppurazioni otitiche.

Oltre a tali numerosi vasi diploici è da ricordarsi specialmente l'esistenza, in corrispondenza della parete anteriore del timpano, di piccole vene sboccanti per i canalicoli carotidei nel plesso venoso-pericarotideo in comunicazione col seno cavernoso.

La vena uditiva interna, che esporta il sangue dal labirinto verso la parte posteriore del seno petroso inferiore o direttamente nel seno trasverso (Iansen), può farsi via di conduzione a germi infettivi.

Lo stesso può dirsi della piccola vena decorrente nell'acquedotto del vestibolo e sboccante pure nel seno petroso inferiore.

Dal sistema mastoideo si diparte pure una vena, di calibro talora assai rilevante, per sboccare direttamente nel seno trasverso.

Date coteste numerose vie vasali non deve recare sorpresa di ritrovere che nella statistica di Körner, fatta su 115 sezioni, la lesione dei seni fosse segnalata 52 volte.

Nei 16 casi da me osservati la lesione dei seni fu riscontrata 11 volte o sotto forma di semplice raccolta perisinusale o di vera tromboflebite.

Occorre però far rilevare che spesso la lesione venosa è preceduta e favorita da una morbosa alterazione dell'osso, che, come vedremo, rappresenta il fattore più importante nella meccanica delle infezioni.

Dei linfatici dell'orecchio, massime per quanto riguarda i rapporti collo spazio subdurale, non si hanno cognizioni di sorta. Una serie di ricerche sperimentali da me fatta in animali, mediante infezioni di sostanza colorante nella cavità timpanica, rimase finora infruttuosa.

(C) MORBOSA DISTRUZIONE DELLE PARETI OSSEE.

Si è già detto che nel trasporto dell'infezione agli organi intracranici tanto per via nasale che auricolare la lesione dell'osso rappresenta un fattore dei più importanti, e spesso il primo passo per una diffusione ulteriore di germi infettivi per vie preesistenti o per via sanguigna.

Da tali lesioni *per continuitatem* traggono pertanto origine non pochi casi di lesioni delle vene diploiche e dei seni nonchè di ascessi sottodurali e encefalici.

Nelle complicazioni derivanti da sinusiti frontali la via di infezione è in $\frac{2}{3}$ dei casi dovuta a una perforazione della parete posteriore. Con ciò ha luogo spesso una adesione della dura madre e la formazione di una fistola conducente a un ascesso del lobo frontale.

Per le lesioni intracraniche procedenti da una etmoidite solo in un terzo dei casi è stata segnalata una perforazione della lamina cribrosa.

In tutti questi casi si ebbe per conseguenza un ascesso nel contiguo lobo orbitale.

Nei casi di sinusite mascellare la distruzione cariosa delle pareti è stata riscontrata da Dreyfuss quattro volte su cinque casi, avendosi per esito in tre casi un ascesso del lobo frontale e in uno, in cui si determinò una carie dell'ala dello sfenoide, un ascesso del lobo temporale.

Dei dodici casi di sinusite sfenoidale seguiti da esito letale in un terzo la sezione mise in evidenza una perforazione delle pareti del seno. Anche in questi casi si ebbe come conseguenza una infezione delle meningi.

Nella diffusione dei processi otitici la lesione ossea è, secondo Körner, un reperto quasi costante. Su 109 casi di complicanze otitiche intracraniche varie, nei quali seguì una accurata sezione, in 86 l'osso si riscontrò ammalato fino in contatto colla dura meninge, in 8 l'osso presentava pure delle lesioni ma queste non arrivavano fino alla dura madre : in 15 l'osso fu riscontrato sano. In questi ultimi casi pertanto (lesione ossea parziale o nulla) l'infezione si diffuse per vie preesistenti o per la sanguigna.

Da ciò si comprende come, avendosi nelle alterazioni dell'osso una lesione *per continuitatem*, si possa fino a un certo punto arguire dalla sede e dalla direzione della lesione otitica alla sede della complicazione intracranica. Se difatti il pus si fa strada verso il lato cerebrale del temporale si ha generalmente una malattia delle meningi o del contiguo lobo temporale. Se invece la lesione ossea raggiunge dapprima la fossa cerebrale posteriore si avrà una infezione delle meningi o del seno trasverso o del cervelletto.

Le lesioni del labirinto finiscono quasi sempre verso la fossa cranica posteriore (Iansen) e ciò perchè, anche ammessa una lesione ossea iniziale, le vie labirintiche preesistenti conducono, come sappiamo, alla fossa cerebellare.

Conosciute per tal modo per quali vie possa l'infezione propagarsi dal naso e dall'orecchio verso il cranio, occorre stabilire alcuni dati che valgano a indicarci il rapporto che tali forme morbose occupano nel campo della patologia in generale.

Credo pertanto opportuno ricercare :

1.° Quale rapporto abbia la mortalità per suppurazioni nasali e auricolari colla mortalità in generale e quale rapporto esista fra coteste due forme di infezione.

2.° Quale rapporto abbia la mortalità per suppurazioni nasali e auricolari col numero in generale di tali forme suppurative.

3.° Quale influenza abbiano nel determinare una diffusione delll'infezione nasale e auricolare verso il contenuto cranico, l'età, il sesso, il lato, le condizioni particolari della regione, la forma della lesione iniziale, la specie dei germi infettivi.

I.

Rapporto della mortalità per suppurazioni nasali e auricolari in confronto colla mortalità in generale e fra di loro.

Per rispondere adeguatamente a una tale questione noi non possiamo che tener conto di quelle statistiche formulate in base a un gran numero di sezioni convenientemente praticate su individui di ogni età e venuti a morte per forme diverse.

Poichè occorre qui di osservare come finora nella pratica comune molte forme di infezioni craniche nasali e auricolari o sfuggono completamente all'indagine o si scambiano con altre forme analoghe da cause completamente diverse. Ogni medico pratico e anche ogni clinico potrebbe fare testimonianza di ciò.

La più attendibile statistica, sulla quale possiamo oggidì basarci, è quella di Pitt formulata su 9000 sezioni fatte in serie fra gli anni 1869 e 1888 al Guy's Hospital. Da tale statistica risultano 57 casi di morte per suppurazioni otitiche, e uno solo per suppurazioni nasali.

Treitel su 6000 sezioni praticate alla Charité di Berlino avrebbe trovato che su 21 casi di ascessi cerebrali 7 conseguivano a suppurazioni auricolari e due a una sinusite frontale.

Si rileva pertanto da tali statistiche che se la mortalità otitica è relativamente frequente—circa 1 su 158 nella statistica di Pitt—quella di origine nasale, senza essere trascurabile, è però notevolmente inferiore.

Compulsando la letteratura speciale di quest'ultimo ventennio noi troviamo confermata tale conclusione pel fatto che, mentre si riscontrano numerosissime le osservazioni di complicanze otitiche, sono rare e quasi accidentali quelle di origine nasale.

Per conto mio mentre posso annoverare nella mia pratica di otto anni circa 16 casi di complicazioni otitiche nei quali mi fu possibile un reperto anatomo-patologico od operativo, non mi occorse di osservare nessun caso di infezione endocrania per la via nasale (*vedi statistica personale*).

Dreyfuss, in una memoria pubblicata nel 1896, è però riuscito a raccogliere cinquanta di questi casi di cui cinque per sinusite mascellare, ventidue per sinusite frontale, dieci per etmoidite, tredici per sinusite sfenoidale. A questi potrebbero aggiungersi altri casi pubblicati da quell'epoca in poi da Luc, Iaboulay, Rafin, Claouè, Plauchu, Botey, Gibson e qualche altro.

Se noi ricerchiamo le cause di questa notevole differenza di mortalità per via nasale e auricolare le possiamo trovare, secondo me, nelle peculiari condizioni fisiologiche e anatomiche delle due regioni.

Quantunque difatti tanto le cavità dei seni nasali che le cavità timpano-mastoidee rappresentino dei diverticoli situati lungo il decorso delle vie aeree, diversi sono però i rapporti che essi hanno col mondo esterno e diverse le condizioni di temperatura e di ambiente che creano allo sviluppo dei germi infettivi provenienti dall'esterno.

È noto che nelle condizioni normali entrano nella corrente aerea per le vie nasali numerosi germi che péro sono in gran parte arrestati nel primo tratto e distrutti per la riconosciuta azione battericida del muco nasale (Wurtz e Lermoyez) tanto che si può ritenere che nelle parti posteriori la mucosa nasale è nell' 86% dei casi in condizioni asettiche (St Clair Thompson). Tale asepsi esiste pure nella tuba e nella cavità timpanica (Lannois).

Quando, per diminuite condizioni di resistenza organica o per l'aumentata virulenza di germi, si stabilisce in una dei tali cavità un processo suppurativo, le condizioni di sviluppo dei microrganismi variano a seconda delle regioni. Tenendo sempre conto dell'azione battericida del muco nasale, che deve attenuarne la vitalità, occorre ricordare come la temperatura delle cavità nasali, in libera comunicazione coll'esterno, è solamente di 30 gradi. Sono forse queste le ragioni del debole potere patogeno del pus e dei batteri riscontrato da Herzfeld e da Hermann in dieci casi di sinusite mascellare. La cavità timpanica invece, come osserva Macewen, è un mezzo ideale per la coltura dei microrganismi patogeni ivi stabilitisi: l'oscurità, la temperatura elevata e costante, l'umidità sono altrettante condizioni favorevoli riunite nella cassa e più ancora nell'antro e nelle cellule mastoidee.

Oltre a tali condizioni di ambiente occorre rilevare che, mentre le cavità nasali e seni accessori sono disposte e scaglionate, per così dire, lungo un piano verticale, le cavità auricolari sono distribuite lungo la base cranica in senso pressochè orizzontale. Tale diversità di disposizione, mentre da una parte favorisce il deflusso dei materiali settici, facilita nell' altro il loro ristagno e lo stabilirsi pertanto di quei processi suppurativi cronici particolarmente pericolosi.

Se finalmente noi ricordiamo, in confronto a quanto esiste per le cavità nasali, l'intimità dei rapporti e le numerose vie che può prestare l'orecchio alla diffusione endocranica noi possiamo comprendere il detto di Körner che "non vi è come l'orecchio alcun punto dell'organismo dove una piccola collezione di pus può facilmente determinare una serie di pericolose situazioni."

II.

Rapporto della mortalità per suppurazioni nasali e auricolari col numero delle suppurazioni nasali e auricolari medesime.

Tale quesito in parte già risolto, per quanto cioè riguarda l'orecchio, dalle statistiche di Bezold, Chauvel, Schwartze e da quella sommaria di Barker che farebbe ascendere a 2 ½ % i casi di morte nei casi di otiti purulente (Gradinigo tenderebbe a portarli fino a 8 %), non può ancora trovare, per quanto riguarda le infezioni per via nasale, una equa risposta.

Il numero per se stesso esiguo delle osservazioni finora raccolte in questo campo, e soprattutto il fatto che molti sinusiti decorrono in modo latente non permettono fino ad oggi delle serie conclusioni. Per quanto riguarda le sinusiti frontali, che meno facilmente sfuggono all'osservazione, Engelmann avrebbe trovato che su 120 casi raccolti da varie fonti si ebbero 5 casi di morte per ascesso cerebrale.

Occorre però ricordare come molti casi descritti sotto il nome di flemmoni orbitali, erisipela della faccia, meningite primaria riconoscono la loro causa in lesioni delle cavità nasali o dei seni.   È questo un punto che i perfezionamenti recenti nei mezzi di indagine e la critica severa dei singoli casi metterà certamente in evidenza.

III.

Le infezioni intracraniche per via nasale e auricolare in rapporto all'età, al sesso, al lato del corpo, alle condizioni particolari della regione, alla forma della lesione iniziale, alla specie dei germi infettivi.

(A) ETÀ.

L'influenza che l'età spiega sulla diffusione di eventuali processi suppurativi trova la sua ragione nel diverso grado di sviluppo delle singole cavità della base craniche alle varie epoche della vita.

Così mentre alla nascita non esiste dei seni nasali che una traccia del mascellare, sotto forma di una piccola depressione in rapporto col meato medio (Zuckerkandl), è già bene sviluppata la cavità timpanica, e l'antro mastoideo ha quasi le dimensioni che avrà nell'adulto.   E mentre in seguito, dei seni nasali, il mascellare solo al nono anno ha la sua forma definitiva, e il frontale raggiunge a 15 o 20 il suo completo sviluppo, il sistema mastoideo inizia assai presto il suo sviluppo tanto che a tre anni si può dire che la mastoide ha già acquistata la sua forma definitiva (Körner).

Tali condizioni anatomiche dànno ragione del fatto che degli individui venuti a morte in conseguenza di sinusiti nasali e nei quali si conosce l'età, la maggior parte appartengono al 3.°, 4.°, e 5.° decennio di vita, e ciò fra un minimo di 2 anni (Ogston) e un massimo di 63.

Le complicazioni intracraniche otitiche prevalgono nell'età giovane. Ciò è in rapporto, oltre che al già citato prematuro sviluppo delle cavità auricolari, e alla maggiore frequenza delle lesioni suppurative auricolari nei giovani (64% secondo Burkner), anche a speciali condizioni proprie dell'osso temporale in tale età.

Tali condizioni sono rappresentate :

(a) dall'esistenza della fessura petro-squamosa attraverso la quale si insinua un prolungamento della dura madre ;

(b) dalla presenza, in corrispondenza di tale fessura, del seno petro-squamoso (Macewen) ;

(c) dall' *Hyatus subarcuatus* sboccante nella cavità cranica sotto il canale semicircolare superiore e contenente vasi sanguigni procedenti dal labirinto.

La maggior frequenza delle complicanze otitiche si ritrova nel secondo decennio di vita. Tale fatto risultante da una statistica di Körner, fatta in base a 246 osservazioni raccolte da varie fonti, è pure confermata dalle mie osservazioni personali.

È molto probabile però, come osserva Hessler, che molti casi che nei bambini passano come forme di meningiti comuni debbano riconoscere una origine otitica, e ciò appunto in grazie delle favorevoli condizioni del temporale ora accennate, e al comune reperto dell'esistenza di germi infettivi nella cavità timpanica in tale età (Ponfik).

(B) SESSO.

Sotto questo riguardo tanto le lesioni per la via nasale come quelle per via auricolare concordano per una prevalenza nel sesso maschile.

Dei 46 casi di complicazioni cerebrali per via nasale, nei quali si fa menzione del sesso, in 27 si tratta di uomini in 19 di donne.

La predominanza del sesso maschile per le complicanze otitiche corrisponde alla maggiore morbilità per suppurazioni otitiche dei maschi (da 57 a 60% nei maschi secondo Burkner).

Tale predominanza si verifica tanto per gli ascessi (61 uomini e 30 donne : Körner) come per le meningiti 69 uomini e 38 donne : Hessler) e ancora più per le sinuflebiti (55 uomini e 15 donne : Hessler). Nei miei 16 casi ne ho avuto ben 13 in maschi e tre soli in femmine.

(C) LATO DEL CORPO,

Se è lecito dai pochi casi finora raccolti di infezione endocranica per via nasale dedurre su questo punto delle conclusioni si dovrebbe segnalare una predominanza per il lato sinistro. Tale fatto è assai manifesto per le lesioni dei seni frontali in cui si ebbe, secondo Dreyfuss, 12 volte a sinistra contro 6 a destra. La stessa predominanza si verifica per le sinusiti sfenoidali.

Per le complicanze cerebrali otitiche si verifica invece il fatto inverso. Che da lesioni suppurative del lato destro fosse più facile la diffusione alla cavità endocranica che non a sinistra era già stato rilevato da Toynbee, Gull e Sutton, R. Meyer e Schwartze, e ciò senza che si possa dimostrare che le lesioni suppurative auricolari di destra sieno più frequenti di quelli a sinistra. Körner crede di trovare la ragione della più facile eventualità di una diffusione dal lato destro nelle condizioni anatomiche del temporale da questo lato, e precisamente nel fatto, d'altronde già noto da tempo agli anatomici (Hernberg), che talvolta tanto il seno trasverso (77 % dei casi) che la fossa giugulare si approfondano maggiormente nel temporale a destra che non a sinistra, creando così una maggiore e più facile superficie di contatto fra le cavità auricolari e le meningi. Körner vorebbe che tale fatto sia più manifesto nei brachicefali, ma ricerche recenti di Schultzke e di Okada avrebbero contraddetto tale rapporto tra la proiezione del seno in avanti e il tipo antropologico.

Per quanto riguarda il lato, nelle mie osservazioni dovrei trovarmi in contraddizione coi dati di Körner in quanto che su 16 osservazioni, 10 volte la lesione era situata a sinistra.

(D) CONDIZIONI PARTICOLARI DELLA REGIONE.

Parrebbe ovvio il pensare che un momento importantissimo per la diffusione verso la cavità cranica di un processo suppurativo dal naso e dall'orecchio debba essere rappresentato da ogni ostacolo al libero scolo del pus verso l'esterno.

L'osservazione ha però dimostrato che tale momento non è né essenziale nè necessario.

In 17 casi di sinusiti frontali a esito letale raccolti da Kuhnt si trovano in 8 indicazioni a questo proposito.   Ora è strano di rilevare che in 5 il canale fronto-nasale era pervio, tanto che Kuhnt, negando ogni importanza alla permeabilità di tale canale, inclina a riferirla piuttosto al grado di virulenza dei germi infettivi.

Un ostacolo all'efflusso del pus si verifica facilmente per le condizioni anatomiche dei seni mascellari e sfenoidali.   Tale fatto d'altronde è ciò che si è verificato nella maggior parte dei casi seguiti da esito letale.   Un ostacolo alla libera uscita del pus si verifica anche più facilmente nelle cavità auricolari e per la loro situazione in un piano orizzontale e sopratutto per le particolari anfrattuosità del sistema mastoideo.   Tale ostacolo è anche maggiormente accentuato per la presenza di granulazioni facili a verificarsi nelle forme croniche.

Ma anche per l'orecchio si può osservare che molte complicazioni intracraniche si verificano pur essendo completamente libera l'uscita del pus verso l'esterno.

(E) FORMA DELLA LESIONE INIZALE.

Quantunque abitualmente si ritenga che una infezione endocranica per via nasale o auricolare consegua più facilmente a una lesione cronica che non a una affezione acuta delle varie cavità, pure per le une e per le altre deve valere l'osservazione che Körner fa a proposito delle varie forme di otiti che cioè le forme croniche sono ritenute più pericolose per la ragione che esse cadono, per la loro lunga durata, più facilmente sotto l'osservazione che non le acute non solo, ma anche perchè le infezioni acute costituiscono per l'individuo un pericolo grave solo per un breve spazio di tempo mentre per le croniche tale pericolo persiste per lungo volgere di anni.

Ciò premesso, constatiamo che dei 22 casi di sinusite frontale raccolti da Dreyfuss, in 13 si trattava di forme croniche, in 7 di acute : due rimasero incerti.   Nei casi di etmoidite prevale la forma acuta.   Le sinusiti sfenoidali e mascellari decorsero per metà circa in forma acuta : le rimanenti ebbero decorso cronico.

Nella determinazione di complicanze cerebrali otitiche predominano indubbiamente le forme croniche.   Una particolare condizione che nelle otiti medie purulente croniche si determina e che favorisce la diffusione di un processo suppurativo verso la cavità cranica è specialmente rappresentato da una sclerosi del sistema mastoideo, nonchè della coesistenza di colesteatoma.

Körner osserva giustamente che è sopratutto nei casi di riacutizzazione di processi suppurativi cronici che si ha ragione di temere una infezione endocranica.

(F) SPECIE DEI GERMI INFETTIVI.

È un capitolo questo che merita ancora di essere confrotato da ulteriori e accurate osservazioni.

Scarsissimi sono infatti i reperti per quanto riguarda le infezioni per via nasale. Dei 22 casi di sinusite frontale e esito letale raccolti da Dreyfuss solo in due si conosce l' esame batteriologico, che mostrò nell'uno (Weichselbaum) il *diplococcus pneumoniae* nel pus delle cavità nasali e delle meningi ; nell'altro (Wallenberg) il pneumococco di Friedländer e diverse forme di bacilli.

Per le etmoiditi solo in un caso (Ewald) l' esame batteriologico dimostrò la presenza dello *staphylococcus piogenes aureus*.

In due casi di sinusiti sfenoidali (Ostmann e Zörkendörfer) si ritrovò il *diplococcus pneumoniae* tanto nel pus nasale che meningeo.

Per quanto riguarda le infezioni procedenti dall'orecchio si può, secondo le ricerche di Moos, Zaufal e altri, ritenere, che tutti i microorganismi che determinano una suppurazione auricolare possono anche infettare il contenuto cranico.

Macewen trovò come determinante delle suppurazioni intracraniche otitiche in generale lo streptococco piogeno o lo stafilococco piogeno aureo ; in alcuni casi anche l'albo e il citreo, ma questi ultimi sempre in unione all'aureo e allo streptococco. Una volta il pus dell'orecchio e dell'ascesso cerebrale conteneva una cultura pure di *bacillus piogenes foetidus;* un' altra volta il *diplococcus pneumoniae*.

Ricerche sperimentali allo scopo di determinare con artificiali infezioni della cavità timpanica una diffusione alla cavità cranica furono recentemente fatte da Chiucini senza però ottenerne risultati positivi.

In 4 casi da me osservati nei quali mi fu possibile praticare un esame batteriologico microscopico e culturale ho notato due volte lo streptococco ; una volta lo stafilococco piogeno aureo e un'altro *il bacillus piogenes foetidus*.

Ulteriori ricerche dimostreranno se e come il modo, di diffusione, il decorso e l'esito di tali lesioni siano diversi per ognuno di cotali germi infettivi.

CONCLUSIONI.

1.—L'infezione endocranica, relativamente frequente per la via auricolare, è rara per la via nasale.

2.—La mortalità otitica da infezione endocranica prévale nel secondo decennio di vita, quella di origine nasale nel terzo quarto e quinto decennio.

3.—Le affezioni dei seni nasali a esito mortale furono riscontrate più frequenti al lato sinistro, le otitiche a destra.

4.—Un ostacolo al libero efflusso del pus, tanto per le lesioni nasali che per le auricolari, non è un fattore essenziale per la determinazione di una infezione endocranica.

5.—In tutti i casi sono le forme suppurative croniche quelle che più facilmente sono seguite da una infezione endocranica.

6.—Le vie d'infezione sono rappresentate da fori o canali preesistenti, da rapporti vascolari sanguigni e linfatici o da una morbosa alterazione delle pareti dei seni nasali o delle cavità auricolari. Questo ultimo fattore è il più importante.

BIBLIOGRAFIA.

ZUCKERKANDL E.—*Normale und pathol. Anatomie der Nasenhöhle.* Wien I. Bd. 2 Aufl. 1893, II Bd. 1892.

MACEWEN W.—*Pyogenic infective diseases of the brain and spinal cord.* Glasgow, 1893.

HERZFELD J. UND HERMANN FR.—*Bacteriologische Untersuchungen etc.* Archiv. für Laryng. u. Rhin. Bd. III. Heft 1-2 p. 143.

KUHNT.—*Ueber die entzündlichen Erkrankungen der Stirnhölen etc.* Wiesbaden, 1895.

R. DREYFUSS.—*Die Krankheiten des Gehirns und seiner Adnexa im Gefolge von Naseneiterungen.* Jena, 1896.

HESSLER H.—*Die Otogene Pyämie.* Jena 1896.

KÖRNER O.—*Die otitischen Erkrankungen des Hirns, der Hirnhäute und der Blutleiter.* Frankfurt ²/M. 1896.

KÖBNER O.—*Die eitrigen Erkrankungen des Schläfenbeins,* Wiesbaden, 1899.

BROCA ET MAUBRAC.—*Traité de Chirurgie cérébrale.* Paris, 1896.

RAFIN M.—*Des complications intracrániennes des inflammations du sinus frontal.* Archives Générales de Médicine, 1897. N. 10 et 12.

OPPENHEIM H.—*Die Encephalitis und der Hirnabscess.* Wien 1897.

secondo decennio di vita, quella di origine nasale nel terzo quarto e quinto decennio.

3.—Le affezioni dei seni nasali a esito mortale furono riscontrate più frequenti al lato sinistro, le otitiche a destra.

4.—Un ostacolo al libero efflusso del pus, tanto per le lesioni nasali che per le auricolari, non è un fattore essenziale per la determinazione di una infezione endocranica.

5.—In tutti i casi sono le forme suppurative croniche quelle che più facilmente sono seguite da una infezione endocranica.

6.—Le vie d'infezione sono rappresentate da fori o canali preesistenti, da rapporti vascolari sanguigni e linfatici o da una morbosa alterazione delle pareti dei seni nasali o delle cavità auricolari. Questo ultimo fattore è il più importante.

Bibliografia.

ZUCKERKANDL E.—*Normale und pathol. Anatomie der Nasenhöhle.* Wien I. Bd. 2 Aufl. 1893, II Bd. 1892.

MACEWEN W.—*Pyogenic infective diseases of the brain and spinal cord.* Glasgow. 1893.

HERZFELD J. UND HERMANN FR.—*Bacteriologische Untersuchungen etc.* Archiv. für Laryng. u. Rhin. Bd. III. Heft 1-2 p. 143.

KUHNT.—*Ueber die entzündlichen Erkrankungen der Stirnhölen etc.* Wiesbaden, 1895.

R. DREYFUSS.—*Die Krankheiten des Gehirns und seiner Adnexa im Gefolge von Naseneiterungen.* Jena, 1896.

HESSLER H.—*Die Otogene Pyämie.* Jena 1896.

KÖRNER O.—*Die otitischen Erkrankungen des Hirns, der Hirnhäute und der Blutleiter.* Frankfurt a/M, 1896

KÖRNER O.—*Die eitrigen Erkrankungen des Schläfenbeins,* Wiesbaden, 1899.

BROCA ET MAUBRAC.—*Traité de Chirurgie cérébrale.* Paris, 1896.

RAFIN M.—*Des complications intracrâniennes des inflammations du sinus frontal.* Archives Générales de Médicine, 1897. N. 10 et 12.

OPPENHEIM H.—*Die Encephalitis und der Hirnabscess.* Wien 1897.

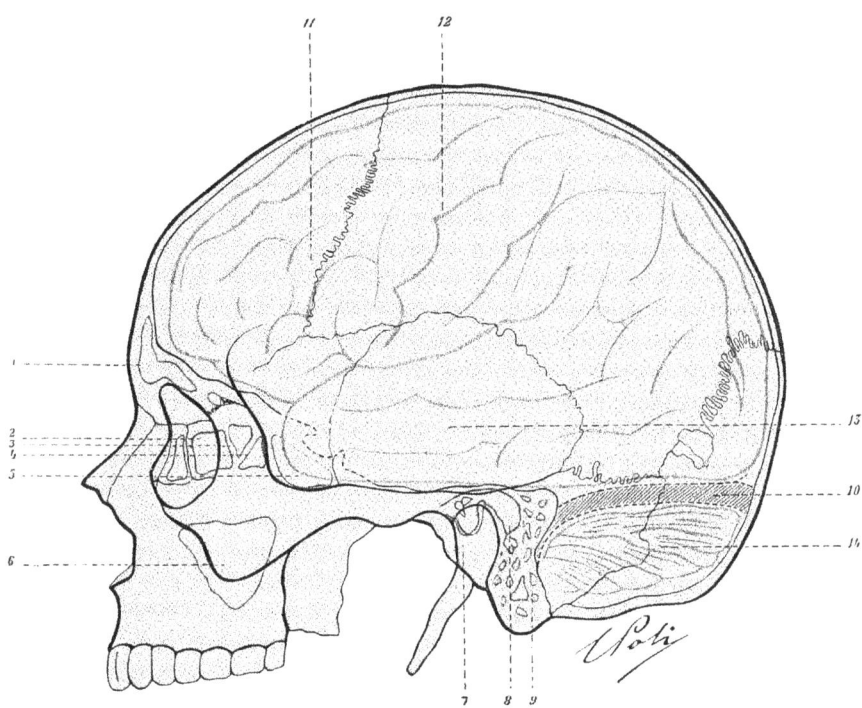

RAPPORTI DEI SENI NASALI E DELLE CAVITÀ AURICOLARI COL
CONTENUTO ENDOCRANICO. *(Figura schematica)*.

1, seno frontale. — 2, cellule etmoidali anteriori. — 3, c. e. medie. — 4, c. e. posteriori.
— 5, seno sfenoidale. — 6, seno mascellare. — 7, cavità timpanica. — 8, antro mastoideo.
— 9, cellule mastoidee. — 10, seno laterale. — 11, lobo frontale. — 12, scissura di Rolando.
— 13, lobo temporo-sfenoidale. — 14, cervelletto.

STATISTICA PERSONALE—Anni 1892-1899.

N. d'Ordine	DATA.	NOME.	Età.	Sesso.	AFFEZIONE PRIMARIA.	LESIONE INTRACRANICA.		VIA DI INFEZIONE.	NOTE BIBLIOGRAFICHE.
						REPERTO OPERATIVO.	REPERTO NECROSCOPICO.		
1	Febb. 1892.	V. Leonardi	17	M.	Otite media purulenta cronica destra.	Non operato.	Pachmeningite limitata alla faccia superiore della rocca : leptomeningite diffusa. Ascesso del lobo temporo-sfenoidale des-tro, a pertosi nei ventricoli laterali.	Osteite del *tegmen tympani*	Pubblicato dal Dott. Laurenti. Gazzetta degli Ospedali, Anno XIII., N. 52.
2	Maggio 1896.	C. Schiappacasse	17	M.	Otite media purulenta cronica sinistra.	Non operato	Trombo-flebite del seno laterale e del seno petro-so inferiore sinistro. As-cessi metastatici polmonali.	Osteite della pa-rete timpanica, postero - supe-riore, e del-l'antro.	Gazzetta degli Ospedali, Anno XIII., N. 94.
3	Giugno 1892.	G. Della Casa.	17	M.	Otite media purulenta cronica sinistra. Colesteatoma.	Trombo-flebite settica del seno laterale sinistro. Apertura del seno ; lega-tura e sezione della vena giugulare profonda	Guarigione.	Usura della parete timpanica, pos-tero - superiore per colestea-toma	Archivio Italiano di Otologia, Vol. VII., fasc. I.
4	Agosto 1896.	E. Novaro.	23	M.	Otite media purulenta cronica sinistra.	Trombo-flebite settica del seno laterale sinistro. Legatura e sezione della vena giugulare profonda, disinfezione del seno.	Meningite basilare : trom-bosi dei seni petroso superiore e inferiore sinis-tro ; emorraggia delle vene rachidee : focolai metas-tatici diffusi.	Osteite della mas-toide e della por-zione limitrofa dell'occipitale.	Idem.
5	Dicem. 1896,	G. B. Riva sordomuto	19	M.	Otite media purulenta cronica sinistra.	Sinuflebite sinistra : piemia : ascesso del cervelletto. Scopertura del seno aper-tura dell'ascesso. Oper-azione radicale della lesione otitica.	Guarigione.	Osteite dell'attico e della parete timpanica pos-tero-superiore.	Idem.
6	Genn. 1897.	E. Noce.	3	M.	Otite media purulenta cronica destra ; mastoidite.	Perisinusite del seno laterale destro.	Guarigione	Osteite della mas-toide.	Gazzetta degli Os-pedali e delle Cliniche. Nu-mero 124, Anno 1897.

Chart illustrating Prof. Poli's Paper-

N. d'Ordine	DATA.	NOME.	Età.	Sesso.	AFFEZIONE PRIMARIA.	LESIONE INTRACRANICA		VIA DI INFEZIONE.	NOTE BIBLIOGRAFICHE.
						REPERTO OPERATIVO.	REPERTO NECROSCOPICO.		
7	Febb. 1897.	R. Pavone.	16	M.	Otite media purulenta cronica sinistra. Colesteatoma.	Sinuflebite : ascesso del lobo temporo-sfenoidale. Scopertura del seno: apertura dell'ascesso.	Constatazione di un ampio ascesso nella parte posteriore del lobo temporo-sfenoidale. La morte avvenne per coma iniziatosi durante l'atto operativo (cloroformio(?))	Usura colesteato-matosa della parete timpanica postero-superiore (adito e antro): Bacillus piogenes foetidus (?) ... cerebrale.	Archivio Italiano di Otologia, Vol. VII, fasc. I.
8	Aprile 1897.	C. Gonin.	24	F.	Otite media purulenta acuta destra da influenza.	Perisinusite del seno laterale destro.	Guarigione.	Osteite della mastoide.	Gazzetta degli Ospedali e delle Cliniche, Nu. 1 oro 124, Anno 1897.
9	Giugno 1897.	L Borusso.	14	M.	Otite media purulenta cronica destra.	Puntura lombare, con esito di liquido purulento fetidissimo.	Leptomeningite cerebruspinale.	Vene del temporale (osteoflebite).	Archivio Italiano di Otologia. Vol. VII, fasc. I.
10	Novem. 1897.	E. Dispa.	42	M.	Otite media purulenta acuta-sinistra: mastoidite	Perisinusite del seno laterale sinistro. Ascesso del collo. Scopertura del seno; apertura dell'ascesso.	Guarigione.	Vene del temporale (osteoflebite).	Gito negli Atti della R. Accademia ... di Genova. Seduta 13 ... bre 1897.
11	Dicem. 1897. Aprile 1898.	Luisita B.	3	F.	Oto-mastoidite acuta sinistra da scarlattina.	Perisinusite del seno laterale sinistro. Ascesso del lobo temporo-sfenoidale sinistro. Ascesso polmonare metastasico. Ai varii esami batteriologici si rilevò la presenza costante dello strepto-cocco p. a.	La sezione non è stata concessa. La morte, avvenuta due mesi dopo l'apertura dell'ascesso intracranico, parve dovesse attribuirsi a un processo di encefalite diffusa.	Osteite della mastoide.	Clinica Medica Italiana, N. 7, Anno 1898.
12	Agosto 1898.	R. Klaus (Pegli)	8	M.	Oto-mastoidite acuta purulenta sinistra.	Trombo-flebite del seno laterale sinistro. Legatura e sezione della vena giugulare profonda: disinfezione del seno.	Sezione non concessa. Nei giorni successivi all'atto operativo si accertarono i sintomi di una diffusione del trombo ai seni della base (seno cavernoso).	Osteite del temporale.	Inedito.

13	Ottobre 1898.	P. Gustavino (Albenga).	34	M.	Oto-mastoidite acuta sinistra.	Carie della mastoide (cellule ampie piene di tessuto di granulazione). Ascesso latente del lobo temporo-sfenoidale sinistro.	Morte subitanea in coma. Sezione non concessa. Probabile rottura dell'ascesso nei ventricoli laterali.	Osteite del temporale.	Inedito.
14	Ottobre 1898.	U. Piccardo	17	M.	Otite media purulenta cronica destra.	Trombo-flebite del seno laterale destro. Legatura e sezione della vena giugulare profonda: disinfezione del seno. Cura radicale della lesione otitica.	Guarigione	Osteite della parete postero-superiore del condotto uditivo e dell'antro.	Atti della R. Accademia Medica di Genova. Seduta 12 Dicembre 1898.
15	Febbr. 1899.	L. Bogliaco (Genova).	9	F.	Otite media purulenta cronica sinistra.	Perisinusite del seno laterale sinistro. Scopertura del seno: Cura radicale della lesione otitica.	Guarigione.	Via venosa: flebite constatata di un vaso che dalla mastoide immette nella doccia del seno laterale.	Inedito.
16	Febbr. 1899.	Chiozza G. (Voltri).	15	M.	Otite media purulenta cronica sinistra.	Trombo flebite del seno laterale destro. Pioemia. Legatura e sezione della vena giugulare profonda: disinfezione del seno.	Trombosi diffusa lungo tutta la giugulare. Ascessi metastatici polmonari.	Osteite della mastoide assai diffusa. Streptococchi.	Inedito.

N.B.—In questa statistica ho tenuto conto solo dei casi nei quali mi fu possibile determinare la via seguita dall'infezione mediante un reperto operativo o necroscopico. Alcuni di tali casi formarono oggetto di particolari pubblicazioni, come appare dalle note bibliografiche.

A CASE OF THROMBOSIS OF BOTH SINUS CAVERNOSI, AS A COMPLICA-
TION OF CHRONIC MASTOIDITIS EX OTORRHŒA, WHICH ENDED IN
RECOVERY.

DR. G. D. COHEN TERVAERT, The Hague.

The case I wish to submit to your discussion and judgment, I think,
offers some interesting features, worthy of your attention, even if you
should not agree with my view, that it is really a thrombosis of the
cavernous sinuses.

It occurred in a youth of sixteen, who had been affected for 8 years
by a slight otorrhœa of the left ear, but whose general health does not
seem to have suffered from that affection. His father is reported to
have died of rheumatic fever, his mother lives and enjoys good health,
so do his five brothers and sisters. At the beginning of November of
last year our patient was admitted to the Hague Town Hospital, for a
sore throat and headache. A whitish exsudation was discovered in
the crypts of both hypertrophied tonsils, while there was no fever
during the first days. When I saw the patient for the first time on
November 17th, the exsudation had quite disappeared, but the evening
before, a rise of the body temperature to 38·5° C. had been noticed. As the
boy showed a slight degree of torticollis, the head being inclined a little
to the left shoulder, we examined the neck with the finger and found
some tenderness on pressure over the mastoid process, without redness
or swelling of the skin. This directed our attention to the left ear, and
here we found a small quantity of thickish, badly smelling matter at the
inner end of the external canal; after having cleansed this it was
obvious that the drum membrane still existed, although it had grown
thicker, and that there was only a minute opening in the membrana
Shrapnelli. The hearing was not very bad in the left ear, but for
various reasons was not examined accurately. As to the psychical
functions we thought we observed somewhat slow cerebration during
those days, or at all events that seemed to be the case, but it is impossible to speak with absolute certainty, as the boy is of a calm and reticent
disposition, as we had opportunity of recognising distinctly later on.
At any rate in those days he was silent and preferred to stay in bed,
did not complain of headache and only once had an attack of vomiting,
owing, according to him, to his having taken coffee, which he was not
accustomed to. The fever, that had been noticed on the evening of
November 16th, and had varied from 37·8—38·6° C. on the 17th, passed
off after a thorough action of the bowels, while an ice bag applied to
the mastoid process improved the local conditions so much that it did
not seem necessary to proceed to the operation immediately. In the
course of November 20th however the aspect changed altogether; in the
morning of that day I had already noticed some redness of the conjunctiva
and a little swelling of the upper lid of the left eye, but I did not think

it of much importance, the boy lying with his left side next to the entrance of the ward, so that a draft from without might have reached him. My surprise was therefore very great on the next morning, when I found both his left upper and under eyelid so enormously swollen and œdematous, that I could scarcely open the eye with my finger. Still I did not fail to perceive that the eyeball protruded a great deal. The day before the temperature had risen to 39·8° C., while no chill had occurred and no abundant perspiration had accompanied the rise of temperature; during my visit it still proved to be 38·3° C. The diagnosis of thrombosis of the left cavernous sinus of course suggesting itself at once, there was now immediate danger, and so we proceeded to the operation at 7 o'clock in the evening. If during the preceding days I had not yet made up my mind which of the two operations, that had to be considered, either the mastoid or the radical one was to be preferred in this case, now with this complication of thrombosis of one or perhaps more of the sinuses of the dura mater, I did not hesitate to choose the one which in itself was the less complicated, as it had to be accompanied by the laying bare, and perhaps the opening, of the sigmoid flexure of the lateral sinus. So I performed Schwartze's classical operation, and working with mallet and chisel I soon hit upon the pus, and with a sharp spoon and bone forceps I made a deep cavity, the innermost part of which consisted of the antrum. Then I opened the groove of the lateral sinus from the mastoid emissarium to the junction between its vertical and lower horizontal portion. The sinus itself looked healthy and showed pulsation, there was only a small granulation on it. Under these circumstances I did not open the sinus, and ended the operation in the ordinary way by packing the wound with iodoform and sterilised gauze. The body temperature, which before the operation had already fallen as low as 37·7, and even reached 36·6 shortly after it, rose again during the night without chill and stood at 39·1 at 7 o'clock in the morning. The œdema of the eyelids and the protrusion of the ball of the left eye had not only remained stationary, but had also appeared on the right side. In the course of that day the temperature did not rise above 38°, while no chill nor any other new symptoms pointed to pyaemia or any other complications. On the next day the right eye was decidedly better, but on the following day the temperature rose again to 38°. I redressed the wound on the 24th. No pus had collected under the dressings, but a minute drop was seen to come from the upper end of the opened groove of the sinus; it increased slowly and at length formed a streak of thick yellow pus, that returned twice after having been washed away. The same occurring the next day, I resolved to loosen the sinus in its groove, but no pus issued from behind; a puncture into the posterior fossa of the cranium through the dura mater forming the posterior wall of the groove was equally without result; so was another puncture in the direction of the sinus transversus. The next day, November 26th, there was no longer any pus on the sinus when redressing the wound.

In the meantime the protrusion had diminished a great deal, and the œdema of the eye-lids had almost entirely disappeared, so that we could proceed to an ophthalmoscopical examination. The vision proved quite normal. There was no impaired function of the muscles of the eye-ball, especially of the rectus externus. It seemed to us that the veins of the left retina were more filled than those of the right eye, but as we are not so very familiar with this mode of examination it is better not to attach too much value to this opinion of ours. During the following days the temperature rose repeatedly, though not often ; twice there was a marked chill, viz.: on the morning of November 27th, and again on the morning of December 1st. The pulse was sometimes frequent and irregular ; there was much salivation, and now and then nausea and vomiting after taking food.

While in the week that now followed, the eye symptoms steadily grew better, suddenly, on December 3rd, the protrusion of the left eye reappeared with a swelling of the upper lid and chemosis conjunctivæ. Now a thorough examination was made by Dr. Hazewinkel, of the Hague Eye Hospital. The eye could still be moved to a small extent, but the mobility seemed to be more impaired in the outward direction than in any other. The pupils of both eyes were of the same size, and gave a prompt reaction to light and accommodation. The vision was normal. The ophthalmoscopical examination proved that the inferior temporal vein of the left eye was wider than that on the right side ; the vessels were not tortuous ; the optic disc looked somewhat paler than it ought to, but was well defined. There was intense pain in the region of the supraorbital nerve. The following days these symptoms increased. There was commencing atrophy of the temporal half of the disc ; no neuro-retinitis. The eye was not anæsthetic and was of normal tension. As a puncture at the inner end of the lower lid gave no pus, this confirmed the oculist's idea that there was no orbital abscess, and that the above symptoms depended exclusively on stasis. We therefore insisted upon the opening of the cranium in the middle fossa, which operation was performed, December 8th, according to Bergmann's method, by Dr. de Zwaan, Surgeon to the Town Hospital. The roof of the antro-attic cavity proving quite healthy the surgeon tried several punctures. especially in the direction of the cavernous sinus: the result was, however, quite negative.

The general health was by no means disturbed by this operation, nor had it any influence on the swelling of the orbit. As, on the contrary, this increased, canthoplasty was executed on December 10th: the next day the pus escaped at a point underneath the caruncle, where the conjunctiva had given way. The swelling and protrusion having nearly subsided some days later, there was a round and hard string to be felt distinctly at the inner and lower corner of the orbit, and it could even be followed up over a short distance in the direction of the inferior ophthalmic vein.

Now all went well till December 16th, when the patient began to complain of severe pain in the right eye, and œdema of the upper lid and outer canthus with chemosis of the conjunctiva and protrusion could be noted, whilst the evening before, the body temperature had risen to 37.6. The chemosis increased rapidly so that the swollen lower fornix conjunctivæ hung as a bag over the everted lower lid. The reaction of the pupil remained unimpaired, and ophthalmoscopical examination proved the fundus quite normal.

On December 19th a puncture, and on December 23rd an incision, were made at the outer and lower corner; but no pus appeared. The cutaneous veins of the right cheek, especially those round the corner of the mouth became distended. On the 28th there was a marked bulging of the inner end of the upper lid of a dark bluish-red colour; now a puncture on this place giving exit to pus, a large incision was made in the conjunctiva at the inner canthus, and was kept open with a drainage tube. This could be removed after some days. The recovery made steady progress, and no relapse occurred; the chemosis of the right eye lasted rather long, and was still to be noticed in April. The vision of both eyes is $^5/_6$ in; the ophthalmoscopic examination reveals no changes. The left ear continuing to discharge a little, and a graunlation occurring from time to time in the opening of Shrapnell's membrane, it is to be expected that excision of the ossicles or perhaps the radical operation may prove inevitable. The wound of the mastoid process is quite healed. Tonsillotomy has been performed. A thorough examination of the accessory sinuses of the nose proved that they are all in the best condition.

SUMMARY.

In going over the principal symptoms we may say that in a patient with chronic suppurative mastoiditis ex otorrhœa, there appears suddenly stasis in the area of the left ophthalmic veins, followed up the next day by the same symptoms in the right eye. After evacuation of the pus out of the mastoid process these symptoms disappear.

This almost simultaneous appearance of venous stasis in both orbits is, I think, the distinctive phenomenon, for it can only admit of the explanation of a common seat being the cause, and this common seat can only be the cavernous sinus, for we know that a thrombosis of one of them rapidly extends to the other through the medium of the intercavernous sinus. And the importance of this symptom, with regard to the diagnosis, cannot be in the least diminished by the almost complete lack of any stasis in the retinal veins, since we know that the central vein of the retina communicates with the cavernous sinus by a venous network, that at the same time has an outflow into the facial vein through the inferior ophthalmic vein. Moreover Jansen, in his masterly paper, has emphasized and even proved by autopsy, that purulent thrombosis of the cavernous sinus is compatible with the absence of any change in the fundus, and of any impairment of the visual acuteness, and of the functions of the extra-ocular muscles.

After an apparent improvement for a week, the left side, and a fortnight later also the right side again exhibit symptoms of obstruction to the venous circulation, which on both sides ends in the signs of orbital phlegmon. This fact again points to the cavernous sinus, all other causes of idiopathic or secondary inflammation of the orbits being absent; there had been no trauma before, nor any surgical operation of the orbit itself, no more had there been any pathological process in the accessory sinuses of the nose, which are known to be the cause of phlegmon of the orbit. But there is more: after evacuation of the pus, when the swelling of the left orbit has subsided, we are able to feel distinctly at the inner and lower corner of the left orbit a round and solid string, that can be nothing but the thrombosed inferior ophthalmic vein or its communication with the facial vein. On the right side we do not find the same, but here we observe in an advanced stage distension of the veins of the cheek, proving the obstruction of the orbital veins by the increased passage through this collateral system.

I need not point out that this distension of the facial veins as a sign of obstruction of the orbital veins proves nothing with regard to the nature of the obstruction, while the observation of the thrombosis of the ophthalmic vein seems to me of the greatest importance. It is true this thrombosis may have occurred subsequent to the inflammation, considered as the primary affection; but when accepting this view we are again at a loss for the origin of the cellulitis; on the contrary, considering the cellulitis as a sequel of the thrombosis there is no difficulty whatever as to the interpretation, viz: primarily there has been thrombosis of the cavernous sinus, the alarming symptoms of which disappeared either by the breaking down of the thrombus or by the substitution of a collateral venous circulation. Recovery might have ensued after this, however it did not, a thrombophlebitis of the left ophthalmic vein set in and ended in a phlegmon of the left orbit. As to the phlegmon of the right orbit, this may have been caused by a so-called ascending phlebitis out of the left orbit, passing through the cavernous sinuses; but I think it more probable that it has been caused directly by the primary thrombosis of the cavernous sinus.

As to the etiology of the thrombosis of the cavernous sinus, two causes have to be considered here, namely, the chronic suppurative inflammation of the left middle ear, and the angina, which indeed occasioned the patient's entering the Hospital. This latter mode of infection seems to me very improbable indeed. Undoubtedly there are well stated instances on record of thrombosis of the cavernous sinus due to angina, but in these cases there has been either a gangrenous angina (cases of Panas,* Blachez,† Mitvalsky‡) or a phlegmonous one (case of Ogle §), at any rate deep-seated and serious affections of the tonsils and pharynx, whilst a superficial and slight exudation, as happened to occur in our patient, is not very likely to be able to clot and infect the blood vessels.

So there remains only the chronic suppuration of the left middle ear as the origin of the infection, and here again several ways come into consideration with regard to the extension from the primary seat to the sinus. The most common way, viz.: through the medium of the air-cells in the mastoid process to the lateral sinus, and from this along the inferior petrosal sinus to the cavernous sinus cannot be made answerable for this, for we found the lateral sinus not thrombosed; no more can the superior petrosal sinus be made answerable, for after having opened the middle fossa we found the tympano-antral roof looking normal and healthy, and so we are led to look on the third and last way, viz.: the plexus of veins and lymphatic vessels in the carotid canal, which plexus communicates by way of the minute canaliculi carotico-tympanici with the veins of the tympanum, and has already been mentioned in this question by several authors, as Körner, Jansen, Meyer, and Preysing. The latter reported last year out of Prof. Körner's clinic a case of phlebitis of the cavernous sinus, which, revealing itself on the first day after a radical operation was diagnosed on account of the triad of symptoms, paralysis of the abducens, exophthalmos, and swelling of both optic discs, and which, like my case, ended in recovery.

In the consideration of his case Preysing says —"In what way the sinus was affected cannot be decided. The carotid sinus, which surrounds the carotid within its bony canal, lies very near to the tympanum and communicates directly with the cavernous sinus. The infection of this latter may have happened in that way. But it is also possible that first one of the petrosal sinuses or the lateral sinus got affected without symptoms, and led the infection on to the cavernous sinus."

As I believe I can in my case exclude participation of the lateral and of both petrous sinuses, I think I have shown it probable that the carotid sinus was the means of infection. As to this I cannot speak with certainty, fortunately, for this certainty is only to be had by a post-mortem examination.

---

* Panas. Traité des Maladies des Yeux. Tome Second. p. 378.
† Blachez. Journ. de Méd. et de Chir., 1880. p. 8.
‡ Mitvalsky. Archives d'Ophthalmologie. Tome Seizième, p. 22. 1896.
§ Ogle. Brit. and Foreign Med. Chir. Rev. p. 509. 1865.

SOME OF THE MOST IMPORTANT DISCOVERIES IN OTOLOGY, MANY OF WHICH HAVE STOOD THE TEST OF THIRTY FIVE YEARS.

DR. LAURENCE TURNBULL, Philadelphia, Pa.

Only those who have studied and practised the scientific treatment of any one speciality for an ordinary lifetime, are competent to give an opinion of the true and the false methods, or speak authoritatively concerning their comparative values. The constant tendency in the profession of medicine is to advance what is either novel or considered a new method of treatment or diagnosis. These measures are brought to the attention of the profession by statements concerning the wonders of certain vaunted drugs or the marvellous results obtained by some form of apparatus or mechanical appliance.

What are a few of the methods, for the diagnosis and treatment of diseases of the ear, which have stood the test of time?

One of the only real and positive discoveries that has withstood this test and can be thoroughly relied upon, is Politzer's method of Inflation of the Tympanum (Middle Ear); so also the Aural Speculum which was one of the very early useful discoveries, but it was not until 1827, that according to Wilde, Newbourg recommended the tubular form, which was modified by Gruber, and is now in general use. This was not of direct service until the introduction by Von Tröltsch, in 1855, of the aural mirror or otoscope. By this scientific instrument, the general practitioner was furnished with a means by which he could with some training, determine the condition of the auditory canal, or the appearance of the membrana tympani, even diagnose changes in topography and pathological conditions.

With the ordinary coal oil lamp, illuminating gas, or a Welsbach lamp, or electricity, we have sufficient light for the examination of the ear, nose, pharynx, and throat. The pure white steady light of the Welsbach makes a most valuable addition to the aural surgeon's armamentarium.

Prior to 1863, the year in which Adam Politzer, of Vienna, published his discovery,* the method of inflating the middle ear or treating obstructions in the Eustachian tube or middle ear, was by auto-inflation or by what was termed the "Valsalva Method." This Valsalvan Method consists in forcing the air in the naso-pharynx and upper air passages through the Eustachian tube, by a strong act of expiration, directing it through the closed nostrils, having the mouth closed. By this method the walls of the Eustachian tube were forced apart and air entered the tympanum. It was found, however, that the "Valsalvan Method" which depended so much for success upon the intelligence of the patient, was of very limited value as a means of diagnosis or treatment, yet we were glad even to attempt to employ it, and it should always be used at the

---

* Wienei Med. Wocienscirift, 1863 No. 6.

commencement, in diagnosing a case, before employing the more forcible "Politzer's Method," or even attempting catheterization of the Eustachian tube.

The "Method of Toynbee" has also been employed as aid in diagnosis, this consists in performing the act of swallowing with closed nostrils, whereby a feeling of fulness in the ears is experienced. This was erroneously attributed by Toynbee to condensation of the air in the middle ear, however, the result was found to be of little value because the air was in reality pumped from the tympanum, and the crackling sound which was thereby heard in the ear meant more or less of a vacuum.

Catheterization of the Eustachian tube:—Although the introduction and use of the Eustachian catheter through the nose into the mouth of the tube was a very early discovery, claimed by both the English and the French, it was von Tröltsch, who was the man, and the translation of his works by D. B. St. John Roosa tells us that he gave us the positive indications for its use. This method of opening and forcing air, by the catheter, through the Eustachian tube and into the middle ear has always been in the hands of the Otologist, and has never been used by the profession, owing to the amount of skill necessary in its execution, furthermore, its manipulation requires much more time, and many and various forms of catheters. Mistakes are not unusual in attempted catheterization, even by the most expert, even by the aid of the mirror and under the most favourable circumstances.

What is the cause of this? Besides congenital anomalies which interfere with the introduction of the catheter, or even make it impossible, there are other obstacles in the nose and naso-pharynx which are often met with. These are due to diseased conditions, or are the result of traumatism, some of the more important of which are:— Deformities due to traumatic affections of the nasal septum, and the turbinated bones; strictures of the nasal cavity from ulceration, caries and cicatricial changes, obstructions such as tumours of all sorts, polypoid growths, etc. These can be seen, it is true, by anterior rhinoscopy and illumination of the nasal cavity, but if the narrowing be situated in the deeper portions posteriorly, these cannot be so easily viewed, except by the aid of what is called posterior rhinoscopy or the examination, per orem, of the post nasal space by means of the small mirror and head mirror. In cases of absolute impermeability of the nostril on either side, the introduction of the catheter through the opposite side or nostril, or by the mouth has been recommended and sometimes accomplished. Several forms of catheter have been devised for this purpose, but they all have the objection that they cause great irritation, choking and even vomiting, rendering their use almost impossible, besides, as a rule, there is a great deal of spasm or reflex resistance on the part of the patient which greatly embarrasses the operator. With nervous children and old people, the procedure is so demoralizing, and the sensation so disagreeable, that it is next to impossible to succeed, indeed in some patients, convulsive cough, dizziness, fainting, with persistent sneezing and bleeding from the nose are the sequels which force us to limit the use of the catheter to a few extraordinary cases, but never to employ it as routine treatment.

The next addition to the catheter was the Politzer rubber bag, by which liquids and vapours of various volatile and nebulized agents were forced into the middle ear. The use of air and vapours is justifiable, and sometimes useful, but the injection of liquids is not safe, except in a few cases, where the tube is patulous and there is a perforation of the membrana tympani. Even with all due care, at times, the point of the catheter is pressed too hard against the wall of the pharynx or the tube, and engages and perforates the mucous membrane, and emphysema ensues. No one except an expert should attempt this procedure, because this form of emphysema has on more than one occasion proved fatal. Not satisfied with the hand bulb, resort has been made to the air pump, as the resistance of the collapsed or partially closed Eustachian tube and the tympanic cavity full of more or less exudate, cannot in a few cases be overcome, and it has been considered necessary to use a force of from ten pounds and upward to overcome this resistance so as to send a stronger current of air through the tube. This form of apparatus has been carried to dangerous and damaging results, and force is not safe nor is it justified by the results obtained. In the single or double bag all the force that is necessary can be obtained, any sort of forcible application should not be made for more than from two to five seconds, nor oftener than once a day.

As the original " Politzer " bag and method ("mein Verfahren ") has been changed and modified and as all these have not been improvements, we will at this point give a description of the Politzer apparatus and method as we have employed it with success from 1863 to the present day.   .

* " The Politzer method of inflating the tympanum through the Eustachian tube."

" The most serviceable instrument for my method is a pyriform balloon (or bag) about the size of the double fist (10 to 12 oz.) which is furnished with a nozzle, upon this a hard rubber nozzle fits and a piece of gum (rubber tubing) about six inches long connects this with a slightly curved tubular hard rubber nozzle. To avoid injury to the mucous-membrane which is frequently bruised or scratched by the immediate impact of the stiff nozzle upon the pituitary membrane, the connection between the balloon and curved nozzle is effected by the

---

* Text Book of " Diseases of the Ear," Am. Ed. 1894, p. 114.

insertion of the short mobile elastic india-rubber tube." We have always used in our practice Politzer's rubber-balloon, from which we usually pump air direct into the outer opening of the Eustachian catheter for catheterization.

The details of the Politzer method are the following. The patient being seated in a chair facing the operator, takes a moderate mouthful of water to facilitate swallowing, this is held in the mouth until the patient is required to swallow when told to do so. The surgeon facing the patient, introduces the curved nozzle of the flexible tube attached to the Politzer bag, about one inch into the nasal orifice of the corresponding side to be inflated, and hugging the floor of the nares. with the left thumb and forefinger compresses both nasal fossæ, closing one side around the nozzle. The patient is next told to swallow, at the same moment the surgeon squeezes the Politzer bag, and suddenly expels the air with his right hand, using more or less force as the case may require. By this condensation of air in the naso-pharynx, it is forced into both middle ears, usually more decidedly in the direction of the side into which the nozzle has been introduced. The closure of the soft palate is effected, and the Eustachian tubes are forced open and a bubbling crackling noise is frequently, though not always, an indication that the air has entered the middle ear.

The air condensed by this method in the naso-pharynx, will, as a rule, enter both tympanic cavities, more powerfully however, on the side where the resistance in the tube and in the tympanic cavity is feebler. Therefore, to concentrate the effect of the current of air upon the diseased ear, when only one is affected, and to prevent the entrance of air into the better ear as much as possible, it is necessary to attempt to create an artificial resistance in its fellow, by hermetically closing the meatus with the finger, or, by pressing the tragus into the meatus. The therapeutic effect of inflation can be increased, closing each meatus alternately, to allow the full power of the air current to act separately upon each tympanic cavity.

The use of the mouthful of water is by no means absolutely necessary in all cases for the application of "Politzer's Method," which is often performed by the simple act of swallowing, or when by Gruber's Method, the patient instead of swallowing, closes the throat by uttering the mono-syllables, hic, haec, hock.

In those affections of the middle ear, where in consequence of the swelling of the mucous membrane, or accumulations of secretion, and of the abnormal cicatricial tension of the membrane or of the ossicles combined, a high degree of deafness often exists, a striking improvement in the hearing will generally follow the application of this method. So convinced are we that this is the most successful mode of treating acute exudative otitis media, that we have kept a careful record of our results, and have found that in one hundred cases of this class, taken indiscriminately in the clinics of two hospitals, the majority of cases have been actually cured, while the others have been improved. In a very few no improvement followed.

When, however, the cases have been neglected, or not properly treated by this method, and connective tissue has developed in the course of the chronic inflammatory process, and thereby caused auchylosis* of the ossicles, or adhesions with the walls of the tympanic cavities have taken place, little improvement follows. In otitis interna, deafness due to the peculiar occupation of the patient, as for instance, boiler makers, or those working in certain machine works or mills where catarrhal diseases of the aural nervous apparatus develop, no improvement can be expected, in fact this method should not be employed.

"Aural Massage" : by successive condensation and rarefaction of the air in the external meatus and middle ear, with or without the electric current.

Aural Massage, by alternately opening and closing the meatus and by moving backward and forward the tragus pressed by the finger into the thus opened and closed meatus, has been recommended and practised for some time for the purpose of giving motion to the membrana tympani, especially when adherent or thickened, and to make passive motion of the ossicles, and is used with some slight benefit. Another method is to open and shut the orifice of the canal by pressure on the tragus, thus tightly closing the meatus, and the force may be increased by greasing the canal. There is also a more perfect method of making massage, by condensation and rarefaction, using the instrument of Siegle (Siegle's Otoscope†), which has for years been employed in the examination of the membrana tympani. This instrument resembles the ordinary hard rubber speculum, but is more elongated, and its outer opening is fitted with an oblique plate of glass. A small nipple projecting from its side marks an opening to which is attached a small rubber tube ending in a mouth piece. The instrument is used by inserting the small specular end into the meatus as far as possible (better after its having been covered with a section of rubber tubing and anointed). The mouth may be applied to the distal end of the connecting tube for suction, or else a small syringe may be used to exhaust the air, or, a valved bulb can be used, and through the oblique glass the movements of the membrana tympani can be watched. All these plans were more or less unsatisfactory until the one devised by Dr. Chas. Delstanche, of Brussels, who has given us two improved instruments. *

Delstauche's instrument for massage, or, as he terms it, his "masseur," consists of a metallic tube enclosing a smaller tube of metal which acts like the valve of a syringe. The recoil of the valve which

---

* Suc1 as has been s1own, by Politzer, to occur between the footplate of the stapes and the oval window or pit or depression in w1ic1 it ests. Comp. Rendus, IVème Congrès d'Otologie, Brussels, 1888. † Siegle's Pneumatic Otoscope or Speculum.

produces the aspiration and condensation is accomplished by a spiral spring between the valve, and the bottom of the metallic tube. The inner tube is graduated in fifths, so that one may determine by a key the amount of power to be employed. Care is necessary in the use of this instrument for fear of rupturing the tympanic membrane thus causing disagreeable complications and to say the least, a great deal of pain, a flow of blood, and an interference with the operation. In order to better condense the air in the tube, the nipple-like process is covered with rubber. This must be withdrawn from time to time, but the to and fro motion may be continued, always examining its effects upon the membrana tympani. The other instrument is termed by Delstanche the "rarefacteur." It is provided with a double valve, and has an advantage over the former instrument in that, without removing it, one may alternately condense and rarefy the air in the external meatus, or rarefy it alone. This instrument is much more powerful and with it we can exhaust the air in the middle ear, especially where there is a sunken membrane, or we may attempt to break up adhesions between the membrana tympani and inner walls of the cavity of the tympanum, or after paracentesis of the membrane, when we wish to withdraw intra-tympanal fluids.

Several other instruments* have been invented and brought forth of late for the same purpose, differing in name, but all of them have the same object in view. They cannot be employed alone, but must serve as an aid to other means. Although they are of value when properly and scientifically applied by the aural surgeon, they are of limited application, and like all good and efficient agents can do much harm as well as good.

Another of these instruments has been termed the "Vibrometer," which combines massage with sound interruptions and is both mechanic and electric, with exhaustion or rarefaction. The first instrument employed was like a violin, the second like a guitar, the third is in the form of a banjo, but so far they have not fulfilled the requirements nor produced the results hoped for.

"Phono-massage" is another form by means of which certain musical sounds may be conveyed into the ear, through tightly fitting rubber tubes, from various musical instruments, or with electro-magnetic machines. There are various forms and contrivances, the main object of which is to impress the nervous patient with the idea of "doing something" more than the more simple method of using the pneumatic speculum, or the ordinary form of auto-massage by the aid of the finger in the auditory canal or on the tragus.

It is not necessary to go into further details, we have found the results borne out in one hundred cases as follows. In only four cases

* Later that devised by Freudenthal, the pneumatic pump of Chevalier Jackson, of Pa., and still later the electric pressure sound of Lester. (Phila. Med. Jour., March 11th, 1899, p. 568.)

FF

was there decided improvement in the deafness, and tinnitus. In several of the cases there was temporary improvement, but in the majority, no permanent or good results, and in some cases the noises were increased.

In two recent cases which we examined, our diagnosis was in the first, deafness from the constant noise of machinery and steam and electric apparatus. This individual has been subjected to "Pneumo-massage" and an "Electro-Metronome" for months with the expecta-tion of a cure, but as a matter of course, little or no benefit resulted.

In the second case our diagnosis was "mill-operative deafness," or chronic paretic neuritis of the auditory nerve in a man who had worked for years in a factory subjected to the noise of all kinds of machinery, yet this man was encouraged to continue "pneumo-massage" treat-ment hoping that his deafness would improve, but on the contrary, after months of treatment by mechanical and electrical massage he was not benefited, his deafness was rather increased, and he could not hear ordinary conversation except in the shop where there were constant and continuous noises. In these two, and in many similar cases which have been reported, there was the usual symptom of "paracousis Willisii" with more or less deafness and chronic middle ear inflammation, in which, if it cannot be improved by the use of Politzer's method, or the methodical exercises of the ear as devised by Urbantschitsch and defended by Brenner, we must rely upon the mechanical assistance from a trumpet or funnel with an elastic tube.

The chronically deaf should be taught "lip-reading" and given a course of instruction in the motion of the lips, and facial expression which greatly facilitates the power of the eye in assisting the defective hearing.

In regard to the surgery of the ear, the following have stood the test for thirty-five years.

The opening of the mastoid and its improved modifications, also by Stacke's operation, also operative interference in chronic suppurative otitis media by the removal of the ossicles, or the removal of the incus in some cases of chronic middle ear inflammation, and in chronic cases the freeing of the stapes dial joint by mobilizing it, using gentle pres-sure and exhaustion.

In the surgery of the ear involving the lateral sinuses and the brain, with or without mastoid complication, great success has been attained, and the full recognition of the mechanical relations of nose and ear, so intimately associated, that we must venture the opinion that every successful Otologist must be a thorough and practical Rhinologist.

The union of the Rhinologist with the Otologist has, in my opinion, given great impulse to the study of our department, and in so far as my experience goes, the benefit to cases of chronic ear and throat disease derived from the removal of spurs and hypertrophies within the nose is little, but in acute tympanic diseases, the benefit has been incalculable, while the removal of post-nasal adenoids for nasal and tubal (Eustachian) interference, and the recognition of "mouth breathing" as a symptom, especially in children, has already proved, and will continue to prove, a boon to the youth of the world that must eventually minimize the tendency to tympanic disease.

DES AMÉLIORATIONS DE L'OUÏE OBTENUES PAR LE TYMPAN ARTIFICIEL DANS L'OTITE MOYENNE SÈCHE OU SCLÉROSE TYMPANIQUE.

DR. VEYRAT, Chambéry, Aix-les-Bains.

Le tympan artificiel, ce petit appareil merveilleux qui, dans les destructions de la membrane tympanique, produit contre la surdité, qui en est la conséquence, de si prompts et si surprenants résultats, peut aussi améliorer l'audition dans certains cas, où, au contraire, la membrane est épaissie, où la caisse du tympan elle-même a subi les plus profondes et les plus définitives altérations.

J'espère démontrer que le tympan artificiel, sous la forme d'une simple petite lamelle de coton, peut avoir des résultats bien appréciables quelquefois contre la surdité progressive et contre les bruits subjectifs qui l'accompagnent, dans l'otite moyenne chronique sèche, ou sclérose tympanique : (processus adhésifs, de Politzer), (sclérose de la caisse, de Tröltsch), (otite sclérémateuse de Duplay), ou otite interstitielle.

La transmission du son dans l'otite sèche est plus ou moins supprimée entre la membrane tympanique et le labyrinthe. La surdité, qui en résulte, tient surtout à l'immobilisation, à la rigidité de la chaine des osselets, et les bruits subjectifs s'expliquent, soit par la pression qu'exerce l'étrier sur la fenêtre ovale, soit par l'extension au labyrinthe du processus scléreux.

Les causes de ces deux symptômes majeurs, surdité et bruits anormaux, seront plus ou moins graves, selon qu'elles dépendront plus ou moins :

De la membrane tympanique qui, épaissie, tendue exagérément, recouverte de dépôts calcaires, ou relâchée par l'atrophie, ne transmettra plus les vibrations sonores ;

De la caisse, où des adhérences, des ligaments en tous sens, des modifications profondes de la muqueuse altéreront les parois ;

De la chaine, où les osselets soudés aux parois de la caisse, soit que la tête du marteau reste fixée à la paroi supérieure, soit que sa longue apophyse soit retenue à la paroi postérieure, où le marteau ossifié à l'enclume et restant immobile, où l'étrier fixé par ses branches à la niche ou par sa base au contour de la fenêtre ovale, rendront rigide ou immobile cet organe essentiel de transmission.

Dans toutes ces modifications si graves, l'audition sera de plus en plus supprimée ; et, cependant, c'est dans quelques-uns de ces cas, que la membrane artificielle viendra apporter une amélioration bien appréciable de l'ouïe, ne devant être repoussée que dans les cas où l'étrier sera définitivement ankylosé, ou lorsque le labyrinthe, continuant la série, sera affecté des mêmes troubles trophiques que la caisse, sa voisine.

Parmi les nombreux cas, où j'ai, depuis vingt ans, employé, avec des résultats divers, le tympan artificiel, je citerai très succinctement les suivants, qui me paraissent plus probants que toute espèce de démonstration :

Première observation.

3 avril 1895.

M. C. est âgé de 49 ans, il est sourd depuis 15 à 16 ans, avec des bourdonnements continus et insupportables. .

Fils de père devenu sourd vers 55 ans. Il a habité longtemps un pays très humide et a eu longtemps de l'inflammation naso-pharyngienne, dont il ne souffre plus aujourd'hui.

Soigné, il y a 12 ans, son audition et les bruits paraissaient s'améliorer sous l'influence des douches d'air ; mais, obligé de partir en voyage, il cessa dès lors tout traitement.

A l'inspection, je trouve :

Oreille gauche : Membrane opaque, grise, épaissie, fortement retirée, très concave, le manche du marteau complètement incliné en dedans.

Au spéculum de Siegle, la membrane paraît immobile, sauf peut-être à la partie supérieure, le malade, du reste, très intelligent, croit sentir un petit mouvement ; le manche du marteau est immobile, la chaîne rigide, l'ankylose est certaine.

Le diapason-vertex rassure sur l'état du labyrinthe. L'épreuve de Gellé est nette et favorable. Le diapason est entendu tout à fait près de l'oreille. La montre nulle. La voix ordinaire à cinquante centimètres.

La douche d'air révèle une trompe libre, mais rétrécie ; elle diminue momentanément les bruits. La montre, après la douche d'air, est perçue au contact ; la voix ordinaire entendu au même point. Le malade me raconte qu'il entend mieux en chemin de fer : il a de la paracousie de Willis.

Le traitement institué fut :—

La douche d'air à fortes pressions, tous les trois jours environ, le massage, les injections diverses. Trois fois je fis la perforation de la membrane, le tout avec peu de succès. Je tentais même la dernière fois un peu de mobilisation, dont souffrit le malade.

Après 40 jours environ, il est assurément mieux, il entend la montre d'une façon persistante au contact, la voix ordinaire à près d'un mètre, la conversation générale est toujours nulle.

J'introduis alors simplement un peu d'huile de vaseline dans la caisse par la sonde d'Itard, et, quelques jours après, j'applique sur le tympan une lamelle de coton imbibée de vaseline liquide, que je fais adhérer le plus possible à toute la périphérie de la membrane naturelle, la tassant légèrement au centre.

Le patient n'éprouve rien d'anormal, ni gêne, ni pesanteur, ni vertige ; il se trouve plutôt mieux. L'audition est sensiblement la même ; les bruits n'ont pas changé. Je le revois deux jours après, il est enchanté et m'annonce que la veille il a entendu sa montre à quelques centimètres de l'oreille, sans qu'il y ait contact en un mot, et, ce qui l'a le plus vivement frappé, il a entendu, se trouvant près d'un jeu de billard, le bruit des billes s'entrechoquant et la voix ordinaire à plus d'un mètre, assure-t-il.

Mais, depuis le matin, l'audition esi redevenue aussi mauvaise et je constate que le tympan artificiel s'est déplacé.

J'applique une nouvelle lamelle, le résultat est immédiat et je constate moi-même l'amélioration annoncée.

Je confie alors à M. C. l'application du petit tympan de coton, lui enseigne la manière de procéder avec la petite pince. Après quelques jours d'essai, il s'en tire très bien.

Il arrive même beaucoup plus sûrement que moi à trouver le point exact de tassement et d'adhésion pour obtenir le maximum d'ouïe. Je le revois encore 15 ou 20 jours après ; l'amélioration non seulement a persisté, mais s'est accrue au point qu'il peut entendre certaines personnes dans la conversation générale, qu'il entend la voix ordinaire à près de trois mètres et que les bruits dont il était continuellement assiégé, ont diminué tellement que souvent il ne les a plus, ne les percevant que lorsqu'il les cherche un instant.

Avant son départ, je conseille à mon client de continuer l'usage quotidien de la poire de Politzer.

Je l'ai revu deux ans après en 1897 et cette année, au mois de mars 1899, l'amélioration s'est maintenue et les bruits ont disparu tout à fait. J'ai fait de nouveau chaque fois quelques instillations de vaseline liquide dans la caisse, ce dont il m'affirme se trouver très bien.

L'oreille droite, dont il entendait peut-être encore un peu il y a 4 ans, s'est paralysée de plus en plus, aussi combien est-il heureux d'avoir conservé son oreille gauche.

Deuxième observation.

12 mai 1896.

Mme Ph., 41 ans, est devenue sourde insensiblement depuis l'âge de 27 ou 28 ans, et a éprouvé, depuis six ou sept ans, des bruits intenses, qui diminuent cependant parfois dans l'oreille droite. Les mêmes symptômes existaient dans l'oreille gauche, où depuis deux ans les bruits ont disparu et la surdité devenue complète.

Pas de sourds dans sa famille. Pharynx en bon état. L'inspection révèle tous les symptômes objectifs de la dégénérescence interstitielle, la membrane est fortement attirée en dedans avec quelques points de relâchement atrophique, synéchies nombreuses, soudure des osselets ankylosés.

La trompe d'Eustache est très ouverte. Les Siegle me paraît cependant favorable et l'épreuve des pressions de Gellé appréciable.

La montre n'est entendue nulle part. Le diapason, entendu près de l'oreille, l'est davantage sur le mastoïde et sur les os de la tête.

La voix ordinaire est entendue à un peu moins d'un mètre.

La conversation générale nulle. Pas de paracousie.

La douche d'air fait diminuer les bruits, mais n'améliore pas l'ouïe.

Du côté gauche, avec une membrane qui, à l'examen, parait normale, la surdité est complète, le labyrinthe est envahi par le processus scléreux.

Après avoir pratiqué pendant quelques semaines la douche d'air avec la sonde d'Itard, injecté de la vaseline liquide, fait le massage sans amélioration soutenue, je fis la section du pli postérieur de la membrane : l'ouïe s'améliora sensiblement et les bruits diminuèrent très notablement, disparurent même quelques heures ; mais ce mieux cessa en quelques jours après la cicatrisation. Je dus abandonner toute autre tentative plus complète qui paraissait indiquée : ma cliente étant à bout de patience et prétendant avoir souffert.

Je continuais quelques instillations d'huile de vaseline et plaçais la membrane artificielle, qui ne produisit un heureux effet qu'après la troisième application, le sixième jour.

Elle entendit alors très nettement la montre au contact, le diapason-vertex très fortement dans l'oreille, et la voix ordinaire très nettement à plus que trois mètres.

Je ne revois ma malade que pendant quelques jours encore ; elle a appris très vite à placer elle-même, à enlever et à remettre au point, la petite lamelle humectée d'huile de vaseline et part très satisfaite.

Je l'ai revue au mois de mars de cette année après trois ans, pendant lesquels elle ne s'est jamais lassée de placer le tympan artificiel et de se servir, au moins deux ou trois fois par semaine, de la poire de Politzer.

L'amélioration s'est maintenue d'une façon appréciable ; les bruits ont à peu près disparu. Je dois ajouter qu'un confrère de son pays a instillé deux fois environ chaque année pendant quelques semaines, de l'huile de vaseline dans la caisse.

TROISIÈME OBSERVATION.

20 avril 1897.

M. B. est un officier de marine en retraite, qui vient à Aix-les-Bains depuis deux ans, pour soigner des rhumatismes. Agé de 64 ans. Il a vécu aux colonies, dans les Indes, et parait encore vigoureux. Pas d'antécédents héréditaires.

Il est devenu sourd depuis dix ans d'une façon progressive, avec des alternatives d'améliorations. Il a des bourdonnements plus forts dans l'oreille gauche qu'à droite.

A l'examen, les deux oreilles sont sensiblement les mêmes ; tou es deux offrent les symptômes objectifs de l'otite moyenne chronique sèche. La membrane naturelle est rétractée fortement en dedans, de chaque côté, plus opaque à gauche qu'à droite, partiellement du moins.

Au spéculum Siegle, peu ou pas de mobilité à gauche, un peu plus à droite. Le diapason-vertex peu différent de chaque côté.

Cependant, à l'épreuve Gellé, il paraît peu interrompu à droite. La montre n'est pas entendue à gauche, elle l'est un peu au contact à droite, et la voix ordinaire parait à peu près également perçue à un demi mètre de chaque côté.

Conversation générale impossible. La douche paraît faire diminuer les bruits, elle est sans résultat pour l'ouïe.

Les trompes d'Eustache sont très perméables, mais rétrécies.

Comme traitement, je pratique la douche d'air douze à treize fois pendant vingt-cinq jours. Les bruits ont notablement diminué, mais l'audition reste la même, quoique le malade se sente mieux et entende à droite la montre au contact, pas du tout à gauche.

Il n'entend pas mieux la voix ordinaire.

M. B. ne veut entendre parler d'aucune opération, j'essaie du massage qui n'amène en huit ou dix jours aucun résultat ; j'instille de l'huile de vaseline pendant quelques jours encore et place la membrane artificielle dans les deux oreilles. Et instantanément l'ouïe est notablement améliorée à droite seulement. Il apprend en quelques jours à l'enlever avec la pince et à la fixer bien au point et je ne le revois que quinze jours après.

Il entend alors la voix basse à 0^m50 centimètres à droite, et la voix ordinaire à plus de cinq mètres ; à gauche il la perçoit facilement à un mètre seulement. Il a pu entendre certaines personnes dans la conversation générale et n'a plus, comme auparavant, de la paracousie qui le gênait beaucoup.

Les bruits sont bien moins forts des deux côtés et très supportables, dit-il.

Je lui conseille de continuer chaque jour les douches d'air par la poire de Politzer.

Je ne l'ai revu qu'en avril dernier. Son audition s'était améliorée au point qu'il ne fait plus usage du tympan artificiel que dans l'oreille gauche, la plus sourde, lorsqu'il veut, prétend-il, mieux entendre dans la conversation générale.

En présence de tels résultats, il n'est pas permis de ne pas utiliser un moyen aussi simple et aussi inoffensif d'améliorer l'ouïe et de diminuer les bruits subjectifs.

Je n'ai, certes, pas la prétention de le donner comme réussissant invariablement, ni de vouloir l'employer comme traitement initial, ni surtout de vouloir le substituer aux délicates et difficiles opérations qu'ont préconisées et pratiquées avec succès tant de maitres illustres ; non : mais il faut savoir s'en servir, lorsque les opérations les plus rationnelles auront échoué, ou ne pourront être pratiquées.

Et ne voit-on pas dans cette variété de processus adhésifs, la plus fréquente dans la pratique otologique, les opérations les plus indiquées et les mieux faites n'avoir qu'un résultat momentané ?

Les effets si prompts de la myringidectomie cesser avec la cicatrisation persistante de l'ouverture ?

La suppression des bruits par la section des plis échouer pour la même cause ?

Les résultats brillants de la ténotomie du muscle du marteau et du marteau lui-même ne pas persévérer toujours ?

Les améliorations réelles obtenues par la mobilisation directe de l'étrier et même par l'excision de cet osselet soumises à des fortunes variables ?

C'est alors que, dans certains cas, le tympan artificiel viendra améliorer, peut-être longtemps encore, des auditions bien compromises, en rétablissant la transmission du son au milieu de ces modifications anatomo-pathologiques si complexes.

Car, il est possible que même dans ces cas, où les altérations scléreuses paraissent le plus étendues, les ondes sonores réunies sur la membrane artificielle puissent arriver jusqu'au labyrinthe, où la plus petite vibration est amplement perçue : il remplacerait dans ce cas la membrane naturelle devenue inutile !

En somme, je crois pouvoir en conseiller l'essai contre la surdité de l'otite moyenne chronique sèche :

Dans les anomalies de tension, lorsque la membrane est insuffisamment tendue, dans les relâchements atrophiques partiels ;

Dans les scléroses, même d'origine catarrhale, si la sécrétion n'existe plus et si la trompe d'Eustache est libre ;

Dans les cas même les plus complexes de synéchies, de soudures, d'ossifications, tant que l'étrier ne sera pas absolument soudé, ankylosé à la fenêtre ovale ;

En ayant soin toutefois de maintenir toujours la trompe d'Eustache très ouverte et même de projeter quelquefois sur les parois de la caisse quelques gouttes de vaseline liquide.

Dans tous les cas où le tympan artificiel réussira, je crois qu'il doit agir par son contact intime à la périphérie osseuse, qui entoure la membrane naturelle et par son adhésion sur celle-ci en conduisant les sons jusqu'à l'air de la caisse, air qui agit assurément dans le phénomène de l'ouïe.

Pourquoi, d'autre part, n'agirait-il pas aussi par les os des parois, alors qu'il est facile de constater par le diapason-vertex, que la perception du son est renforcée après l'introduction de la membrane artificielle ?

DES INJECTIONS INTERSTITIELLES DE SUBLIMÉ CORROSIF DANS LE TRAITEMENT DES LUPUS DU NEZ.

DR. VEYRAT, Chambéry, Aix-les-Bains.

Il m'a été donné, dans ces dernières années, de soigner trois cas très nets de Lupus primitif de la muqueuse nasale, avec extension à la peau du nez, de pouvoir en suivre la marche, de les revoir après de longs intervalles, d'en constater les récidives et de n'obtenir leur guérison complète après le raclage et les cautérisations galvaniques que par des injections profondes et répétées de sublimé corrosif dans les nodules lupiques eux-mêmes.

Les résultats que j'ai obtenus à la suite de ces injections, m'encouragent à présenter au Congrès de Londres les trois observations suivantes :

PREMIÈRE OBSERVATION.

22 juillet 1897.

Mlle R...., âgée de 14 ans, est une fillette que j'avais soignée trois ans auparavant pour la Rhinite hypertrophique bilatérale, qui parut guérie après quelques semaines, sous l'action de douches nasales d'eau boratée tiède avec le syphon de Weber, et de quelques badigeonnages.

Elle revient aujourd'hui, avec un nez déformé, augmenté de volume, à plaques bleuâtres, indolentes, la narine gauche complètement oblitérée par des croûtes jaunâtres qui adhèrent au rebord extrême de l'aile du nez. J'enlève les croûtes après quelques lotions et je trouve au-dessous une surface rougeâtre, recouverte de petites saillies ulcérées, grosses comme des grains de chénevis, bourgeonnantes, mais molles et non saignantes, qui siègent sur la partie cartilagineuse de la cloison. Une ulcération plus grande et unique, surélevée, existe aussi à l'extrémité antérieure du cornet inférieur, très gonflé au-dessus. Dans la narine droite, la muqueuse un peu granulée paraît saine.

Les antécédents sont très bons : père et mère forts et en bonne santé ; cinq frères ou sœurs bien portants.

J'institue un traitement général des plus reconstituants, et je pratique sous la chloroformisation un raclage des plus complets, suivi de galvano-cautérisation, pansement iodoformé, etc.

Une amélioration telle se produit, que je la crois guérie et l'envoie passer le mois d'août à Moûtiers-Salins (Savoie), dont les eaux chlorurées sodiques m'ont toujours donné d'excellents résultats chez les scrofulo-tuberculeux.

Elle en revient très bien portante ; mais le nez n'a pas repris un aspect normal ; la muqueuse n'est pas ulcérée, mais reste hypertrophiée, par places surtout, et je conseille des injections d'eau naphtolée.

Je ne revois ma jeune malade qu'en février 1898 ; les parents ont négligé de me l'amener plus tôt.—De nouvelles croûtes obstruent toute la narine gauche, et je trouve au-dessous et aux mêmes places des exulcérations plus volumineuses et plus nombreuses avec bourgeons charnus, exubérants, inégaux, à peine saignants, sans sensibilité ui fétidité.

Dès le lendemain et pendant le sommeil anesthésique, je procède à un nouveau raclage, aussi complet que possible, suivi de galvano-cautérisation, et je fais un pansement iodoformé. Tout va bien pendant un mois, lorsque de nouvelles croûtes apparaissent sur l'aile du nez, près du sillon naso-génien gauche ; au-dessous, je trouve une petite exulcération. Nouveau raclage et légère cautérisation avec la créosote étendue. Nouvelle amélioration ; la fillette est très bien portante, devient vigoureuse, la menstruation s'établit franchement.

Je revois Mlle R... un bon mois après. La famille s'inquiète d'une bosselure bleuâtre qui existe sur le lobule, et de quelques saillies de même aspect sur l'aile du nez qui est toujours déformé. La muqueuse du reste n'a pas repris l'aspect qu'on lui trouve dans la narine droite ; elle est toujours hypertrophiée.

Je pratique alors quatre petites injections, de une à deux gouttes chacune, dans chaque nodosité et deux, sous la muqueuse de la cloison, avec une solution de sublimé corrosif au centième. Les suites en sont pénibles et même très douloureuses : gonflement énorme, inflammation de la peau du voisinage ; mais, sous l'action de sachets de glace renouvelés et entretenus sur le nez, la douleur violente disparaît rapidement et tout rentre dans l'ordre après quatre jours. Je recouvre alors le nez de gaze imbibée d'huile iodoformée, et le dixième jour, le nez a repris son état normal. Un nouveau nodule se manifeste huit jours après vers l'aile du nez ; je fais deux nouvelles injections interstitielles de sublimé ; quinze ou vingt jours après, deux nouvelles nodosités bleuâtres, molles, indolentes apparaissent vers le sillon naso-génien et sont traitées par de nouvelles injections et la guérison est définitivement assurée. La muqueuse du nez a repris son aspect rosé ; il n'y a plus le moindre gonflement ; et, deux mois après la dernière injection, n'offrant plus la moindre tache, ui la moindre cicatrice, la peau du nez est aussi nette d'un côté que de l'autre. Depuis cette époque, un an s'est écoulé sans récidive ; la guérison parait complète et définitive.

Deuxième observation.

Hôtel Dieu de Chambéry, 10 Janvier 1898.

M. P...., 30 ans, ouvrier tanneur. Père et mère bien portants ; sept frères ou sœurs vivants et en bonne santé. A eu des gourmes dans son enfance, a été chétif jusqu'à 18 ans, a pris jusqu'à cet âge de huile de foie de morue. Sujet aux rhumes de cerveau et aux maux de gorge. A fait dans de bonnes conditions son service militaire et s'est bien porté jusqu'en août 1894. Depuis cette époque, dit-il, il a toujours eu le nez bouché. Pas de traces de syphilis. Larynx et poumons sains. Pas de fétidité de l'haleine. Le nez n'est pas effondré à la base ; il est déformé et bosselé, parsemé de boursouflures bleuâtres, surtout du côté droit. Les deux narines sont obstruées par des croûtes jaunes verdâtres. Audessous, je trouve 9 à 10 ulcérations saillantes sur la partie cartilagineuse, de la cloison du côté droit ; une ulcération recouvre la partie inférieure cutanée de la cloison et une surface rougeâtre, couverte de saillies bourgeonnantes, va rejoindre la muqueuse du côté gauche. Sur le rebord de l aile droite existe aussi une petite ulcération qui s'engage vers la joue dans le pli naso-génien. Rien au-delà du tiers antérieur de la muqueuse. La cloison est perforée. Un traitement antisyphilitique fut institué et l'on fit en même temps des cautérisations à l'acide lactique, puis à une solution alcoolique de chlorure de zinc.

Après six semaines, il n'avait donné aucun résultat. Je le remplace par un traitement général reconstituant, et, sous la chloroformisation, l'arrière cavité des fosses nasales ayant été tamponnée, je pratique le raclage aussi complet que possible, avec les curettes de Volkmann, de toute la muqueuse exubérante et je cautérise le fond des plaies avec le galvano-cautère ; les ulcérations de la peau subissent le même sort. Je n'eus pas à recommencer, sauf à faire quelques attouchements avec une solution concentrée de créosote dans l'alcool et la glycérine sur de petites ulcérations du sillon naso-génien. Mais la peau du nez reste inégale, le lobule et le côté gauche sont mamelonnés par de petites élevures bleuâtres, le nez est plus gros du côté gauche. Je pratique une première fois six injections d'une à deux gouttes de solution de sublimé au centième, suivies d'application de glace et plus tard pansement iodoformé. Le gonflement disparaît rapidement et après quinze jours, je puis faire quatre ou cinq nouvelles injections dans les nodules qu'on aperçoit toujours sous la peau, et deux d'une seule goutte sous la muqueuse au bas de la cloison. Je les renouvelais en moindre quantité une troisième fois vingt-cinq jours après. Alors seulement, et, malgré un abcès qui se déclara près du sillon naso-génien, tout marcha rapidement vers la guéri on ; la cicatrisation de la muqueuse s'acheva sans sténose de la narine, grâce au pansement iodoformé. Et le nez lui-même, quoique recouvert de petites cicatrices blanchâtres, très peu visibles, a repris au bout d'un mois un aspect très acceptable. Le malade quitte mon service de l'Hôtel-Dieu dans les premiers jours de juin 1898, guéri et bien portant. Depuis un an, il n'a pas eu la moindre récidive.

Troisième observation.

15 novembre 1897.

Mlle C..., 33 ans. Bien portante. Trois sœurs vivantes, mariées et en bonne santé Père décédé à 65 ans, mère vivante et bien portante. N'a fait aucune maladie sérieuse, tout en restant chétive. N'a pas eu de gourmes dans son enfance ; mais depuis longtemps est sujette à des rhumes de cerveau. Pharynx, larynx et poumons en bon état. Elle me raconte qu'elle avait la mauvaise habitude d'introduire souvent le doigt dans le nez et qu'un jour, à la suite d'une petite excoriation qu'elle se fit dans la narine gauche, des croûtes se formèrent sur ce point et se renouvelèrent continuellement. Elle vit alors un médecin qui lui fit faire des lavages antiseptiques et cautérisa l'ulcération d'abord au nitrate d'argent, puis à l'acide lactique. Les croûtes cessèrent, puis reparurent. Entre temps, il avait prescrit un traitement antistrumeux et reconstituant. Depuis un an, elle ne fait plus qu'ôter les croûtes et se tonifier. Elle se présente à moi avec la narine gauche absolument obstruée par des croûtes jaunâtres qui recouvrent une partie du lobule du nez et l'aile gauche, et en partie l'entrée de la narine droite par laquelle l'air eut encore passer. Sous les croûtes, je trouve à gauche, une surface rougeâtre et jaunâtre à la fois, parsemée de bourgeons fongueux, mous, peu saignants qui re-couvrent toute la partie cartilagineuse de la cloison.   Les cornets sont très gonflés, mais la muqueuse y parait saine.   La fosse nasale droite présente aussi, mais sur une petite étendue et sur la partie antérieure de la cloison, deux ou trois ulcérations saillantes et audessus, des granulations d'un rouge plus vif.   La cloison n'est pas perforée.   Sur le rebord de l'aile gauche du nez, une ulcération unique existe et une autre plus large sur le lobule du nez qui a beaucoup augmenté de volume.   Le nez est du reste, à gauche surtout, très mamelonné par des sailles bleuâtres et molles.   Je continue un traitement des plus reconstituants, et peu après je pratique sous l'anesthésie un premier raclage aussi complet que possible, suivi d'une légère cautérisation galvanique sur le fond des plaies.   Pansement à l'iodoforme.   Quinze jours après de nouvelles croûtes apparaissent sur les ulcérations de la peau du lobule et de l'aile du nez que j'avais ménagées, pour éviter les cicatrices de la brûlure.   Je les racle de nouveau et les touche quelques fois à la créosote en solution alcoolique ; je panse à l'iodoforme et j'obtiens, en dix ou douze jours la cicatrisation.   Mais le nez a gardé sa forme mamelonnée, les nodosités bleuâtres qui existent sur la partie gauche du nez et sur le lobule existent toujours et affectent ma malade.   Je pratique alors une première fois, le 6 janvier 1898, cinq injections interstitielles de ma solution de sublimé au centième sous ces nodosités, vrais nodules lupiques et une sur la muqueuse de la cloison, en un point suspect. Douleur inflammation, gonflement énorme, tout est calmé par la glace et la suppuration évitée sous l'action de l'huile iodoformée.

Le 27 janvier, trois injections de deux à trois gouttes sont de nouveau néces-saires sur le nez, et autant le 19 février.   Dès lors, le nez reprend peu à peu sa forme normale, quelques petites cicatrices s'établissent sur les anciennes ulcérations, mais sont à peine visibles ; aucune nodosité n'existe encore.   Je conseille de continuer quelques lavages antiseptiques au moindre coryza, de relever, le plus possible la nutri-tion générale déprimée et je revois ma malade tous les deux ou trois mois jusqu'aux premiers jours de mai dernier.   Depuis quatorze mois, il n'y a eu aucune récidive.

Après ces résultats, je me crois autorisé à conclure que, pour éviter ou éloigner le plus possible les récidives dans les lupus du nez, on devra, après la destruction complète du processus lupique par le raclage et la galvano-cautérisation ou autre, poursuivre sous la muqueuse et sous la peau le germe morbide, tant que des saillies bleuâtres, des nodosités molles, révélant les nodules lupiques, reparaîtront sur la cloison ou sur la peau du nez.   Pour cela, les injections interstitielles de sublimé corrosif au centième semblent être le mode le plus actif pour arrêter la reproduction des bacilles et en débarrasser le terrain contaminé.

En relevant en même temps par tous les moyens les forces de l'or-ganisme, la muqueuse nasale, ce terrain si favorable à l'envahissement tuberculeux, deviendra plus résistante et l'économie plus forte dans sa lutte contre l'invasion du parasite.

CURABILITY OF CHRONIC SUPPURATIVE OTITIS MEDIA.

MR. F. FAULDER WHITE, Coventry.

The attitude of the medical profession in England towards suppura-tive otitis media is still unsatisfactory ; patients are still being told

that there is no cure for running ears and that it is dangerous to meddle
with them.   On the other hand some aural surgeons recommend extensive perforations of the bone.   In uncomplicated cases, I believe these
operations to be generally unnecessary, and most will admit that they
are dangerous and do not always effect a cure.

The importance of this disease was not at one time at all generally
recognized.   In my student days, cases of so-called simple otorrhœa
were never admitted to the hospital wards.   They were treated as out-
patients, being usually given a bottle of mild lotion with which to
syringe the ear.

Now of one thing I am firmly persuaded, that to effect the cure of
these cases requires regular and frequent skilled attendance and that
when that is given, good results may be obtained without operation.
For some years past I have been in the habit of admitting cases of
suppurative otitis to the wards of the Coventry Hospital for treatment,
by frequent washings with antiseptic solutions.   Other cases are
attended to by a trained nurse twice a day in the out-patient department.   In private practice too, I prefer to carry out the treatment
myself and not to leave it to some friend of the patient.   The fact that
this point has not usually been insisted on is sufficient to account for
many failures in treatment.

I think it not unlikely that I shall be told that the syringe has
been tried over and over again, and that some pronounce douching to
be of little use : I am aware of that.

While attending the Section of Otology at the 1895 meeting of the
B.M. Association, I heard Professor Macewen's paper, in which he
challenged Otologists with their failure in this disease.   I have noted
the practical failure of vicarious syringing in the work of an aural
department of a large London Hospital.   As a practitioner, I have
seen many cases of long standing that had been syringed without any
good result by trained and untrained attendants.   Notwithstanding
this, I have for a long time held that the mechanical and vital difficulties attending the treatment of suppurative otitis by antiseptic
irrigation are generally surmountable by care and perseverance.   And
experience has confirmed that opinion.   The principle of my treatment
is simple, namely to purify the diseased parts and to arouse the dormant
vitality of the poisoned tissues.

Considering the size of the cavities affected, the meatus may be
compared to a very large drainage tube provided that there is a large
perforation in the membrane.   This is fortunately present in the
majority of cases, but when there is only a small one I believe the right
course is to enlarge the opening, and this I have done in a few cases
with some success.

Although our special interest in the middle ear inclines us, perhaps,
to magnify its area, I would lay stress on the fact, that the cavities

affected in suppurative otitis media are really quite small, and the intercommunicating passages or spaces comparatively large. So long as disease is confined to these spaces, and has not affected the bone, I believe it may be reached, and consequently influenced, by injections through a large perforation. Even when the bone is affected, a cure will sometimes follow simple irrigation. I recently reported a case in which there was exfoliation of the modiolus of the cochlea with complete recovery. Anyone who has treated many poisoned wounds with hot baths or fomentations must have observed how wonderfully the tissues are thereby assisted in throwing off the poison, and though we cannot place a poisoned ear permanently under similar conditions, we adopt the same principle of treatment and obtain the same results by using hot antiseptic irrigations. I do not use the brass or glass syringe, but prefer the india rubber Higginson. By means of this we can inject an almost continuous stream of fluid with a minimum of shock to the tender parts. As a stimulating disinfectant I know nothing so good as the silico-fluoride of potassium. I use the saturated solution diluted with from one to six parts of hot water. This solution is well tolerated by the tissues. I have used it extensively in surgery, and believe it to be preferable to corrosive sublimate, which probably depresses tissue vitality.

I do not think that I need, before this assembly of experts, go into minor details of treatment, but I should like to draw your attention to one or two points.

The usual foul-smelling case is ordered irrigation with a quart of this solution three or four times a day, and in a few days a marked diminution in the offensive odour is generally to be noted. At this stage I never use strong astringents as any check to the process of elimination is especially to be avoided. The practice of treating these cases with absolute alcohol or dry dressings before a course of irrigation has disinfected the ear is in my opinion a dangerous one and likely to cause absorption of poison instead of elimination. I have seen more than one case of cerebral abscess that had been treated in this way and I would no more apply dry dressings to a foul ear than I would to a whitlow or poisoned wound.

I occasionally get cases of long standing in which the odour remains for weeks and even months, but when the patient perseveres, I have generally been able to make a cure and I have often remarked that the general health improves before the cure is complete. This, I believe is due to the fact that the treatment favours elimination of poison and puts an end to absorption.

I have recently seen a pamphlet by a Lecturer on Otology denouncing irrigation, but the fact is, we cannot do without the syringe if we wish to cure suppurative otitis. I am confident that when irrigation is persevered with, good results will generally be obtained. I have had several cases that had been under the care of skilled specialists and which only got well after a course of irrigation. Otologists would not denounce the douche if they had the opportunity of seeing their patients daily and attending to the treatment themselves. The arguments against the use of the syringe are not very conclusive. Douching a suppurating ear has been likened to watering plants, but though the growth of germs may be encouraged by stagnant moisture, the injection of a quart of antiseptic fluid has a very different effect. We might perhaps find theoretical objections to the use of hot baths for poisoned wounds. I attach much more importance to practical results than to theoretical objections. A rather more reasonable objection has been made to the douche, the possibility of germs being carried to healthy parts of the ear. I may say at once that I am not at all concerned about this problematical danger, problematical so far as the douche is concerned though it is real enough when one takes up the chisel or the drill. For when the antiseptic fluid is injected with a proper gentleness by means of a Higginson's syringe, there is little fear of opening up cavities previously shut off from the middle ear.

Perhaps the best answer to the objection, is the fact that out of the large number of cases I have treated by irrigation, I cannot recall one in which there was any evidence of extension of mischief while under treatment. I have too, kept a sharp look out for such extension of trouble, knowing how often the bone itself becomes diseased in neglected cases.

In conclusion, I must apologize if I have appeared to lay down the law to a body of experts. If I have spoken freely, my excuse is that I have devoted much time and labour to the treatment of suppurative otitis media and have arrived at the conclusion, which is largely based on results, that, in spite of the teachings and practice of some Otologists, we have in antiseptic irrigation the best hope of curing this troublesome disease. The large majority of cases will yield to irrigation if that be carried out with energy, gentleness, and perseverance.

INDEX OF SUBJECTS.

———

A

PAGE.

Abscess of the face   187
Absence and occlusion of external meatus   40
Acoustic exercises in deaf-mutes   195
Acoustic phenomena in fluid media   17
Addresses by President. &c. 1-8-273
Adeno-carcinoma of meatus   294
Adenoid vegetations : a factor in ear diseases   54
    ,:   ,,   operation on   116
    ,,   ,,   precocious involution on the Riviera ...   47
Anatomy of facial nerve in its relation to mastoid operations   108
   ,,   ,, frontal sinus and anterior ethmoid cells   107
   ,,   ,, internal and middle ear; stereoscopic views of ... 114-115
   ,,   ,, organ of Corti...   115
   ,,   ,, petro-squamosal sinus   160
Anterior abscess of mastoid and furunculosis of meatus ...   188
Aortic insufficiency as a cause of tinnitus   238
Artificial ear-drums in sclerosis   459
Attic, chronic suppurations of   126
Aural practice in India   306
Aural and nasal routes of intra-cranial infections   429
Aural epilepsy   407
Auricle, malformation of, with atresia of meatus ... ... · · 403

B

Beetlers' hearing-power   296
Blue diaphanousness of the membrana tympani   43

C

Cerebral abscess of nasal origin in a case of otitis media ...   406
Cerebral affections of otitic origin, *see Intracranial complications*

PAGE.

Chronic catarrhal deafness, prognosis in   257
  „   „   otitis, see *Otitis media catarrhalis*
  „   „   inflammation of pharynx, treatment of   ...   170
Condition of ears, throat, and nose in old people   304
Contagiousness of acute otitis media   127
Corrosive sublimate injections in lupus of nose   464
Cortical auditory centre   276
Corti, organ of, see *Anatomy*
Curability of otitis media suppurativa chronica   467

D

Deaf-mutes, acoustic exercises for   195
Deafness due to tumour of medulla and pons   378
Delegates to Congress, list of   7
Dewey's decimal system of notation applied to otological
    bibliography   366
Differential diagnosis between cerebral tumour, cerebral
    abscess, and hydrocephalus internus...   384
Diminished bone conduction as a contra-indication for ossicu-
    lectomy ...   . · ...   375

E

Ear complications of ozæna   217
Ear diseases caused by adenoid vegetations   54
  „   „   pneumatic treatment of   254
  „   „   rheumatic   121
  „   „   tubercular   20-34
Election of Officials   10
Endocranial complications see *Intracranial*
Epilepsy ab aure laesa   407
Ethmoid cells and frontal sinus, anatomy of   107
Évidement pétro-mastoïdien, in treatment of chronic dry
    catarrh of middle ear   176
Exostosis of meatus externus   219
External meatus, see *Meatus*
Eustachian obstruction treated by graduated bougies...   ...   415
Extraction of stapes   221-261

F

Facial abscess   187
Facial nerve, topography of, in relation to mastoid operations   108
Fenestra ovalis, operation on, in cases of ankylosis   240
Fibro-angioma of meatus externus   412
Fifth meeting...   126
Fluid media, acoustic phenomena in   17

PAGE.

Fourth meeting 107
Frontal sinus and ethmoid cells, anatomy of 107
Furunculosis of meatus, and anterior mastoid abscess... ... 188

H

Hanging-head position in operating on adenoid growths ... 116
Hearing-centre, cortical 276
Hearing-power in Beetlers 296
   ,,   ,,   measurement and notation of ... 11-15-16-281-290
High-pressure massage 251
Hydrorrhœa nasalis... 410

I

Inaugural meeting 1
Increase in the study of Otology 373
India, aural practice in 306-328
Indications for opening the mastoid in chronic suppurative
   otitis media 61-66-72-84-92-94
Instruments shown 115-406
Intra-cranial complications of ear disease 138-151-265-286-340-394-446
   ,,   ,,   infections *via* ear and nose... 429
Intra-dural abscess at the site of the saccus endolymphaticus 392
Intra-tympanic injections of pilocarpine for middle-ear catarrh 246

L

Labyrinth, transparent preparations of 115
Lateral sinus thrombosis, *see Intracranial complications*
Lenval prize award 272
   ,,   ,, jury 273
Letters and telegrams read by Secretary 7-11-61
Local application of remedies in treatment of chronic middle-
   ear catarrh 293
Lupus of nose treated by interstitial injections of corrosive
   sublimate... 461

M

Massage, vibratory 223
Mastoid abscess and furunculosis of meatus 188
   ,, diseases, their course and treatment 418
   ,, opening of, in chronic suppurative otitis media
                      61-66-72-84-92-94-147-265-331
   ,, operations, relations of facial nerve to 108
   ,, process, primary inflammation of 208
Measurement of hearing power, *see Hearing*
Meatus externus, adeno-carcinoma of 294

PAGE.

Meatus externus, atresia of, with malformation of auricle 403
　　,,　　　　,,　　congenital absence and acquired occlusion of 40
　　,,　　　　,,　　exostosis of 219
　　,,　　　　,,　　fibro-angioma of 412
　　,,　　　　,,　　sarcoma of 295
Meetings.— Inaugural 1
　　,,　　　　Second 11
　　,,　　　　Third 61
　　,,　　　　Fourth 107
　　,,　　　　Fifth 126
　　,,　　　　Sixth 199
　　,,　　　　Closing 270
Membrana tympani, blue diaphanousness and varix of ... 43
Middle ear, inflammation, see Otitis.
　　,,　　　,,　　tuberculosis of 20-34
Mobilization of ossicles in non-suppurative otitis media ... 343
　　,,　　　　,, stapes 351

N

Nasal and aural routes of intracranial infections 429
　,, hydrorrhœa 410
　,, lupus, treatment by injections of corrosive sublimate ... 464
Native Indian remedies for ear diseases 306-328

O

Obstruction of Eustachian tubes treated with graduated
　　bougies 415
Officials, election of 10
Old people, the condition of ears, larynx, and nose in 304
Operative treatment of mastoid inflammation 147
Operation on the fenestra ovalis in ankylosis 240
Optical method of acoumetry 16
Organization Committee of Seventh International Otological
　　Congress 270
Ossiculectomy contra-indicated by diminished bone conduction 375
Otitis media acuta, contagiousness of 127
　　,,　　　,,　co-existing with cerebral abscess of nasal origin 406
　　,,　　　,,　non-suppurativa, early mobilization of ossicles in 343
　　,,　　　,,　　,,　　　,,　　local treatment of 293
　　,,　　　,,　　,,　　　,,　　treatment by pilocarpine ... 246
　　,,　　　,,　　,,　　　,,　　　,,　　　,,　petro-mastoid
　　operation 176
Otitis media sicca, artificial ear-drums in 459
　　,,　　　,,　causing retropharyngeal abscess 414
　　,,　　　,,　suppurativa chronica, curability of 467

PAGE.

Otitis media suppurativa intracranial complications of, 138-151-265
                                                                286-340-394-446
,,   ,,   ,,   operation for, 61-66-72-84-92-94-147-265-331
Otological bibliography, decimal notation of   366
Otology, discoveries in   452
    ,,   section of, at general medical congresses   237
    ,,   the study of   373
Ozæna, ear complications of   217

P

Panotitis, with cerebral complications   151
Petro-squamosal sinus, its anatomy, etc.   160
Pharynx, catarrh of, new treatment of   170
Pilocarpine injections in catarrhal middle ear disease   246
Pneumo-massage under high pressure   251
Pneumatic treatment of diseases of the ear   254
Primary inflammation of mastoid process   208
Prognosis in chronic catarrhal deafness   257

R

Resolution regarding sections of otology and laryngology at
    general medical congresses   237
Retro-pharyngeal abscess of otitic origin   414
Rheumatic diseases of the ear   121
Riviera, influence of climate of, on adenoids   47

S

Saccus endolymphaticus, abscess at site of   392
Sarcoma of meatus externus   295
Second meeting   10
Septic pneumonia, etc., of otitic origin   286
Sixth meeting   199
Stapes extraction and mobilization of   221-261-351
Stereoscopic views of middle ear, labyrinth, etc.   114-115
Suppuration (chronic) of attic   126

T

Thrombosis of lateral sinus, etc., see *Intracranial Complications*
Tinnitus due to aortic insufficiency   238
Transparent preparations of labyrinth   115
Tuberculosis of middle ear   20-34
Tumour of brain co-existing with otorrhœa; differential
    diagnosis between cerebral tumour, cerebral abscess and
    hydrocephalus internus   384
Tumour of medulla and pons causing deafness, etc.   378

PAGE.

Tympanic mucous membrane, therapy of   199

V

Vibratory massage, in treatment of deafness   223
Varix, etc., of membrana tympani...   43

INDEX OF AUTHORS.

ALT, Ferdinand, 276
AVOLEDO, Pietro, 187
BABER, Cresswell, 7-43-103-275
BALLINGER, W. L., 208
BAR, Louis, 188
BARATOUX, J., 281
BARR, Thomas, 100-286
BENNI, C. H., 275
BOBONE, T., 47
BONNIER, Pierre, 290
BRIEGER, O., 20-40-99-146
BRONNER, Adolph, 293
CHEATLE, Arthur H., 160-275-294
COHN, Felix, 235
CONNAL, Galbraith, 295
COOSEMANS, E., 296
COSTINIU, A., 195-304
CURSETJI, J. J., 306
DADYSETT, H. J., 328
DELIE, 151
DENCH, E. B., 103-147-151
DE SANTI, Philip, 104-331-340
DIDSBURY, 198
EEMAN, 59-98-114-238
FARACI, Giuseppe, 100-186-240-246-343-351
FISCHENICH, Fr., 246
GARNAULT, Paul, 198-245-261
GOLDSTEIN, M. A., 199-236

GRADENIGO, Giuseppe, 15-16-60-96-146-250-366-373
GRANT, Dundas, 15-235-240-375
GRAY, Albert A., 378
GRAZZI, Vincenzo, 8-59-170-198-274
GUYE, A. A., 94
HAIGHT, Allen T., 54
HARTMANN, Arthur, 40-43-107-124
HEIMAN, Th., 146-198-208
HESSLER, 384
HOLINGER, J., 42-104
HOLMES, C. R., 102-260
HORNE, W. Jobson, 392
HOVELL, T. Mark, 102
JACKSON, Chevalier, 254
JANSEN, 95
JONES, Hugh E., 394-403
JOYCE, Robert Dwyer, 108
KATZ, L., 114
KAYSER, Richard, 17-20
KEIPER, Geo. F., 406
KNAPP, Herman, 59-84-106-120-151-170-246
KOEBEL, 406
KUEMMEL, 39-98
LACROIX, P., 217
LANNOIS, M., 407
LAURENS, Georges, 265

LEDERMAN, 105-120-207

LERMOYEZ, Marcel, 127-147

LUC, 72-106-145

LUCAE, A., 20-92-223-236

MacCORMAC, Sir William, 8

MACEWEN, William, 66-105

MALHERBE, Aristide, 176-187

McBRIDE, P., 40-95

MELZI, Urbano, 410-412-414

MENDOZA, Suarez de, 101-186-415

MÉNIÈRE, E., 126

MILBURY, Frank S., 418

MILLIGAN, 34-102

MINK, P. J., 251

MOURE. E. J., 94-138

NOYES, Henry, 97

NUVOLI, 245-254

OSTMANN, 223-236

POLI, Camillo, 429

POLITZER, Adam, 10-15-39-61-221-234-245-272-275

PRITCHARD, Urban, 1-8-105-273 275

ROHRER, F., 43-234

RUDLOFF, P., 116

RUTTEN, 219

SCATLIFF, J. M. E., 236

SCHMIEGELOW, E., 11-15

SNOW, Sargent, 257

TAYLOR, Lewis, 260

TERVAERT, G. D. Cohen, 446

TURNBULL, Laurence, 452

TURNER, Aldreu, 108

UCHERMANN, V., 121-125

VEYRAT, Ernest, 459-464

WHITE, Faulder, 105-467

Lightning Source UK Ltd.
Milton Keynes UK
UKHW010909161218
334046UK00007B/304/P